Radical and Reconstructive Gynecologic Cancer Surgery

Robert E. Bristow, MD, MBA
The Philip J. DiSaia Prestigious Chair in Gynecologic Oncology
Professor and Director, Division of Gynecologic Oncology
Vice-Chair for Clinical Affairs, Department of Obstetrics and Gynecology
University of California, Irvine–Medical Center and School of Medicine
Orange, California

Dennis S. Chi, MD
Deputy Chief and Fellowship Program Director
Gynecology Service, Department of Surgery
Co-Director, Pelvic Reconstructive Surgery, Department of Surgery
Memorial Sloan Kettering Cancer Center
New York, New York

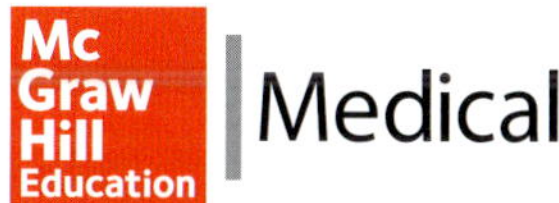

New York Chicago San Francisco Athens London Madrid Mexico City
Milan New Delhi Singapore Sydney Toronto

Radical and Reconstructive Gynecologic Cancer Surgery

1 2 3 4 5 6 7 8 9 0 CTP/CTP 19 18 17 16 15 14

ISBN 978-0-07-180809-5
MHID 0-07-180809-4

Notice

Medicine is an ever-changing science. As new research and clinical experience broaden our knowledge, changes in treatment and drug therapy are required. The authors and the publisher of this work have checked with sources believed to be reliable in their efforts to provide information that is complete and generally in accord with the standards accepted at the time of publication. However, in view of the possibility of human error or changes in medical sciences, neither the authors nor the publisher nor any other party who has been involved in the preparation or publication of this work warrants that the information contained herein is in every respect accurate or complete, and they disclaim all responsibility for any errors or omissions or for the results obtained from use of the information contained in this work. Readers are encouraged to confirm the information contained herein with other sources. For example and in particular, readers are advised to check the product information sheet included in the package of each drug they plan to administer to be certain that the information contained in this work is accurate and that changes have not been made in the recommended dose or in the contraindications for administration. This recommendation is of particular importance in connection with new or infrequently used drugs.

This book was set in Adobe Caslon Pro by Cenveo® Publisher Services.
The editors were Alyssa Fried and Harriet Lebowitz.
The production supervisor was Rick Ruzycka.
Project Management was provided by Vastavikta Sharma, Cenveo Publisher Services.
The copyeditor was Sherri Damlo.
China Translation and Printing Services was the printer and binder.

This book is printed on acid-free paper.

Library of Congress Cataloging-in-Publication Data

Radical and reconstructive gynecologic cancer surgery / editors, Robert E. Bristow, Dennis S. Chi.
p. ; cm.
Includes bibliographical references and index.
ISBN 978-0-07-180809-5 (hardcover : alk. paper)—ISBN 0-07-180809-4 (hardcover : alk. paper)
I. Bristow, Robert E., editor. II. Chi, Dennis S., editor.
[DNLM: 1. Genital Neoplasms, Female—surgery. 2. Reconstructive Surgical Procedures. WP 145]
RG104.6
616.99'465059—dc23

2014021875

To my wife, Michelle, and children, Jackson, Chloe, and Haley, for your love, patience, and support; to my colleagues and mentors for your guidance in learning the art of being a perpetual student of surgery; and to all women suffering from gynecologic cancer, whose courage, determination, and grace inspire us to always do better.

Robert E. Bristow, MD, MBA

To my wife, Hae-Young, and our children Jessica, Stephanie, and Andrew, for your patience, encouragement, and love; to my mother, who is my first and best mentor; and to all our patients who have entrusted their care and lives in our hands motivating us to keep on fighting to make a difference.

Dennis S. Chi, MD

Contents

Contributors

Sonsoles Alonso, MD
Department of Gynecologic Oncology
MD Anderson Cancer Center
Madrid, Spain
Chapter 13: Bladder and Ureteral Substitution and Augmentation

Bernard H. Bochner, MD, FACS
Attending Surgeon, Urology Service
Vice Chairman, Department of Surgery
Memorial Sloan Kettering Cancer Center
Kimmel Center for Prostate and Urologic Cancers
New York, New York
Chapter 12: Continent Diversions

Patrick J. Boland, MD
Attending Orthopedic Surgeon
Orthopedic Service, Department of Surgery
Memorial Sloan-Kettering Cancer Center
New York, New York
Orange, California
Chapter 10: Extended Pelvic Resection

Mary S. Brady, MD, FACS
Attending Surgeon
Memorial Sloan-Kettering Cancer Center
New York, New York
Chapter 20: Bioprosthetic and Prosthetic Materials in Abdominal Wall Reconstruction and Hernia Repair

Robert E. Bristow, MD, MBA
Professor and Director
Division of Gynecologic Oncology
Department of Obstetrics and Gynecology
University of California, Irvine—Medical Center
Orange, California
Chapter 5: Radical Vulvectomy

Luis M. Chiva, MD, PhD
Head of Department, Gynecologic Oncology
MD Anderson Cancer Center
Madrid, Spain
Adjunct Professor of University of Texas
Chapter 13: Bladder and Ureteral Substitution and Augmentation

Michael W. Chu, MD
Institute of Reconstructive Plastic Surgery
New York University Medical Center
Department of Plastic & Reconstructive Surgery
New York, New York
Chapter 17: Rectus Abdominis Flaps and Pudendal Thigh and Related Flaps

David Cibula, MD, PhD
Professor, Gynecologic Oncology Centre
Department of Obstetrics and Gynecology 1st Medical Faculty
Charles University, General University Hospital
Prague, Czech Republic
Chapter 3: Radical Hysterectomy with En Bloc Vaginectomy or Pelvic Lymphadenectomy

Atreya Dash, MD
Associate Professor
Department of Urology
University of Washington
Seattle, Washington
Chapter 6: Radical Cystectomy

John P. Diaz, MD
Associate
Gynecologic Oncology Service
South Miami Gynecologic Oncology Group
Miami Cancer Institute
Baptist Health South Florida
Miami, Florida
Chapter 4: Fertility-Sparing Radical Abdominal Trachelectomy

Timothy F. Donahue, MD
Fellow, Urology Service
Department of Surgery
Memorial Sloan Kettering Cancer Center
Kimmel Center for Prostate and Urologic Cancers
New York, New York
Chapter 12: Continent Diversions

Elizabeth A. Dubil, MD
Division of Gynecologic Oncology
Walter Reed National Military Medical Center
Bethesda, Maryland
Chapter 2: Surgical Anatomy and Instrumentation

John C. Elkas, MD, JD
Division of Gynecologic Oncology
Mid-Atlantic Pelvic Surgery Associates
Annandale, Virginia
Chapter 2: Surgical Anatomy and Instrumentation

Ricardo E. Estape, MD
Director of Robotic Surgery
Gynecologic Oncology Service
South Miami Gynecologic Oncology Group
Miami Cancer Institute
Baptist Health South Florida
Miami, Florida
Chapter 4: Fertility-Sparing Radical Abdominal Trachelectomy

Jeffrey M. Fowler, MD
Department of Obstetrics & Gynecology
Division of Gynecologic Oncology
Wexner Medical Center
The Ohio State University
Columbus, Ohio
Chapter 18: Gracilis, Tensor Fascia Lata, Vastus Laterlis, Rectus Femoris, and Gluteus Maximus Flaps.

Julio Garcia-Aguilar, MD, PhD
Chief, Colorectal Service/Department of Surgery
Stuart H.Q. Quan Chair in Colorectal Surgery
Memorial Sloan-Kettering Cancer Center
New York, New York
Chapter 7: Abdominoperineal Excision of the Rectum

John P. Geisler, MD
Professor, Department of Obstetrics and Gynecology
Division of Gynecologic Oncology
University of Toledo College of Medicine and Life Sciences
Toledo, Ohio
Chapter 14: Colorectal Anastomosis, Colostomy, and Small Bowel Anastomosis

Vivian E. von Gruenigen, MD
Chair, Department of Obstetrics and Gynecology
Summa Akron City Hospital
Systems Medical Director of Women's Health Services
Summa Health System
Akron, Ohio
Chapter 21: Rehabilitation, Quality Of Life, and Symptom Management

Michael Höckel, MD, PhD
Department of Gynecology
University of Leipzig
Leipzig, Germany
Chapter 9: (Laterally) Extended Endopelvic Resection

Matias Jurado, MD, PhD
Head of Department of Gynecologic Oncology
University Of Navarre
Navarre, Spain
Chapter 13: Bladder and Ureteral Substitution and Augmentation

Beman Khulpateea, MD
The Women's Institute for Gynecologic Cancer & Special Pelvic Surgery
Coopersburg, Pennsylvania
Chapter 15: The Ileal Pouch Anal Anastamosis

Edward M. Kobraei, MD
Division of Plastic and Reconstructive Surgery
Massachusetts General Hospital
Harvard Medical School
Boston, Massachusetts
Chapter 16: Skin Grafts, Omental Flaps, Advancement and Rotational Flaps

Fernando Lapuente, MD
Department of Gynecologic Oncology,
MD Anderson Cancer Center
Madrid, Spain
Chapter 13: Bladder and Ureteral Substitution and Augmentation

Hak J. Lee, MD
Urologic Oncology Fellow
University of California, San Diego Medical Center
San Diego, California
Chapter 6: Radical Cystectomy

Javier F. Magrina, MD
Department of Gynecology
Mayo Clinic in Arizona
Phoenix, Arizona
Chapter 8: Pelvic Exenteration

Paul M. Magtibay, MD
Department of Gynecology
Mayo Clinic in Arizona
Phoenix, Arizona
Chapter 8: Pelvic Exenteration

Kelly J. Manahan, MD
Professor and Chair, Department of Obstetrics and Gynecology
Division of Gynecologic Oncology
University of Toledo College of Medicine and Life Sciences
Toledo, Ohio
Chapter 14 : Colorectal Anastomosis, Colostomy, and Small Bowel Anastomosis

Evan Matros, MD
Attending Surgeon
Plastic and Reconstructive Surgery
Memorial Sloan-Kettering Cancer Center
New York, New York
Chapter 19: Tissue Rearrangement Techniques and Regional Flaps

Michele L. McCarroll, PhD
Assistant Professor
Human Performance and Exercise Science
Bitonte College of Health and Human Services
Youngstown State University
Youngstown, Ohio
Chapter 21: Rehabilitation, Quality Of Life, and Symptom Management

Colleen M. McCarthy, MD, MS
Memorial Sloan-Kettering Cancer Center
New York, New York
Chapter 17: Rectus Abdominis Flaps and Pudendal Thigh and Related Flaps

David G. McKeown, MD
Orthopaedic Service, Department of Surgery
Memorial Sloan-Kettering Cancer Center
New York, New York
Chapter 10: Extended Pelvic Resection

G. Scott Rose, MD
Division of Gynecologic Oncology
Mid-Atlantic Pelvic Surgery Associates
Annandale, Virginia
Chapter 2: Surgical Anatomy and Instrumentation

G. Dante Roulette, MD
Gynecologic Specialist
Summa Health System
Akron, Ohio
Chapter 21: Rehabilitation, Quality Of Life, and Symptom Management

Ritu Salani, MD
Department of Obstetrics & Gynecology
Division of Gynecologic Oncology
Wexner Medical Center
The Ohio State University
Columbus, Ohio
Chapter 18: Gracilis, Tensor Fascia Lata, Vastus Laterlis, Rectus Femoris, and Gluteus Maximus Flaps.

Jaspreet S. Sandhu, MD
Associate Attending Surgeon, Urology Service
Memorial Sloan Kettering Cancer Center
New York, New York
Chapter 11: Incontinent Urinary Diversions

John O. Schorge, MD
Department of Obstetrics and Gynecology
Massachusetts General Hospital
Harvard Medical School
Boston, Massachusetts
Chapter 16: Skin Grafts, Omental Flaps, Advancement and Rotational Flaps

Jordan Siegel, MD
Department of Urology
University of California, Irvine—Medical Center
Orange, California
Chapter 6: Radical Cystectomy

David F. Silver, MD
Director of Gynecologic Oncology
The Women's Institute for Gynecologic Cancer & Special Pelvic Surgery
Coopersburg, Pennsylvania
Chapter 15: The Ileal Pouch Anal Anastamosis

Rudy S. Suidan, MD
Pelvic Reconstruction Clinical Research Fellow
Gynecology Service, Department of Surgery
Memorial Sloan-Kettering Cancer Center
New York, New York
Chapter 10: Extended Pelvic Resection

Krishnansu S. Tewari, MD, FACOG, FACS
Professor and Director of Research
Division of Gynecologic Oncology
Department of Obstetrics and Gynecology
University of California, Irvine—Medical Center
Orange, California
Chapter 1: History of Radical and Reconstructive Surgery for Gynecologic Cancer

Pankaj Tiwari, MD
Department of Plastic Surgery
Wexner Medical Center
The Ohio State University
Columbus, Ohio
Chapter 18: Gracilis, Tensor Fascia Lata, Vastus Laterlis, Rectus Femoris, and Gluteus Maximus Flaps.

Laszlo Ungar, MD
Professor
Department of Obstetrics, Gynecology and Gynecologic Oncology
St. Stephen Hospital
Budapest, Hungary
Chapter 4: Fertility-Sparing Radical Abdominal Trachelectomy

Theresa Y. Wang, MD
Memorial Sloan-Kettering Cancer Center
New York, New York
Chapter 17: Rectus Abdominis Flaps and Pudendal Thigh and Related Flaps

Cindy Wei, MD
Fellow
Plastic and Reconstructive Surgery
Memorial Sloan-Kettering Cancer Center
New York, New York
Chapter 19: Tissue Rearrangement Techniques and Regional Flaps

Jonathan M. Winograd, MD
Division of Plastic and Reconstructive Surgery
Massachusetts General Hospital
Harvard Medical School
Boston, Massachusetts
Chapter 16: Skin Grafts, Omental Flaps, Advancement and Rotational Flaps

Katherine L. Wood, MD
Resident, Department of Obstetrics and Gynecology
University of Toledo College of Medicine and Life Sciences
Toledo, Ohio
Chapter 14 : Colorectal Anastomosis, Colostomy, and Small Bowel Anastomosis

Xiaohua Wu, MD, PhD
Professor and Chair
Department of Gynecologic Oncology
Fudan University Shanghai Cancer CenterShanghai, China
Chapter 4: Fertility-Sparing Radical Abdominal Trachelectomy

Donghua Xie, MD
Fellow, Urology Service
Department of Surgery
Memorial Sloan Kettering Cancer Center
New York, New York
Chapter 11: Incontinent Urinary Diversions

Preface

The effective surgical management of advanced and recurrent gynecologic cancer includes a complex array of extirpative and reconstructive operative procedures and requires an integrated multidisciplinary team approach. This text is intended for surgeons and students of surgery performing radical and ultraradical operations for gynecologic cancers and related tumors affecting the female pelvis. It fills an unmet need in the surgical educational literature as a crossdisciplinary single source of information. The book is organized into 3 main parts.

Part I covers the historic evolution of radical pelvic surgical procedures and provides an anatomic review of pertinent pelvic and abdominal visceral, vascular, and bony structures as a foundation for the detailed descriptions and illustrations of the surgical procedures that follow. ***Part II*** consists of the extirpative (resection) procedures organized by system physiology and anatomic region as a combination textbook and surgical atlas. The detailed illustrations are complemented by operative photographs, emphasizing the practical or "how-to" aspects of each procedure. ***Part III*** includes comprehensive coverage of the full range of reconstructive procedures and surgical options available to optimize patient outcome as well as a chapter on rehabilitation, quality-of-life issues, and symptom management.

The contributors to this text include a multidisciplinary international team of leading surgical educators from the disciplines of surgical oncology, gynecologic oncology, urologic oncology, colorectal surgery, and plastic and reconstructive surgery.

Robert E. Bristow, MD, MBA
Dennis S. Chi, MD

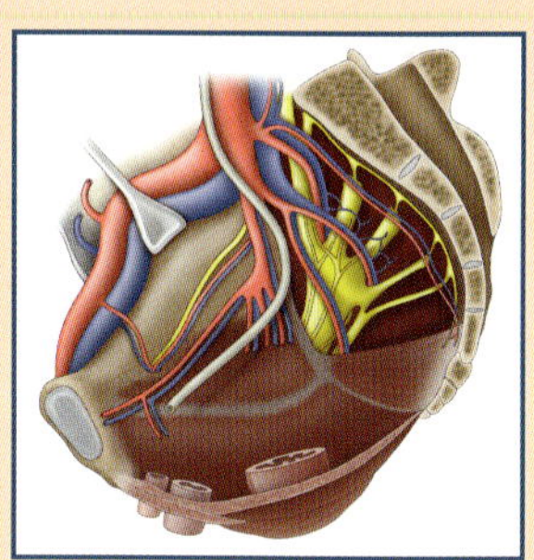

Part I

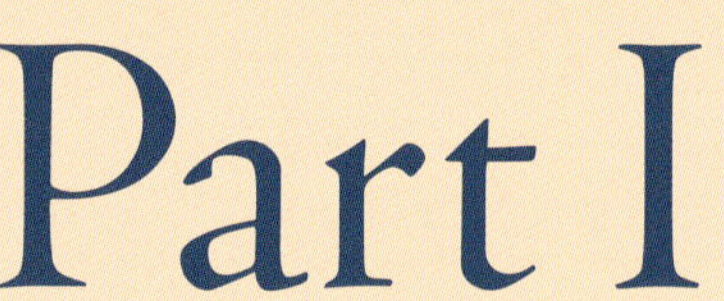

Overview

Chapter 1. History of Radical and Reconstructive Surgery for Gynecologic Cancer

Krishnansu S. Tewari, MD, FACOG, FACS

EXTIRPATIVE PROCEDURES

Radical Hysterectomy

The evolution of the radical hysterectomy encompasses nearly 2500 years and is among the most fascinating stories in surgical oncology. Some writings on cervical cancer have survived from antiquity. Hippocrates of Cos (460–370 BC) attempted trachelectomy but noted that nothing he did could eradicate the disease.[1] In the mid-fifth century, Byzantine physician Aëtius of Amida used vaginal irrigation with herbal compounds to relieve pain caused by cervical cancer.[1] Ambroise Paré recommended cervical amputation, which was performed in 1652 by Tulpius.[1] Father of American gynecology J. Marion Sims (1813–1883) used galvanocaustic loops to amputate and cauterize a cervical cancer.[2]

John Hunter (1728–1793), founder of the Royal College of Surgeons of England, was 19 years of age when he traveled from Glasgow to London to study and subsequently work with his brother William Hunter, a graduate of Edinburgh University.[1] Although J. Hunter had no formal medical training, he became the leading anatomist and one of the country's finest surgeons through self-education and training. Among his many prosected specimens are specimens of advanced cervical cancer demonstrating the natural history and route of spread locally within the pelvis.

The spectacular rise of the Johns Hopkins Hospital and School of Medicine began in the late 1890s with the recruitment of 40-year-old William Osler (1849–1919; later Sir William) and 31-year-old Howard Atwood Kelly (1858–1943), both members of the University of Pennsylvania faculty. They joined famous surgeon William Halstead (aged 37 years) and distinguished pathologist William H. Welch (1850–1934; aged 38 years) to form the nucleus that spearheaded the development of Johns Hopkins into the world class institution it is today.

John Goodrich Clark (1867–1927) completed his training at the University of Pennsylvania and interned at a local Philadelphia hospital for 2 years before coming to Johns Hopkins.[3] Originally he had been granted a residency position with Osler; however, upon arriving in Baltimore, Maryland, he was told that position had been committed to another physician. Osler sent him to Kelly who had an opening in gynecology. Thus, but a quirk of fate, Clark became a gynecologist rather than an internist.

Kelly assigned Clark to develop a more radical surgical approach for the treatment of cervical cancer. At a pathologic examination of 20 cases of cervical cancer treated by hysterectomy, Clark found that the disease had extended beyond the margins of resection in 15 cases.[3] Influenced by the surgical doctrines of Halsted, he began considering an en bloc radical hysterectomy for cervical cancer. Clark was familiar with the combined operation described in 1894 by the German surgeon A. Mackenrodt who extensively used actual cautery to destroy the local growth at its primary site before dissecting free the upper vagina and suturing it over the cervix.[4] He credited Mackenrodt's procedure as the first step toward wider extirpation of the pelvic tissues along with the uterus.

The year 1895 turned out to be critical in the development of the surgical attack on cervical cancer. In March, the German surgeon Reis presented the anatomic theory of what would become the modern radical hysterectomy, calling for systematic removal of pelvic lymph nodes.[5] Independently, Clark at Johns Hopkins,[6] Rumpf in Berlin,[7] and Wilhelm Latzko (1863–1945)[8] in Vienna performed the first radical hysterectomies. Clark had his case on April 26, 1895, when he was just a second-year resident and the sole author of a manuscript that described the operation. He wrote, "The faults common to all methods of removal of the uterus are (1) the broad ligaments are cut too close to the uterus, and (2) too small portions of the vagina are removed."[6]

Citing the unacceptable surgical mortality of abdominal surgery, Austrian surgeon Friedrich Schauta (1849–1919) advocated a vaginal approach to radical hysterectomy.[9] Schauta made use of the experience of the Czech surgeon

K. Pawlik who performed his first simple vaginal hysterectomy in a patient with cervical cancer in 1880 and, then, in 1889 reported 3 radical vaginal hysterectomies.[10] Although Pawlik is credited as having performed the very first radical vaginal hysterectomy, Schauta was the first to systematically perform it. His first extensive radical vaginal hysterectomy was performed in 1901. The German Chair of Gynecology at the Berlin Charite, Walter Stoeckel (1871–1961), extensively modified Schauta's operation,[11] and the Austrian gynecologist Isodor Alfred Amreich (1885–1972)[12] extended the radicality of the procedure for the treatment of more advanced cervical and endometrial carcinomas.

Although Schauta was already a professor in Innsubruck at 32 years of age and would soon develop an international reputation during his lifetime, he had the misfortune of having to live in the shadow of his pupil, the Viennese surgeon Ernst Wertheim (1864–1920).[13-15] Wertheim was critical of the vaginal procedure for its failure to include an assessment of the lymph nodes. An intense rivalry developed between Schauta and Wertheim regarding the operative approach and their disagreement caused considerable antagonism between them.

Ultimately, Wertheim would modify and popularize the operation, describing his abdominal radical hysterectomy in a 1900 manuscript.[13] Wertheim advocated removal of the adjacent medial portion of the parametria and the upper part of the vagina and any adjacent enlarged pelvic lymph nodes. He was extremely disciplined and demanding with a difficult disposition, nervously performing surgery without surgical gloves for fear of losing sensitivity in his fingertips. His published experience was impressive in magnitude, follow-up, and descriptions of complications. In 1912, Wertheim published a monograph that included more than 500 cases, with an overall mortality rate of 10%.[15] Due to the influenza pandemic, Wertheim died on February 15, 1920, at 56 years of age. Schauta had died 1 year earlier and the 2 men were buried side-to-side.

In 1944, the surgical approach to treatment of early-stage cervical cancer was revisited by Joe Vincent Meigs (1892–1963) of Harvard Medical School and the Massachusetts General Hospital.[16-18] He initiated a full-scale research program and visited surgeons in Europe and was impressed with the logic of Wertheim's procedure. Acknowledging the 1934 report by Frederick J. Taussig (1872–1943) of Washington University Medical School, in which a survival benefit was obtained when pelvic lymphadenectomy was added to standard radiotherapy for cervical cancer,[19] Meigs developed a modified Wertheim operation to include more extensive removal of the parametria and complete bilateral pelvic lymphadenectomy. In his initial series of 47 patients, he observed positive lymph nodes in 17%.[20] The series was extended to include 100 patients in which the operative mortality rate was 1%, with 5-year survival rates of 81.1% for stage 1 and 61.8% for stage 2 cancers.[21] Although fistulas remained a significant obstacle to widespread endorsement of radical hysterectomy, the mortality associated with the procedure was virtually eliminated with the availability of antibiotics, blood transfusion, and specially trained gynecologic surgeons. It is ironic that the operation is often called the Wertheim operation in the United States, where as many European surgeons refer to it as the Meigs operation.

Two decades earlier on the other side of the world, Wertheim's operation was further modified in 1921 by renowned Japanese surgeon Hidakazu Okabayashi.[22-24] He did not propose his operation as a new technique but more as a modification of the operation performed by his teacher, Professor Takayama, who had perfected the original Wertheim procedure by operating on 200 cases each year.[22] Okabayashi placed emphasis on the extended radicality of extirpation of the parametrium. His 1932 film of the procedure was discovered in 2007 and demonstrates an even more radical operation, with a complete separation of the deep layer of the vesicouterine ligament, thus enabling the surgeon to perform an extensive resection of the parametrium and the lateral paravaginal tissue.[25] This essential step enabled the surgeon to completely separate the bladder from the uterus and the lateral side of the cervix and vagina, allowing sufficient transection of the vagina at the required level, as necessary.

Since its publication in 1974, the operative classification of Piver, Rutledge, and Smith has been used widely to assess the radicality of an abdominal cervical cancer operation.[26] This system describes 5 classes of radical (or extended) hysterectomy, classes I to V. Class II or modified radical hysterectomies with bilateral pelvic lymphadenectomy are indicated for microinvasive carcinomas (International Federation of Gynecology and Obstetrics [FIGO] IIA, occult IB1), while class III or Wertheim-Meigs radical hysterectomy with bilateral pelvic lymphadenectomy is the standard treatment for patients with early stage, visible lesions (FIGO IB1–IB2; some IIA1). The Piver classification was not designed to accommodate vaginal radical hysterectomy, nerve-sparing, or minimally invasive procedures.

In 1961, Kobayashi from Tokyo University modified Okabayashi's radical hysterectomy and identified the principles for prevention of bladder dysfunction.[27] Kobayashi preserved the pelvic splanchnic nerves by separating the vascular part and the neural part of the cardinal ligament during resection of the parametrial tissues.[27] In recent years, the nerve-sparing radical hysterectomy has been expertly rendered by Okabayashi's direct descendent and successor, Fujii.[28]

Radical Trachelectomy for Fertility Preservation

Daniel Dargent (1937–2005) was the French pioneer of both the radical trachelectomy to preserve fertility and the use of the sentinel node concept for surgical staging in cervical cancer. Dargent resurrected the anatomic principles of Schauta's radical vaginal hysterectomy and combining that with the surgical modality of laparoscopy, he performed the first successful systematic conservative surgical approach for invasive cervical cancer in 1994.[29] The radical vaginal trachelectomy, involving the removal of the cervix, surrounding parametria, and upper vagina, was preceded by laparoscopic bilateral pelvic lymphadenectomy.[30] In a seminal paper published in 2000, Dargent reported on a series of 56 patients scheduled for the procedure, of whom 47 successfully underwent it.[31] The disease distribution ranged from IA1 to IIB. At a mean follow-up of 52 months, 2 recurrences (4%) were observed. Subsequent pregnancies resulted in 25% late miscarriages and 13 healthy livebirths. Dargent's operation has emerged as the standard of care for women with early cervical cancer who wish to preserve fertility.

Pelvic Exenteration

In his colorful remembrance of Alexander Brunschwig (1901–1969), Boronow notes that, although his immigrant parents from the Alsace Lorraine area gave him little in the way of material things, they gifted him with superb intellect.[32] Following the 1935 publication of the first report of a successful 2-stage procedure for radical en bloc resection of the duodenum and head of the pancreas for a growth of the ampulla of Vater by Whipple, Parsons, and Mullins,[33] the first "one-stage" Whipple was published by Brunschwig in 1939.[34] He was appointed Chief of Gynecology at the Memorial Hospital for Cancer and Allied Disease in New York in 1947, where he turned his attention to the problem of cervical cancer. He noted that treatment was primarily with radiation therapy and local failures were frequent, as were fistulae, both from uncontrolled cancer and from radiation injury. Brunschwig hypothesized that ultra-radical dissection of organs in the pelvic area may eradicate recurrent cervical cancer. It was in his sentinel publication in 1948,[35] which contained his first 22 cases, that Brunschwig carefully described the en bloc removal of the uterus, cervix, vagina, parametria, the entire internal iliac complex, rectum, bladder, and sometimes, the distal ureters. Bilateral pelvic and aortocaval lymphadenectomies typically preceded the extirpative phase, and creation of a wet colostomy, and occasionally vaginal reconstruction, immediately followed. This concept was met with an enormous credibility gap. His colleague Hugh Barber recalled, "Many in high places regarded this as a thoughtless form of mutilation, with limited chance of success for palliation, much less cure. The criticism was frequent, harsh, and bitter. Even the moral right to carry out such extensive surgery was questioned. Dr. Brunschwig had an extremely sensitive nature and was easily hurt. It took every measure of his strength, courage, and dedication to continue."[32] The operation was regarded as "the most radical surgical attack so far described for pelvic cancer" and, at the time of Brunschwig's initial publication, the operative mortality rate was 23%. Brunschwig himself described the procedure as "brutal and cruel, but one that saved lives."[32] His technique for fecal and urinary diversion was the so-called "wet colostomy" (bilateral ureterocolostomy) and Boronow recalls that, when scrubbing with him, he would select the naval as the site for the stoma.[32] During his time, operations were often glorified by names that seem oddly out of place in today's politically correct world.[32] Brunshwig's total pelvic exenteration was called the "All-American"; an anterior exenteration was a "North American," and a posterior exenteration was, *of course*, a "South American."[32] With improvements in critical care, antibiotics, hyperalimentation, thromboembolism prophylaxis, and advances in surgical technique (subjects that Brunschwig published extensively on),[36-38] the morbidity and mortality rates have dramatically improved, with current operative mortality rates below 5%, major perioperative complication rates of 30% to 44%, and overall 5-year survival rates as high as 60%.

In 1952 Hugh R. K. Barber (1918–2006) became the first gynecologic trainee at what is now Memorial Sloan Kettering Cancer Center, to be accepted into their 2-year postresidency program in general surgical oncology. It was during this time that Barber met Brunschwig. The 2 men developed a special bond and exhaustively studied pelvic exenteration. Together they coauthored 9 pivotal manuscripts that covered the prognostic significance of preoperative nonvisualization of the kidney, fistulae, secondary and tertiary rediversion of the urinary tract, resection of the bony pelvis, excision of major blood vessels at the periphery of the pelvis, added resections of the small bowel, and pelvic exenteration for extensive visceral necrosis, recurrent endometrial cancer, and locally advanced/recurrent ovarian cancer.[39-47]

Radical Vulvectomy

At the turn of the twentieth century, vulvar cancer was considered incurable, with less than 25% of patients surviving after local excision. Topical therapies, cautery, and local excision all proved inadequate. Furthermore, the social and sexual standards of the time made it difficult for patients and physicians to openly discuss vulvar complaints. To treat what many referred to as a horrible disease, radical vulvectomy and bilateral inguinal femoral lymphadenectomy were combined utilizing one continuous incision; their use was popularized by pioneers including Kehrer,[48] Basset,[49] Taussig,[50,51] Way,[52] and Twombly.[53] During this period, en bloc dissection of regional nodes with a wide margin was an important principle in cancer surgery.

Kehrer reported on 3 patients treated by radical vulvectomy and bilateral lymph node dissection in 1912,[48] and Stoekel provided fair illustrations together with a complete review of the existing literature in 1947.[54] Peham and Amreich's *Operative Gynecology*, which was published in 1934,[12] contained the most elaborate and complete illustrations of radical vulvectomy during those formative years. Among the prevailing concepts of the time were that continuity of the lymphatics of the vulva made the location of the primary tumor irrelevant and that procedures involving partial vulvectomy or those allowed for primary closure were inadequate. Adding to these concepts were the poor results obtained with radiation, and what emerged was the surgical principle of removing the tumor with all of the skin and lymphatic channels of the vulva and the lymph nodes of the groin and pelvic nodes at risk.

En bloc radical vulvectomy with an inguinal and pelvic lymphadenectomy, as described by Way in 1948,[55] was adopted and resulted in a 5-year survival rate of 74%, as reported by Morley in 1976.[56] This success rate convinced most surgeons to use this operation regardless of tumor size. Major morbidity included poor wound healing and long-term lower extremity lymphedema. Back in the 1940s, Frederick J. Taussig (1872–1943) had modified Basset's procedure for smaller lesions, making oblique incisions across the middle of Poupart's ligament in each groin but a block dissection in continuity with the vulva was not carried out. This *triple incision technique* was designed to decrease morbidity but was not routinely used until Hacker reported his experience with 100 patients in 1981.[57] His team found that when using the triple incision technique, as described by Taussig for patients with clinical stage 1 disease, the 5-year survival rate was 97%.

RECONSTRUCTIVE PROCEDURES

Separation of Urinary and Fecal Streams

Wet colostomy provides the constant threat of ascending urinary tract infection from reflux of intestinal contents. Recurrent infection in the ureter and kidney may lead to progressive hydronephrosis, with resulting ureterointestinal anastomotic obstruction and metabolic abnormalities due to intestinal resorption of urinary constituents. Acute pyelonephritis following pelvic exenteration may also be fatal. Bricker was a proponent of separation of the urinary fecal streams and, in 1950, described implanting the ureters into an isolated loop of terminal ileum.[58] This ileal conduit for urinary drainage is exteriorized through the right lower quadrant and the fecal sigmoid colostomy is implanted in the left lower quadrant of the abdomen. This method eliminates the complications of reflux fecal infection of the urinary tract and also provides for prompt urinary drainage via a small segment of bowel, thus minimizing intestinal absorption of urinary constituents.

Abdominoperineal Resection and Low Anterior Resection

William Ernest Miles (1869–1947) described the abdominoperineal resection in 1908 at a time when radical surgical procedures were being developed for cancers of the breast, head and neck, and cervix.[59] This procedure left patients with a permanent colostomy. In 1939, Claude F. Dixon (1893–1968) introduced the low anterior resection.[60,61] This was the first operation to allow patients with rectal cancer to avoid definitive stoma. While initially performed only in patients with tumors of the upper third of the rectum, the trans-anal coloanal anastomosis extended the possibility of sphincter preservation, even to patients with very low rectal cancers. In the early 1940s, Henry E. Bacon began to use the pull-through procedure,[62] a technique first described in the late 1880s. This procedure has now been adapted for the ultra-radical surgical management for cervical cancer (ie, pelvic exenteration) and for ovarian cancer (ie, cytoreduction).

Urinary Diversion

Urinary diversion to the sigmoid colon was first described in 1855 and was performed by an end-to-end anastomosis between the ureter and sigmoid colon (*ureterosigmoidostomy*). Because of pyelonephritis caused by reflux of urine into the sigmoid colon, in 1911, Coffey created an antireflux mechanism using an oblique submucosal passage of the ureter into the sigmoid colon.[63] Coffey's procedure was most commonly used until 1950, when Bricker described the first successful *ileal conduit*.[58] This noncontinent form of urinary diversion is typically constructed by isolating a 15- to 20-cm segment of distal ileum, with the ureters implanted using a direct anastomosis technique.

The development of continent urinary reservoirs was predicated by the Gilchrist procedure. In 1950, Gilchrist et al[64] used an ileocecal segment and the right colon in tubular form as the reservoir and the terminal ileum served as the efferent limb. The continence mechanism was created by the ileocecal valve and less active peristalsis of the terminal ileum. In designing the *Indiana pouch* in 1987, Rowland et al[65] from the University of Indiana modified the Gilchrist procedure first by plicating the ileocecal valve and tapering the efferent limb to create the continent mechanism. The pouch is created using a 25- to 30-cm segment of cecum and ascending colon. Detubularization of the right colon increases the capacity and lowers the pressure in the Indiana pouch. The ureters are implanted in the tenia using a tunneled antireflux method to limit pyelonephritis. The pouch has a cutaneous diversion that requires catheterization of an abdominal stoma with no need for an external appliance.

The *Miami pouch* was developed at the University of Miami in 1988 by Bejany and Poitano.[66] The pouch is constructed by a bowel segment which includes the distal ileum to the midtransverse colon, incorporating a detubularized colonic pouch. The continence mechanism is created by a tapered ileum and pursestring sutures placed to reinforce the ileocecal valve. The ureterocolonic anastomosis is not tunneled and is nonrefluxing.

The *Kock pouch* is another continent ileal urinary reservoir and was described in 1982 by Kock et al.[67] This pouch is a high capacity, low-pressure reservoir and functionally simulates the natural bladder. It is constructed from a long segment of distal ileum formed into a U-shape. Intussusception of the distal and proximal segments form 1-way nipple valves. The ureters are anastomosed into the afferent limb, and the afferent nipple valve provides a reflux mechanism. The efferent nipple valve functions as the continence mechanism and is brought out to the skin flush with the abdominal wall stoma.

Vaginal Reconstruction

Early attempts at filling the pelvic cavity and reconstructing the vagina involved using simple skin grafts that had varying rates of success. The split-thickness skin graft was found to be useful in covering skin defects following skinning vulvectomy for carcinoma in situ, simple vaginectomy for extensive carcinoma in situ, congenital absence of the vagina, and vaginal distortion secondary to prior radiation or surgery.[68,69] However, when there has been major loss of skin and subcutaneous tissue of the vulva, groin, or vagina, full-thickness skin grafts were felt to be superior. Defined arterial and fasciocutaneous flaps were more reliable than cutaneous flaps. Pioneers in this field recognized that the type of flap required is dependent on size, contour, depth of the deformity, proximity of the deformity to the potential donor site, presences of necrosis and infection, and the requirement for a new blood supply as occurs in an irradiated bed. In most cases, the myocutaneous flap was found to provide the most reliable source of a fresh new blood supply.

The first compound skin–muscle flaps were designed by Owens using the sternomastoid muscle.[70] One of the first myocutaneous flaps for vaginal reconstruction incorporated the *bulbocavernosus muscle* but was limited by its small size and poor cosmetic results. The *gracilis myocutaneous flap* was first used by Orticochea to cover an ankle defect and for total penile reconstruction.[71,72] In 1976, McCraw and Massey first described the surgical procedure for the use of gracilis myocutaneous vaginal reconstruction following pelvic exenteration.[73,74] Although this flap contains an expendable muscle, and for the most part contains nonirradiated tissue, the gracilis is a small-caliber vessel, and rotation of the flap into the pelvis can place the vessels under significant tension that results in vascular compromise and flap necrosis in up to 20% of cases. The *rectus abdominal myocutaneous flap* contains a large-caliber vessel that can be mobilized so that it is tension-free after rotation of the flap into the pelvis. The inferiorly based rectus abdominis myocutaneous flap to fill the pelvic defects was first reported by McGraw et al[75] in 1988 and then by Benson et al[76] in 1993.

SUMMARY

The development of radical and extensive extirpative operations was borne out of the need to clear the margins of locally advanced pelvic carcinomas and to manage the consequences of suboptimal radiotherapy, which often resulted in pelvic failure. Understandably, these procedures were accompanied by significant morbidity, leading to deterioration in quality of life as a consequence of recurrent pyelonephritis, permanent colostomy, sexual dysfunction, and psychological sequelae due to a perceived mutilated body image. Fortunately, the evolution of restorative and reconstructive procedures has kept pace with innovations and refinements of surgical technique, yielding notably improved quality of life and sexual function, significantly lessened medical sequelae, and a remarkable decrease in surgical morbidity paralleling survivorship gains.

REFERENCES

1. Hall DP. Our surgical heritage: Europe: Vincenz Czerny. *Am J Surg*. 1964;107:922.
2. Sims JM. The treatment of epithelioma of the cervix uteri. *Am J Obstet*. 1879;12:451-489.
3. Mikuta JJ. A history of the centennial of the first radical hysterectomy and its developer – Dr. John Goodrich Clark. *J Pelvic Surg*. 1995;1:3-7.
4. Eastman JR. Gynecology in Berlin: A. Mackenrodt. *JAMA*. 1897;29:737-738.
5. Ries E. Eine neue operations methode des uterus carcinomas. *Z Geburtshilfe Gynakol Stuttgart*. 1897;37:518.
6. Clark JG. A more radical method of performing hysterectomy for cancer of the uterus. *Bull Johns Hopkins Hosp*. 1895;6:120.
7. Rumpf H. Sitzung der Berliner Gesselschaff. *Geb u Gyn Centr f Gyn*. 1895;31:849
8. Latzko W, Schiffmann J. Klinisches und anatomisches zur Radikaloperation des Gebarmutterkrebses. *Zbl Gynakol*. 1919;34:689-705.
9. Shauta F. Die operation des gebarmutterkrebes mittels des Schuchardt schen paravaginal schnittes. *Montasschr Z Geburtschilfe Gynakol*. 1902;15:133.
10. Schuchardt K. Eine neue methode der gebarmutterexstirpation. *Zentralbl Chir*. 1893;20:1121.
11. Staude C. Ueber total extirpation des carcinomatosen uterus mittelst doppelseitiger scheidenspaltung. *Monatschr f Geburtsli u Gynak*. 1902;3:73.
12. Von Peham H, Amreich I. *Gyankologische Operationslehre*. Berlin/Basel: Verlag S. Karger; 1930.
13. Wertheim E. Zur frage der radikal operation beim uterus kebs. *Arch Gynecol*. 1900;61;627.
14. Wertheim E. Discussion on the diagnosis and treatment of carcinoma of the uterus. *Br Med J*. 1905;2:689.
15. Wertheim E. The extended abdominal operation for carcinoma uteri. Based on 500 operated cases. Translated by Grad H. *Am J Obstet Dis Women Child*. 1912;66:169-232.
16. Dursun P, Gultekin M, Ayhan A. The history of radical hysterectomy. *J Lower Gen Tract Dis*. 2011;15:235-245.
17. Meigs JV. Carcinoma of the cervix: The Wertheim operation. *Surg Gynecol Obstet*. 1944;78:195.
18. Meigs JV. The Wertheim operation for carcinoma of the cervix. *Am J Obstet Gynecol*. 1945;49:542.
19. Taussig FJ. Iliac lymphadenectomy with irradiation in the treatment of cancer of the cervix. *Am J Obstet Gynecol*. 1934;28:650.
20. Meigs JV. Radical hysterectomy with bilateral pelvic lymph node dissections. Report of 100 cases operated on 5 years or more. *Am J Obstet Gynecol*. 1951;62:854-870.
21. Meigs JV. Radical hysterectomy with bilateral dissection of the pelvic lymph nodes for cancer of the cervix (the Wertheim, Reis, Clark, Wertheim-Meigs operation). *Surg Clin North Am*. 1956;1083-1116.
22. Okabayashi H. Abdominale systematische Panhysterektomie fur karzinom des uterus. *Surg Gynecol Obstet*. 1921;33:136-156.
23. Okabayashi J. Radical abdominal hysterectomy for cancer of the cervix uteri. *Surg Gynecol Obstet*. 1921;33:335-341.
24. Yagi J. Extended abdominal hysterectomy with pelvic lymphadenectomy for carcinoma of the cervix. *Am J Obstet Gynecol*. 1955;69:33-47.
25. Fujii S. Original film of the Okabayashi's radical hysterectomy by Okabayashi himself in 1932, and two films of the precise anatomy necessary for nerve-sparing Okabayashi's radical hysterectomy clarified by Shingo Fujii. *Int J Gynecol Cancer*. 2008;18:383-385.
26. Piver MS, Rutledge F, Smith JP. Five classes of extended hysterectomy for women with cervical cancer. *Obstet Gynecol*. 1974;44:265-272.
27. Kobayashi T. *Abdominal Radical Hysterectomy with Pelvic Lymphadenectomy for Cancer of the Cervix*. 2nd ed. Tokyo: Nanzando; 1961:86.
28. Fujii S, Takakura K, Matsumura N, et al. Anatomic identification and functional outcomes of the nerve-sparing Okabayashi radical hysterectomy. *Gynecol Oncol*. 2007;107:4-13.
29. Dargent D, Brun JL, Roy M, Mathevet P. La trachelectomie elargie: une alternative a l'hysterectomie. Radicale dansu traitment des cancerws in filtrants. *J Ob Gyn*. 1994;2:285-292.
30. Dargent D, Mathevet P. Shauta's vaginal hysterectomy combined with laparoscopic lymphadenectomy. *Baillieres Clin Obstet Gynaecol*. 1995;9:691-705.
31. Dargent D, Martin X, Sacchetoni A, Mathevet P. Laparoscopic vaginal radical trachelectomy: a treatment to preserve the fertility of cervical carcinoma patients. *Cancer*. 2000;88:1877-1882.

32. Boronow RC. Remembering Alexander Brunschwig, MD (1901-1969). *Gynecol Oncol*. 2008;111(2 suppl):S2-S8.
33. Whipple AO, Parsons WG, Mullins CR. Treatment of carcinoma of the ampulla of Vater. *Ann Surg*. 1935;102:763-769.
34. Brunschwig A. Resection of head of pancreas and duodenum for carcinoma–pancreatoduodenectomy. *Surg Gynecol Obstet*. 1937;65:681.
35. Brunschwig A. Complete excision of pelvic viscera for advanced carcinoma: A one-stage abdominoperineal operation with end colostomy and bilateral ureteral implantation into the colon above the colostomy. *Cancer*. 1948;1:177-183.
36. Brunschwig A, Daniel W. Pelvic exenterations for advanced carcinoma of the vulva. *Am J Obstet Gynecol*. 1956;72:489-496.
37. Brunschwig A, Daniel W. Pelvic exeneration operations: With summary of sixty-six cases surviving more than five years. *Ann Surg*. 1960;151: 572-576.
38. Brunschwig A. Hemipelviectomy in combination with partial pelvic exenteration for uncontrolled recurrent and metastatic cancer of the cervix, five year survival. *Surgery*. 1962;52:299-304.
39. Barber HR, Roberts S, Brunschwig A. Prognostic significance of preoperative nonvisulaizing kidney in patients receiving pelvic exenteration. *Cancer*. 1963;16:1614-1615.
40. Brunschwig A, Barber HR. Extended pelvic exenteration for advanced cancer of the cervix. Long survivals following added resection of involved small bowel. *Cancer*. 1964;17:1267-1270.
41. Barber HR, Brunschwig A. Pelvic exenteration for extensive visceral necrosis following radiation therapy for gynecologic caner. *Obstet Gynecol*. 1965;25:575-578.
42. Barber HR, Brunschwig A. Pelvic exenteration for locally advanced and recurrent ovarian cancer. Review of 22 cases. *Surgery*. 1965;58:935-937.
43. Barber HR, Brunschwig A. Urinary tract fistulas following pelvic exenteration. *Obstet Gynecol*. 1966;28:754-763.
44. Barber HR, Brunschwig A. Excision of major blood vessels at the periphery of the pelvis in patients receiving pelvic exenteration: Common and/or iliac arteries and veins 1947 to 1964. *Surgery*. 1967;62:426-430.
45. Barber HR, Burnschwig A. Treatment and results of recurrent cancer of corpus uteri in patients receiving anterior and total pelvic exenteration 1947–1963. *Cancer*. 1968;22:949-955.
46. Brunschwig A, Barber HR. Secondary and tertiary rediversion of the urinary tract. A study based upon 72 cases among 840 pelvic exenterations for advanced cancer. *JAMA*. 1968;203:617-620.
47. Brunschwig A, Barber HR. Pelvic exenteration combined with resection of segments of bony pelvis. *Surgery*. 1969;65:417-420.
48. Kehrer E. Diagnose und therapie des vulva-karzinoms. *Zentralbl f Gynak*. 1912;36:1151-1155.
49. Basset A. Traitement chirurgical operatoire de l'epithelima primitif du clitoris indications-technique-resultats. *Rev Chir*. 1912;46:546.
50. Taussig FJ. Cancer of the vulva: An analysis of 155 cases (1911–1940). *Am J Obstet Gynecol*. 1940;40:764-779.
51. Taussig FJ. Results in treatment of lymph node metastasis in cancer of the cervix and the vulva. *Am J Roentgenol*. 1941;45:813-818.
52. Way S. Carcinoma of the vulva. *Am J Obstet Gynecol*. 1960;79:692-697.
53. Twombly GH. The technique of radical vulvectomy for carcinoma of the vulva. *Cancer*. 1953;6:516-530.
54. Stoeckel W. Classification of carcinoma of the cervix. Z Geburtshilfe Gynakol 1951;134:235-236.
55. Way S. The anatomy of the lymphatic drainage of the vulva and its influence on the radical operation for carcinoma. *Ann Roy Coll Surg Engl*. 1948;3:187-209.
56. Morley GW. Infiltrative carcioma of the vulva: Results of surgical treatment. *Am J Obstet Gynecol*. 1976;124:874-878.
57. Hacker NF, Leuchter RS, Berek JS, et al. Radical vulvectomy and bilateral inguinal lymphadenectomy through separate groin incisions. *Obstet Gynecol*. 1981;58:574-579.
58. Bricker EM. Bladder substitution after pelvic evisceration. *Surg Clin North Am*. 1950;30:1511-1521.
59. Miles WE. A method of performing abdomino-perineal excision for carcinoma of the rectum and of the terminal portion of the pelvic colon. *Lancet*. 1908;2:1812-1813.
60. Dixon CF. Surgical removal of lesions occurring in the sigmoid and recto-sigmoid. *Am J Surg*. 1939;46:12-17.
61. Dixon CF. Anterior resection for malignant lesions of the upper part of the rectum and lower part of the sigmoid. Read before the American Surgical Association, Quebec, Canada, May 27, 1948. *Ann Surg*. 1948;128:425-442.
62. Bacon HE. Abdominoperineal proctosigmoidectomy with sphincter preservation; five-year and ten-year survival after pull-through operation for cancer of rectum. *JAMA*. 1956;160:628-634.
63. Hopkins MP, Lowery A. Urinary conduits and continent urinary diversions. *CME J Gynecol Oncol*. 2003;8:290-297.
64. Gilchrist RK, Merricks, JW, Hamlin HH, Rieger IT. Construction of a substitute bladder and urethra. *Surg Gynec Obstet*. 1950;90:752-760.
65. Rowland RG, Mitchell ME, Bihrle R, et al. Indiana continent urinary reservoir. *J Urol*. 1987;137:1136-1139.
66. Bajany D, Politano VA. Stapled and nonstapled tapered distal ileum for construction of a continent colonic urinary reservoir. *J Urol*. 1988;140:491-494.
67. Kock NG, Nilson AE, Nilsson LO, et al. Urinary diversion via a continent ileal reservoir: Clinical results in 12 patients. *J Urol*. 1982;128: 469-475.
68. McIndoe AH, Bannister JB. An operation for the cure of congenital absence of the vagina. *Br J Obstet Gynaecol*. 1938;45:490-494.
69. Garcia J, Jones HW Jr. The split thickness graft technic for vaginal agenesis. *Obstet Gynecol*. 1977;49:328-332.
70. Owens N. A compound neck pedicle designed for repair of massive fascial defects. *Plast Reconstr Surg*. 1955;15:369-389.
71. Orticochea M. The musculo-cutaneous flap method: An immediate and heroic substitute for the method of delay. *Br J Plast Surg*. 1972;25 :106-110.
72. Orticochea M. A new method of total reconstruction of the penis. *Br J Plast Surg*. 1972;25:347-366.
73. McCraw JB, Massey FM. Vaginal reconstruction with gracilis myocutanous flaps. *Plast Reconstr Surg*. 1976;58:176-183.
74. Becker DW, Massey FM, McCraw JB. Myocutaneous flaps in reconstructive pelvic surgery. *Obstet Gynecol*. 1979;54;178-183.
75. McGraw J, Kemp G, Given F, Horton CE. Correction of high pelvic defects with the inferiorly based rectus abdominal myocutanous flap. *Clin Plast Surg*. 1988;15:449-454.
76. Benson C, Soisson AP, Carlson J, et al. Neovaginal reconstruction with a rectus abdominis myocutaneous flap. *Obstet Gynecol*. 1993;81:871-875.

Chapter 2. Surgical Anatomy and Instrumentation

Elizabeth A. Dubil, MD
G. Scott Rose, MD
John C. Elkas, MD, JD

SURGICAL ANATOMY

The complexities of radical extirpative surgery for locally advanced and recurrent pelvic cancer and the associated procedures necessary for successful functional and cosmetic reconstruction require a thorough understanding of anatomy that extends from the upper abdomen to the thigh. This chapter is not intended as an exhaustive anatomic discourse but rather as a summary of the relevant anatomic considerations important to the various operative procedures detailed in the chapters that follow.

Pelvis

1. Pelvic viscera

The true pelvis is bounded by the pelvic floor inferiorly and the pelvic brim superiorly and is defined by an imaginary line connecting the sacral promontory, the upper margin of the pubic symphysis, and the arcuate and pectineal lines (Figure 2-1). The pelvis contains the urinary bladder, rectosigmoid colon, uterus, adnexa, and a portion of the vagina, and important vasculature and lymphatic structures. The uterus is a centrally located organ between the bladder anteriorly and the rectosigmoid colon posteriorly. The muscular upper portion of the uterus is the fundus, while the tapered more fibrous component is the cervix, which directly communicates with the vagina. The fallopian tubes arise from the lateral, superior portion of the uterine corpus anterior to the utero-ovarian ligaments. The utero-ovarian ligaments suspend the ovaries and contain anastomoses between the uterine and ovarian vessels. The adnexa are classically lateral to the uterus; however, they may be found between the uterus and the rectosigmoid colon along the pelvic sidewall.

The only portion of the uterus not covered with serosa is the anterior cervix, which is covered by the bladder. The posterior portion of the bladder not only covers the anterior cervix, but it also overlies the proximal vagina. The anterior portion of the bladder lies against the pubic symphysis and abdominal wall, and the lateral and inferior portions lie against the obturator internus and levator ani muscles, respectively. The ureters are smooth muscle, retroperitoneal structures that drain urine from the kidney and enter the pelvis at the level of the bifurcation of the common iliac artery, medial to the infundibulopelvic ligament. They cross the common iliac vessels anteriorly and course laterally, under the infundibulopelvic ligaments while descending into the pelvis, running posterior to the ovary and deep to the broad ligament before traversing through the cardinal ligament and under the uterine artery approximately 2 cm lateral to the cervix. The ureters then curve anteromedially to enter the back of the bladder at the vesicoureteric junction.

The sigmoid colon is a short "S" curving of the descending colon just before the rectum. It is normally approximately 40 cm in length and is distinguished from the descending colon and rectum because it features a traditional mesentery and is not retroperitoneal. The sigmoid mesocolon fixes the sigmoid loop at the junction between the iliac colon and rectum; however, it can have a considerable range of motion. The sigmoid colon gradually transitions to the rectum just cephalad to the level of the posterior pelvic cul-de-sac, also known as the peritoneal reflection, and is defined by both a loss of appendices epiploicae and attenuation of the taenia coli. The posterior cul-de-sac, or pouch of Douglas, is formed by the posterior cervical and proximal vaginal peritoneum and the rectal peritoneum. The rectum is approximately 12 cm long, terminates at the anorectal ring, and transitions to the anal canal, which signifies the end of the gastrointestinal tract. The proximal one-third of the rectum is covered by peritoneum along the anterior and lateral portions. The middle third of the rectum is covered anteriorly by peritoneum, and the distal one-third is entirely retroperitoneal.

2. Ligaments and potential spaces

The term *ligament*, when used in the pelvis, refers to one of several membranous peritoneal folds that support the visceral organs and can contain vasculature, nerves, and smooth muscle. Five paired ligaments suspend the uterus. The round

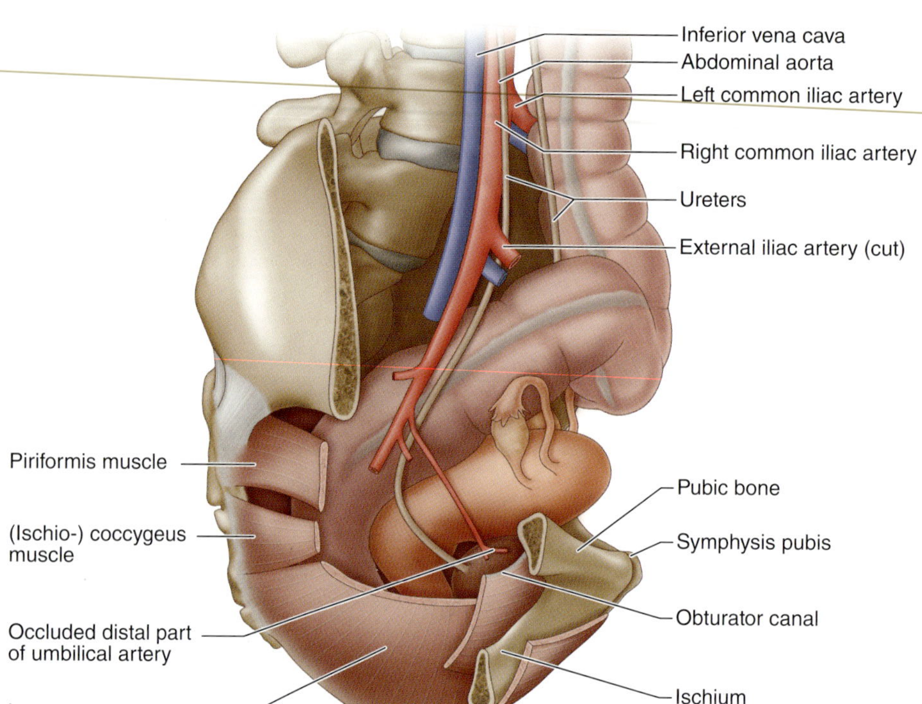

Fig. 2-1. Pelvis lateral view, right paramedian section.

ligaments are extension of the uterine muscle that extend from the anterior fundus to the pelvic retroperitoneum lateral to the epigastric vessel and pass into each inguinal canal, where they continue to the labia majora and mix with the tissue of the mons pubis. The artery of Sampson runs in the round ligament. The broad ligaments are large folds of peritoneum that connect the lateral aspect of the uterus to the pelvic sidewalls and floor. The paired cardinal (Mackenrodt's) ligaments are located at the base of the broad ligament and attach the cervix to the pelvic sidewall (Figure 2-2). Each cardinal

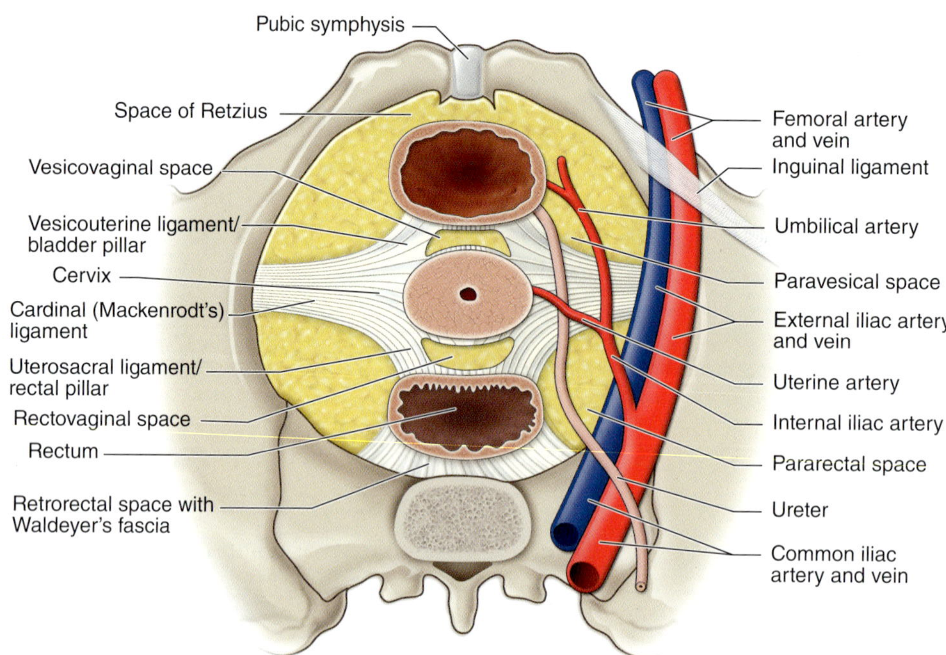

Fig. 2-2. Potential spaces and ligaments of the pelvis.

ligament contains the uterine, inferior vesicle, vaginal, middle rectal arteries and veins, and associated lymphatics. The posterior portion of cardinal ligament also contains major components of the autonomic nerve supply to the bladder and rectum. The uterosacral ligaments arise from the inferior portion of the posterior uterus and attach to the front of the sacrum, "sandwiching" the rectum at the rectal pillars. The ovaries are suspended to the uterus by the utero-ovarian ligaments and to the pelvic sidewall by the infundibulopelvic ligaments, which contain the respective gonadal artery and vein.

There are 8 potential spaces (2 paired lateral spaces and 4 unpaired midline spaces) in the pelvis that are filled with fatty or areolar tissue and that are important in radical pelvic surgery, as they provide relatively bloodless cleavage planes during dissection (see Figure 2-2). The ***retropubic space of Retzius*** is bounded anteriorly by the pubic symphysis and posteriorly by the bladder. Laterally, it merges with the ***paired paravesical spaces***, with the point of delineation being the umbilical artery. The paravesical space is typically developed by first dividing the round ligament and extending the peritoneal incision superiorly, inferiorly, and parallel to the infundibulopelvic ligament. The paravesical space is then entered between the superior vesicle artery or umbilical artery and the external iliac vein. The boundaries of each paravesical space are the pubic symphysis anteriorly, the superior vesicle artery and umbilical artery medially, the obturator internus muscle and external iliac vein laterally, and the cardinal ligament posteriorly. The cardinal ligament is the demarcation between the paravesical spaces and the ***paired pararectal spaces***. The boundaries of each pararectal space include the cardinal ligament anteriorly, the rectum medially, the internal iliac artery laterally, and the sacrum posteriorly. The pararectal spaces merge posteriorly with the ***retrorectal or presacral space***. The retrorectal space is defined by the posterior rectal fascia anteriorly, the pararectal spaces laterally, and Waldeyer's fascia along the anterior sacrum posteriorly. The ***rectovaginal space*** is bounded by the vagina anteriorly, the uterosacral ligaments laterally, and the rectum posteriorly. Lastly, the vesicouterine space continues inferiorly as the ***vesicovaginal space*** is defined by the posterior portion of the bladder anteriorly, the vesicouterine ligaments (bladder pillars) laterally, and the cervix (proximal) and vagina (distal) posteriorly.

3. Vascular anatomy and lymphatic drainage

The primary blood supply to the pelvis and lower extremities comes from the common iliac arteries, which arise from the bifurcation of the aorta at the level of L4 to L5 and extend laterally, where they divide across the sacroiliac joints to form the external and internal (hypogastric) iliac arteries (Figure 2-3). Each external iliac artery gives rise to an inferior epigastric artery, immediately proximal to the inguinal ligament, before it crosses under the ligament and becomes the femoral artery, which supplies the lower extremity. The inferior epigastric artery occasionally arises from the femoral artery and it supplies the lower portion of the rectus abdominis muscle and anastomoses with the superior epigastric artery, which arises from the internal thoracic artery. Preservation of the inferior epigastric artery is required for use of the rectus abdominis muscle for myocutaneous flap reconstructive surgery. The external iliac artery also gives rise to the deep circumflex artery at the level of the inferior epigastric artery. The deep circumflex iliac artery ascends obliquely behind the inguinal ligament to the anterior superior iliac spine, where it anastomoses with a branch of the lateral femoral circumflex artery.

The external iliac veins enter the pelvis inferior to the corresponding arteries; however, the right common iliac vein lies lateral to the right common iliac artery, while on the left side this relationship is reversed. In a small percentage of cases (22%), an accessory obturator vein enters the external iliac vein near its midpoint, which can be prone to tearing during dissection of the overlying obturator lymph nodes.

Each internal iliac (hypogastric) artery bifurcates into anterior and posterior divisions approximately 4 to 5 cm distal to the common iliac bifurcation. The posterior division typically gives rise to 3 parietal arteries: the iliolumbar, lateral sacral (superior and inferior branch), and the superior gluteal arteries. The anterior division of the internal iliac artery gives rise to 3 parietal and 3 or 4 visceral arteries. The visceral branches are the umbilical, uterine, and middle rectal arteries; a separate vaginal artery may also be present. The umbilical artery gives rise to the superior and inferior vesicle arteries before traversing toward the umbilicus and becoming obliterated. The parietal branches of the anterior division of the internal iliac artery are the obturator, internal pudendal, and inferior gluteal arteries. The venous drainage of the internal iliac system is variable and typically forms a large plexus deep within the lateral pelvis.

The major blood supply to the uterus is via the uterine artery, which gives off an inferior vaginal branch and an ascending branch that anastomoses superiorly with a descending branch of the ovarian artery. The ovarian arteries are unique in that they arise as paired visceral branches from the anterolateral surface of the aorta 2 to 3 cm below the renal arteries. The ovarian venous system does not mirror its arterial partner. The left ovarian vein enters the left renal vein lateral to the aorta, whereas the right ovarian vein enters the anterolateral portion of the vena cava just inferior to the renal vein.

The blood supply to the bladder originates at the umbilical artery, which gives rise to the superior and inferior vesicle arteries. The venous drainage of the bladder does not follow the arterial supply, instead draining the bladder neck through a large plexus of veins, which also forms anastomoses with the dorsal vein of the clitoris and vaginal plexus veins. Venous drainage continues from the bladder neck through the bladder pillars and into the cardinal ligament. The blood supply to the ureter comes from multiple small branches that arise along its path from the abdomen to the deep pelvis and have multiple anastomoses in the ureteral adventitia. The vascular supply to the abdominal ureter consists of branches to its medial aspect arising from the aorta, common iliac artery, and ovarian vessels, whereas the pelvic ureter receives its blood supply along its lateral aspect via branches from the internal iliac, uterine, and vesicle arteries.

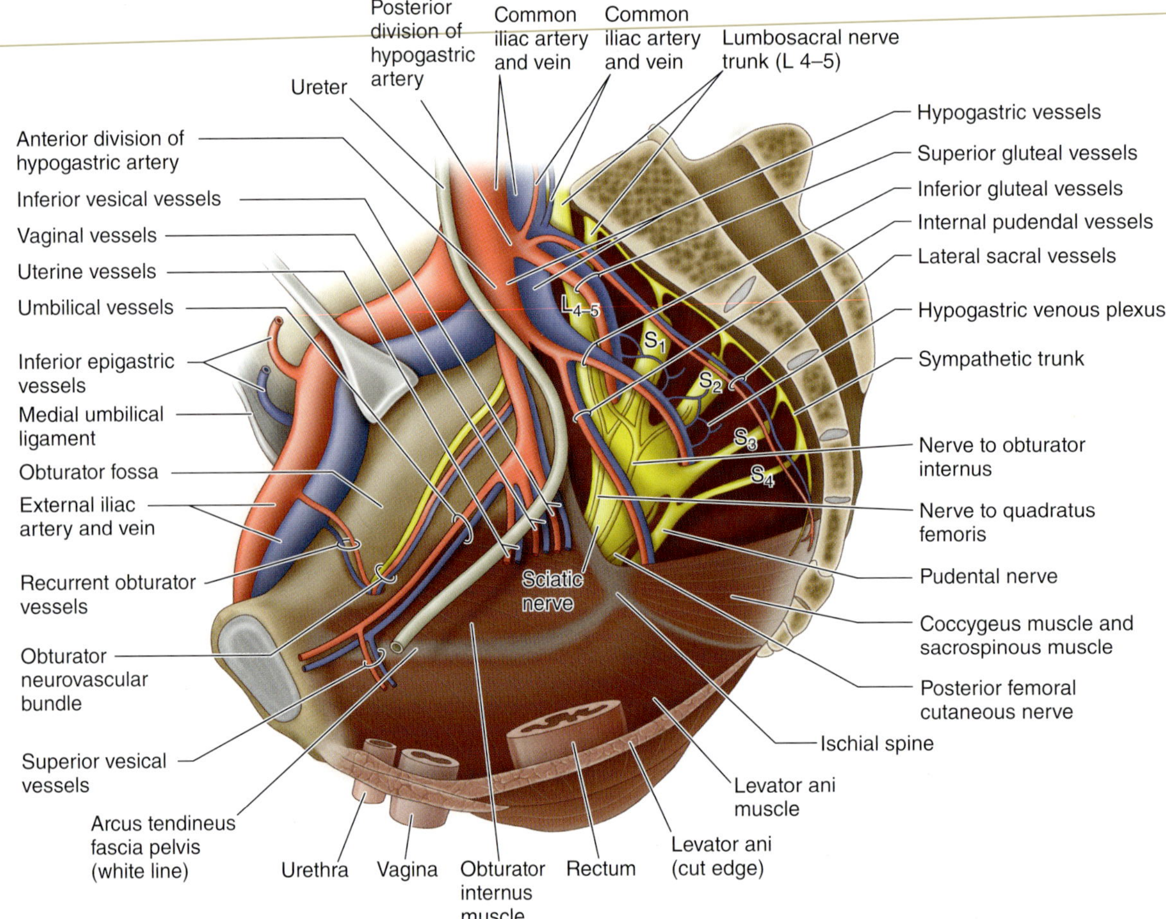

Fig. 2-3. Pelvic vasculature.

The blood supply to the upper vagina comes from descending branches of the uterine arteries. A separate vaginal artery can arise directly from the anterior division of the internal iliac artery or from the pudendal artery. The lower portion of the vagina is supplied by the inferior rectal artery or the inferior pudendal artery.

The rectum receives vascular supply from multiple sources including the inferior rectal artery (a branch of the internal pudendal artery), the middle rectal artery, the median sacral artery, and the superior rectal artery, which is a branch of the inferior mesenteric artery (IMA; Figure 2-4). The middle sacral artery arises from the posterior aspect of the aorta just above the aortic bifurcation and also gives off lateral sacral arteries. The critical point of Sudeck is represented by the bifurcation of the IMA into the superior rectal artery and the lowest sigmoid artery and has the potential for poor perfusion states if used for surgical anastomosis in the presence of hypotension.

The lymphatic drainage of the pelvic viscera can follow multiple routes, depending on the primary site of origin. Lymphatic drainage from the ovaries, fallopian tubes, and uterine fundus usually follow the ovarian veins directly to the abdominal aorta lymphatics (para-aortic, para-caval, and aorto-caval lymph nodes). The proximal vagina, cervix, lower uterine segment, and occasionally, the uterine fundus typically drain through the lymphatics of the broad ligament to the pelvic lymph node group, which is composed of the obturator, internal iliac, and external iliac nodal chains. Jackson's node refers to the distal-most external iliac lymph node. There is a separate lymphatic drainage pathway via the round ligament to the external iliac and inguinofemoral lymph nodes. The pelvic lymph node group drains to the common iliac lymph nodes and then to the aortic and caval node chains.

Vulva, Groin, and Anterior Thigh

Topographically, the vulva consists of the mons pubis, the paired labia majora and labia minora, clitoris, urethra, vaginal introitus, paired Bartholin's glands, paired paraurethral (Skene's) glands, the perineum, anus, and perianal tissue (Figure 2-5). Underlying the labia majora are the labial fat pads, which cover the superficial perineal compartment. The superficial perineal compartment contains the crura of the clitoris, the vestibular bulbs, and 3 paired muscles. The bulbocavernosus muscle immediately lies laterally to the lower vaginal wall, while the ischiocavernosus muscle runs

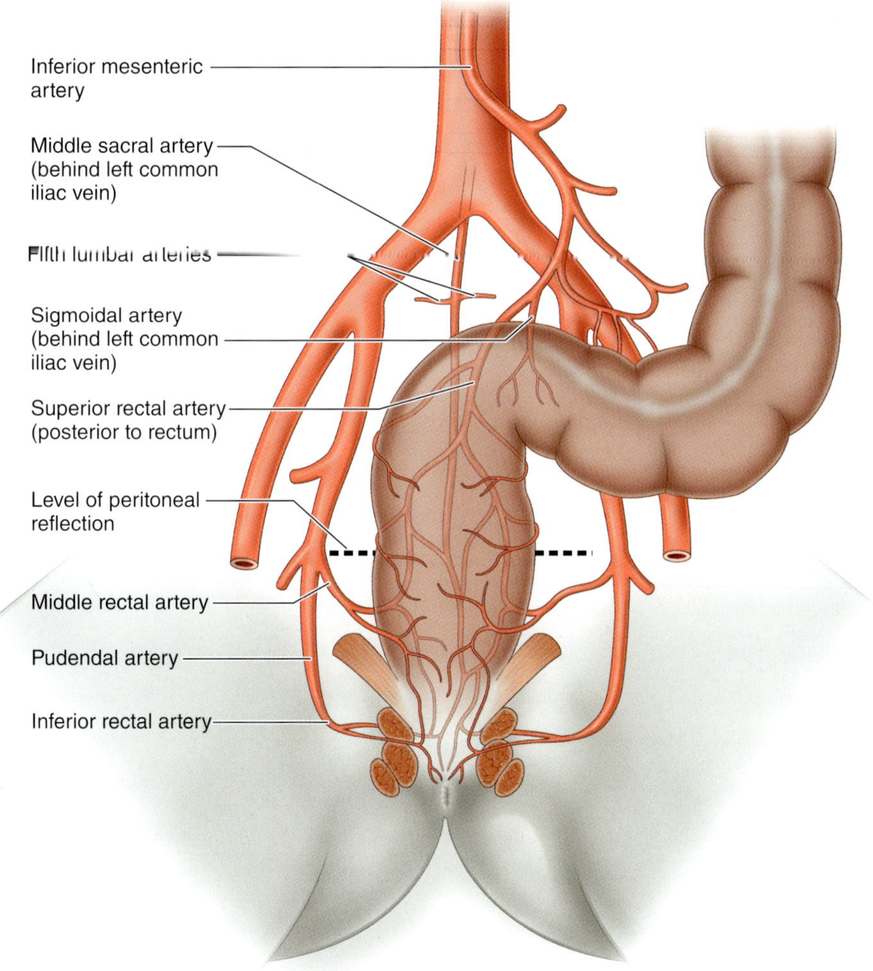

Fig. 2-4. Vascular supply to the rectum. Multiple anastomoses between the inferior mesenteric artery and internal iliac arterial systems, along with the middle sacral artery, to supply the rectum.

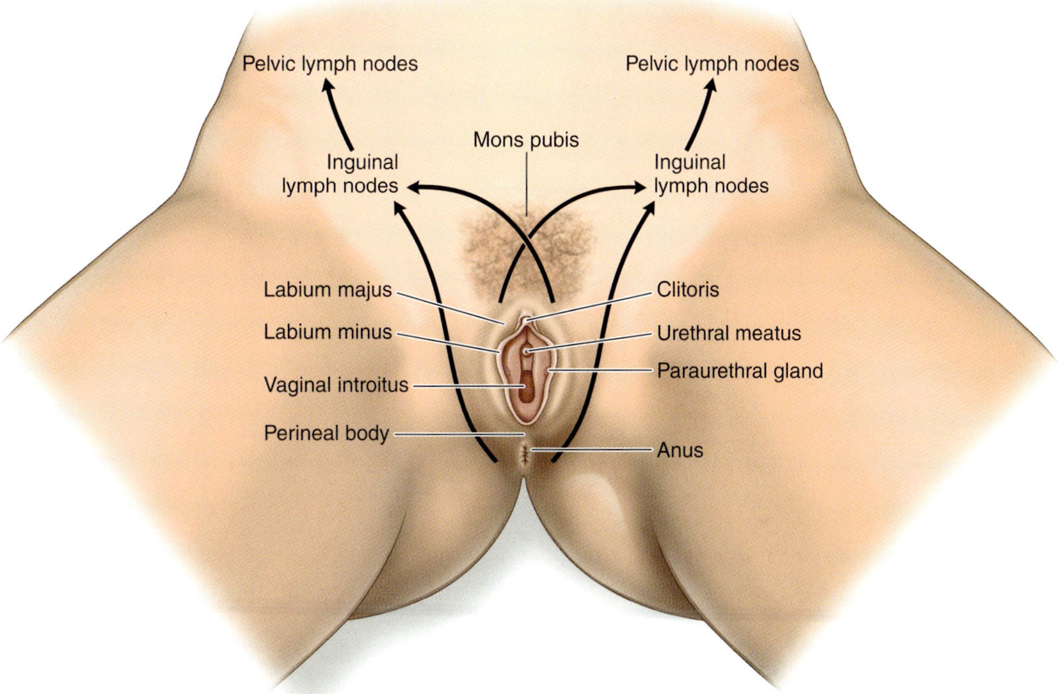

Fig. 2-5. Topographic anatomy of the vulva.

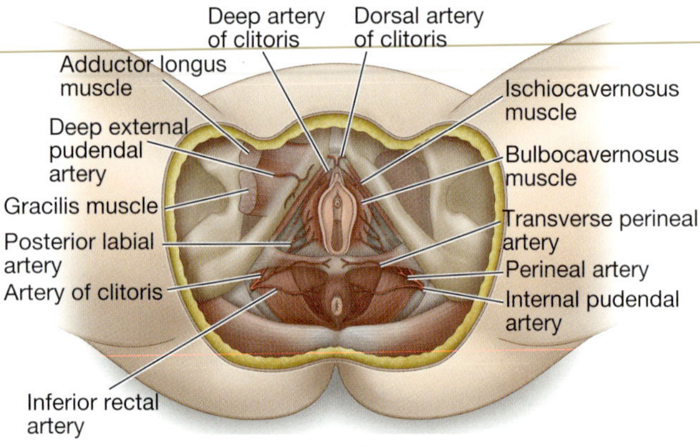

Fig. 2-6. Vascular and deep muscular anatomy of the vulva.

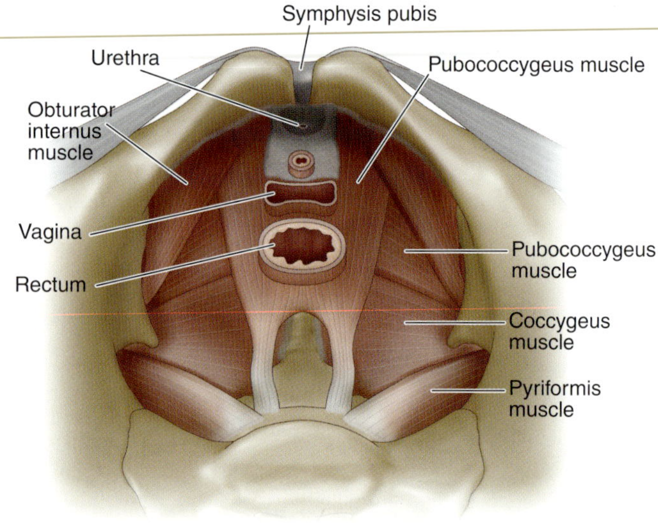

Fig. 2-7. Musculature of the pelvic floor.

along the medial margin of the pubic ramus (Figure 2-6). The perineal membrane is a tough connective tissue structure that traverses these 2 muscles. The ischiocavernosus muscles cover the clitoral crura and attach to the inferior pubic rami. The bulbocavernosus muscles cover the vestibular bulbs and run from the perineal body to the clitoris, passing around the vaginal introitus and urethral meatus. The superficial transverse perineal muscles run from the anterior ischial tuberosities to attach to the central tendon of the perineum. Cephalad to the superficial perineal space is the deep perineal space, which contains the deep transverse perineal muscle, and is delineated by the inferior and superior fascia of the urogenital diaphragm. The superior surface of the urogenital diaphragm is contiguous with the inferior surface of the levator ani muscle. The levator ani muscle (iliococcygeus, pubococcygeus, and puborectalis muscles) arises from the inner surface of the lesser pelvis and unites with its contralateral component in the midline, fusing with the bulbocavernosus and external anal sphincter muscles, to form the majority of the floor of the pelvic cavity (Figure 2-7). In combination with the coccygeus muscle, the levator ani muscle forms the pelvic diaphragm.

The vulva has 2 main sources of vascular support. The pudendal artery arises from the internal iliac (hypogastric) artery, which reaches the vulva via the pudendal (Alcock's) canal, and gives off the inferior rectal artery (within the ischiorectal fossa) and the perineal artery (see Figure 2-6). As it traverses the vulva superiorly, the internal pudendal artery becomes the clitoral artery. The second major blood supply to the vulva arises from the common femoral arteries, which give rise to the superficial external pudendal arteries (supplying the anterior and medial vulva) and the deep external pudendal arteries (supplying the labia majora and labial fat pads). The venous drainage of the vulva generally follows the arterial system except for the superficial and deep external pudendal veins, which drain into the greater saphenous vein rather than the femoral vein.

The principal lymphatic drainage pathway of the vulva is to the inguinofemoral lymph nodes, bounded by the femoral triangle (see below), and courses from posterior to anterior, across the mons pubis, to the superficial inguinal lymph nodes (see Figure 2-5). The superficial inguinal lymph nodes drain into the deep inguinal (femoral) lymph nodes, which are tributaries to the pelvic lymph nodes. Lymphatic pathways draining the midline vulvar structures (clitoris, anterior labia minora, and perineal body) lead to both right and left groin node basins. As a result, lateralized vulvar lesions (> 2 cm from the midline) are usually treated with a unilateral lymph node excisional procedure, while midline lesions require bilateral groin assessment. The superficial inguinal lymph nodes are almost always the primary node basin for cancers of the vulva and usually total 8 to 10 lymph nodes. The deep femoral nodes usually consist of 3 to 5 nodes, are located beneath the cribriform fascia, and are generally thought to represent the secondary node basin before drainage into the deep pelvic nodes occurs. The most proximal deep femoral node, Cloquet's node, is located in the femoral canal just beneath the inguinal ligament.

The inguinal ligament demarcates the superior border of the femoral triangle and is formed by the aponeuroses of the anterior abdominal wall muscles extending from the anterior superior iliac spine to the pubic tubercle. The femoral triangle is laterally defined by the medial border of the Sartorius muscle; the medial border of the triangle is formed by the lateral border of the adductor longus muscle (Figure 2-8). The Sartorius muscle originates at the anterior superior iliac spine and inserts on the medial tibial condyle, while the adductor longus muscle (the most superficial of the three thigh adductor muscles) arises from the front of the pubic bone and inserts on the body of the femur (linea aspera). The important structures within the femoral triangle, crossing from the pelvis beneath the inguinal ligament to enter the anterior thigh, moving from lateral to medial can be recalled by the

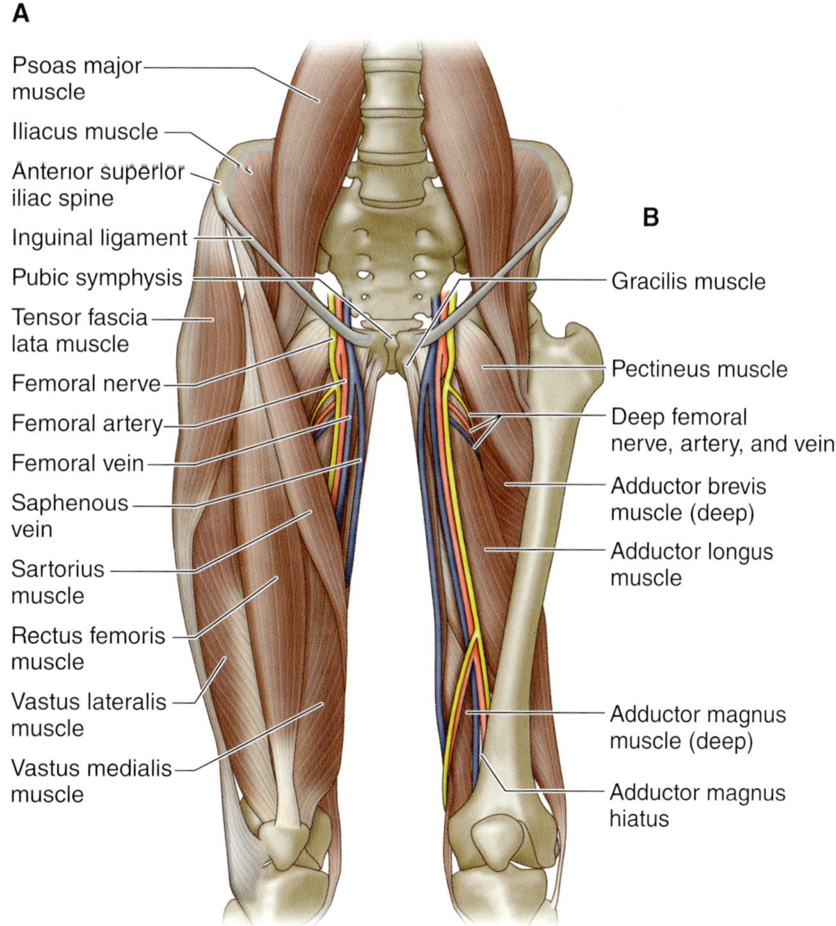

Fig. 2-8. Musculature and vasculature of the groin and anterior thigh, including the femoral triangle.

pneumonic N-A-V-E-L indicating the ***n***erve (femoral nerve), ***a***rtery (femoral artery), ***v***ein (femoral vein), ***e***mpty space, and ***l***ymphatic space. The iliopsoas and pectineus muscles form the floor of the femoral triangle. The femoral nerve lies on Iliopsoas muscle beneath the Iliopsoas fascia.

The muscles of the anterior thigh relevant to reconstructive surgery of the pelvis and vulva include those that function in extension of the leg and flexion/adduction of the thigh and individually are considered expendable. The gracilis muscle is the most superficial muscle of the medial thigh, originates from the symphysis pubis and pubic arch, and inserts into the upper medial tibia. The quadriceps femoris includes the four main extensor muscles of the anterior thigh. The rectus femoris is situated in the middle of the anterior thigh and arises from the anterior inferior iliac spine and acetabulum, while the vastus lateralis, the largest part of the quadriceps femoris, arises primarily from the greater trochanter. Both muscles insert into the patella and can be raised as myofascial or myocutaneous flaps to fill vulvar defects. The vastus medialis and intermedius muscles arise from the body of the femur and are generally not used in pelvic reconstruction.

Abdomen

1. Abdominal wall

The abdominal wall is composed of skin, Camper's and Scarpa's fascia, the external oblique muscles, internal oblique muscles, transversus abdominis muscles and aponeurosis, the transversalis fascia, rectus abdominis muscles, pre-peritoneal fat, and the parietal peritoneum (Figure 2-9). The 3 flat muscles of the abdomen attach to the lower costal cartilage, iliac crest, lateral two-thirds of the inguinal ligament, thoracolumbar fascia, and the linea alba, which is the collection of their aponeuroses. The rectus abdominis muscles extend from the pubic symphysis and pubic crest to the xiphoid process and lower costal cartilage. Each rectus abdominis muscle is enclosed within a sheath of fascia composed of the aponeuroses of the 3 flat abdominal wall muscles. The arcuate line is the transition point, usually midway between the pubic bone and the umbilicus, where the aponeurosis of each internal oblique muscle bifurcates around the ipsilateral rectus abdominis muscle. Below the arcuate line, the aponeuroses of all muscles pass anterior to the rectus. Above the arcuate line, the anterior

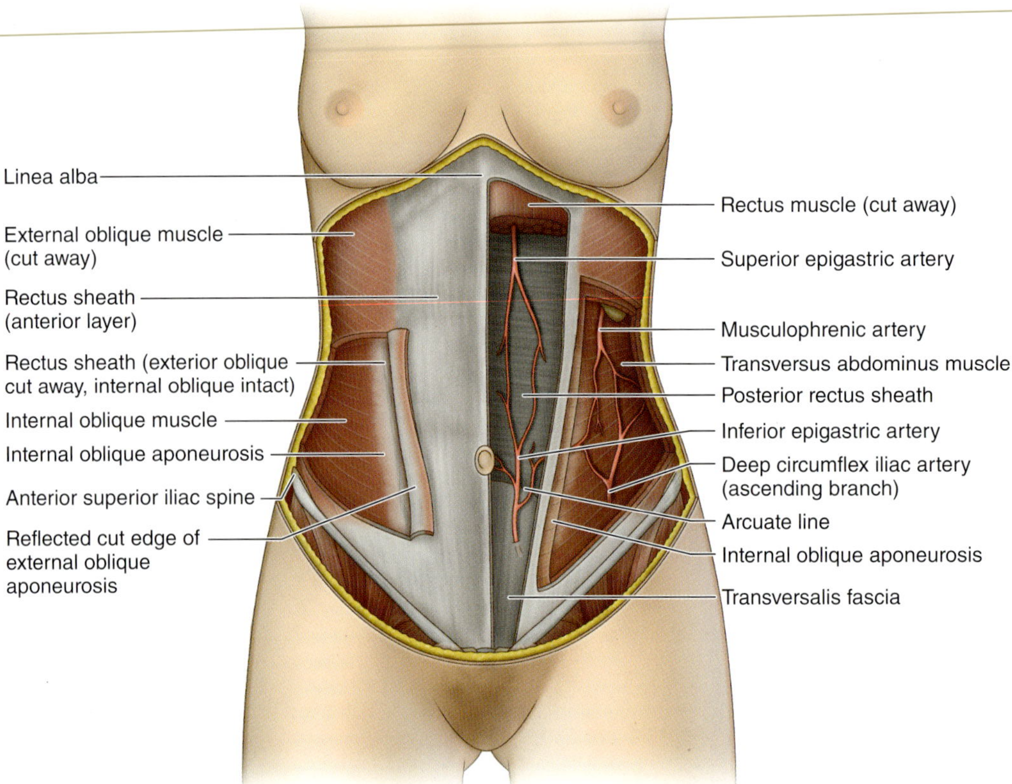

Fig. 2-9. Abdominal wall.

rectus sheath is formed by the external oblique aponeuroses and one-half of the bifurcated internal oblique aponeuroses, while the posterior rectus sheath consists of the other one-half of the bifurcated internal oblique aponeuroses and the aponeuroses of the transversus abdominis. The pyramidalis muscle attaches to the linea alba and the pubic symphysis and is frequently sacrificed in abdominal entry without consequence. The blood supply to the lateral portion of the abdominal wall comes from the lumbar arteries and the deep circumflex artery.

2. Abdominal viscera

The stomach connects the esophagus and the duodenum and rests on the transverse mesocolon. The blood supply to the stomach is via the celiac axis, directly by the left gastric, and indirectly by the right gastric artery and right gastroepiploic artery (via the gastroduodenal artery), which arise from the hepatic artery, as well as the short gastric arteries and the left gastroepiploic artery from the splenic artery. The gastric veins follow the course of the arteries and empty into the splenic vein, the superior mesenteric vein, or directly into the portal vein.

The small intestine extends from the pylorus of the stomach to the cecum. The duodenum connects the stomach to the jejunum is "C" shaped, and hugs the head of the pancreas. It is divided into 4 sections for description purposes only. The first portion travels left to right from the pylorus. This proximal portion of this section has a mesentery and is attached to the omentum and hepatoduodenal ligament. The second portion runs parallel to the inferior vena cava (IVC), in front of the right kidney and ureter. The third and fourth portions are retroperitoneal and run from right to left beneath the superior mesenteric artery (SMA) and ascend, respectively. The ligament of Treitz connects the duodenum to the diaphragm and marks the duodenal to jejunal transition. The first and second portions of the duodenum are supplied by the gastroduodenal artery; the third and fourth sections are supplied by the inferior pancreaticoduodenal artery, a branch of the SMA. Venous drainage follows the arterial supply, eventually draining into the portal system.

There is no anatomic demarcation between the jejunum and the ileum; however, the jejunum is generally of larger diameter and has a thicker wall with more prominent plicae circularis, while the ileum characteristically has more pronounced fat along its mesenteric border. The vascular supply to the small bowel is exclusively derived from the SMA, which lies behind the neck of the pancreas and arises directly from the aorta (Figure 2-10). The SMA gives off the inferior pancreaticoduodenal artery, the middle colic artery, right colic artery, and ileocolic arteries, which supply the head of the pancreas, duodenum, ascending and proximal transverse

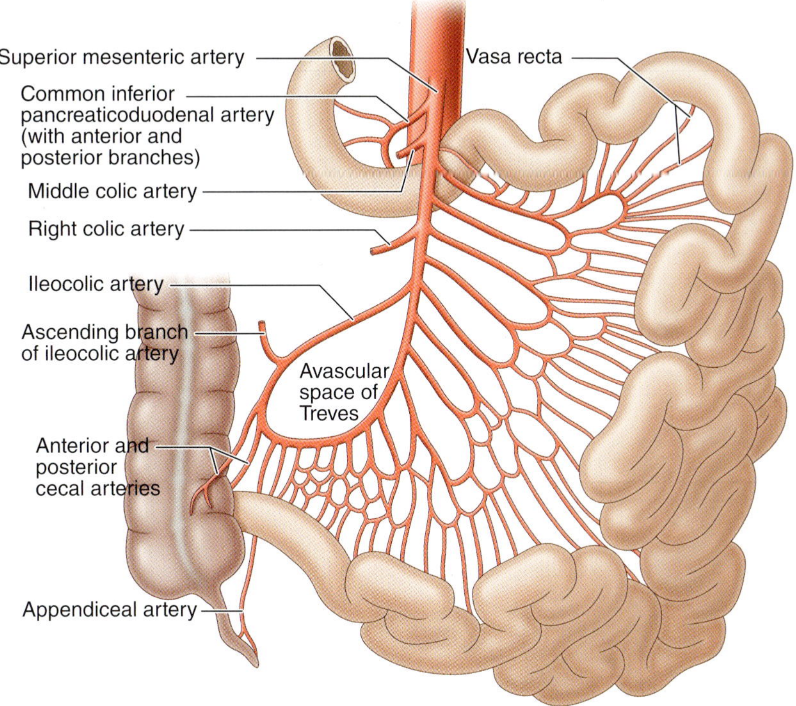

Fig. 2-10. Anatomy of the small bowel and arterial supply.

colon, cecum, appendix, and terminal ileum. The intestinal arteries (jejunal and ileal) arise from the SMA and supply the remainder of the small bowel. The intestinal arteries arise in multiple branches from the SMA and form arcades through the mesentery, giving rise to smaller parallel vasa recti that do not anastomose. The intestinal arteries can support a length of bowel approximately 6 to 8 cm distal to their point of entry into the bowel wall. The avascular space of Treves is the mesenteric area demarcated by the terminal ileal arteries and the ileocolic artery; the associated terminal ileum has an inconsistent blood supply and should not be incorporated into a bowel anastomosis. The venous drainage parallels the arterial supply, with the superior mesenteric vein joining the splenic vein to form the portal vein. The lymphatic drainage also parallels the venous system, originating in the mesenteric lymph nodes and terminating in the cisterna chyli.

The large bowel starts at the cecum and terminates at the anus (Figure 2-11). The colon consists of the ascending, transverse, descending, and sigmoid colon. There are 3 thickened longitudinal muscles that run the length of the colon from the appendix to the rectum referred to as taenia coli (taenia omentalis, taenia libera, and taenia mesocolic). The cecum is a blind pouch attached to the ileum and the ascending colon, and it does not have a mesentery. The appendix arises from the cecum, inferior to the ileocecal junction and has its own mesoappendix. The ascending colon runs from the ileocecal junction to the hepatic flexure and is retroperitoneal. The white line of Toldt is a peritoneal reflection that runs parallel to the ascending colon and descending colon and is a useful dissection entry point for mobilization of the colon. The transverse colon runs from the hepatic to splenic flexures and is intraperitoneal with its own mesentery. The descending colon begins at the splenic flexure, is retroperitoneal, and terminates at the pelvic brim where it transitions to the sigmoid colon. The arterial supply to the large bowel is from branches of the SMA and the inferior mesenteric artery (IMA; see Figure 2-11). The SMA gives rise to the ileocolic artery (cecum and appendix), the right colic artery (ascending colon), and the middle colic artery (transverse colon). The IMA branches into the left colic artery, sigmoidal arteries, and the superior rectal arteries, which supply the descending colon, sigmoid colon, and rectum, respectively. The marginal artery of Drummond is an anastomosis between the various branches of the SMA and the IMA that provides continuity of vascular support throughout the length of the colon. The area of the colonic mesentery between the middle colic artery and the left colic artery is known as the avascular space (or arc) of Riolan. Griffiths point is a watershed area at the communication of the ascending left colic artery with the middle colic artery through the marginal artery of Drummond at the splenic flexure. The vascular anastomosis at Griffiths point may be absent or tenuous in approximately 50% of cases; consequently, the splenic flexure is at risk for vascular compromise if used in an intestinal anastomosis. The venous drainage of the colon follows the arterial pattern except for the inferior mesenteric vein, which drains into the splenic vein, both of which then join the superior mesenteric vein to form the portal vein. The lymphatic drainage of the

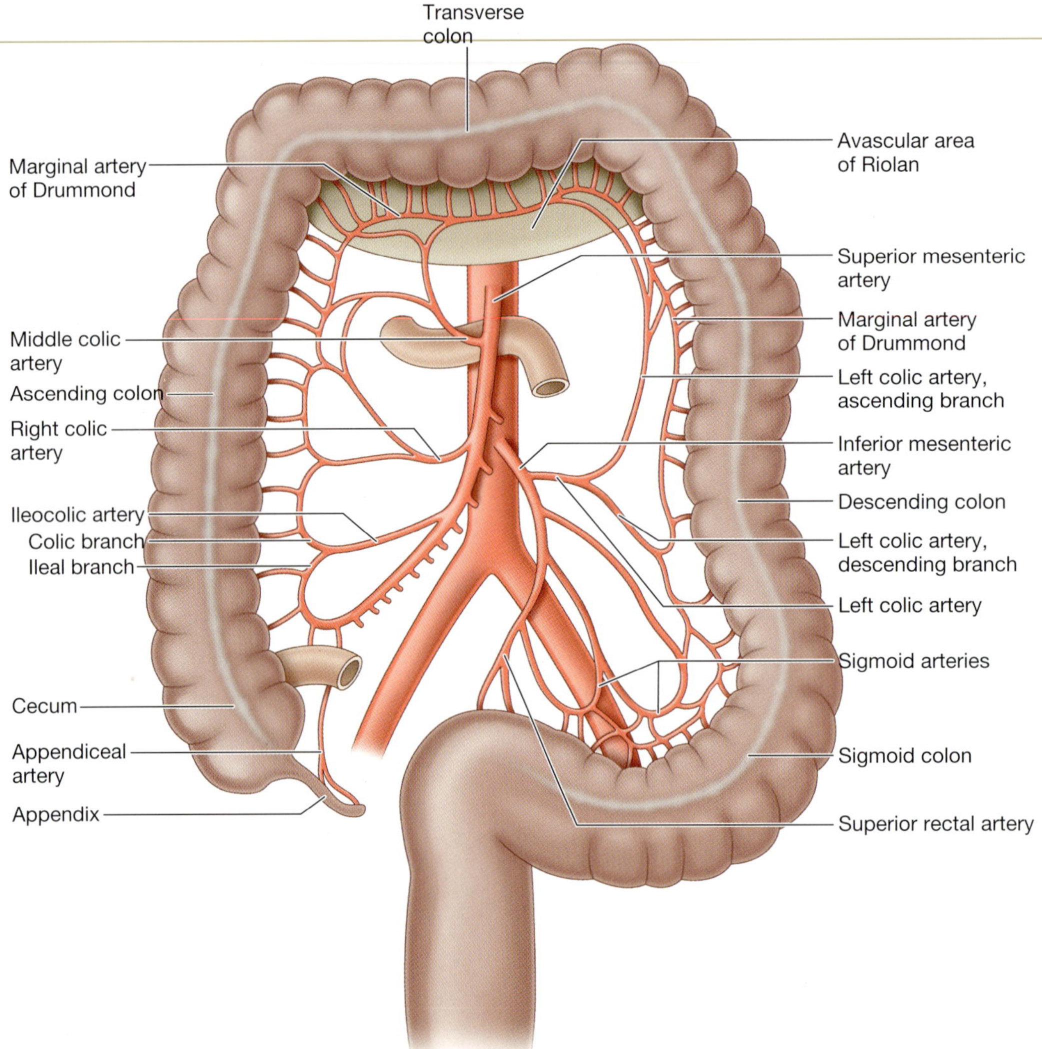

Fig. 2-11. Anatomy of the colon and arterial supply.

small bowel, ascending colon, and transverse colon is via the superior mesenteric lymph nodes. The descending colon and sigmoid colon drain to the inferior mesenteric nodes. Both lymphatic bundles are preaortic nodes and terminate in the cisterna chyli.

The greater omentum drapes from the greater curvature of the stomach over the transverse colon and doubles back toward the posterior abdominal peritoneum. The vascular supply to the omentum is provided by the right gastroepiploic artery (a branch of the gastroduodenal artery) and the left gastroepiploic artery (a branch of the splenic artery). The gastrocolic ligament is the portion of the omentum that connects the anterior transverse colon to the greater curvature of the stomach. The gastrocolic ligament is frequently fused with the transverse mesocolon, putting the middle colic artery at risk of injury during dissection in this area.

The liver is a large wedge-shaped organ under the right diaphragm that consists of 4 lobes (right, left, quadrate, and caudate lobe), and it is covered by a fibrous sheath called Glisson's capsule. Although divided into 4 lobes, the surgical anatomy of the liver is delineated by the functional anatomy and classified into 8 segments called Couinaud's segments. The spleen is located underneath the left diaphragm and is covered by peritoneum, except at the hilum, and is attached by 2 main ligaments: the gastrosplenic and lienorenal. Surgery on the liver or spleen is rarely indicated as part of radical pelvic cancer surgery and, as such, a detailed discussion of their anatomy is beyond the scope of this chapter.

3. Abdominal retroperitoneal structures

Behind the peritoneum in the abdomen lie the kidneys, ureters, adrenal glands, and crucial vasculature and lymphatic structures. The kidneys are symmetrical organs that lie at the level of T12 to L3, with their upper poles tilted medially. The left kidney is typically higher than the right. They are encapsulated organs, capped by the adrenal glands, and surrounded by perinephric fat (Gerota's fascia). The ureter arises from the renal pelvis and descends through the abdomen and pelvis to the bladder. The abdominal ureter runs along the psoas muscle with the ovarian vessels before passing over the iliac vessels and into the pelvis. The adrenal glands sit atop the kidneys and are enveloped in the renal fascia.

The pancreas is a delicate gland positioned anterior to the aorta and vena cava. It is divided into a head, neck, body, and tail, which start just right of midline and taper into the hilum of the spleen. Along the anterior surface, the right half of the pancreas is in contact with the transverse colon with only loose areolar tissue intervening. The narrow tail lies within the lienorenal ligament and extends to the splenic hilum. The arterial supply to the pancreas comes from the superior pancreaticoduodenal artery, a branch of the gastroduodenal artery, and the inferior pancreaticoduodenal artery, a branch of the SMA. Branches from the splenic artery also supply the body and tail of the pancreas. The venous drainage is either to the splenic vein or directly to the portal vein along the common bile duct.

The abdominal aorta enters the abdomen through the aortic hiatus of the diaphragm. It descends in the midline before bifurcating at the L4 to L5 level. The aorta has 6 paired and 4 unpaired branches. The first branches are the inferior phrenic arteries, which arise posteriorly just below the level of the diaphragm and supply the diaphragm. The celiac and superior mesenteric arteries are the next branches that arise anteriorly in close proximity to each other and supply a large portion of the gastrointestinal tract. Posteriorly, at the same level, are the suprarenal and renal arteries. The suprarenal arteries supply the adrenal glands. The renal arteries divide into several branches, which supply the inferior adrenal glands and the ureter before terminating at the kidneys. The right renal artery passes behind the IVC, renal vein, head of the pancreas, and descending duodenum. The left renal artery is generally higher than the right and passes behind the left renal vein, body of the pancreas, and splenic vein. Just below the level of the renal arteries, the ovarian arteries arise anteriorly and course over the ureters. The inferior mesenteric artery is the last anterior branch of the aorta and has a variable location, although it is commonly found 3 to 4 cm above the bifurcation of the aorta and supplies the colon and rectum. The terminal branches of the aorta are the common iliac arteries, between and just superior to which the median sacral artery can usually be found, which supplies the rectum and anus. Throughout the lumbar region, the aorta also gives off paired, posterior lumbar arteries supplying the abdominal wall and spinal cord.

The IVC ascends through the abdomen on the right side of the aorta before exiting the abdomen through the central tendon of the diaphragm. Inferiorly, it branches below the level of the aortic bifurcation and thus passes below the right common iliac artery. Tributaries to the IVC are the 3 hepatic veins, the right adrenal, paired renal, right ovarian, and lumbar veins. The left adrenal and left ovarian veins typically drain into the left renal vein. The "fellow's vein" is a small vein draining from the overlying lymph node bundle directly into the IVC just above the bifurcation. The lymphatic drainage of the mid-abdomen runs along the common iliac vessels and the anterior and lateral portion of the aorta. There are additional lymphatics between the aorta and the vena cava, as well as on the surface of the vena cava. All the lymphatics of the pelvis and abdomen join to form the cisterna chyli in the abdomen, which continues into the chest before emptying into the jugular vein.

SURGICAL INSTRUMENTATION

Surgical proficiency requires a well-planned approach with an appreciation for and knowledge of the instruments available. The surgeon should understand the advantages and limitations of each instrument before selecting which will best assist a procedure.

Retractors

Abdominal exposure for radical and reconstructive surgery for gynecologic cancer is usually best achieved via a midline vertical incision to gain access to the pelvis and the upper abdomen. There are 2 major types of retractors to assist with exposure, fixed and nonfixed. Two of the most commonly employed fixed retractors in gynecologic surgery are the Bookwalter (Codman and Shurtleff, Inc., Raynham, Massachusetts) and the Omni (Omni-Tract Surgical, St. Paul, Minnesota) retractors, as they both have a fixed arm attaching the retractor to the operating table, which provides consistent exposure to maximize patient safety while minimizing surgeon fatigue. The Bookwalter retractor has a fixed arm that attaches to the operating table and an oval, circular, or hinged ring that allows for the addition of various retractor blade attachments (eg, Deaver, Richardson, malleable blade) in multiple locations around the incision (Figure 2-12). The Omni retractor has a fixed arm attaching it to the operating table and two bent arms rather than a fixed ring for attaching

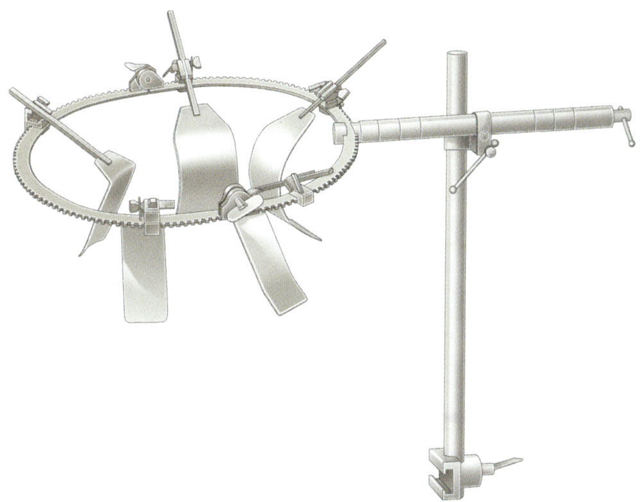

Fig. 2-12. Bookwalter retractor.

additional blade retractors. A hinged arm extension is also available if retraction is needed from an additional angle. The Omni retractor is helpful when operating on patients who are obese because the extent of lateral retraction is not limited by the width of a retractor ring. Nonfixed retractors are stabilized by the principle of counter-pressure on the abdominal wall incision. Two examples of nonfixed retractors are the Balfour (Sklar Surgical Instruments, West Chester, Pennsylvania) and the O'Connor–O'Sullivan (Medline Industries, Chicago, Illinois). With both fixed and nonfixed retractors care must be taken when placing the lateral blades so the femoral nerve is not compressed, because it runs under the psoas muscle along the lateral abdominal wall.

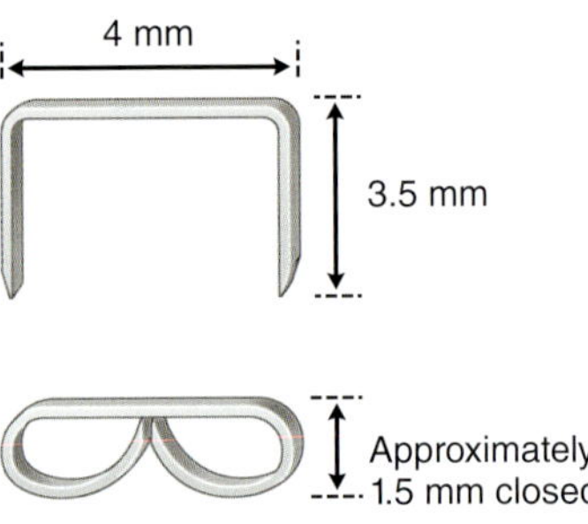

Fig. 2-13. Surgical staple dimensions: open and closed.

Vascular Clamps

Vascular clamps are used to control hemorrhage caused by damage to large caliber vessels, such as the iliac arteries or veins and the aorta and IVC. The clamps can be applied above and below the area of injury to facilitate repair of the defect, but must be done so without causing additional damage. If dissection and application of clamps cannot be performed in a safe manner, then direct pressure above and below the injury suffices. Commonly used vascular clamps include the DeRing Handle Bulldog (straight, curved, 90 or 45 degree), Glover (sharply curved), Debakey peripheral (straight or 45-degree), and the Lambert-Kay aortic clamps (Medline Industries, Chicago, Illinois).

Automated Stapling Devices

Contemporary stapling devices are most commonly used in radical pelvic surgery to close a segment of intestinal tract, either distal to the point of division or due to an enterotomy or colostomy, or to create anastomosis. There are also various staples for vascular pedicles. These procedures can be performed using hand-sewn suture techniques; however, automated stapling devices afford greater simplicity, increased speed, and comparable efficacy. A large case series reporting the use of automated stapling devices used for end-to-end anastomosis in radical gynecologic surgery in 49 patients reported 2 anastomotic breakdowns, and both patients had previously undergone radiation therapy.[1] It has been shown in animal models that some benefit may be derived from the improved blood flow.[1-3]

There are 3 basic categories of automated stapling devices: linear, curved, and circular, and most are offered in open (laparotomy) or laparoscopic versions. Typical variations of these basic stapler types include the addition of a cutting component, different angles of the stapling head, and multiple sizes. All stapling devices utilize the same basic principle of compressing an inverted U-shaped staple into a B-shape in the closed position, thereby securing the approximated tissue edges into place (Figure 2-13). This design is critical to allow the tissue to be secured without constriction of the vascular supply to the staple line. The exceptions to this rule are stapling devices designed for vascular pedicles. There are many types of linear stapling devices offered from 2 main manufacturers. Covidien (Mansfield, Massachusetts) manufactures the thoracoabdominal (TA), gastrointestinal anastomosis (GIA), and the Roticulator staplers, while Ethicon (Cincinnati, Ohio) manufactures the Proximate, Proximate-cutter, Proximate Access, and Endo-Surgery Linear Cutter stapling devices (Table 2-1).

The GIA stapler places a double- or triple-staggered row of titanium staples with a linear knife blade that transects tissue between the rows of staples. The GIA stapler comes in multiple cartridge lengths with various staple sizes for different tissue thicknesses (Figure 2-14). The appropriate staple size selected is dependent on the desired compression thickness of the tissue to be stapled. The 2.0-mm cartridge can comfortably compress 0.75 to 1.0 mm tissue; the 2.5-mm cartridge can comfortably compress 1.0 to 1.5 mm of tissue; the 3.5-mm cartridge can comfortably compress 1.5 to 2.0 mm of tissue; and the 4.8-mm cartridge can compress 2.0 mm of tissue. Staples are composed of titanium for most versions. The GIA stapling device also can deploy absorbable copolymer Lactomer staples with the same features as Polysorb suture in a 75-mm device with 1.5-mm staples. Each GIA stapler can be used up to 8 times, with a new cartridge and knife blade for each firing. All laparoscopic GIA staplers can be introduced through a 12-mm trocar sleeve, unless at 4.8-mm staple is chosen, which needs a 15-mm sleeve. The Endo GIA stapler compresses tissue as it is fired, with technology to consistently control tissue gap while the staple line is laid down and the tissue transected. The proximate linear staplers and linear cutting staplers allow adjustment of staple height versus multiple sizes of loads.

The TA stapler places a double row of titanium staples and does not transect tissue between the rows of staples, which is in contrast to the GIA. The TA stapler is offered in 30-mm, 45-mm, 60-mm, and 90-mm cartridge lengths (Figure 2-15). The 30-mm length also comes with a vascular load, which has 3 rows of staples. The 2.0-mm staple cartridge can comfortably compress 0.75 to 1.0 mm of tissue and is used for vascular pedicles. The 3.8-mm staple cartridges can comfortably compress 1.5 mm of tissue, and the 4.8-mm cartridge can compress 2.0 mm of tissue. The TA stapler can be fired up to 8 times in

Table 2-1. Examples of linear stapling devices.

Stapler	Length (mm)	Staple height (mm)	Rows	Comments
TA				
Open staplers	30, 45, 60, 90	3.5, 4.0	2	
	30VB	2.5	3	
Laparoscopic staplers	30	2.5, 3.5	3	
Proximate	30, 60, 90	Single height adjustable to 1.0 or 1.5	2	
	30V	3.1	3	
Gastrointestinal Anastomosis				
Open staplers	50	3.8[a]	4	
	60	2.5, 3.8[a], 4.8	4	
	75	1.5	4	Lactomer absorbable staples
	80, 100	3.8, 4.8	4	
	90	3.5[a]	4	
Laparoscopic staplers	30	2.0, 2.5[a], 3.5, 4.8[b]	6	Four rows if noncutting stapler
	45	2.0, 2.2, 3.5, 4.8[b]	6	
	60	2.5, 3.5, 4.8[a,b]	6	CO_2 gas-powered, 4 rows if noncutting stapler
Proximate Cutter	55, 75, 100	2.5, 3.8, 4.2, 4.5	4	
Endosurgery Linear Cutter	55, 100	Single height adjustable to 1.5, 1.8, or 2.0	6	
Roticulator	30	3.5, 4,8	2	
	30VB	2.5	3	
	55	3.5, 4,8	2	
	55 poly	4.3, 5.0	2	Lactomer absorbable staple

[a]This size also offered in a noncutting stapler.
[b]15-mm shaft; all others 12-mm.

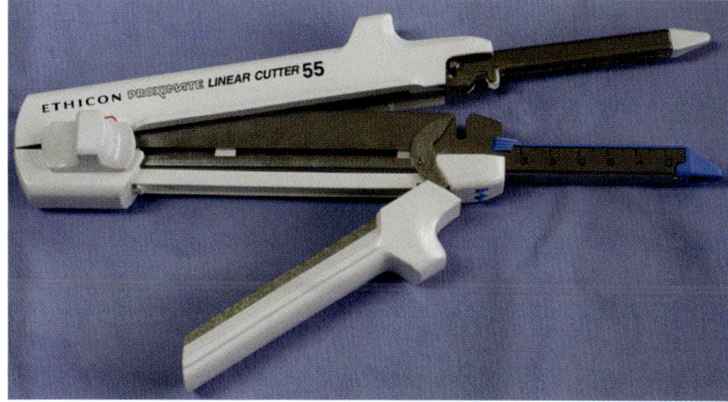

Fig. 2-14. Gastrointestinal anastomosis stapling device.

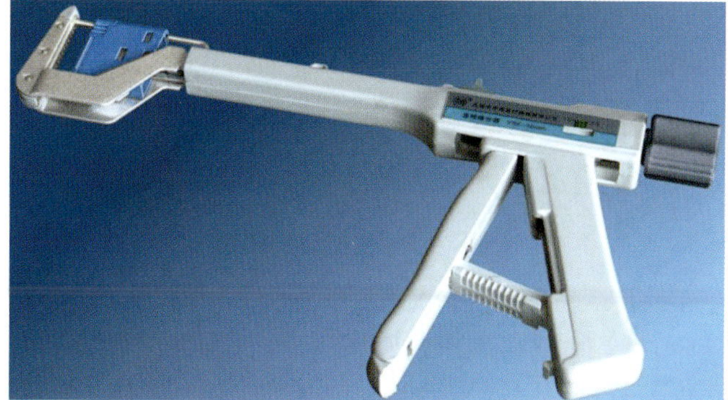

Fig. 2-15. Thoracoabdominal stapling device.

1 surgery. The Roticulator (Covidien, Mansfield, Massachusetts) is a linear stapler that has the ability to rotate its shaft 320 degrees and articulate a hinged cartridge 120 degrees, thus allowing for greater flexibility of application. It comes in 30- and 55-mm lengths and places a double staggered row of 3.5- or 4.8-mm titanium staples, or a triple row of 2.5-mm staples in its vascular version. This device also can deploy absorbable copolymer Lactomer staples in the 55-mm length version. The Proximate Access comes in a 55-mm length and allows for 30 degrees of flexion and 80 degrees of rotation. The Contour (Ethicon, Somerville, New Jersey) curved stapler/cutter lays down 4 rows of titanium staples and cuts between the 4 rows of staples in a 40-mm line with a width of 30 mm. It is fashioned for use in the lower pelvis.

The circular end-to-end anastomosis (CEEA) stapler lies down a double row of titanium staples and has a self-contained cutting blade to excise the inverted internal ring of tissue (Figure 2-16). The CEEA stapler is typically offered in 3.5-mm and 4.8-mm staple sizes based on desired tissue compression thickness. The Covidien CEEA comes in 21-mm, 25-mm, 28-mm, 31-mm, 33-mm, and 34-mm cartridge sizes that indicate the outer diameter of the stapler cartridge. The smaller 3 sizes only accommodate 3.5-mm staples and the others come in both 3.5 and 4.8 mm. The Ethicon circular stapler comes in 21-mm, 25-mm, 29-mm, and 33-mm sizes and had adjustable compressed staple heights of 1.0 mm and 2.5 mm. The functional anastomotic luminal diameter will be approximately 10 mm smaller than the outer diameter of the stapler cartridge.

The success of an intestinal anastomosis is dependent on several patient factors, such as nutritional status, infection and inflammation due to tumor, and use of medications such as steroids. However, many surgical factors should be abided when performing anastomosis, such as elimination of tension, maintenance of adequate blood supply, gentle handling of the tissue, and creation of a line that does not leak or bleed (but also does not cause a luminal stricture or devascularization from too much tissue compression). One innovation that has been developed in an effort to prevent staple line anastomotic leak is the use of reinforcement material along the staple line to redistribute the tension more evenly and seal the narrow spaces between the staples as well as the staple holes.[1,2]

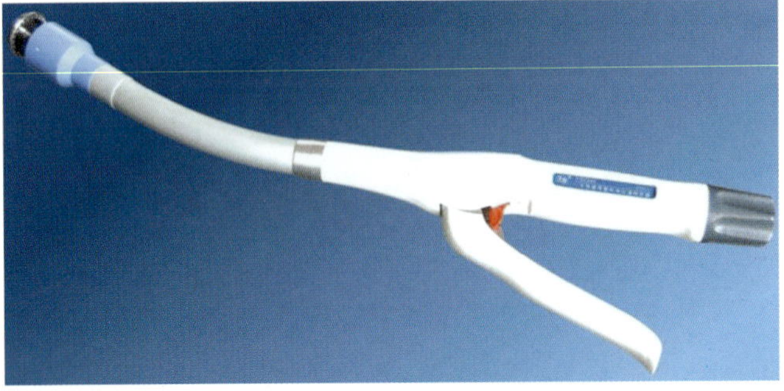

Fig. 2-16. Circular end-to-end anastomosis stapling device.

Material that have been used as a buttress include the Gore Seamguard (Gore Medical, Flagstaff, Arizona), a nonabsorbable and absorbable sleeve placed over each arm of the stapler prior to firing, and Peristrips dry with Veritas (Synovis Surgical Innovations, Deerfield, Illinois) collagen matrix, an absorbable product made from bovine pericardium attached to the stapler with a gel.

Energy Sources

1. Electrosurgery

The use of energy in surgery has been around since man discovered that heated stones could be applied to wounds to stop bleeding. Electrosurgery, sometimes referred to as electrocautery, as we know it began with fulguration in the early 1900s in which high frequency, low amperage current was applied to superficial cancers by Simon Pozzi.[3] Modern electrosurgical units, of which the Bovie (Valleylab, Boulder, Colorado) is the most well known, generate and alternating current of adjustable frequency in either a monopolar or bipolar fashion. Monopolar energy passes electrons from an active electrode through the patient in the path of least resistance to a dispersive electrode pad, which completes the circuit. Bipolar energy has a return electrode integrated into the device, and thus electrons pass between their electrodes, delivering current to the target tissue in between. Waveforms can be modified to delivery continuous current (known also as "cut" mode), interrupted current ("coagulation" mode), and a blended version. The continuous flow of energy leads to rapid buildup of heat and subsequent vaporization without significant heat transfer. The interrupted flow results in less current exposure over time, which is lower-energy, translating into a coagulum of tissue. How the electrode of a unipolar device is held in relation to the tissue also effects tissue reaction, with arcing of current cutting at continuous flow and fulgurating with interrupted flow.

2. Vessel sealers

Bipolar devices are used for their coagulative effects. Devices such as the Ligasure (Valleylab, Boulder, Colorado) and Enseal (Ethicon, Cincinnati, Ohio) are examples of biopolar electrothermal devices that function in both the sealing and cutting of vessels. These devices function by denaturing and reforming the collagen in the vessel walls and have a self-contained surgical knife for dividing the pedicles after vessel sealing. The electrosurgical circuit for the Ligasure device is a tissue response generator that senses the impedance of the tissue bundle held within the forceps. The circuitry of the generator automatically adjusts for an appropriate amount of energy to be delivered to the tissue, thereby effectively sealing vessels up to 7 mm in diameter. The device has a curved jaw and 180-degree rotating shaft that allows for access into the deep pelvis. The electrode length is 36 mm and its cutting length of 34 mm. It uses an audible activation tone that changes from a continuous tone to one short tone when the seal cycle is complete.

The Enseal device comes with a curved or straight jaw is 20 mm in length, and has a 360-degree rotating shaft. It can seal vessels up to 7 mm in diameter. The Enseal uses a temperature-controlling polymer that expands and causes local disruption in conduction over a temperature of 100°C. This allows heat to be delivered to thicker tissue in the jaws without overheating and causing thermal spread in the thinner areas. The thermal spread is 1 mm. The Enseal uses an I-Blade that compresses the jaws together as the blade travels down the jaw.

The Harmonic ACE (Ethicon, Cincinnati, Ohio) and the Gyrus PK (Olympus, Southborough, Massachusetts) are vessel sealers that can cut a pedicle, but which utilize different energy forms. The Gyrus PK uses radiofrequency energy to seal, coagulate, and cut tissue. The current delivered is adjusted based on tissue resistance. The Harmonic ACE uses ultrasonic vibration to coagulate, coapt, and cut tissue. It can seal and transect vessels up to 5 mm in diameter. The low-frequency energy causes tissue shear and denaturing of proteins, resulting in the coagulum without much collateral tissue damage.

3. Argon beam coagulator and the PlasmaJet system

The argon beam coagulator (Conmed, Utica, New York) is a device that delivers energy to tissue by a column of ionized argon gas, which contacts the tissue as a current via a stream of gas. Individual arc tunnels are formed within the target tissue. It is thought that because of the formation of these arc tunnels, more uniform distribution of current occurs within the tissue, resulting in a more uniform coagulative effect with less thermal injury. The argon gas also functions to improve visualization of the operative field by displacing blood and debris. The gas flows at 4 to 7 L/minute, with a voltage of 5000 to 9000 and 4 to 10 mm of thermal spread. Typical settings are 70 to 80 W for cauterizing small caliber vessels and 110 to 120 W for dissecting through thicker tissue (eg, pelvic sidewall). The PlasmaJet system (Theale, Berkshire, UK) also utilizes argon gas. The manufacturer purports that the system delivers a neutral stream of energy, which acts similarly in that it clears debris from the operating field and creates coagulative necrosis of underlying tissue; however, the gas flow is less than 0.4 L/minute, with a voltage of 30 to 60 and a reported thermal spread of 0.5 to 2 mm.

REFERENCES

1. Yo LS, Consten EC, Quarles van Ufford HM, Gooszen HG, Gagner M. Buttressing of the staple line in gastrointestinal anastomoses: overview of new technology designed to reduce perioperative complications. *Dig Surg*. 2006;23(5-6):283-291.
2. Choi YY, Bae J, Hur KY, Choi D, Kim YJ. Reinforcing the staple line during laparoscopic sleeve gastrectomy: does it have advantages? A meta-analysis. *Obes Surg*. 2012;22(8):1206-1213.
3. Massarweh NN, Cosgriff M, Slakey DP. Electrosurgery: history, principles, and current and future uses. *J Am Coll Surg*. 2006;202(3):520-530.

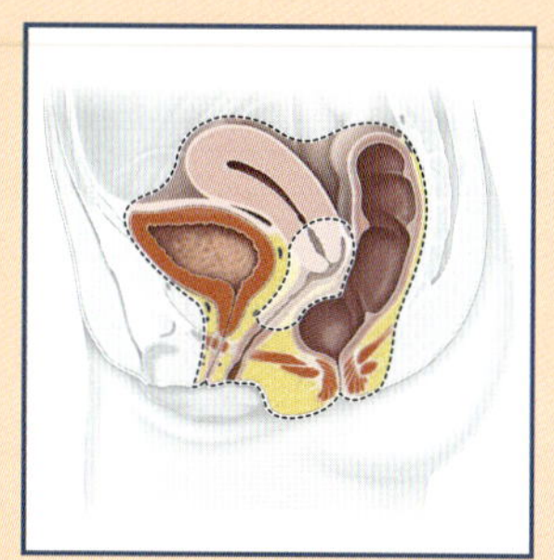

Part II

Extirpative Operations

Chapter 3. Radical Hysterectomy With En Bloc Vaginectomy or Pelvic Lymphadenectomy

David Cibula, MD, PhD

BACKGROUND

Radical hysterectomy with en bloc total vaginectomy is rarely performed in gynecologic oncology; however, both radical hysterectomy and vaginectomy are separately considered classic procedures. The first hysterectomy with resection of lateral parametria was described in 1895 by Clark.[1] However, lymphadenectomy was not part of this procedure. Three years later, Wertheim performed the first radical hysterectomy in combination with pelvic lymphadenectomy in Austria.[2] Wertheim's early mortality rate was about 30%, but this decreased quickly in time, with a cumulative experience of 10% in his report of 500 operations published in 1911.[3] In parallel to the abdominal approach to radical hysterectomy, Schauta developed a vaginal technique, which was first published in 1908.[4] Both approaches, abdominal and vaginal, form the current basis for the radical surgical treatment of cervical cancer. The surgical principles were modified during the twentieth century by many other surgeons; Amreich made meaningful contributions to the vaginal approach, while Wertheim's abdominal procedure has been expanded upon by Latzko, Okabayashi, and Meigs.[5]

INDICATIONS AND CLASSIFICATION

Indications

The most frequent contemporary indication for radical hysterectomy with en bloc vaginectomy is early-stage (FIGO I–II) vaginal cancer, provided the disease is localized to the proximal part of the vagina and is invading into the paracolpium and parametrium.[6,7] This procedure is also indicated for the clinical scenario with combined pathology consisting of early-stage cervical cancer (FIGO I-IIA) and vaginal intraepithelial neoplasia (VaIN). VaIN is often multifocal, and an underlying invasive cancer is reported in nearly one-third of cases.[8] Although more conservative treatment modalities are usually preferred, especially in patients who are younger, partial or total vaginectomy is a treatment of choice in women who are not sexually active, in recurrent lesions, or in multifocal dispersive lesions involving the entire vagina. Less common indications described in the literature include cervical embryonal rhabdomyosarcoma,[9] recurrent endometrial cancer in the upper vagina,[10] or clear cell carcinoma of the cervix or vagina.[11-13]

Considering radical hysterectomy as an individual procedure, the indications are not entirely uniform. One commonly accepted indication for radical hysterectomy is the treatment of cervical cancer stage IB1, in which radical hysterectomy has been associated with excellent oncologic outcomes. Primary surgical treatment is also feasible and has a satisfactory oncologic outcome, according to available data, for locally advanced cervical cancer tumors of stages IB2, IIA, and selected patients with stage IIB disease.[14,15] However, the major limitation of the surgical approach in locally advanced stages is the high proportion of patients with lymph node involvement, which may be as high as 40% for patients with stage IIB disease, and is a requirement for adjuvant radiotherapy.[16] The requirement for 2 treatment modalities—extensive surgical procedure and adjuvant radiotherapy—is associated with a substantial increase in the risk of postoperative morbidity. An alternative treatment modality for bulky cervical tumors or tumors with parametrial invasion is primary chemoradiation. There are no data available comparing directly the morbidity and oncologic outcome of surgery and radiotherapy.

Radical hysterectomy with or without vaginectomy may be indicated for other disease processes, depending on the extent of local disease. The role of parametrial resection with hysterectomy is not well established in locally advanced endometrial cancer. Radical hysterectomy is fully advocated only in tumors invading into the parametria, while, in stage II endometrial cancer with the invasion limited to cervical stroma, a survival benefit of radical hysterectomy over simple hysterectomy has not been established.[17] In clinical practice, most patients with endometrial cancer and stage II disease are referred for adjuvant radiotherapy, which likely abolishes any benefit from surgical removal of parametria. Radical hysterectomy may also be a necessary part of the debulking procedure in ovarian cancer surgery if there is an invasion of carcinomatosis into the broad ligament and lateral parametria. Radical hysterectomy is occasionally required to ensure satisfactory excision of non-oncologic disease process such as severe endometriosis or extensive tubo-ovarian abscess.

Classification

Even though radical hysterectomy with en bloc vaginectomy is performed in 1 step and results in 1 specimen removed en bloc, in terms of procedure performance it essentially consists of 2 different surgeries: radical hysterectomy and vaginectomy. Therefore, both procedures must be separately classified.

The key parameter for differentiating among the types of radical hysterectomy is the extent of parametrial resection. Due to the location of autonomic nerves in the caudal parts of the parametria, it is largely the vertical (deep parametrial) resection that determines late morbidity, particularly bladder and rectal dysfunctions.[18-21] The extent of resection should be precisely defined for all 3 parts of the parametria (ventral, lateral, dorsal) in 3 planes (sagittal, frontal, and transverse). The classification system described in this chapter is based on the proposal published by Querleu and Morrow[22] and later extended into three dimensions.[23] Five types of the procedure (A, B, C1, C2, D) coincide with other common historical types of radical hysterectomy (Table 3-1). Because type A corresponds with the extrafascial hysterectomy and type D, aiming at the resection of internal iliac vessels, is rarely used; differentiating between types B, C1, and C2 is clinically the most relevant.

The type B procedure corresponds with modified radical hysterectomy. The main resection margin is located ventrally and laterally at the ureter. Identification of autonomic nerves is not required, because the nerves remain unexposed in the parametria and the hypogastric plexus is fully preserved. The ureter is identified in the parametrium, unroofed, dissected from the cervix and laterally displaced. The objective of this type of radical hysterectomy is the resection of just a small initial part of the medial leaf of the ventral parametria and 1 to 1.5 cm of the lateral and dorsal parametria.

The major intention of the type C1 procedure is to remove adequate parts of the ventral, lateral and dorsal parametria, while concurrently preserving the major autonomic nerves comprised of the inferior hypogastric plexus and splanchnic nerves. The inferior hypogastric plexus runs in the lateral part of the dorsal parametrium, laterally around the cervix below the ureter at the level of the vaginal fornix and ventrally in the infra-ureteral part of the ventral parametrium towards the urinary bladder.[18-20] It receives branches of the splanchnic nerves localized at the bottom of the lateral pararectal space and in the caudal part of the lateral parametrium below the parametrial veins. The surgical margins of this nerve sparing procedure must therefore be kept above the course of nerve structures in the ventral, lateral and dorsal parametrium. The radicality of the C2 procedure is substantially different, with the aim being to remove the majority of all three parametrial components. The resection margins are extended caudally to the sacral bone and ventrally to the urinary bladder wall. As a consequence, major branches of the autonomic nerves are sacrificed during the C2 type procedure.

The classification of the vaginectomy procedure is simpler than radical hysterectomy. Considering the anatomic relationship of the vagina to other organs such as the urinary bladder, the rectum and the urethra, no option exists for increasing the radicality of resection in the sagittal plane. The length of the resected vagina can be adjusted, either described by the length of the proximal vagina that should be excised (eg, 3-cm excision of proximal vagina), as a proximal vaginectomy (proximal one-half of the vagina), or as a total vaginectomy (complete excision of the vagina to the introitus). In cases in which other associated organs must be removed together with the vagina (urinary bladder, rectum, urethra) the procedure is more accurately classified as pelvic exenteration.

Table 3-1. Querleu-Morrow classification system and corresponding historic types of radical hysterectomy.

Q-M classification system	Corresponding types
A	Extrafascial hysterectomy
B	Modified radical hysterectomy Class 2 radical hysterectomy
C1	Nerve sparing radical hysterectomy
C2	Class 3 radical hysterectomy Classical/standard radical hysterectomy
D	Laterally extended parametrectomy

PREOPERATIVE PREPARATION

Box 3-1 KEY SURGICAL INSTRUMENTATION

- Monopolar pencil (Bovie)
- Bipolar forceps
- LigaSure Impact Instrument (Covidien, Mansfield, Massachusetss) *or* Enseal Super Jaw Curved (Ethicon, Somerville, New Jersey)
- LigaSure 5-mm Blunt Tip Instrument (Covidien, Mansfield, Massachusetss) *or* Enseal G2 Curved (Ethicon, Somerville, New Jersey)

Clinical Staging

Radical hysterectomy alone or in combination with vaginectomy is a demanding procedure, which may have serious long-term consequences for the patient. Therefore, prior to undertaking surgery, all efforts should be made to exclude distant metastases, which, if present, will dictate an alteration in treatment strategy. Positron emission tomography scanning is currently the most accurate method in detecting extrapelvic tumor spread from cervical cancer. Preoperative imaging is helpful for local staging of disease in the pelvis to exclude invasion into other surrounding organs, including the urinary bladder, ureters, rectum, and large vessels. In case of their involvement, exenterative surgery is required to achieve complete tumor removal; however, primary chemoradiation is the typical treatment of choice. Magnetic resonance imaging (MRI) is considered to be the gold standard in local staging due to high soft-tissue contras.[24] Recently, it has been shown that ultrasonography may have comparable accuracy with MRI, particularly in local staging of cervical cancer.[25-27] The accuracy of ultrasonography is improved with the use of power Doppler, which may help to detect abundant tumor vascularization and dynamic examination, enabling the differentiation of tumor or organ borders due to its movement aroused by the pressure of the probe inserted transvaginally, transrectally, or on the abdominal wall. Although cystoscopy and proctoscopy are commonly recommended for exclusion of adjacent organ invasion from the cervix, these procedures cannot identify the tumor involvement into the organ walls until the whole thickness of the wall has been permeated and in most cases they do not bring any additional information beyond MRI or ultrasonography. If a lesion is present in the vagina, then vaginoscopy is important to allow exact description of the lesion location.

Performance Status, Body Mass Index, and Nutritional Status Assessment

There are no strict requirements for an upper age limit or performance status for radical hysterectomy with vaginectomy. At the same time, one must be cognizant that this surgery is always challenging for the surgeon and can be associated with major complications for the patient. Therefore, a preoperative Gynecologic Oncology Group performance status 0 or 1 is required in our department. Technical difficulty can be further increased by various factors, including the size of the tumor, its localization (ie, its attachment to pelvic diaphragm or to large vessels), and obesity. A high body mass index (BMI) does not mean that surgery is contraindicated, but rather that the risks and feasibility should be carefully considered in combination with other factors. In patients with significant visceral obesity, it is usually more favorable to perform a larger part of the operation (complete vaginectomy) from a perineal approach.

In patients with vaginal cancer or locally advanced cervical cancer, significant nutritional deficiency is only rarely manifested. However, severe malnutrition is associated with significantly increased morbidity; therefore, a comprehensive assessment of nutritional status is an essential part of preoperative preparation. Different laboratory tests and scoring systems are used for the assessment; the authors use serum albumin (< 3 g/dL) and Malnutrition Universal Screening Tool score in their department. Preoperative total parenteral nutrition for 5 to 7 days may be considered for patients who are severely malnourished.[28]

Antibiotic Prophylaxis, Bowel Preparation, Thromboembolic Prophylaxis

Antibiotic prophylaxis is justified in all patients with cancer who are candidates for radical pelvic surgery and should be administered no longer than 30 minutes prior to incision. The choice of the regimen should be directed according to the epidemiological situation in each particular institution. In general, ampicillin or a second-generation cephalosporin is used as first-line prophylaxis, while doxycycline or clindamycin can be used in patients with penicillin allergy. A single dose is sufficient, but only if the procedure does not last beyond 3 hours or there is no excessive blood loss (> 1500 mL); in such cases, the dose should be repeatedly administered at appropriate intervals on the basis of the half-life of the antibiotic.

Bowel surgery is not a routine part of radical hysterectomy with vaginectomy; however, when the dorsal parametria or posterior vaginal wall has been affected, then the dissection of the tumor may be associated with a risk of rectum perforation. For this reason, mechanical bowel preparation was previously recommended for all patients scheduled for vaginectomy or type C2 radical hysterectomy. This practice is largely being abandoned according to critical analyses of available data showing that bowel preparation is not required, even in patients with anticipated bowel procedure.[29] Preoperative bowel preparation has not been shown to reduce the risk of anastomotic leak or contamination of the surgical field and may have adverse events, including renal failure.

In general, patients with pelvic cancer undergoing surgery are at increased risk of deep venous thrombosis and pulmonary embolism. Thromboembolic prophylaxis must be employed in all candidates for surgery, including both mechanic and pharmacologic methods. Most often, the combination of compression stocking and low-molecular weight heparin dosed according to BMI, starting 2 hours prior to surgery and continuing at least 7 days postoperatively. Occasionally, an inferior vena cava filter should be preoperatively placed for a patient with a recent or current thromboembolism.

Preoperative Procedure Description

Each part of the procedure and its extent (radicality) should be carefully specified prior to the procedure. The preoperative plan should contain a description of the following:

a. Lymph node staging (ie, pelvic lymphadenectomy/sentinel lymph node (SLN) biopsy/low or complete paraaortic lymphadenectomy/removal of bulky pelvic nodes)
b. Procedure on adnexa (ie, bilateral salpingo-oophorectomy (BSO)/adnexa transposition)
c. Type of parametrectomy (B, C1, C2)
d. Length of vaginal resection (ie, proximal vaginectomy, total vaginectomy)
e. Any reconstructive procedures

SURGICAL PROCEDURE

Box 3-2 MASTER SURGEON'S PRINCIPLES

- Develop the potential pelvic spaces first before beginning resection
- Carefully plan the radicality of resection for all 3 parts of the parametria (ventral, lateral, dorsal) in both dimensions (horizontal and vertical)
- Perform an adequate caudal bladder dissection before opening the ureteral tunnel in the lateral parametria
- Consider the perineal approach for vaginectomy in patients who are obese or in patients with a demanding abdominal dissection

Procedure Performance

The patient is positioned in the low dorsal lithotomy position using Allen-type stirrups to facilitate vaginal exposure should a perineal phase of the operation be required. The abdominal approach is initiated through a low vertical midline or transverse incision, depending on the anticipated scope of resection and patient body habitus. A self-retaining retractor is placed and the pelvis and abdomen are explored to exclude the presence of extrapelvic metastatic disease.

Radical hysterectomy with en bloc vaginectomy usually begins with pelvic lymphadenectomy, with or without previous sentinel lymph node biopsy, to ascertain the pelvic lymph node status as well as to define the anatomy of the central pelvis and sidewalls. The ureters are identified and tagged, and the paired paravesical and pararectal spaces are developed using a combination of blunt and sharp dissection to expose the external and internal (hypogastric) vascular systems (Figure 3-1). In Figure 3-1, the uterus is retracted medially to show the right lateral parametria stretching between the paravesical and pararectal spaces. The uterine artery and superior vesicle artery are skeletonized, doubly suture ligated, and divided at their origin, just proximal to the continuation of the umbilical ligament. In this fashion, the vessels and associated parametrium are completely resected at their origin from the internal iliac artery, reflected medially, and the remaining attachments divided along the medial aspect of the internal iliac vein up to the sacral bone. Thus, the paravesical and pararectal spaces are unified; the combined space resulting from connecting the paravesical and pararectal spaces is shown in Figure 3-2, which illustrates complete resection of the lateral parametria from the pelvic sidewall (surgical resection is the blue dotted line). Next, the vesicovaginal space is further developed and the urinary bladder is sharply dissected from the cervix and upper vagina deep into the anterior pelvis. Figure 3-3 demonstrates the position of the distal ureter running within the ureteral tunnel in the lateral parametria and the ureteral entrance into the bladder ventrally, running on the ventral vaginal wall. For a complete ventral parametrial resection, the ureter must

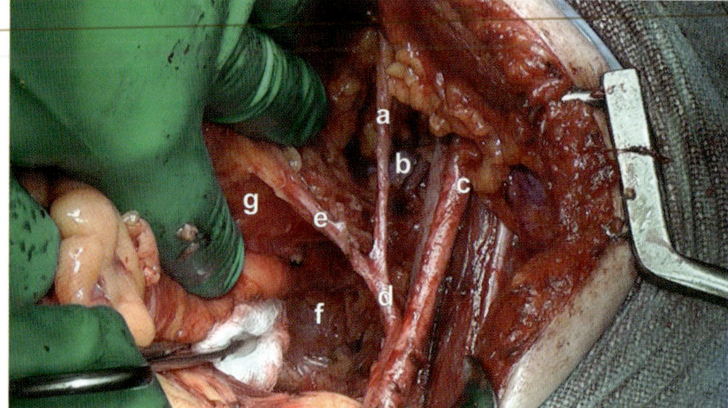

Fig. 3-1. Opening of the paravesical and pararectal spaces. **(A)** Umbilical ligament. **(B)** Opened paravesical space. **(C)** External iliac artery and vein. **(D)** Internal iliac artery. **(E)** Superior vesical artery and below it stretched right lateral parametrium containing uterine artery and vein, parametrial veins and splanchnic nerves in its caudal part. **(F)** Opened pararectal space. **(G)** Uterus pulled medially.

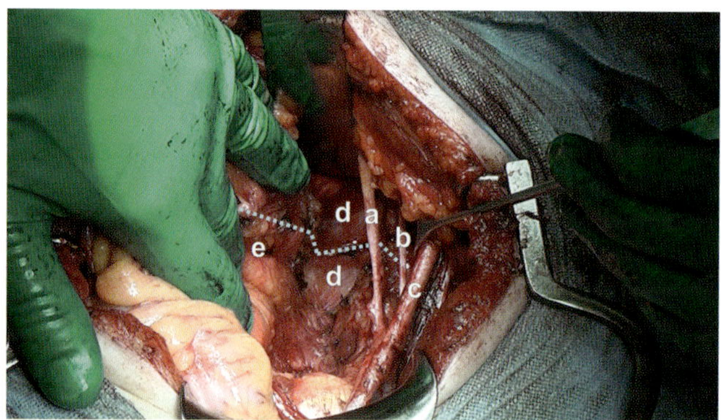

Fig. 3-2. Resection of the right lateral parametrium. **(A)** Umbilical ligament. **(B)** obturator nerve. **(C)** External iliac artery and vein pulled laterally toward the psoas muscle. **(D)** Connected space of former paravesical and pararectal fossa. **(E)** Uterus and retracted lateral parametrium pulled medially. Dotted line = medial and lateral resection line of the lateral parametrium.

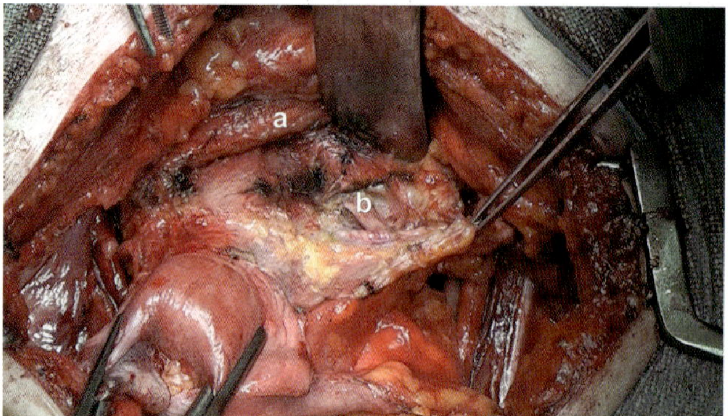

Fig. 3-3. Dissection of the urinary bladder. **(A)** Urinary bladder. **(B)** Distal ureter between right lateral parametrium and its entrance into the bladder, running on the anterior vaginal wall.

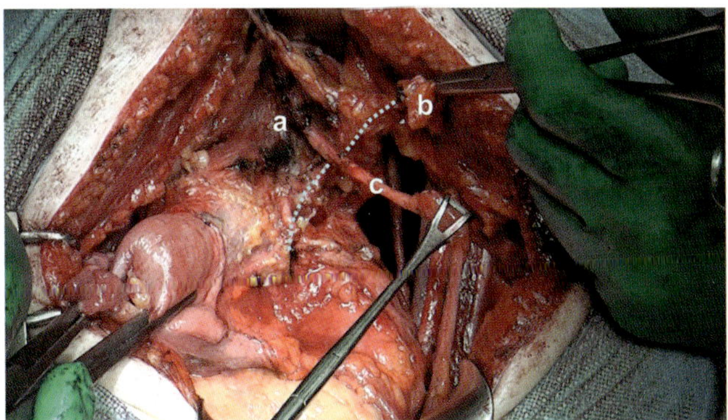

Fig. 3-4. Dissection of the distal ureter. **(A)** Urinary bladder. **(B)** Lateral parametrium grasped and pulled laterally after having divided it above the ureter. **(C)** Ureter dissected from the lateral and ventral parametria, freed up to its entrance into the bladder.

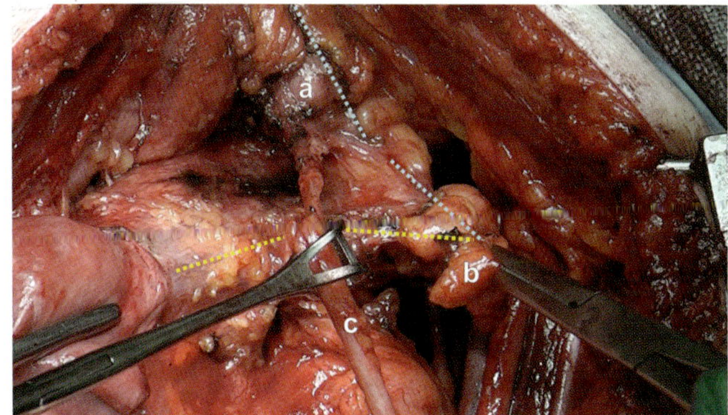

Fig. 3-6. Resection of the ventral parametrium. **(A)** Lateral wall of the urinary bladder. **(B)** Separated ventral and lateral parametrium pulled dorsally and laterally. Blue dotted line = ventral and dorsal resection line on the ventral parametrium, yellow dotted line = medial and lateral resection line on the lateral parametrium.

be completely dissected from the cervix as well as from the ventral parametria. Figure 3-4 demonstrates the completely freed ureter and the resection line on the lateral parametria as it is opened above the ureter. In the next step, the ureter is retracted, and the ventral parametrium is skeletonized and resected on the bladder wall, which is best identified by palpation (Figure 3-5). After mobilization and resection of the ventral parametrium, the ureter is completely free from its surrounding attachments, the lateral bladder wall is exposed, and the lateral margins of resection are clearly defined (Figure 3-6).

Attention should now be directed toward posterior pelvic dissection. The uterus is drawn anteriorly, and the cul-de-sac of Douglas sharply incised to expose the upper portion of the rectovaginal space. The rectovaginal space is developed using a combination of blunt and sharp dissection. The rectum is dissected completely from its attachments to the dorsal parametrium on both sides and mobilized from the posterior vaginal wall deep into the pelvis (Figure 3-7). In this case, the dorsal parametria are completely resected at their attachments to the pararectal ligaments. After resection of the dorsal and lateral parametria from the pelvic sidewalls and the rectum, the uterus can then be drawn sharply anteriorly revealing the bottom of the pararectal spaces delineated by the sacral bone and the levator ani muscles (Figure 3-8). At this stage of the operation, resection of the lateral paravaginal tissue can be adjusted to the extent of disease—in this case, with an adequate free margin below the tumor, at the level of about half of the vagina. Once adequate clearance of disease has been assured, the paravaginal tissue is resected horizontally from the pelvic sidewall up to the vaginal wall, with the ureter reflected laterally (Figure 3-9).

In many instances, it is more convenient to complete the vaginectomy from the perineal approach at this point. Attention is directed toward the perineal phase of the operation, and the Allen-type stirrups are adjusted accordingly to allow for vaginal exposure. A circumscribing incision

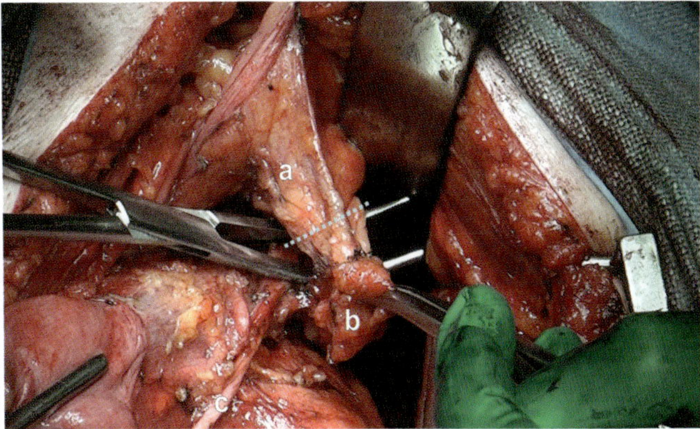

Fig. 3-5. Resection of the ventral parametrium. **(A)** Lateral wall of the urinary bladder. **(B)** Lateral and ventral parametrium pulled dorsally. Dotted line = future resection line on the ventral parametrium.

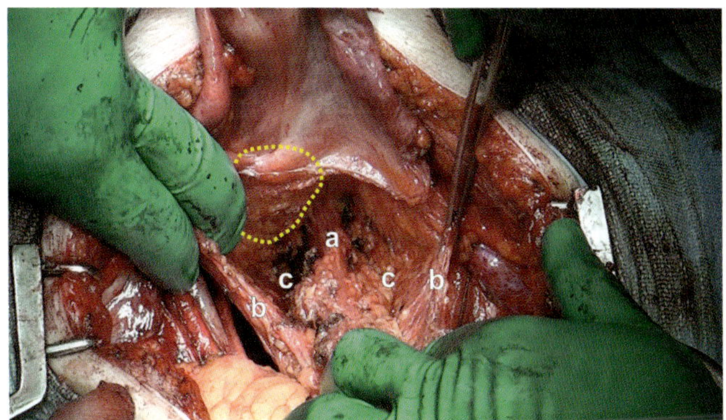

Fig. 3-7. Dissection of the rectum. **(A)** Rectum. **(B)** Dorsal parametria comprising of sacrouterine ligament, meso ureter, and inferior hypogastric nerve plexus. **(C)** Opened medial pararectal spaces (between rectum and sacrouterine ligaments). Dotted line = location of the cervical cancer.

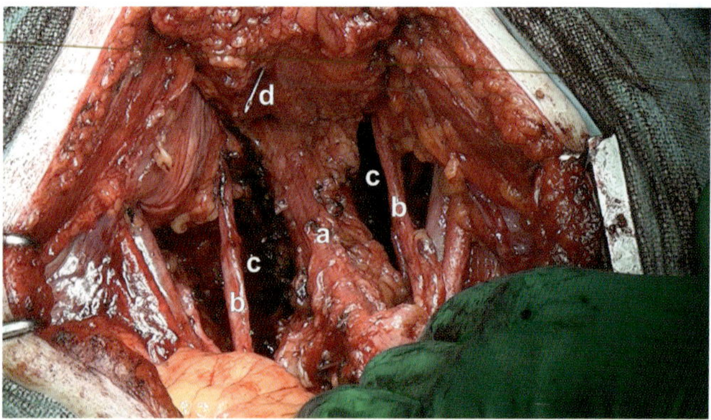

Fig. 3-8. Resection of dorsal parametria. **(A)** Rectum. **(B)** Ureters. **(C)** Space after complete resection of dorsal and lateral parametria, bottom of the space formed by the pelvic diaphragm. **(D)** Needle indicates the level of vagina attachment to the cervix.

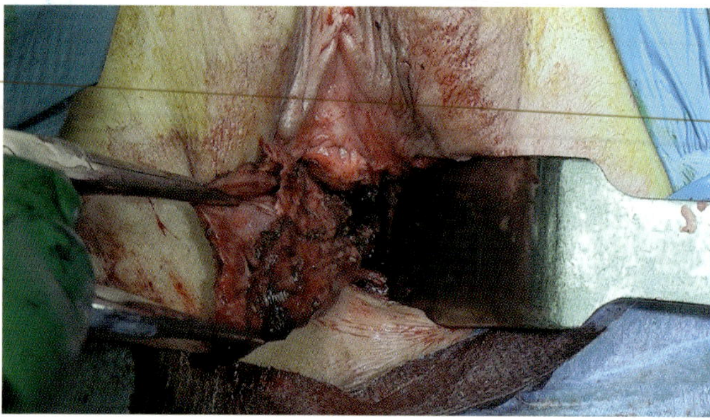

Fig. 3-10. Perineal phase of vaginectomy.

is made around the vaginal introitus. The vagina is carefully dissected from the urethra, bladder, rectum and paravaginal tissue until reaching the level of the abdominal resection (Figure 3-10). The specimen is removed en bloc. Figure 3-11 shows the pelvis after the specimen has been removed and Figure 3-12 demonstrates preserved external genitalia with perineal closure. The final radical hysterectomy with en bloc vaginectomy specimen demonstrates a centrally located tumor with free margins, large parametria on both sides, together with lateral paracolpium resected above the pelvic diaphragm at about the lower third of the vaginal length, and complete excision of the vagina (Figure 13-13).

Variations of Radical Hysterectomy With En Bloc Vaginectomy and Vaginal Reconstruction

All types of radical hysterectomies can be performed in combination with total vaginectomy (see Table 3-1). The technique described in this chapter represents a type C2 procedure with the objective being to remove the maximum extent of the lateral, dorsal and ventral parametria. The nerve-sparing (type C1) radical hysterectomy, together with vaginectomy, has been described by others, in which the autonomic nerves are preserved aiming at faster recovery of bladder functions following the procedure.[20,30] Similarly, the type B procedure, with minimal resection of lateral and dorsal parametria, can be combined with vaginectomy. It is necessary to emphasize that the extent of parametria and paracolpos resection in the proximal part of the vagina in types B and C1 is very limited; therefore, these procedures must only be performed in patients with small lesions without significant invasion to the parametrium, paracolpos, or both.

Radical parametrectomy in combination with vaginectom[31,32] is a treatment option for women when:

1. Simple hysterectomy has been inadvertently performed for locally advanced cervical cancer
2. A recurrence of cervical cancer, *or*
3. A primary vaginal carcinoma is localized in the upper vagina

The procedure is identical to that described for radical hysterectomy; however, it is technically more demanding, in particular dissection of the urinary bladder, and it is associated with higher intraoperative and postoperative morbidity rates.

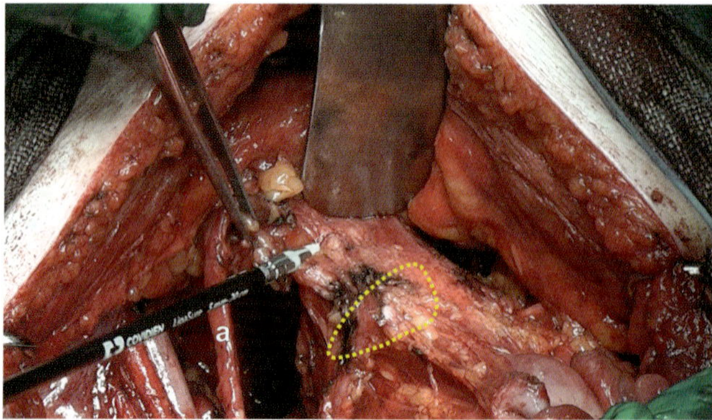

Fig. 3-9. Resection of the paracolpium (paravaginal tissue). Dotted line = location of the cervical cancer in the cervix and left lateral parametrium.

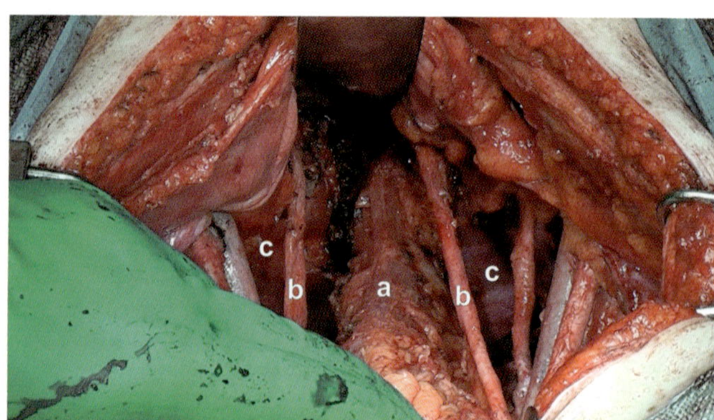

Fig. 3-11. Pelvis after removal of the specimen. **(A)** Rectum. **(B)** Ureters. **(C)** Pelvic muscle diaphragm.

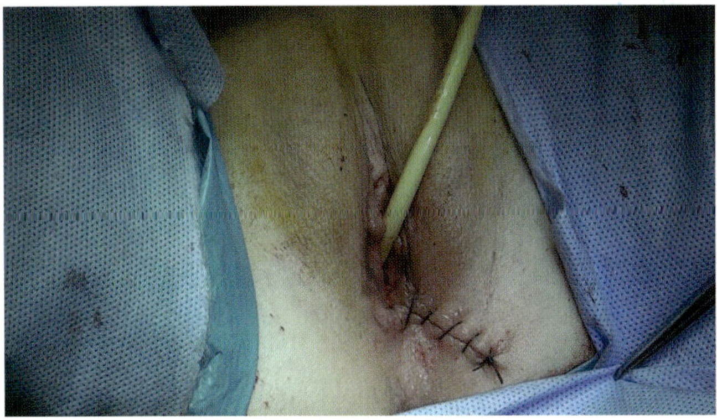

Fig. 3-12. Preserved external genitalia and perineal repair.

Partial Vaginectomy

Vaginal pathology is most commonly located in the proximal/upper part, which allows for partial preservation of the vagina. Partial vaginal preservation may also decrease postoperative morbidity. The length of resected vagina can be easily adjusted during the procedure, and the extent of resection should be clearly defined pre-operatively. The surgical approach, whether vaginal or abdominal, for vagina resection is chosen according to the anatomic conditions, including the BMI of the patient, tumor size and localization, and the extent of vaginal resection. The upper half or two-thirds of the vagina (down to the pelvic muscle floor) can, in most cases, be easily dissected from the abdominal approach as a continuation of the radical hysterectomy, while the lower one-third to one-half is more easily accessible from the perineal approach. The perineal approach may also help to identify the required distal resection margins in the vagina.

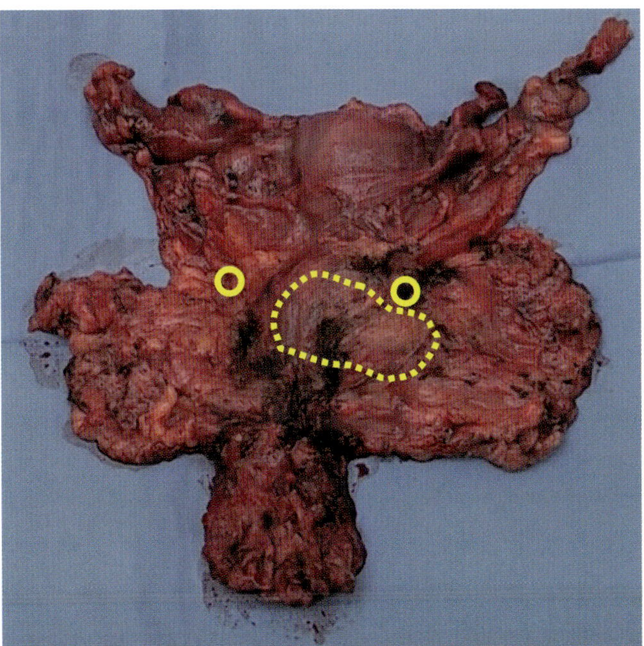

Fig. 3-13. Final en bloc specimen. Dotted line = location of the cervical cancer, circles = former position of both ureters.

Resection of the Pelvic Floor Muscle

Should the pathologic process spread laterally to the paracolpos at the distal third of the vagina, it may infiltrate into the pelvic diaphragm (levator ani muscle). Achievement of free surgical margins unavoidably requires resection of the pelvic muscle floor. The technique is analogous to the infralevator pelvic exenteration (Chapter 8). Resection of the pelvic floor is associated with a higher risk of intraoperative bleeding. Empty pelvic syndrome postoperatively occurs more often when the pelvic diaphragm has been resected.

Vaginal Reconstruction

In patients who are sexually active, total vaginectomy should ideally be performed during the same procedure together with vaginal reconstruction. The rectus abdominis myocutaneous (RAM) flap, described in Chapter 17, remains the most often used technique and is associated with good functional outcomes and low morbidity.[33] The flap is easy to harvest and transpose to the pelvis. Besides preservation of the possibility for vaginal intercourse, use of the RAM flap may also help prevent empty pelvis syndrome. Alternative techniques for vaginal reconstruction include sigmoid colon vaginoplasty or the bilateral gracilis myocutaneous flap.[33,34] Although some reported experiences with preservation of sexual life have been very optimistic, other authors have reported maintenance of sexual activity only in a minority of patients with a longer interval from the vaginal reconstruction.[35]

POSTOPERATIVE CARE

Box 3-3 PERIOPERATIVE MORBIDITY

- The risk of ureteral, urinary bladder, and rectal intra-operative injury is proportional to the radicality of resection
- Intraoperative hemorrhage
- Delayed spontaneous voiding recovery is common

Radical hysterectomy combined with total vaginectomy is an extensive surgical experience for all patients. In addition to standard perioperative management, there are some specific measures related to this procedure. Although it has been well demonstrated in colorectal surgery, as well as in patients undergoing radical hysterectomy, that prophylactic pelvic drainage does not decrease postoperative complication rate, it is recommended in this procedure to place a passive drainage due to high risk of fluid or hematoma collection.[36-38] Drains can be extracted soon after the surgery, typically the first or second postoperative day. Due to the high risk of loss of bladder sensation and voiding difficulties after the procedure, it is recommended to insert a suprapubic catheter at the end of the procedure. Placement of a suprapubic catheter is associated with a lower risk of urinary tract infections, shorter postoperative hospital stay, and earlier successful trial of voiding in patients following radical hysterectomy than with the classic transurethral catheter.[39] The major benefit of suprapubic drainage is the possibility of beginning with spontaneous voiding training early after the surgery. The suprapubic catheter is kept in place until sufficient voiding recovery, usually considered as post-voiding residuum less than 80 mL throughout the day.

The small number of cohorts of patients reported in literature do not allow for a systematic evaluation of the intraoperative and postoperative morbidity of radical hysterectomy with en bloc vaginectomy. The main intraoperative risks are associated mostly with radical parametrectomy, including urinary bladder and ureteral injuries, parametrial bleeding, rectal injury, or large vessel laceration. Both urinary bladder and rectal injuries are the most common intraoperative complications of vaginectomy.

FAST TRACK SURGERY

Cumulative evidence published recently suggests that so-called fast track management may lead to faster recovery and decreased postoperative hospital stay in patients following procedures for benign conditions and colorectal cancer, as well as in cases of gynecologic oncology surgery.[40] This multidisciplinary approach includes multiple elements in preoperative preparation (eg, optimization of hemoglobin levels, management of preexisting morbidities, assessment of nutritional status and eventual nutrition support, comprehensive patient information about expected postoperative management and discharge planning, possible admission on day of surgery, adequate preoperative hydration, reduced starvation, none or reduced oral bowel preparation), intraoperative management (eg, avoidance of nasogastric tube, preference of epidural anesthesia, use of epidural postoperative analgesia, individual and restricted fluid management), and postoperative management (eg, planned and fast mobilization, rapid hydration and nutrition, individual and restricted fluid intake, absence of drains or their early extraction, early removal of catheters, preference of oral analgesia and restriction of systemic opiate-based analgesia, discharge on planned day).

LONG-TERM OUTCOMES

Box 3-4 DELAYED COMPLICATIONS

- Empty pelvis syndrome
- Urinary bladder dysfunction
- Anorectal dysfunction
- Sexual dysfunction

The so-called "empty pelvis syndrome" is one of the most frequent reasons of postoperative complications, and occurs mainly after pelvic exenteration but may also occur following radical hysterectomy and vaginectomy, especially if combined with pelvic floor muscle resection. Empty space in the depth of pelvis following the removal of a large specimen may cause the retention of blood, fluid, and tissue debris, as well as abscess formation and adhesions of the small bowel onto pelvic walls and sacral bone, with a high risk of chronic infection and/or bowel or bladder fistulas. These serious morbidities can be prevented—or at least minimized—by filling the cavity with an omental flap, myocutaneous flap, or artificial material (absorbable mesh). In our department, the best experiences have been seen with use of the vertical RAM, which is easy to harvest and allows for a massive replacement of tissue. RAM is associated with low morbidity due to a reliable blood supply and can be easily used for vaginal reconstruction if harvested as a myocutaneous flap.

Another frequent symptom in the early and late postoperative periods is the impairment of spontaneous voiding.[41-43] Time to spontaneous voiding recovery is related to radicality of parametria resection; it is shorter following the nerve-sparing type of parametrectomy. It is hypothesized that perivesical edema, autonomic denervation, and loss of urinary bladder support all play a role in etiology. Spontaneous voiding is typically restored in a majority of patients within 1 month following surgery; however, rarely, in cases with an extensively radical parametrectomy, a longer period of time may be required or may extend indefinitely, relegating the patient to a lifetime self-catheterization.

Long-term urinary bladder dysfunction is among the most frequent and best-documented types of late morbidity. The frequency and severity of bladder dysfunction increases with the extent (radicality) of the parametrial resection.[18-21] According to some authors, bladder dysfunction is also strongly associated with the length of vaginal resection.[44] This is in accordance with our experience, in which concomitant vaginectomy increases the frequency and severity of urinary bladder symptoms. The most frequently reported bladder problems include urinary incontinence, impairment of bladder sensation, or voiding with abdominal straining.[19,41,44,45] Preservation of the autonomic nerves in the nerve-sparing type of parametrectomy does not eliminate postoperative bladder symptoms; however, it does significantly decrease the severity and frequency of their manifestation.

Anorectal dysfunction are less common in the late postoperative period; however, these symptoms may have a significant negative influence on a patient's quality of life.[19,46-48] Among the most frequent symptoms are constipation and flatulence incontinence, occurring mainly in cases with extensive resection of the dorsal parametria or extensive vaginectomy.

Another potential late complication associated with radical hysterectomy with en bloc vaginectomy is sexual dysfunction. The etiology of sexual dysfunction is multifactorial—psychological, functional, and anatomic changes all play a role. Shortening of the vagina has a negative effect on the quality of postoperative vaginal intercourse. As a consequence of adnexectomy, surgical menopause is associated with climacteric symptoms that reduce libido, insufficient lubrication, and dyspareunia. A diagnosis of cancer, as such, is associated with anxiety and fear that sexual activity can cause disease recurrence. The main sexual problems following radical hysterectomy are sexual desire disorder, objective arousal disorder, and dyspareunia.[49-53]

In general, oncologic outcomes are excellent after the primary surgical treatment of early stages of cervical and vaginal cancers. The goal of primary surgery, as well as salvage procedures, for recurrent disease is always the achievement of radical resection with free-tissue margins so that adjuvant radiotherapy may be avoided. The combination of radical surgery, together with adjuvant radiotherapy, significantly increases the risk of major complications, such as bladder dysfunction and ureteral, bladder, or rectal fistulas.

SUMMARY

Radical hysterectomy, combined with total vaginectomy, is a rare procedure in gynecologic oncology. Most often, it is indicated for early-stage vaginal cancer if it is localized in the proximal vagina, or if there is simultaneous cervical cancer with multifocal VaIN lesions in the vagina. Rarely, it is performed for recurrent disease. Involvement of surrounding organs should be carefully excluded preoperatively, because such a condition may either change the treatment modality or lead to performance of exenterative procedure. Complete tumor excision with free surgical margins should be the aim of such a radical procedure so that adjuvant radiotherapy can be avoided. The combination of radical surgery with adjuvant radiotherapy increases serious early and late postoperative morbidities. All types of radical hysterectomy can be performed in combination with vaginectomy. The radicality of the parametria resection and length of vaginal resection should be preoperatively planned. Oncologic outcomes of surgical treatment are excellent for the treatment of early-stage cervical or vaginal cancer without lymph node involvement. Postoperative morbidity is mostly related to the type of parametrectomy (parametria resection). Simultaneous vaginectomy increases the frequency and severity of complications. Impairment of spontaneous voiding and symptoms of empty pelvis syndrome are the most frequent early postoperative complications. Urinary bladder dysfunction, including urinary incontinence, impairment of bladder sensation, and voiding with abdominal straining, are the most frequent late postoperative complications. Anorectal dysfunction is less frequently manifested and mainly consists of constipation or flatulent incontinence.

ACKNOWLEDGMENT

This chapter was supported by Charles University in Prague (UNCE 204024) and Ministry of Health of the Czech Republic (MH CZ - DRO VFN 64165).

REFERENCES

1. Clark JG. A more radical method of performing hysterectomy for cancer of the uterus. *Bull Johns Hopkins Hosp*. 1895;6:120.
2. Wertheim E. Zur frag der radikaloperation beim uteruskrebs. *Arch Gynakol*. 1900;61:627.
3. Wertheim E. The extended abdominal operation for carcinoma uteri (based on 500 operative cases). *Am J Obstet Dis Women Child*. 1912;66:169-232.
4. Schauta F. *Die erweiterte vaginale Totalexstirpation des Uterus beim Kollumkarzinom*. Wien: Verlag von J. Safar; 1908.
5. Meigs JV. The Wertheim operation for carcinoma of the cervix. *Am J Obstet Gynecol*. 1945;49:542.
6. Ling B, Gao Z, Sun M, at al. Laparoscopic radical hysterectomy with vaginectomy and reconstruction of vagina in patients with stage I of primary vaginal carcinoma. *Gynecol Oncol*. 2008;109(1):92-96.
7. Benedetti Panici P, Bellati F, Plotti F, at al. Neoadjuvant chemotherapy followed by radical surgery in patients affected by vaginal carcinoma. *Gynecol Oncol*. 2008;111(2):307-311.
8. Frega A, Sopracordevole F, Assorgi C, et al. Vaginal intraepithelial neoplasia: a therapeutical dilemma. *Anticancer Res*. 2013;33(1):29-38.
9. Raspagliesi F, Ditto A, Martinelli F. Nerve-sparing radical vaginectomy: two case reports and description of the surgical technique. *Int J Gynecol Cancer*. 2009;19(4):794-797.
10. Nezhat F, Prasad Hayes M, Peiretti M, Rahaman J. Laparoscopic radical parametrectomy and partial vaginectomy for recurrent endometrial cancer. *Gynecol Oncol*. 2007;104(2):494-496.
11. Hill EC, Galante M. Radical surgery in the management of clear cell adenocarcinoma of the cervix and vagina in young women. *Am J Obstet Gynecol*. 1981;140(2):221-226.
12. Jones WB, Koulos JP, Saigo PE, Lewis JL Jr. Clear-cell adenocarcinoma of the lower genital tract: Memorial Hospital 1974–1984. *Obstet Gynecol*. 1987;70(4):573-577.
13. Robboy SJ, Young RH, Welch WR. Atypical vaginal adenosis and cervical ectropion. Association with clear cell adenocarcinoma in diethylstilbestrol-exposed offspring. *Cancer*. 1984;54(5):869-875.
14. Cibula D, Pinkavova I, Dusek L, et al. Local control after tailored surgical treatment of early cervical cancer. *Int J Gynecol Cancer*. 2011;21(4):690-698.
15. Höckel M, Horn LC, Manthey N, et al. Resection of the embryologically defined uterovaginal(Müllerian) compartment and pelvic control in patients with cervical cancer: a prospective analysis. *Lancet Oncol*. 2009;10(7):683-692.
16. Cibula D, Abu-Rustum NR, Dusek L, et al. Prognostic significance of low volume sentinel lymph node disease in early-stage cervical cancer. *Gynecol Oncol*. 2012;124(3):496-501.
17. Wright JD, Fiorelli J, Kansler AL, et al. Optimizing the management of stage II endometrial cancer: the role of radical hysterectomy and radiation. *Am J Obstet Gynecol*. 2009;200(4):419.
18. Landoni F, Maneo A, Cormio G. Class II versus class III radical hysterectomy in stage IB-IIA cervical cancer: a prospective randomized study. *Gynecol Oncol*. 2001;80(1):3-12.
19. Cibula D, Velechovska P, Sláma J, et al. Late morbidity following nerve-sparing radical hysterectomy. *Gynecol Oncol*. 2010;116(3):506-511.
20. Raspagliesi F, Ditto A, Fontanelli R, Zanaboni. Type II versus type III nerve sparing radical hysterectomy: comparison of lower urinary tract dysfunctions. *Gynecol Oncol*. 2006;102(2):256-262.
21. Cibula D, Sláma J, Velechovská P. Factors affecting spontaneous voiding recovery after radical hysterectomy. *Int J Gynecol Cancer*. 2010;20(4):685-690.
22. Querleu D, Morrow CP. Classification of radical hysterectomy. *Lancet Oncol*. 2008;9(2):297-303.
23. Cibula D, Abu-Rustum NR, Benedetti-Panici P. New classification system of radical hysterectomy: emphasis on a three-dimensional anatomic template for parametrial resection. *Gynecol Oncol*. 2011;122(2):264-268.
24. Mitchell DG, Snyder B, Coakley F, Reinhold C, Thomas G, Amendola M, et al. Early invasive cervical cancer: tumor delineation

by magnetic resonance imaging, computed tomography, and clinical examination, verified by pathologic results, in the ACRIN 6651/GOG 183 Intergroup Study. *J Clin Oncol.* 2006;24(36):5687-5694.

25. Fischerova D, Cibula D, Stenhova H, Vondrichova H, Calda P, Zikan M et al. Transrectal ultrasound and magnetic resonance imaging in staging of early cervical cancer. *Int J Gynecol Cancer.* 2008;18(4):766-772.
26. Testa AC, Ludovisi M, Manfredi R, Zannoni G, Gui B, Basso D et al. Transvaginal ultrasonography and magnetic resonance imaging for assessment of presence, size and extent of invasive cervical cancer. *Ultrasound Obstet Gynecol.* 2009;34(3):335-344.
27. Epstein E, Testa A, Gaurilcikas A, Di Legge A, Ameye L, Atstupenaite V, et al. Early-stage cervical cancer: tumor delineation by magnetic resonance imaging and ultrasound - a European multicenter trial. *Gynecol Oncol.* 2013;128(3):449-453.
28. National Collaborating Centre for Acute Care. *Nutrition Support in Adults Oral Nutrition Support, Enteral Tube Feeding and Parenteral Nutrition.* London: National Collaborating Centre for Acute Care; 2006.
29. Wells T, Plante M, McAlpine JN; Communities of Practice Groups on behalf of the Society of Gynecologic Oncologists of Canada. Preoperative bowel preparation in gynecologic oncology: a review of practice patterns and an impetus to change. *Int J Gynecol Cancer.* 2011;21(6):1135-1142.
30. Li Y, Chen Y, Xu H, Wang D, Wang Y, Liang Z. Laparoscopic nerve-sparing radical vaginectomy in patients with vaginal carcinoma: surgical technique and operative outcomes. *J Minim Invasive Gynecol.* 2012;19(5):593-597.
31. Fleisch MC, Hatch KD. Laparoscopic assisted parametrectomy/upper vaginectomy LPUV)-technique, applications and results. *Gynecol Oncol.* 2005;98(3):420-426.
32. Magrina JF, Walter AJ, Schild SE. Laparoscopic radical parametrectomy and pelvic and aortic lymphadenectomy for vaginal carcinoma: a case report. *Gynecol Oncol.* 1999;75(3):514-516.
33. McArdle A, Bischof DA, Davidge K, Swallow CJ, Winter DC. Vaginal reconstruction following radical surgery for colorectal malignancies: a systematic review of the literature. *Ann Surg Oncol.* 2012;19(12):3933-3942.
34. Yin D, Wang N, Zhang S. Radical hysterectomy and vaginectomy with sigmoid vaginoplasty for stage I vaginalcarcinoma. *Int J Gynaecol Obstet.* 2013;2:132-135.
35. Løve US, Sjøgren P, Rasmussen P, Laurberg S, Christensen HK. Sexual dysfunction after colpectomy and vaginal reconstruction with a vertical rectus abdominis myocutaneous flap. *Dis Colon Rectum.* 2013;56(2):186-190.
36. Yeh CY, Changchien CR, Wang JY, et al. Pelvic drainage and other risk factors for leakage after elective anterior resection in rectal cancer patients: a prospective study of 978 patients. *Ann Surg.* 2005;241(1):9-13.
37. Lopes AD, Hall JR, Monaghan JM. Drainage following radical hysterectomy and pelvic lymphadenectomy: dogma or need? *Obstet Gynecol.* 1995;86(6):960-963.
38. Jensen JK, Lucci JA III, DiSaia PJ, Manetta A, Berman ML. To drain or not to drain: a retrospective study of closed-suction drainage following radical hysterectomy with pelvic lymphadenectomy. *Gynecol Oncol.* 1993;51(1):46-49.
39. Wells TH, Steed H, Capstick V, Schepanksy A, Hiltz M, Faught W. Suprapubic or urethral catheter: what is the optimal method of bladder drainage after radical hysterectomy? *J Obstet Gynaecol Can.* 2008;30(11):1034-1038.
40. Sidhu VS, Lancaster L, Elliott D, Brand AH. Implementation and audit of 'Fast-Track Surgery' in gynaecological oncology surgery. *Aust N Z J Obstet Gynaecol.* 2012;52(4):371-376.
41. Charoenkwan K, Pranpanas S. Prevalence and characteristics of late postoperative voiding dysfunction in early-stage cervical cancer patients treated with radical hysterectomy. *Asian Pacific J Cancer Prev.* 2007;8(3):387-389.
42. Pikaart DP, Holloway RW, Ahmad S, et al. Clinical-pathologic and morbidity analyses of types 2 and 3 abdominal radical hysterectomy for cervical cancer. *Gynecol Oncol.* 2007;107(2):205-210.
43. Fujii S, Takakura K, Matsumura N, et al. Anatomic identification and functional outcomes of the nerve sparing Okabayashi radical hysterectomy. *Gynecol Oncol.* 2007;107(1):4-13.
44. Benedetti-Panici P, Zullo MA, Plotti F, Manci N, Muzii L, Angioli R. Long-term bladder function in patients with locally advanced cervical carcinoma treated with neoadjuvant chemotherapy and type 3-4 radical hysterectomy. *Cancer.* 2004;100(10):2110-2117.
45. Pieterse QD, Maas CP, Ter Kuile MM, et al. An observational longitudinal study to evaluate miction, defecation, and sexual function after radical hysterectomy with pelvic lymhadenectomy for early-stage cervical cancer. *Int J Gynecol Cancer.* 2006;16(3):1119-1129.
46. van Dam JH, Gosselink MJ, Drogendijk AC, Hop WCJ, Schouten WR. Changes in bowel function after hysterectomy. *Dis Colon Rectum.* 1997;40(11):1342-1347.
47. Barnes W, Waggoner S, Delgado G, et al. Manometric characterization of rectal dysfunction following radical hysterectomy. *Gynecol Oncol.* 1991;42(2):116-119.
48. Sood AK, Nygaard I, Shahin MS, Sorosky JI, Lutgendorf SK, Rao SSC. Anorectal dysfunction after surgical treatment for cervical cancer. *J Am Coll Surg.* 2002;195(4):513-519.
49. Bergmark K, Avall-Lundqvist E, Dickman PW, Henningsohn L, Steineck G. Vaginal changes and sexuality in women with a history of cervical cancer. *N Engl J Med.* 1999;340(18):1383-1389.
50. Donovan KA, Taliaferro LA, Alvarez EM, Jacobsen PB, Roetzheim RG, Wenham RM. Sexual health in women treated for cervical cancer: characteristics and correlates. *Gynecol Oncol.* 2007;104(2):428-434.
51. Park SY, Bae DS, Nam JH, et al. Quality of life and sexual problems in disease-free survivors of cervical cancer compared with the general population. *Cancer.* 2007;110(12):2716-2725.
52. Jensen PT, Groenvold M, Klee MC, Thranov I, Petersen MA, Machin D. Early-stage cervical carcinoma, radical hysterectomy, and sexual function. A longitudinal study. *Cancer.* 2004;100(1):97-106.
53. Vrzackova P, Weiss P, Cibula D. Sexual morbidity following radical hysterectomy for cervical cancer. *Expert Rev Anticancer Ther.* 2010;10(7):1037-1042.

Chapter 4. Fertility-Sparing Radical Abdominal Trachelectomy

John P. Diaz, MD,
Ricardo E. Estape, MD,
Xiaohua Wu, MD, and
Laszlo Ungar, MD

BACKGROUND

There are an estimated 42,910 new cases of cervical carcinoma in the United States and the European Union annually.[1,2] Approximately 28% of all cervical carcinomas are diagnosed in women younger than 40 years of age.[3] Women throughout the developed world are postponing childbearing for professional, economic, and other personal reasons. This postponement of childbearing accompanied with the comparatively young age at which many women are diagnosed with cervical carcinoma has posed new challenges in the management of this disease.

The standard surgical management for early-stage cervical carcinoma is a radical abdominal hysterectomy and pelvic (with or without paraaortic) lymph node dissection. This treatment obviously eliminates the possibility of future conception. In recent decades, there has been an increased emphasis on tailoring treatment to provide fertility-sparing options without compromising oncologic outcomes. The radical vaginal trachelectomy with laparoscopic pelvic lymphadenectomy is a fertility-preserving procedure first described in 1994 by Dargent et al.[4]

Subsequently, numerous investigators have reported their experience with this technique. In addition to the vaginal approach, a fertility-sparing abdominal radical trachelectomy, and a minimally invasive approach have been described in the literature.[5,6] These procedures have received widespread acceptance as fertility-sparing surgical options for select patients with early-stage invasive carcinomas of the cervix.[7]

INDICATIONS AND CLINICAL APPLICATIONS

Appropriate candidates for fertility sparing radical trachelectomy for patients with cervical cancer are those with stages IA1 with lymphovascular invasion, IA2, and IB1 disease. In other words, the tumor should be confined to the cervix without spread to the vagina, parametria, or the lower uterine segment, such that the radical trachelectomy can completely encompass the malignancy with negative surgical margins. Patients who will most likely need postoperative adjuvant whole pelvic radiation therapy following surgery (such as those with suspicious pelvic nodes or possible parametrial invasion) are not ideal candidates for the procedure. There should be no evidence of metastatic disease.

The patient must have a strong desire to preserve her fertility and must be of an age in which future fertility is a reasonable possibility. The procedure has been successfully performed on patients with squamous, adeno, and adenosquamous histologies but is not recommended for small-cell carcinoma or sarcomas due to their overall poor prognosis.

ANATOMIC CONSIDERATIONS

The uterus is a fibromuscular organ. It has 2 portions: an upper muscular corpus and a lower fibrous cervix. The cervix is generally 2 to 4 cm in length and divided into 2 portions: the portio vaginalis, which is the part protruding into the vagina, and the portio supravaginalis, which lies above the vagina and below the corpus. The adnexa is comprised of the fallopian tubes and ovaries. The fallopian tubes are bilateral tubular structures that connect the endometrial cavity to the peritoneal cavity. The ovaries are bilateral, white, flattened oval structures that store ova. The lateral pole of the ovary is attached to the pelvic wall by the infundibulopelvic ligament, which contains the ovarian artery and vein. Medially, it is connected to the uterus through the utero-ovarian ligament. The round ligaments are extensions of the uterine musculature and represent the homologue of the gubernaculum testis. They begin as broad bands that arise on each lateral aspect of the anterior corpus, pass lateral to the deep inferior epigastric vessels and enter each internal inguinal ring, terminating in the labia majora. The midline uterus is connected to the pelvic sidewall by a double layer of peritoneum. Within the upper 2 layers of the broad ligament, lies the fallopian tubes, round ligaments, and ovaries. The cardinal and uterosacral ligaments are at the lower margin of the broad ligament.

The blood supply to the genital organs comes from the ovarian arteries and uterine and vaginal branches of the internal iliac arteries. A continuous arterial arcade connects these vessels on the lateral border of the adnexa, uterus, and vagina. The blood supply of the upper adnexal structures comes from the ovarian arteries that arise from the anterior surface of the aorta. They connect with the upper end of the marginal artery of the uterus. The uterine artery originates from the internal iliac artery. It joins the uterus near the junction of the corpus and cervix. The uterine artery gives off small branches to form the marginal artery. The ureter passes laterally under the uterine artery at the level of the internal cervical os.

Lymphatic drainage of the cervix is primarily to the obturator, internal, and external iliac lymph nodes. However, lymphatic drainage has been documented to the presacral and lower paraaortic lymph nodes.

There are several planes and potential spaces that must be understood to facilitate the performance of a radical trachelectomy. The vesicovaginal spaces are bound caudally by the fusion of the junction of the proximal one-third and distal two-thirds of the urethra with the vagina, ventrally by the urethra and bladder, cephalad by the peritoneum, forming the vesicocervical reflection. The paravesical spaces are paired spaces adjacent to the bladder. The medial border is the bladder and obliterated umbilical artery. The lateral border is the obturator internus. The pararectal spaces are paired spaces adjacent to the rectum. The space is bordered medially by the ureter, uterosacral ligament, and rectum. The lateral border is the hypogastric vessels and pelvic sidewall. The rectovaginal space is caudally bordered by the apex of the perineal body, laterally by the uterosacral ligament, ureter, and rectal pillars, and ventrally by the vagina, and dorsally by the rectum.

PREOPERATIVE PREPARATION

Box 4-1 KEY SURGICAL IMENTATION

- Collin-Buxton–type clamp
- Zeppelin clamps
- Wertheim clamp
- Free Ferguson needle
- #1 Prolene suture

Although preoperative imaging is not part of standard International Federation of Obstetrics and Gynecology (FIGO) staging, many authorities recommend a preoperative magnetic resonance imaging (MRI) of the pelvis prior to planned radical trachelectomy. MRI can help assess tumor size, potential parametrial invasion, and the amount of disease-free tissue above the malignancy that will be needed for uterovaginal reconstruction. Computed tomography, positron emission tomography, and vaginal and rectal ultrasonography have all been utilized to preoperatively evaluate the carcinoma.

Prior to the procedure, the patient should have the standard tests and evaluations for a major abdominal surgical procedure. In most institutions, patients are extensively counseled preoperatively that if negative surgical margins cannot be achieved as determined on frozen section pathologic analysis, then standard radical hysterectomy will be performed.

SURGICAL PROCEDURE

Box 4-2 MASTER SURGEON'S PRINCIPLES

- Create your surgical spaces and mobilize your ureter prior to the initiation of the trachelectomy
- Care is taken not to destroy the uterine cornua or the utero-ovarian pedicle
- Care is taken not to injure the fallopian tube or disrupt the utero-ovarian ligament
- The knot for the permanent cerclage should be posteriorly tied and placed prior to the reconstruction

Fertility-Sparing Radical Abdominal Trachelectomy

The aim of the radical abdominal trachelectomy is to resect the cervix, the upper 1 to 2 cm of the vagina, parametrium, and paracolpos in a similar manner to type 3 radical hysterectomy, but instead sparing the uterine fundus. We will describe an open procedure; however, similar surgical principles can be applied to a laparoscopic or robotic surgical approach. To better demonstrate and magnify the anatomic planes and structures, some of the operative pictures provided in this chapter are from a robotic radical abdominal trachelectomy.

First, after laparotomy or trocar site placement, bilateral, complete pelvic lymphadenectomy is performed in a similar manner to patients undergoing a radical abdominal hysterectomy. The limits of nodal dissection are the deep circumflex iliac vein caudally and the proximal common iliac artery cephalad (Figure 4-1). Any suspicious lymph nodes are sent for frozen-section analysis. A fertility-sparing approach should be abandoned if positive lymph nodes are identified. Sentinel lymph node identification is also a reasonable option and may allow for pathologic ultrastaging of these sentinel nodes.[8] The removal of para-aortic and sacral nodes is also considered for lesions stage IB1 or greater.

Developing the Paravesical and Pararectal Spaces

The radical abdominal trachelectomy is initiated by developing the paravesical and pararectal spaces and dissecting the bladder caudal to the mid-vagina. The paravesical space is medially lined by the bladder and vagina, laterally by the external iliac vessels and the obturator fossa, posteriorly by the cardinal ligament, and anteriorly by the pubic ramus (Figure 4-2). The paravesical space is opened by dissection between the

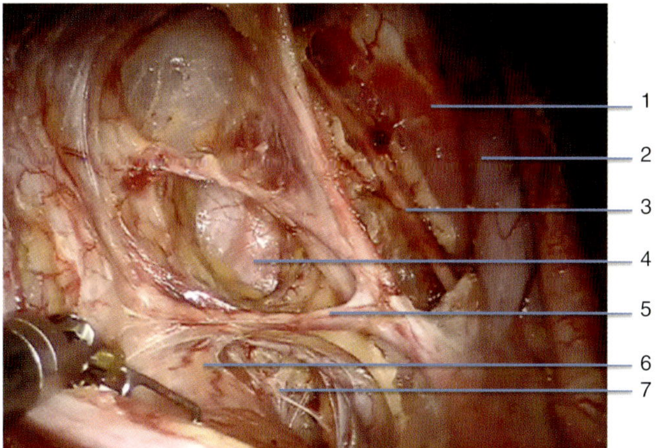

Fig. 4-1. Retroperitoneal anatomy. **(1)** Psoas muscle (right). **(2)** External iliac artery and vein (right). **(3)** Obturator nerve (right). **(4)** Paravesical space (right). **(5)** Uterine artery (right). **(6)** Ureter (right). **(7)** Pararectal space (right).

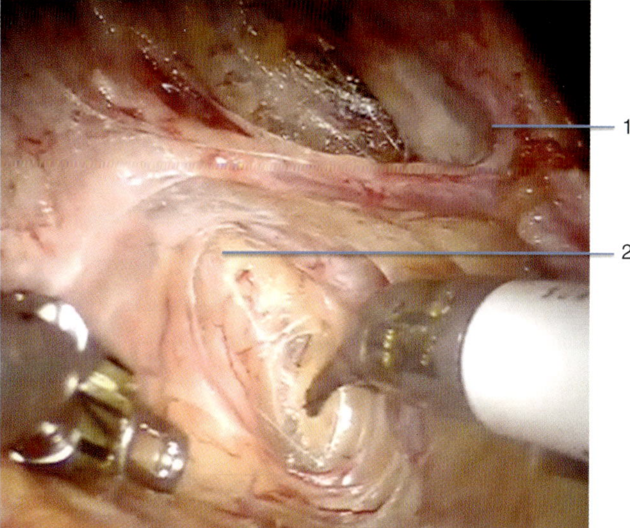

Fig. 4-3. Pararectal space (left). **(1)** Left umbilical artery. **(2)** Left paravesical space.

umbilical artery at the lateral border of the bladder and the external iliac vein. The pararectal space is laterally lined by the hypogastric artery, medially by the rectum, posteriorly and superiorly by the sacrum, and inferiorly by the cardinal ligament Figure 4-3). This space is developed using blunt dissection between the ureter and the hypogastric artery.

The round ligaments are divided, and large Kelly clamps are placed on the medial round ligaments to manipulate the uterus (in the case of minimally invasive cases, a uterine manipulator will have already been placed at the beginning of the procedure). The uterus is manipulated with clamps at the round ligaments; alternatively, a Collin-Buxton–type clamp can be utilized (Figure 4-4). Care should be taken not to destroy the cornu or the utero-ovarian pedicles. The infundibulopelvic ligaments with ovarian blood support are to be kept intact. Care should also be taken not to injure the fallopian tubes or disrupt the utero-ovarian ligament.

Anterior Colpotomy

The uterine vessels are then ligated and divided at their origin from the hypogastric vessels (Figure 4-5). Alternatively, a uterine artery sparing approach can be utilized (Figure 4-6). The parametria and paracolpos with uterine vessels are medially mobilized with the specimen, and complete ureterolysis is performed, similar to type 3 radical abdominal hysterectomy (Figure 4-7). The posterior cul-de-sac peritoneum is incised (Figure 4-8) and the uterosacral ligament divided (Figure 4-9); similarly, the parametrial and paracolpos are divided. A Wertheim clamp is placed at the desired length of

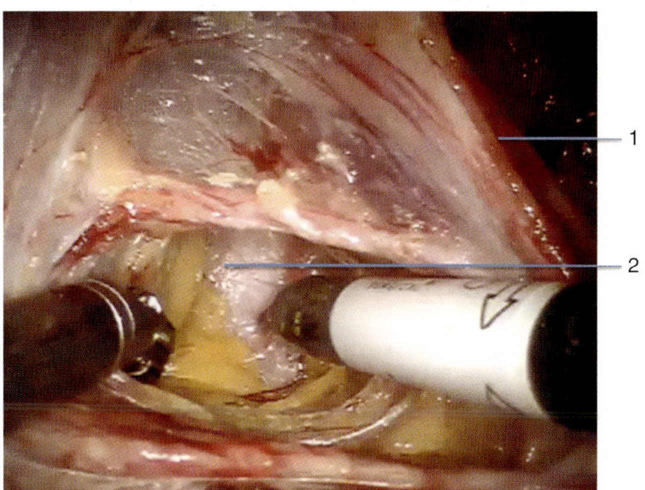

Fig. 4-2. Paravesical space (left). **(1)** Left umbilical artery. **(2)** Left paravesical space.

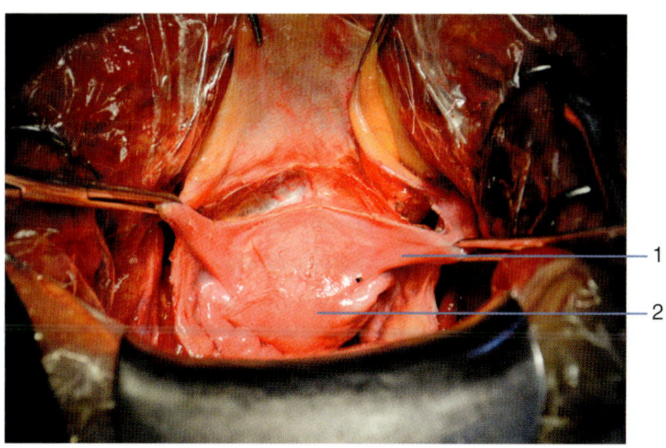

Fig. 4-4. **(1)** Round ligament (right). **(2)** Uterine fundus.

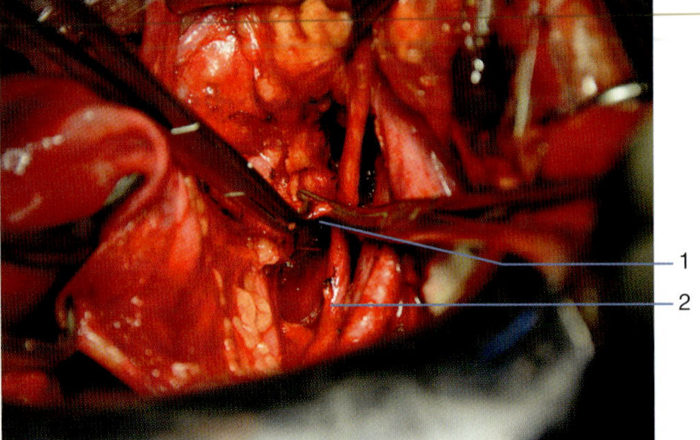

Fig. 4-5. Ligation of uterine artery. **(1)** Uterine artery (right). **(2)** Hypogastric artery (right).

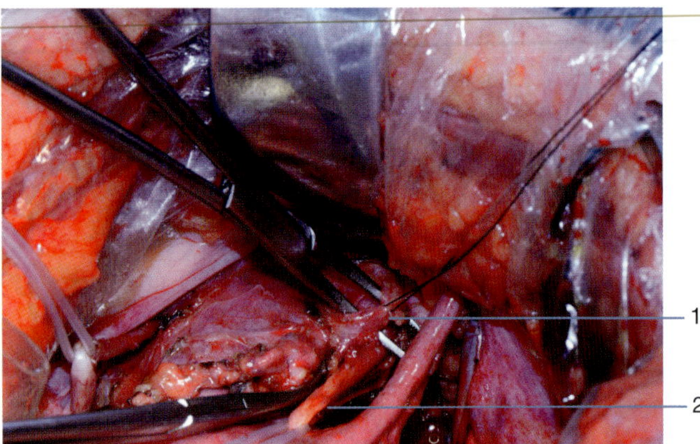

Fig. 4-7. Ureterolysis. **(1)** Uterine artery (right). **(2)** Ureter (right).

the vagina. Vaginectomy is performed (Figure 4-10), and the specimen is completely separated from the vagina and placed in the mid-pelvis, keeping its attachments to the utero-ovarian ligaments. The preservation of the utero-ovarian ligaments allows blood supply to the retained uterine fundus and is one of the key steps in differentiating radical trachelectomy from radical hysterectomy (Figure 4-11).

Completing the Radical Trachelectomy

The lower uterine segment is then estimated and clamps are placed at the level of the internal os. Using a knife, radical trachelectomy is completed by separating the fundus from the isthmus or upper endocervix at approximately 5 mm below the level of the internal os (Figure 4-12). The uterine fundus with preserved attachments to the utero-ovarian ligaments is placed in the upper part of the pelvis. The specimen, consisting

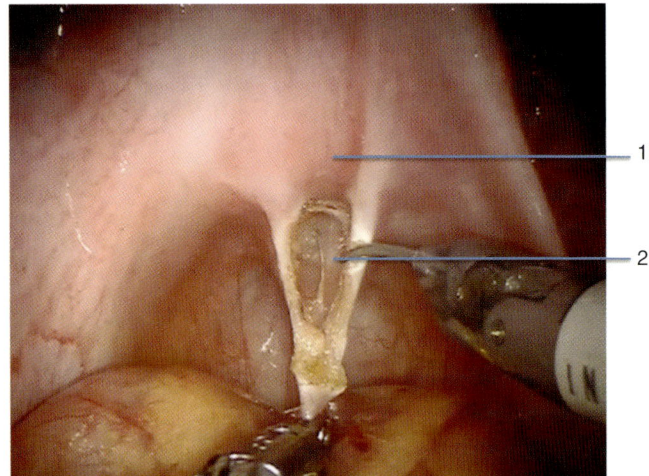

Fig. 4-8. Creation of the rectovaginal space. **(1)** Cervix. **(2)** Rectovaginal space.

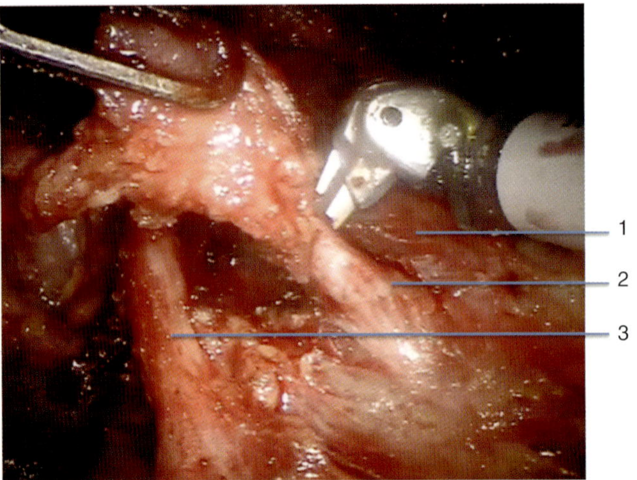

Fig. 4-6. Uterine artery sparing approach. **(1)** Trachelectomy specimen. **(2)** Uterine artery (left). **(3)** Ureter (left).

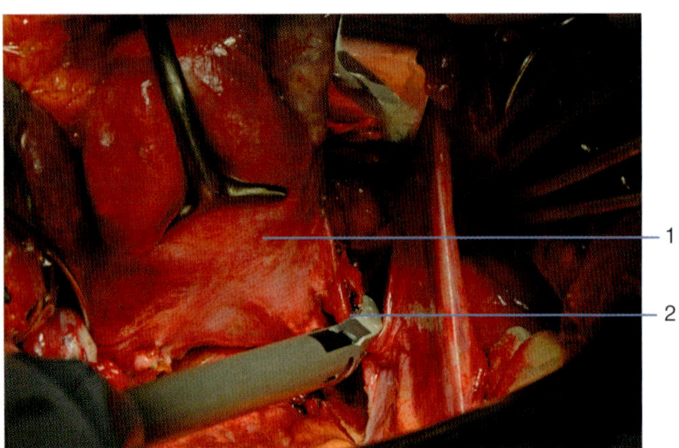

Fig. 4-9. Division of the uterosacral ligaments. **(1)** Radical trachelectomy specimen. **(2)** Uterosacral ligament (right).

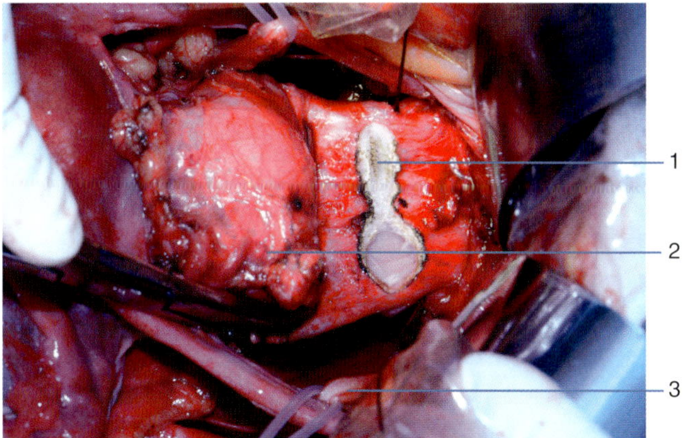

Fig. 4-10. Amputation of the radical trachelectomy specimen from the vagina. **(1)** Vaginal incision allowing for adequate vaginal margin. **(2)** Radical trachelectomy specimen. **(3)** Ureter (right).

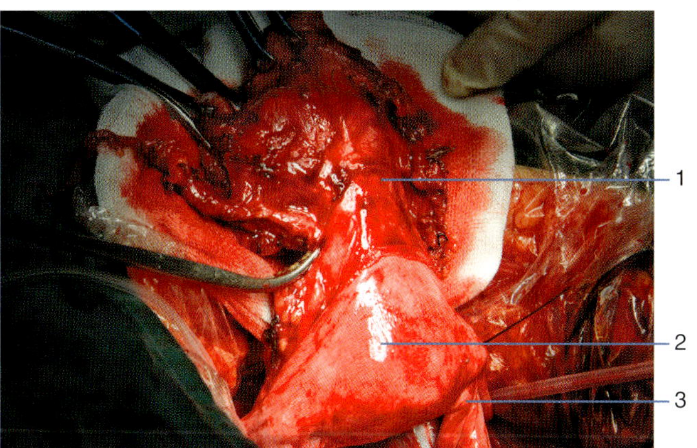

Fig. 4-11. Radical trachelectomy specimen with preservation of blood supply. **(1)** Radical trachelectomy specimen. **(2)** Uterine fundus. **(3)** Uteroovarian ligament (right).

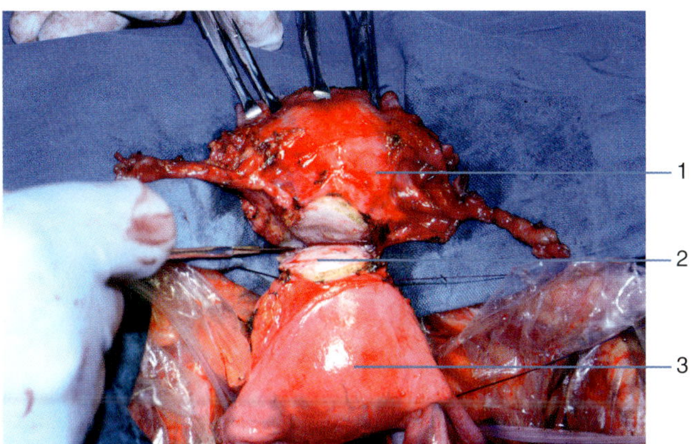

Fig. 4-12. Amputation of the radical trachelectomy specimen from the vagina. **(1)** Radical trachelectomy specimen. **(2)** Proximal cervical stump. **(3)** Uterine fundus.

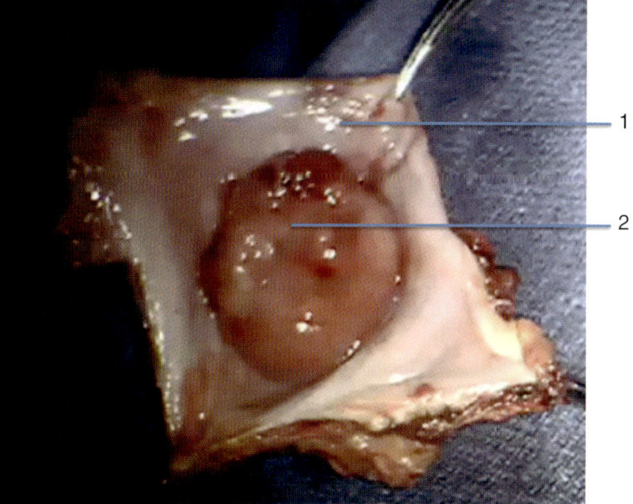

Fig. 4-13. Radical trachelectomy specimen. **(1)** Vaginal margin. **(2)** Cervical carcinoma.

of radical trachelectomy and parametria with suture marking the vaginal cuff at 12 o'clock, is sent for frozen-section evaluation of its endocervical margin (Figure 4-13).

An alternative approach is to separate the uterine fundus from the cervix prior to the colpotomy, pack the fundus with the intact utero-ovarian blood supply in the upper pelvis, place retraction clamps on the cervix, and proceed with the radical trachelectomy.

Verifying Margins Prior to Reconstruction

The uterine fundus is inspected, and a gentle curettage of the endometrial cavity is performed in addition to a shave disc margin on the remaining cervical tissue. Both specimens are sent for frozen-section analysis. The frozen-section analyses are performed to ensure that the reconstructed complex of the uterus to the vagina is disease free. If clinically indicated, a frozen-section analysis is also obtained on the distal vaginal margin. If a positive margin is identified, then either an extra margin of tissue is obtained or in the case of a positive endocervical margin a completion hysterectomy performed.

Placing a Cerclage

If all frozen sections tested are all benign and at least a 5 mm clear margin is obtained on the endocervical edge, a permanent cerclage with #1 Prolene (or #0 Ethibond) may be placed prior to the reconstruction (Figure 4-14). The knot is tied posteriorly.

Reconstruction

The reproductive tract is then reconstructed by suturing the lower uterus to the upper vagina. Six to eight #2-0 interrupted absorbable sutures are placed from the vagina to the lower uterus in a circumferential manner. Generally, for better visualization it is easier to start posteriorly, placing the back row of

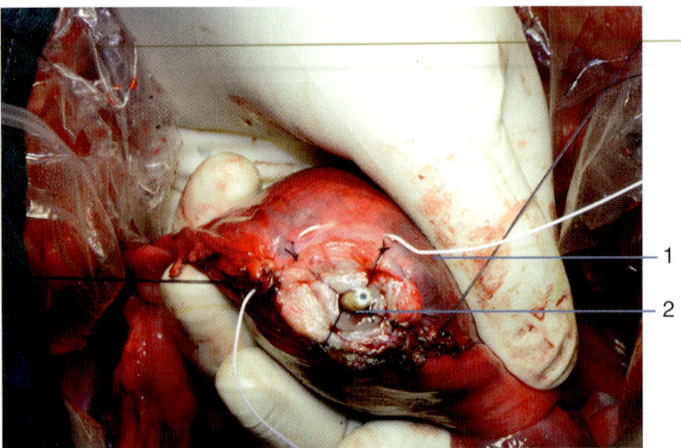

Fig. 4-14. Cerclage placement. **(1)** Cerclage placed in proximal cervical stump. **(2)** Foley catheter to prevent cervical stenosis.

sutures without tying them down until the entire row of sutures is placed, then tying them down prior to beginning the front row of sutures. Figure 4-15 shows the placement of an anterior suture prior to securing the sutures. No drains are placed. Some authors advocate the use of cystourethroscopy with bilateral temporary ureteral catheterization just prior to the performance of radical trachelectomies to improve ureteral identification and minimize trauma, but most feel that this is optional.

POSTOPERATIVE CARE

Box 4-3 PERIOPERATIVE MORBIDITY

- Urinary retention
- Bleeding from the cut edge of the uterine fundus
- Lymphocyst formation
- Lymphedema

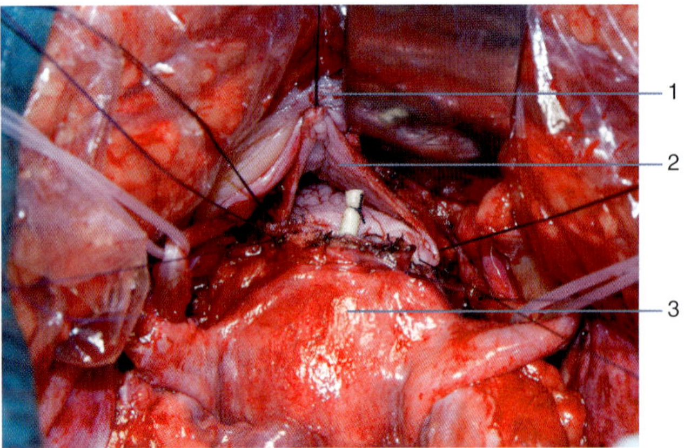

Fig. 4-15. Reconstruction of vagina to uterine fundus. **(1)** Anterior vaginal sutures. **(2)** Proximal vagina. **(3)** Uterine fundus.

Standard antibiotic and thromboembolic prophylaxis, as would be given for radical hysterectomy, are prescribed. Foley catheter drainage is identically managed to those undergoing radical hysterectomy. The length of time the catheter is left in depends on multiple factors such as type of approach (open or minimally invasive), type of pain relief prescribed (epidural vs not), and surgeon preference. In general, no matter how long the catheter has been in, a postvoid residual is checked to make sure there is no urinary retention. If the patient does have a component of urinary retention, then this almost always resolves over time. The patient is then sent home with the urinary catheter and another trial of void is attempted in approximately 2 weeks.

Other potential perioperative morbidity includes bleeding from the cut edge of the uterine fundus, lymphocyst formation, and lymphedema. In cases of heavier than expected vaginal bleeding, a pelvic examination is key to determining the source. This may need to be performed in the operating room. The bleeding should be controlled with local measures; however, in severe and extremely rare cases, the uterine fundus may need to be removed to control the bleeding. Lymphocysts are generally identified as incidental findings after pelvic lymphadenectomy; however, in rare cases, they can cause ureteral hydronephrosis and/or pelvic pain. If there is suspicion that the lymphocyst is infected or causing clinical manifestations, then it should be percutaneously drained and appropriate testing, such as bacterial cultures, performed. Following this procedure, the incidence of lymphedema has not been specifically studied but is thought to be low. In patients with lower extremity lymphedema, early initiation of physical therapy and the use of compression stockings have been associated with better outcomes.

Long-Term Outcomes

Box 4-4 DELAYED COMPLICATIONS

- Cervical/isthmic stenosis
- Infertility
- Second trimester miscarriage

1. Premature rupture of membrane

The most frequent delayed complication following a fertility-sparing approach is cervical stenosis. This may be prevented with utilization of an intrauterine cannula placed at the time of the radical trachelectomy. Another approach to attempt to prevent stenosis is to encourage the use of vaginal dilators to stretch the vaginal fornices after the reconstruction site is completely healed. Despite these efforts, occasionally, patients will develop stenosis that cannot be dilated in the office and they need to be returned to the operating room for dilatation of the uterovaginal reconstruction and even excision of tissue surrounding the opening.

Numerous studies have reported oncologically similar outcomes in women with early-stage cervical cancer treated with fertility sparing surgery as compared with standard radical hysterectomy. In the published literature, there have been more than 485 patients who have undergone radical abdominal trachelectomy. In all 16 patients (3.8%) experienced a recurrence following radical abdominal trachelectomy. Two patients (0.4%) died from cervical cancer following this fertility-sparing approach.[9]

Obstetric outcomes have been well documented, with more than 229 live births being reported. The most concerning obstetric outcome is prematurity. Second-trimester miscarriage and premature rupture of membranes with subsequent premature labor are complications associated with radical trachelectomies. However, nearly 70% of the reported births occurred after 36 weeks, while only 8.8% occurred prior to 32 weeks gestation. Cesarean section is recommended after 37 weeks. These pregnancies should be considered high-risk and a maternal-fetal medicine specialist should be involved in the obstetric care of the patient.

MIS APPLICATIONS

The abdominal approach to the fertility-sparing radical trachelectomy has allowed for this technique to be rapidly adopted. As our experience with minimally invasive surgery, particularly robotic-assisted surgery, has grown in the field of gynecologic oncology, so has the application of this platform to fertility-sparing surgery. Several institutions have published their initial experience with robotic-assisted fertility-sparing radical trachelectomy.[6] The same surgical principles of the abdominal approach can be applied to the robotic platform.

SUMMARY

Cervical cancer affects a segment of women for whom fertility preservation is a priority. It is important to understand the eligibility criteria and surgical techniques as they apply to this disease. Thorough oncologic, reproductive, and psychologic counseling is needed before offering young patients with cervical cancer a fertility-sparing option. A multidisciplinary approach, including a gynecologic oncologist, maternal-fetal medicine specialist, as well as a reproductive endocrinologist, is recommended to maximize patient comprehension and fertility outcomes.

REFERENCES

1. Siegel R, Naishadham D, Jemal A. Cancer statistics, 2013. *CA Cancer J Clin.* 2013;63:11-30.
2. Arbyn M, Autier P, Ferlay J. *Ann Oncol.* 2013;18(8):1423-1425.
3. Watson M, Saraiya M, Benard V, et al. *Cancer.* 2008;113(10):2855-2864.
4. Dargent DB, Roy M, Remy I. Pregnancies following radical trachelectomy for invasive cervical cancer. *Gynecol Oncol.* 1994;54.
5. Ungar L, Palfalvi L, Hogg R, et al. Abdominal radical trachelectomy: a fertility preserving option for women with early cervical cancer. *Br J Obstet Gynaecol.* 112;3:366-369.
6. Nick AM, Frumovitz MM, Soliman PT, et al. Fertility sparing surgery for treatment of early-stage cervical cancer: open versus robotic radical technique. *J Min Invasive Gyencol.* 116(5):569-572.
7. Diaz JP, Sonoda Y, Leitao MM, et al. Oncologic outcome of fertility-sparing radical trachelectomy versus radical hysterectomy for stage IB1 cervical carcinoma. *Gynecol Oncol.* 2008;111(2):255-260.
8. Diaz JP, Gemignani ML, Pandit-Taskar N, et al. Sentinel lymph node biopsy in the management of early-stage cervical carcinoma. *Gynecol Oncol.* 2011;120(3):347-352.
9. Pareja R, Rendon GJ, Sanz-Lomana GM, Monzon O, Ramirez PT. Surgical oncological, and obstetrical outcomes aftter abdominal radical trachelectomy – a systemic literature review. *Gynecol Oncol.* 2013;131(1): 77-82. doi: 10.1016/j.ygyno.2013.06.010. Epub 2013. Review. PMID: 23769758.

Chapter 5. Radical Vulvectomy: En Bloc Radical Vulvectomy, Separate Incision Radical Vulvectomy, Wide Radical Excision of the Vulva, and Inguinofemoral Lymphadenectomy

Robert E. Bristow, MD, MBA

BACKGROUND

Radical vulvectomy has 2 major variations: en bloc radical vulvectomy and bilateral inguinal lymphadenectomy and the technique with separate vulvar and groin incisions. Historically, all cases of vulvar cancer were treated by the classic en bloc radical vulvectomy popularized by Taussig and Way in the 1940s and 1960s.[1-3] This procedure demonstrated superior outcomes compared with simple vulvectomy and, as a result, became the therapeutic approach for virtually all cancers of the vulva. Advances in the understanding of disease etiology, natural history, and prognostic factors precipitated changes in practice focusing more on individualization of care and paralleled the more contemporary realization that it is possible to adhere to the important principles of wide excision of the primary tumor and diagnostic/therapeutic removal of groin lymph nodes without performing radical vulvectomy with bilateral inguinal lymphadenectomy on all patients.[4-6] In addition, recent advances in irradiation therapy combined with sensitizing chemotherapy have greatly reduced the requirement for radical vulvectomy as primary treatment of locally advanced vulvar cancer.[7] Today, radical vulvectomy using separate groin incisions or radical wide excision is the preferred technique for most cases of locally advanced disease not amenable to treatment with chemoradiation, because this approach is associated with less risk of wound breakdown and overall morbidity.

INDICATIONS AND CLINICAL APPLICATIONS

The surgical management of vulvar cancer has evolved over the past 3 decades. Contemporary surgical treatment principles include tailoring the radicality of resection of the primary lesion (eg, wide radical excision), more conservative techniques for assessing regional lymph nodes (eg, unilateral lymphadenectomy, sentinel node biopsy), and the liberal use of reconstructive surgical techniques to restore anatomy and function. The main indication for radical vulvectomy is invasive squamous carcinoma of the vulva stages II to IVA: non-lateralized T2 lesions (> 2 cm in maximal diameter), T3 lesions (adjacent spread to the lower urethra, vagina, or anus), and T4 lesions (spread to the upper urethra, bladder or rectal mucosa, or pubic bone) not amenable to radical wide excision or combined chemoradiation. Additional indications may include extensive Paget's disease of the vulva with an underlying adenocarcinoma, advanced adenocarcinoma of the Bartholin's gland with infiltration of vulvar soft tissues, locally advanced vulvar melanoma (without evidence of regional or distant spread), and extensive verrucous carcinoma of the vulva (generally not treated with radiation therapy, which may aggravate the disease and lead to dedifferentiation). Extensive hydradenitis suppurativa not amenable to more conservative resection may also be managed by radical vulvectomy, although there is no requirement for formal node dissection.

The wide radical excision of the vulva procedure arose from the move toward individualized treatment for patients with vulvar cancer. In properly selected patients, radical wide excision has been associated with similar recurrence and survival outcomes as radical vulvectomy while offering a substantial reduction in morbidity and improved quality of life and self-image. Radical wide excision as an alternative to radical vulvectomy is generally indicated for malignant tumors up to 2 cm in diameter without clinically apparent nodal involvement. For lateralized lesions (> 2 cm from the midline), radical wide excision is combined with unilateral inguinofemoral lymphadenectomy or sentinel lymph node biopsy. The procedure of choice for midline lesions, lesions of the anterior vulva or mons pubis, and cases with microscopically positive ipsilateral groin nodes is bilateral inguinofemoral lymphadenectomy.

Inguinal lymphadenectomy is primarily indicated for the diagnostic assessment, treatment (resection of gross adenopathy), or both of squamous carcinoma of the vulva. Recent data indicate that sentinel lymph node biopsy may be a safe and accurate alternative to inguinal lymphadenectomy for patients with stage I and II squamous tumors. Inguinal lymphadenectomy is also indicated for patients with invasive adenocarcinoma of the vulva and vulvar melanoma as well as patients with invasive cancer of the lower one-third of the vagina. Rarely, inguinal lymphadenectomy is performed for the purpose of resecting gross lymph node metastases and surrounding subclinical nodal disease as part of the therapeutic approach in selected patients with advanced ovarian or endometrial cancers.

Both radical wide excision and radical vulvectomy, with or without groin node dissection, may be incorporated as a part of a larger procedure for an extensive locally recurrent gynecologic cancer involving multiple pelvic viscera and structures (eg, extended pelvic exenteration with vulvar resection).

ANATOMIC CONSIDERATIONS

The topographic, vascular, and lymphatic anatomy of the vulva is described in Chapter 2. Traditionally, radical vulvectomy is defined by a visibly normal tissue resection margin of at least 2 cm in all directions; the deep margins of resection are the pubic aponeurosis anteriorly, the pubic rami and superficial perineal fascia laterally, and the levator ani muscles/ischiorectal fossa/anal sphincter posteriorly. From an anatomic perspective, primary closure of the en bloc radical vulvectomy defect requires extensive undermining of the surrounding tissues of the lower anterior abdominal wall and medial thigh or coverage with 1 or more of the vulvovaginal reconstructive techniques described in Chapters 16, 17, and 18. At least one study has suggested that a 1-cm margin of uninvolved tissue prior to pathologic processing may be adequate, and this is particularly applicable to the areas of the perineal body/rectovaginal septum and introitus/urethra, where a 2-cm surgical margin may be impractical due to the proximity of underlying or juxtaposed structures to be retained.[8] For wide radical excision procedures, the scope of the operation is tailored to the location of the lesion with the anatomically relevant deep margins of resection outlined above.

PREOPERATIVE PREPARATION

Box 5-1 KEY SURGICAL INSTRUMENTATION

- Basic vaginal surgery tray
- Allen Universal Stirrups (Allen Medical Systems, Cleveland, OH)
- Electrosurgical unit (Bovie)
- Weitlaner and skin hook retractors

In preparation for radical vulvar surgery, all patients should undergo a comprehensive history and physical examination, focusing on areas that may indicate a reduced capacity to tolerate major surgery. The vagina and cervix should be thoroughly evaluated to exclude a synchronous lesion or metastatic lesion. Routine laboratory testing should include a complete blood count, serum electrolytes, age-appropriate health screening studies, and electrocardiography for women 50 years of age or older. Preoperative computed tomography (CT) or combined positron emission tomography/CT imaging of the abdomen and pelvis is advisable, particularly if the groin nodes are clinically suspicious. Chest radiography should be obtained, or, alternatively, CT scanning can be extended to include the chest.

Enemas should be administered the evening before surgery. Prophylactic antibiotics (cephazolin 1 g, cefotetan 1–2 g, or clindamycin 800 mg) are administered prior to incision, and thromboembolic prophylaxis (eg, pneumatic compression devices and/or subcutaneous heparin) should be initiated prior to surgery.

SURGICAL PROCEDURE

Box 5-2 MASTER SURGEON'S PRINCIPLES

- A minimum of 1 to 2 cm of visibly disease-free surgical margins should be sought in all dimensions
- Achieving a satisfactory deep surgical margin can be challenging with posterior vulvar lesions involving the perineal body and/or posterior vaginal wall because of the proximity to the rectum/anus
- Preservation of the greater saphenous vein during inguinofemoral lymphadenectomy reduces the risk of lower extremity lymphedema

Either general or regional anesthesia is acceptable. The patient should be positioned in the dorsal lithotomy position using Allen-type stirrups, with the buttocks protruding slightly over

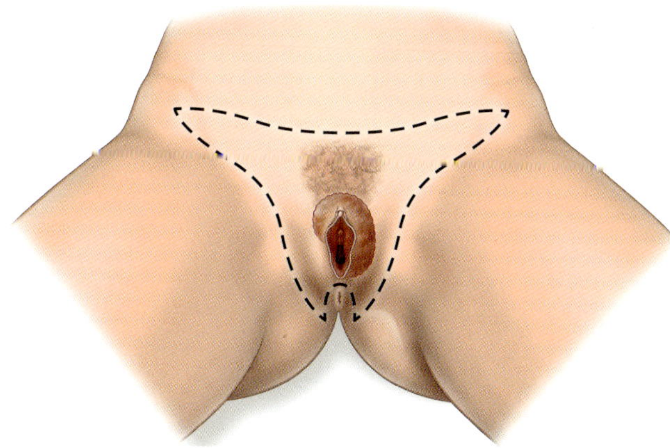

Fig. 5-1. En bloc radical vulvectomy. Extent of the incision encompassing the entire vulva and a "horn" of contiguous skin and subcutaneous tissue overlying each groin.

the edge of the operating table. The vulva, vagina, and thighs are prepped and a transurethral catheter placed.

En Bloc Radical Vulvectomy

Traditional en bloc radical vulvectomy includes removal of the vulva, mons pubis, and a contiguous "horn" of skin and underlying fatty tissue extending from the vulva over each groin (Figure 5-1). The procedure is initiated by starting anteriorly, with the patient's thighs flexed at a 15° angle in the Allen stirrups; the legs are repositioned into hyperflexion later to facilitate the posterior dissection. The cephalad skin incision is curvilinear and connects a point 2 cm medial and 2 cm inferior to each anterior superior iliac spine and extends along the superior border of the mons pubis. Bilateral vulvar incisions are created by extending downward along the groin crease into the labiocrural folds on each side. Using the knife blade, the skin of anterior portion of the specimen is incised down to the mid-point of the vulva. The electrosurgical unit (ESU) is utilized for deeper dissection. Lateral incisions are carried into the posterior vulva and directed medially and anteriorly to the anus, tailored to the extent of disease.

The anterior curvilinear incision is extended into the deep tissues between the lower abdominal wall and upper border of the mons pubis, through Camper's fascia and Scarpa's fascia, exposing the lower border of the anterior rectus sheath fascia and inguinal ligaments. An advancement flap of anterior abdominal wall skin and subcutaneous fat is then raised superiorly from the anterior rectus sheath to facilitate incision closure. This flap can be extended as far as the umbilicus if necessary. Working inferiorly, the subcutaneous tissue is dissected off of the underlying symphysis pubis, and the lateral incisions of each groin are carried into the subcutaneous tissue and extended down to the labiocrural folds, exposing the femoral triangle on each side (Figure 5-2). The superficial epigastric and external pudendal vessels are ligated with 2-0 or 3-0 delayed absorbable suture and divided as they are encountered. At this point, the bilateral inguinofemoral lymphadenectomy is performed (see below).

Following completion of the inguinofemoral lymphadenectomy, the anterior portion of the specimen is undermined along the fascia of the anterior abdominal wall and medial thigh. Closed suction drains are placed in each groin and brought out through separate incisions in the lateral

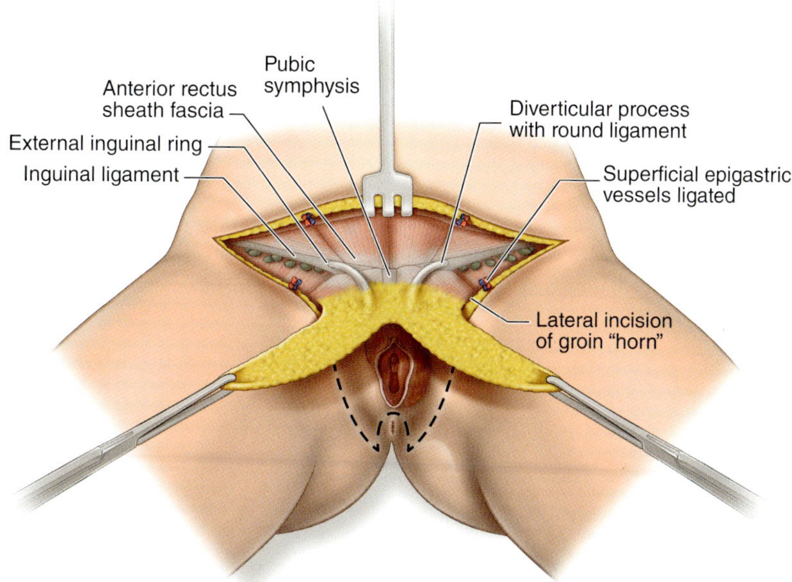

Fig. 5-2. En bloc radical vulvectomy. Anterior incision exposing abdominal wall and groin node dissection beds.

abdominal wall. The groin incisions are closed in layers using interrupted simple stitches of 3-0 delayed absorbable suture. The skin can be closed with staples or a series of vertical mattress sutures of 2-0 or 3-0 delayed absorbable sutures. The legs are repositioned into hyperflexion (45° or more) to provide exposure for the lower vulvar dissection. The labiocrural fold incisions are extended lateral to the labial fat pads, past the perineal body, and then directed medially around the anus to meet in the midline. The specimen is drawn sharply downward and separated from the symphysis pubis until the lower border of the pubic arch is reached. The dissection is taken down to the pubic aponeurosis and the suspensory ligament of the clitoris, the clitoral shaft, and clitoral vessels clamped, divided, and the pedicle(s) secured with 1-0 delayed absorbable suture ligatures.

The lateral incisions are developed down to the pubic arches and, working medially, the specimen is dissected from the inferior urogenital diaphragm. The inferior pudendal vessels are ligated with 2-0 or 3-0 delayed absorbable suture and divided. The inner vulvar incision is created by circumscribing the urethra and vaginal introitus. The dissection is carried inferiorly along the inferior fascia of the urogenital diaphragm and around the urethra, which is identified by palpating the Foley catheter. The specimen is reflected inferiorly and dissected off of the perineal body (Figure 5-3). The posterior dissection is completed by working from lateral to medial, carefully dissecting the deep vulvar tissue from the external anal sphincter and meeting in the midline at the posterior fourchette.

Primary closure of the en bloc radical vulvectomy defect requires that the incision margins be approximated in a tension-free fashion, which is especially important in the areas of the urethra and vagina. If the defect cannot be closed without tension, then one of a variety of rotational or pedicle-based flaps can be utilized (Chapters 17 and 18). The anterior extent of the defect was closed following completion of the inguinal lymphadenectomy. The thighs are taken out of hyperflexion and the lateral margins of the defect are undermined along the fascial investments of the anterior and medial thighs. The distal vaginal wall can be undermined for a short distance circumferentially, but extensive dissection around the urethra should be minimized. The wound is closed in layers with deep sutures of 2-0 or 3-0 delayed absorbable suture to obliterate dead space. Closed suction drains can be placed prior to closing the deep tissue layer and brought out through separate stab incisions. Anterior to the urethra, the skin edges are reapproximated in a vertical direction. Closure of the skin and superficial fat is best accomplished by a series of interrupted vertical mattress stitches of 2-0 delayed absorbable sutures (Figure 5-4). If a tension-free closure cannot be obtained in the periurethral region, then the area should be left open, dressed with Vaseline-impregnated gauze, and allowed to heal by secondary intention.

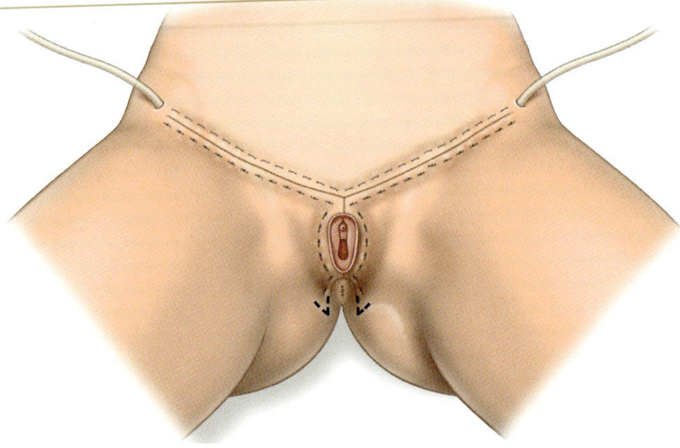

Fig. 5-4. En bloc radical vulvectomy. Primary closure.

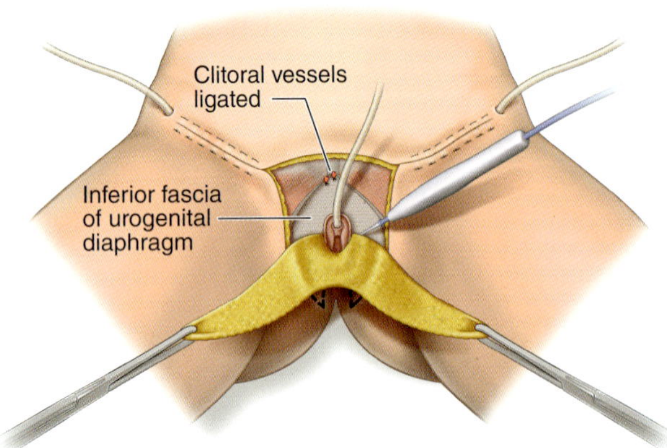

Fig. 5-3. En bloc radical vulvectomy. Vulvectomy phase after closure of groin defects. The specimen is dissected from the symphysis pubis and reflected into the posterior vulva.

Separate Incision Radical Vulvectomy

Separate incision radical vulvectomy and bilateral groin lymph node dissection accomplish the same surgical objective as the en bloc procedure without removing the skin overlying each groin or a bridge of skin and subcutaneous fat between the central vulvar resection and each groin node dissection (Figure 5-5).

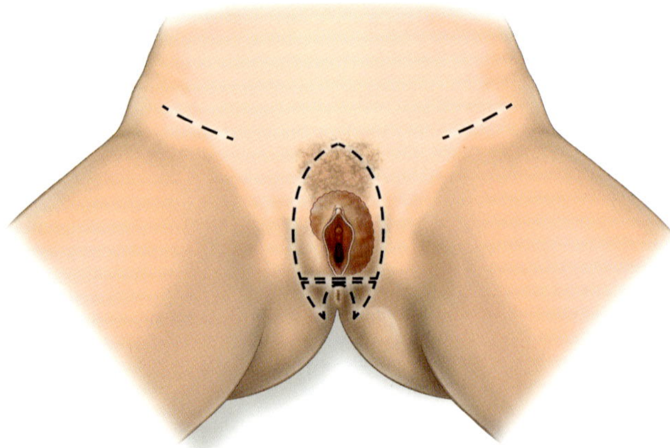

Fig. 5-5. Separate incision radical vulvectomy. Lines of incision.

For separate incision radical vulvectomy, bilateral groin lymph node dissections are performed first (see below); the incisions are closed and the legs repositioned before proceeding to the vulvectomy. The outer and inner surgical margins of dissection to encompass the central vulvar resection described above are outlined with a surgical marking pen. The knife blade is used to make the oval-shaped outer skin incision, which extends from an anterior apex in the mons pubis laterally through the skin of the labia majora and medially to meet in the midline at the perineal body. The ESU is used for the remainder of the dissection. With the exception of removing the "horns" of tissue in the en bloc radical vulvectomy, the dissection and closure for separate incision radical vulvectomy is the same as described for radical en bloc vulvectomy.

Radical Wide Excision of the Vulva

Although the scope of resection should be tailored to the anatomy and lesion topography of each individual patient, there are 3 major variations of wide radical excision of the vulva: lateral, anterior, and posterior types (Figure 5-6). Radical wide excision of the vulva includes a 1- to 2-cm resection margin of visibly disease-free tissue in all dimensions. Lateralized lesions can be accompanied by unilateral inguinal lymphadenectomy, while anterior or posterior lesions at or crossing the midline require a bilateral inguinal lymphadenectomy. A wide radical excision of the vulva is illustrated for an anterior lesion replacing the clitoris with extension into the left hemi-vulva (ie, anterior-lateral wide radical excision; Figure 5-7).

The outer skin incision consists of a curvilinear triangular incision over the mons pubis, extending through the labia major bilaterally (inclusive of the labia minora) to the level of the perineal body on the left and to the mid-vulva on the right. Anteriorly, the shaft, glans, and prepuce of the clitoris are included in the scope of resection. The outer incision is created using the knife blade and the dissection taken into the subcutaneous tissue using the ESU (Figure 5-8). The inner incision is designed around the introitus and between the urethral meatus and the prepuce of the clitoris.

Anteriorly, the dissection is carried down to the aponeurosis over the symphysis pubis. The suspensory ligament of the clitoris is divided using the ESU. The clitoral shaft and associated vessels are clamped, divided, and the pedicle secured with a transfixion stitch of 2-0 delayed absorbable suture. Using Allis clamps to provide traction on the specimen and counter-traction on the vulva, the ESU is used to extend the lateral incisions into the subcutaneous tissue. The lateral dissection on either side includes the entire labial fat pad, which is resected with the specimen and mobilized medially to expose the deep margin of resection, the adductor fascia, and pubic ramus (Figure 5-9). The lateral incisions on either side are carried medially along the deep perineal fascia and joined to the inner incision line previously demarcated and the specimen excised (Figure 5-10).

Primary closure of the defect requires that the incision margins be approximated in a tension-free fashion, which is especially important in the areas of the urethra and vagina.

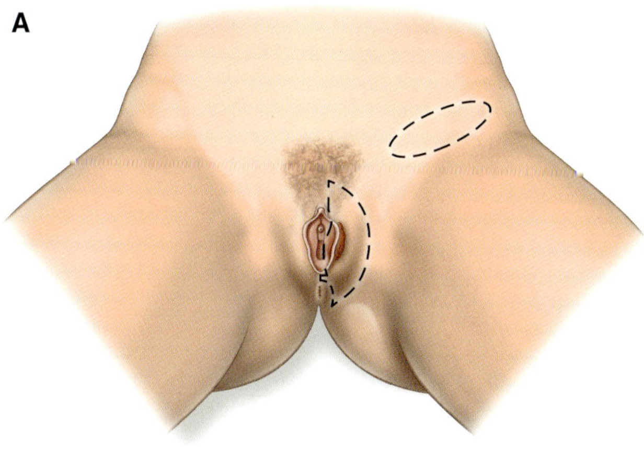

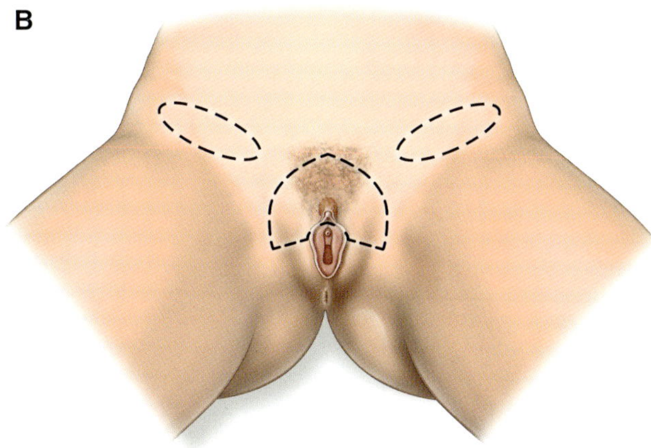

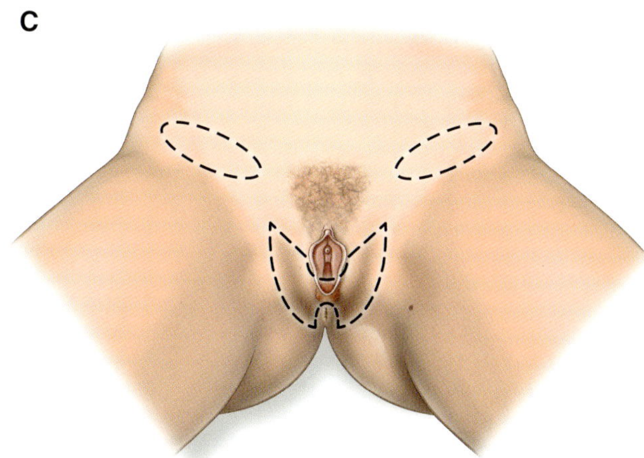

Fig. 5-6. Wide radical excision of the vulva: Types of resection are: **(A)** Lateral excision with unilateral inguinal lymphadenectomy, **(B)** anterior excision, or **(C)** posterior excision with bilateral inguinal lymphadenectomy.

The thighs are taken out of hyperflexion and the lateral margins of the defect are undermined along the fascial investments of the anterior and medial thighs. The distal vaginal wall can be undermined for a short distance circumferentially, but extensive dissection around the urethra should be minimized.

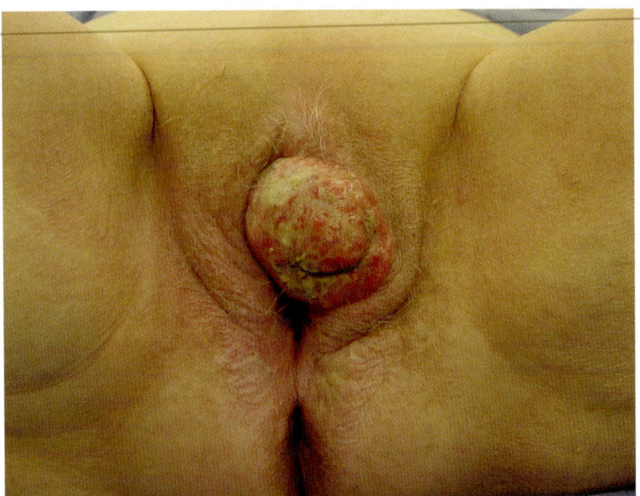

A

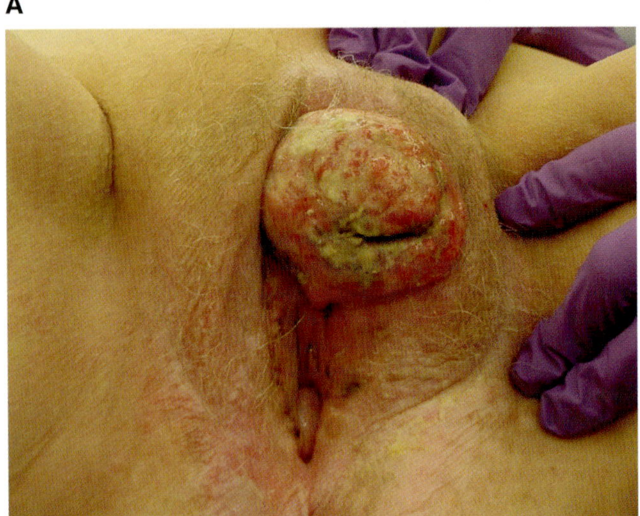

B

Fig. 5-7. **(A)** Wide radical excision of the vulva. Squamous cell carcinoma of the anterior and left lateral vulva. **(B)** The clitoris has been replaced by tumor.

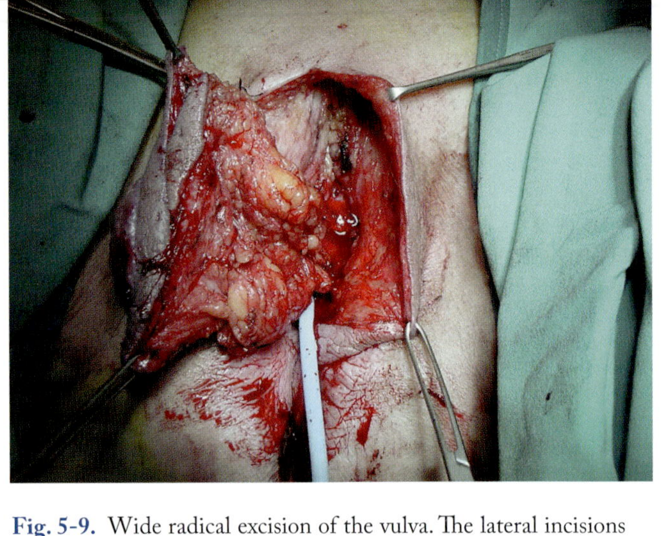

Fig. 5-9. Wide radical excision of the vulva. The lateral incisions are extended to the pubic rami and adductor fascia and the labial fat pads reflected medially as the specimen is dissected from the deep perineal fascia; the base of the clitoris and clitoral crura have been suture ligated and divided.

A closed suction drain is placed in the deep subcutaneous space and brought out through a separate stab incision in the posterior lateral vulva. Once adequate mobility of the remaining vulvar tissue has been achieved, the defect is closed as an inverted "Y" in layers, with deep sutures of 2-0 or 3-0 delayed absorbable suture to obliterate dead space. Anterior to the urethra, the skin edges are reapproximated in a vertical direction. Closure of the skin and superficial fat is best accomplished by a series of interrupted vertical mattress stitches of 2-0 delayed absorbable suture (Figure 5-11).

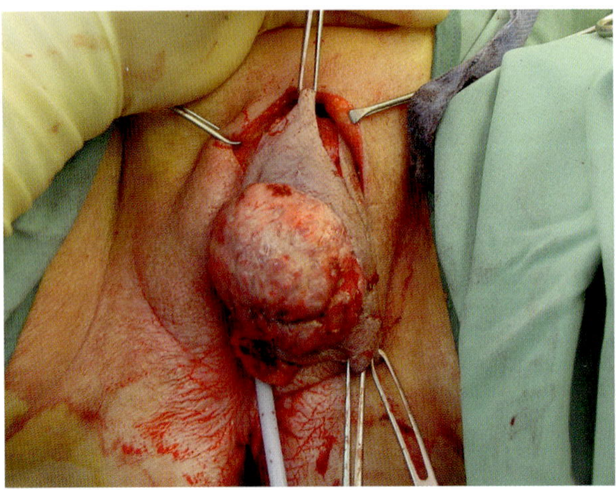

Fig. 5-8. Wide radical excision of the vulva. The anterior and lateral incisions are extended into the subcutaneous tissue.

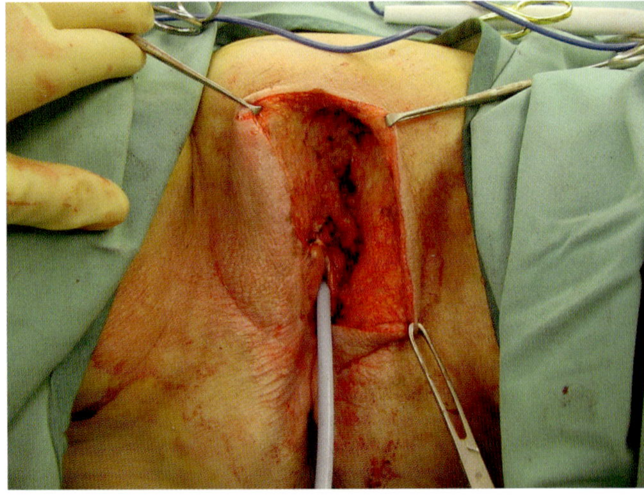

Fig. 5-10. Wide radical excision of the vulva. Completed resection.

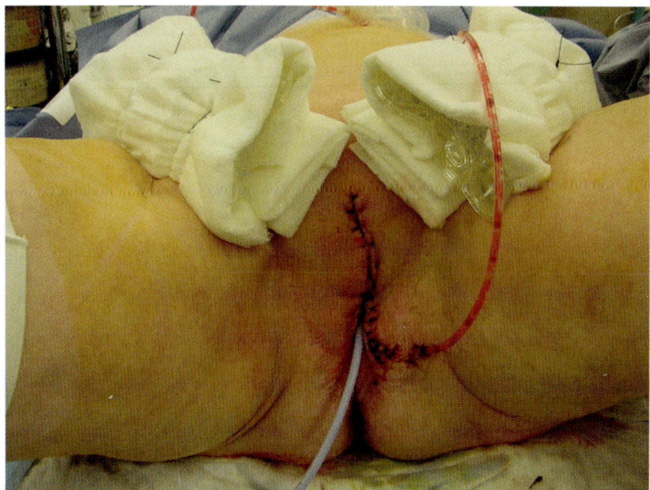

Fig. 5-11. Wide radical excision of the vulva: closure of the defect in an inverted "Y" using a series of vertical mattress sutures. Bilateral inguinofemoral lymphadenectomy has been completed and the pressure dressings applied to the surgical sites.

Radical wide excision of posterior vulvar lesions can be challenging for 2 reasons:

1. The close proximity of lesions involving the perineum and posterior vaginal wall to the anus and anterior rectal wall make attainment of a 1- to 2-cm deep surgical margin of resection difficult.
2. The surrounding tissue mobility is relatively more limited on the posterior vulva, so that primary closure of posterior-based defects often requires the use of myocutaneous flaps (Figure 5-12) or Z-plasty (Figure 5-13).

Inguinofemoral Lymphadenectomy

The patient should be positioned in the dorsal lithotomy position using Allen-type stirrups with the thighs externally rotated and flexed at 15° or less to optimize exposure to the groin. For en bloc radical vulvectomy, the groin dissection incision is incorporated into the primary resection. For separate incision radical vulvectomy and wide radical excision, an 8- to 10-cm incision is drawn with a marking pen in the groin crease, 1 to 2 cm below the inguinal ligament, midway between the anterior superior iliac spine and the ipsilateral pubic tubercle (Figure 5-14). It may also be useful to mark the anatomic area of the femoral triangle by tracing a line from the anterior superior iliac spine to the medial femoral condyle (sartorius muscle) and a line from the pubic tubercle to the lateral femoral condyle (adductor longus muscle). The knife blade is used to create the groin incision, which should be carried to a depth of approximately 1 cm. The initial incision must be deep enough to facilitate the creation of the upper and lower skin/subcutaneous tissue flaps (but which must not be so thin that they become devascularized).

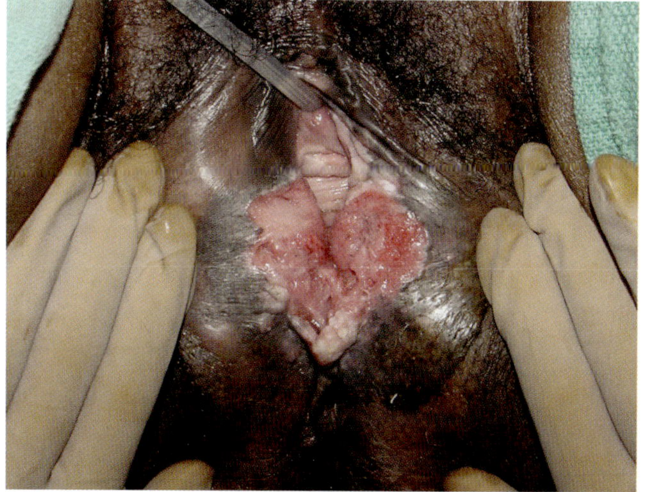

A

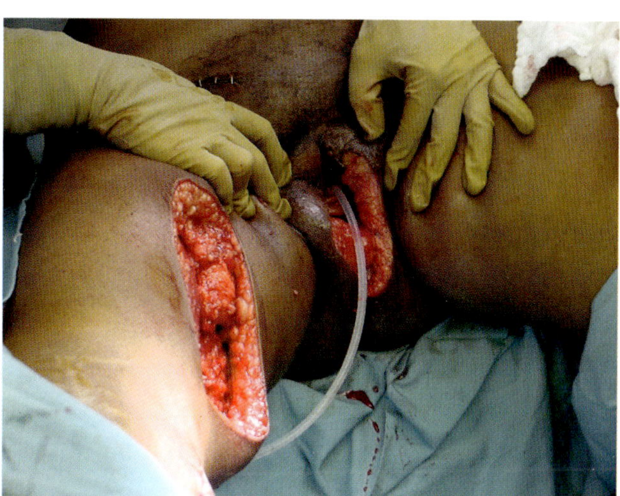

B

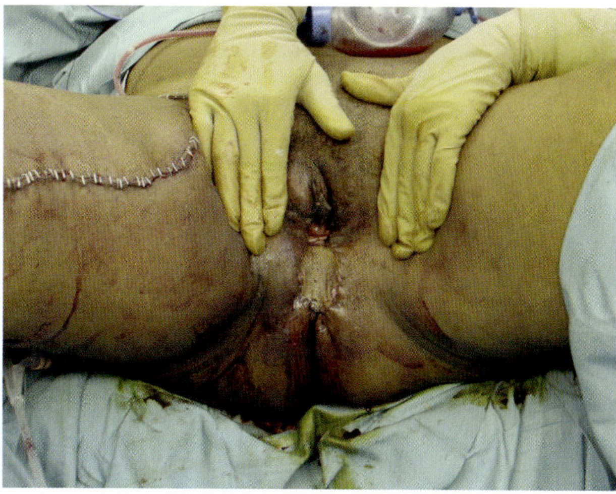

C

Fig. 5-12. **(A)** Squamous cell carcinoma of the posterior vulva. **(B)** Wide radical excision of the posterior vulva with harvesting of gracilis myocutaneous flap. **(C)** Gracilis flap rotated into posterior vulvar defect.

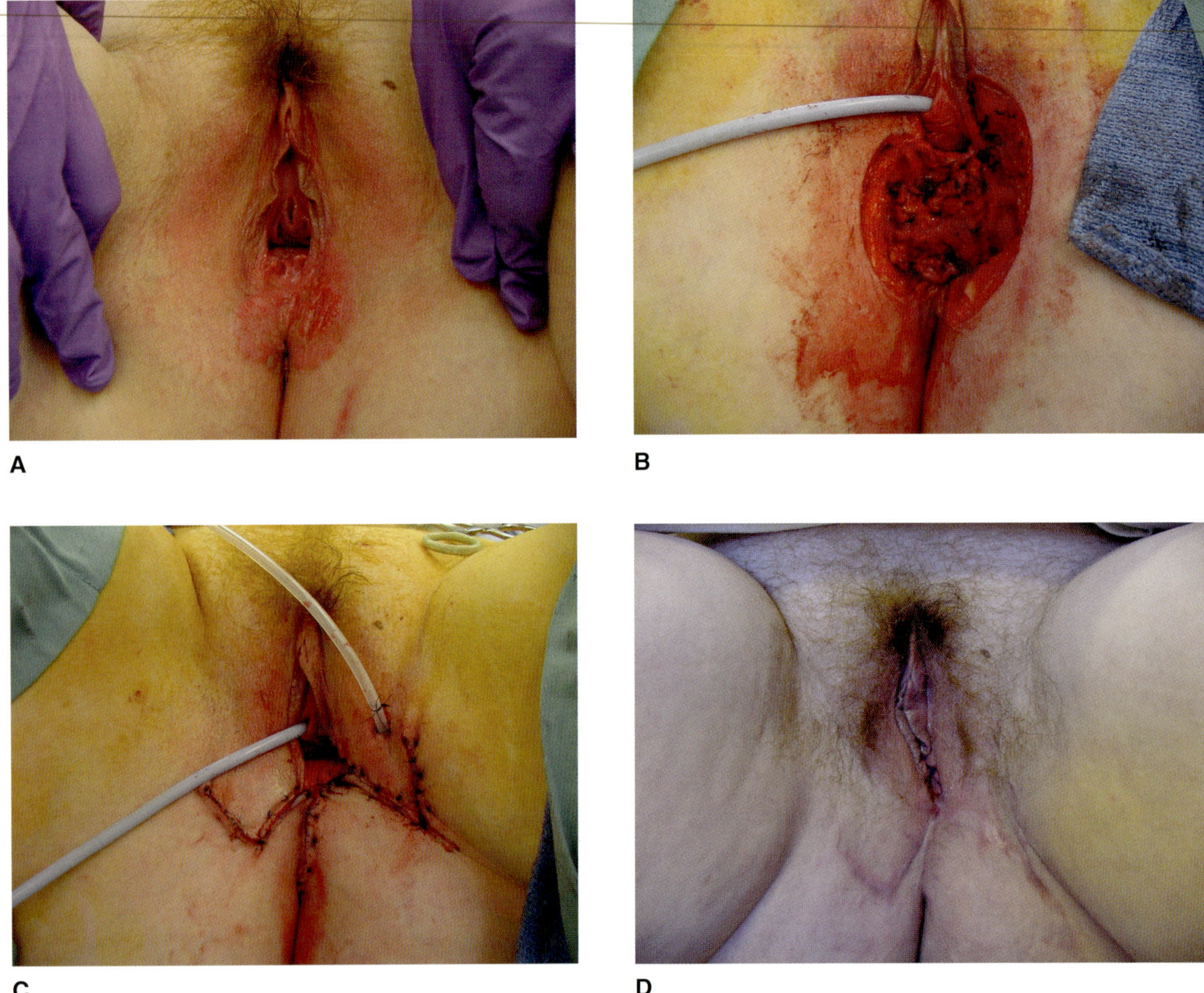

Fig. 5-13. **(A)** Squamous cell carcinoma of the posterior vulva. **(B)** Posterior vulvar defect after wide radical excision. **(C)** Closure of posterior defect using bilateral Z-plasty flaps. **(D)** Appearance 6 weeks postoperatively.

The skin and associated subcutaneous tissue are undermined using either the ESU or sharp scissor dissection. Superiorly, the tissue is undermined for an extent at least 2 to 3 cm above the superior margin of the inguinal ligament. The superficial epigastric vessels are clamped, divided, and ligated with 3-0 delayed absorbable suture as they are encountered. Inferiorly, the flap is raised for a distance of 8 to 10 cm and encompasses the area of the femoral triangle. The lateral borders of the node dissection are defined by creating tunnels in the subcutaneous tissue underneath the preoperative markings delineating the medial and lateral margins of the femoral triangle. The subcutaneous tunnels are developed with either gentle finger dissection or a long Kelly clamp placed along the anatomic margin and just above the fascia lata (Figure 5-15).

The node dissection begins at the superior margin of the femoral triangle, where the fat pad is elevated off of the inguinal ligament. The dissection proceeds systematically, working from superior to inferior and from lateral to medial. The superficial circumflex iliac vessels are located at the superior-lateral margin of the dissection and clamped, divided, and ligated. At the superior-medial margin of the dissection, the superficial external pudendal vessels are identified, clamped, divided, and ligated.

As the dissection proceeds into the center of the femoral triangle, the surgeon must be cautious of the neural and vascular structures in this area. A useful pneumonic for the location of the femoral nerve, femoral artery, and femoral vein is N-A-V-E-L, ie, proceeding from lateral to medial for ***n***erve, ***a***rtery, ***v***ein, ***e***mpty space, and ***l***ymphatic space. The specimen

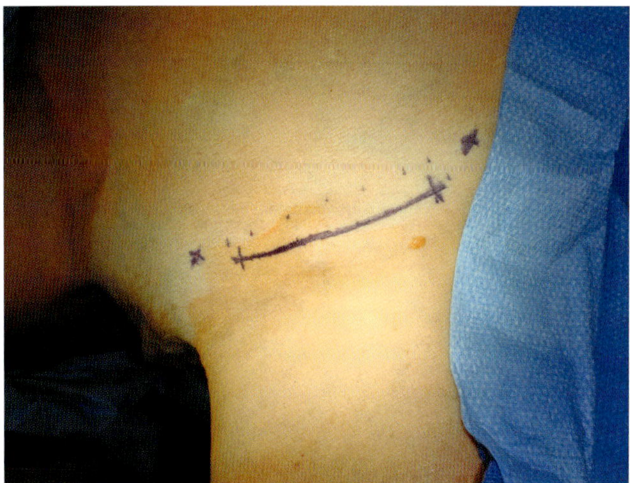

Fig. 5-14. Incision marking for left inguinofemoral lymphadenectomy. Xs mark the pubic tubercle (medial) and anterior superior iliac spine (lateral).

is reflected medially off of the iliopsoas muscle (the femoral nerve runs deep to this structure) and the lateral margin of the cribriform fascia incised, exposing the underlying femoral vessels. The femoral branch of the genitofemoral nerve runs parallel to the iliopsoas muscle along its medial margin and should be preserved. The deep femoral nodal tissue beneath the cribriform fascia is left attached to the superficial specimen and resected en bloc. As the specimen is reflected medially off of the femoral artery, the femoral vein is identified and traced distally. The great saphenous vein enters the medial surface of the femoral vein and should be carefully dissected from within the superficial and deep nodal fat pad and, if at all possible, preserved (Figure 5-16). Preservation of the great saphenous vein during inguinal lymphadenectomy has been shown to reduce both short- and long-term complications without compromising treatment outcomes. The deep external pudendal artery is identified passing just beneath the great saphenous vein as it enters the femoral vein. This arterial branch can be ligated with a 3-0 delayed absorbable suture either medial or lateral to the great saphenous vein, whichever location is more convenient. The most proximal of the deep femoral nodes, Cloquet's node, is located within the femoral canal, just medial to the femoral vein, and should be removed if present and submitted separately for pathologic analysis. The nodal fat pad is raised until the medial margin of dissection, the adductor longus muscle, is reached. The dissection then proceeds toward the inferior margin, or apex, of the femoral triangle, gently stripping the nodal tissue from the underlying femoral vessels. Once the apex is reached, a long Kelly clamp is placed across the distal aspect of the specimen; the pedicle is divided and secured with a ligature of a 3-0 delayed absorbable suture and the specimen removed (Figure 5-17).

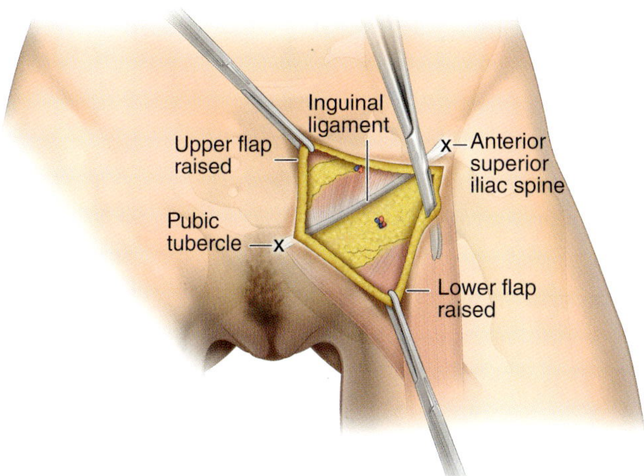

Fig. 5-15. Left inguinofemoral lymphadenectomy. The superficial epigastric vessels are ligated and divided, and the lateral and medial boundaries of dissection are defined by suing a long Kelly clamp or finger dissection.

The nodal dissection bed is inspected for hemostasis, and a closed-suction drain is placed and brought out through a separate stab incision in the lower lateral abdominal wall. The groin defect is closed in layers. The fatty tissue of the superior and inferior skin flaps is reapproximated using a series of interrupted stitches of 3-0 delayed absorbable suture. The skin incision can be closed with a series of vertical mattress stitches of 3-0 delayed absorbable suture or surgical clips. Placement of a pressure dressing may reduce the incidence and severity of postoperative lymphocyst formation and is left to the discretion of the surgeon.

POSTOPERATIVE CARE

Box 5-3 PERIOPERATIVE MORBIDITY

- Wound breakdown with potential infection and tissue necrosis occur in as many as 60% of patients undergoing en bloc radical vulvectomy
- Thromboembolic events and lower extremity lymphedema are the most common complications in the early postoperative period
- Elderly patients undergoing radical vulvectomy are susceptible to myocardial infarction and cerebrovascular accidents

In the earliest reports, operative mortality was as high as 20%; however, in more recent studies this risk is 1% to 2%. Radical vulvectomy, whether en bloc or separate incision, with bilateral inguinal lymphadenectomy is associated with a substantial risk (75%) of early postoperative complications, most notably wound breakdown and infection, thromboembolic events, urinary tract infection, and lower extremity lymphedema. Because of the extensive nature of the en bloc resection, elderly

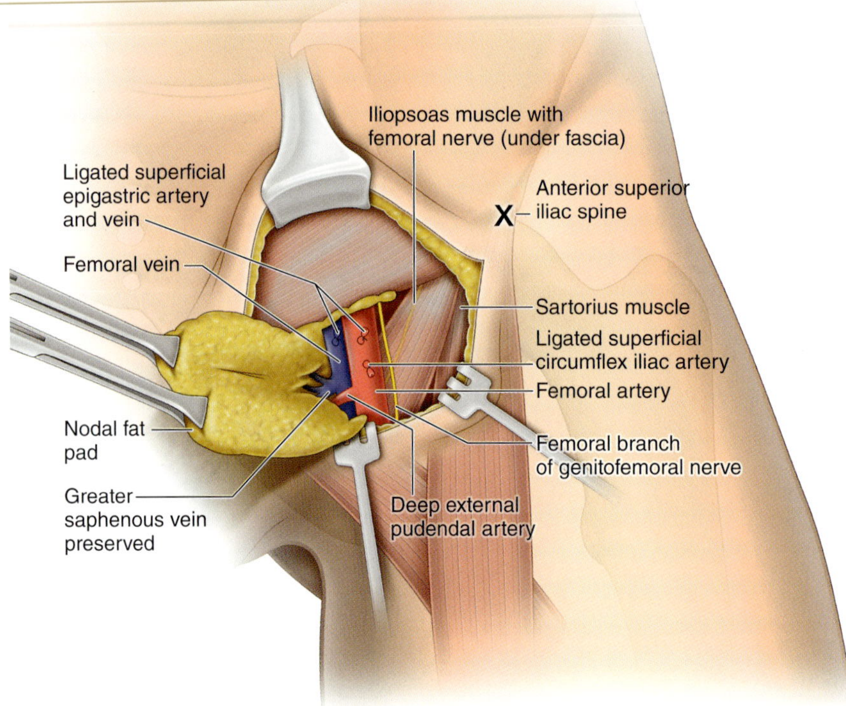

Fig. 5-16. Left inguinofemoral lymphadenectomy. The nodal fat pad is mobilized medially exposing the femoral vessels and great saphenous vein.

patients or those with pre-existing cardiovascular disease are prone to myocardial infarction and cerebrovascular accidents.

If there are no concerns about disrupting the vulvar closure, then ambulation should be initiated as early as possible in the postoperative period. To reduce tension on the incision lines, the patient should be positioned with the hips slightly flexed while in bed. As with simple vulvectomy, sitz baths should be avoided, and the vulvar area should be kept clean and dry. Routine thromboembolic prophylaxis should include both mechanical and pharmacologic measures until the patient is fully ambulatory. Pharmacologic prophylaxis should be continued for a period of several weeks thereafter. The Foley catheter is removed once the patient is ambulatory but may be continued for 7 days if there has been extensive periurethral dissection. Diet can be advanced as tolerated. Forced constipation is unnecessary unless there has been a significant posterior (perianal) dissection and avoidance of fecal contamination is desirable. Because of the risk of lymphedema of the lower extremities, it is advisable to have the patient fitted for antiedema stockings in the immediate postoperative period.

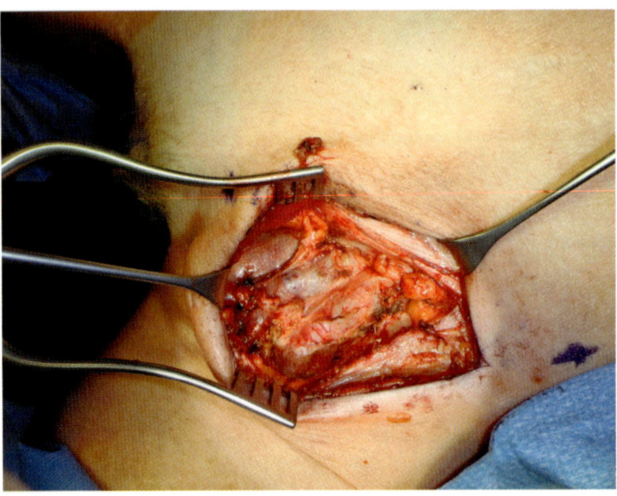

Fig. 5-17. Completed left inguinofemoral lymphadenectomy.

LONG-TERM OUTCOMES

Box 5-4 DELAYED COMPLICATIONS

- Late complications related to radical vulvectomy include sexual dysfunction, pelvic relaxation, and bladder or bowel dysfunction
- The main late complication related to the inguinal lymphadenectomy is chronic lower extremity lymphedema, which can be minimized by preservation of the great saphenous vein

Contemporary 5-year survival rates for stages III to IV vulvar cancer range from 20% to 70%, depending on the presence or absence of prognostic factors such as age, tumor size, lymph node status, and surgical margins of resection.[9] When radical vulvectomy is combined with a larger extirpative procedure (eg, exenteration), survival determinants depend on the primary tumor site, completeness of resection, and the nature and extent of prior treatment.

Late complications associated with radical vulvectomy include sexual dysfunction, pelvic floor relaxation (eg, cystocele and rectocele), urinary incontinence, and chronic lower extremity lymphedema. Depending on the extent of resection, varying degrees of lymphedema can be expected in as many as 70% of patients.[10] The more limited excision procedure with wide radical excision is associated with a lower—but still substantial—risk of long-term lymphedema (25%–40%). Rarely, osteomyelitis of the pubic bone can occur following radical vulvectomy.

SUMMARY

Radical en bloc or separate incision vulvectomy with inguinofemoral lymphadenectomy is not commonly performed today. This is because primary surgical treatment for vulvar cancer has been largely replaced by the more conservative operation of wide radical excision in combination with a targeted assessment of groin node status or primary chemoradiation therapy. Nevertheless, radical resection of the vulva may be the only feasible surgical treatment option for patients with extensive primary disease not amenable to conservative initial treatment or those with recurrent gynecologic cancer involving the vulva who have failed definitive primary treatment (eg, irradiation). Advances in reconstructive procedures to restore the anatomic appearance and function have significantly improved patient outcomes, but the risk of significant morbidity associated with radical vulvar resection, such as lymphedema, remains high.

REFERENCES

1. Taussig FJ. Cancer of the vulva: an analysis of 155 cases. *Am J Obstet Gynecol.* 1940;40:764-770.
2. Way S. Carcinoma of the vulva. *Am J Obstet Gynecol.* 1960;79:692-699.
3. Way S, Hennigan M. The late results of extended radical vulvectomy for carcinoma of the vulva. *J Obstet Gynaecl Br Commonw.* 1966;73:594-598.
4. DiSaia PJ, Creasman WT, Rich WM. An alternative approach to early cancer of the vulva. *Am J Obstet Gynecol.* 1979;133(7):825-829.
5. Berman ML, Soper JT, Creasman WT, Olt GT, DiSaia PJ. Conservative surgical management of superficially invasive stage I vulvar carcinoma. *Gynecol Oncol.* 1989;35(3):352-356.
6. Burke TW, Stringer CA, Gershenson DM, Edwards CL, Morris M, Wharton JT. Radical wide excision and selective inguinal node dissection for squamous cell carcinoma of the vulva. *Gynecol Oncol.* 1990;38(3):328-334.
7. Moore DH, Ali S, Koh WJ, et al. A phase II trial of radiation therapy and weekly cisplatin chemotherapy for the treatment of locally-advanced squamous cell carcinoma of the vulva: a Gynecologic Oncology Group study. *Gynecol Oncol.* 2012;124(3):529-533.
8. Heaps JM, Fu YS, Montz FJ, Hacker NF, Berek JS. Surgical-pathologic variables predictive of local recurrence in squamous cell carcinoma of the vulva. *Gynecol Oncol.* 1990;38(3):309-314.
9. Tabbaa ZM, Gonzalez J, Sznurkowski JL, Weaver AL, Mariani A, Cliby WA. Impact of the new FIGO 2009 staging classification for vulvar cancer on prognosis and stage distribution. *Gynecol Oncol.* 2012;127(1):147-152.
10. Podratz KC, Symmonds RE, Taylor RF. Carcinoma of the vulva: analysis of treatment failures. *Am J Obstet Gynecol.* 1982;143(1):340-351.

Chapter 6. Radical Cystectomy

Jordan Siegel, MD,
Hak J. Lee, MD, and
Atreya Dash, MD

BACKGROUND

Initial reports of cystectomy are attributed to Bardenheuer et al of Cologne in 1887, with the first female cystectomy being performed by Pawlik in Czechoslovakia around the same time. The modern steps of the radical cystectomy with pelvic lymph node dissection were described by Whitmore and Marshall in 1962.[1] Further refinements have taken place over the years, with Schlegel and Walsh describing the nerve-sparing approach in 1987.[2] With the advent of minimally invasive surgery, the first laparoscopic radical cystectomy (LRC) was described by Parra et al in 1992,[3] and, in 2003, Menon et al[4] demonstrated the feasibility of robotic-assisted radical cystectomy. Both of these new techniques have proven to have oncologic equivalency when compared with the open technique. In addition, the minimally invasive approach offers improved perioperative outcomes (lower blood loss, shorter hospital stay, and morbidity), although long-term outcomes have shown only small benefits with limited follow-up.[5]

INDICATIONS AND CLINICAL APPLICATIONS

The most common indication for cystectomy worldwide is invasive bladder cancer in the form of urothelial carcinoma, or squamous cell carcinoma, as is more common in areas with endemic schistosomiasis infection.[6] In addition, bladder cancer involvement of reproductive organs has been shown to occur in 7.5% of females, with the vagina (3.8%) and cervix (0.7%) being the most commonly involved.[7]

However, in the setting of gynecologic malignancy involvement of adjacent pelvic organs, such as the bladder, is less common. The most common scenario is cervical cancer, with involvement of adjacent organs occurring in fewer than 5% of North American patients.[8] Cystectomy for gynecologic malignancy is a treatment often done for recurrent disease with about one-half of the patients having undergone previous treatment, either chemotherapy or radiotherapy. Less common indications for cystectomy include intractable hematuria, end-stage bladder secondary to radiation injury, neurologic disease, or refractory fistula disease.

ANATOMIC CONSIDERATIONS

The bladder is an ovoid, muscular organ with a capacity of 400 to 500 mL. The bladder occupies the anterior pelvis and is juxtaposed to the posterior border of the symphysis pubis, separated only by the potential retropubic space of Retzius. The paired paravesical spaces laterally bound the bladder. The bladder and adjacent structures define the inner surface of the lower abdominal wall, which includes the median umbilical fold (urachus), the paired medial umbilical folds (obliterated umbilical arteries), and the paired lateral umbilical folds (inferior epigastric vessels). The internal anatomy of the bladder includes the base or trigone (defined by the internal urethral orifice and both ureteral orifices), a ventral wall, and a dorsal wall. The ventral and dorsal walls meet at the bladder apex, where the urachus begins its course toward the umbilicus. In women, the bladder base rests on the anterior cervix and proximal anterior vagina. As such, radical cystectomy in the female patient includes removal of the bladder and surrounding fat, the uterus and adnexa (unless previously removed), and a portion of the proximal anterior vaginal wall (Figure 6-1). Radical cystectomy may or may not include urethrectomy. While it is similar in theory to an anterior pelvic

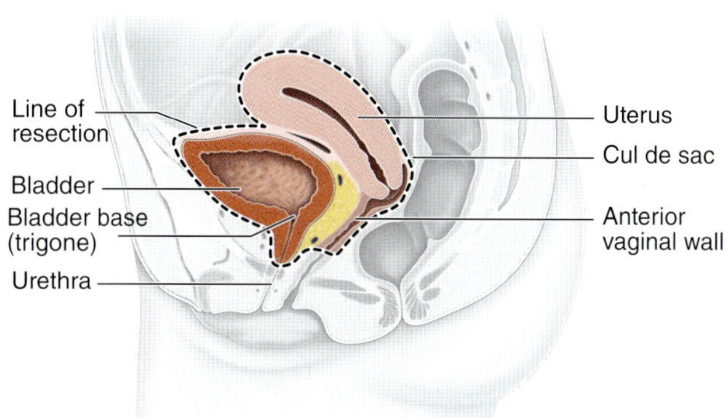

Fig. 6-1. Radical cystectomy in the female patient: the scope of resection incorporates the bladder and surrounding fat, the uterus and adnexa, and a portion of the anterior vaginal wall. Urethrectomy may or may not be included.

exenteration, the scope of pelvic sidewall and vaginal resection with radical cystectomy is comparatively less radical than with a classic exenterative surgery (Chapter 8). The bladder has a dual blood supply by way of the superior vesicle pedicle, which carries the superior vesicle artery, and the inferior vesicle pedicle, which carries the inferior vesicle artery. Both pedicles arise from the anterior division of the internal iliac (hypogastric) artery. The inferior vesicle artery supplies the bladder base and proximal urethra. The innervation of the bladder is via the vesicle plexus (anterior part of the inferior hypogastric plexus), which runs with the arteries of the bladder base.

PREOPERATIVE PREPARATION

Box 6-1 KEY SURGICAL INSTRUMENTATION

- A major open tray with a long and fine instrument tray
- Bookwalter or Omni abdominal retractor
- 7-French ureteral diversion stents × 2
- Jackson-Pratt or other abdominal drain
- Tenotomy and Potts scissors
- Smooth Gerald forceps
- Short and long Allis clamps
- Regular, long handle, and right angle clip appliers
- Optional: hemostatic device (eg, LigaSure [Covidien, Mansfield, Massachusetts])
- Suture:
  - Ureteral anastomosis: 4-0 monocryl on RB-1 needle
  - Stoma: 3-0 delayed absorbable suture on SH needle
  - Ureteral stents: 3-0 chromic on SH needle
  - Fascial closure: 1 Ethibond (Ethicon, Somerville, New Jersey) or 1 PDS

Preoperative preparation for radical cystectomy should include relevant imaging studies to accurately define the extent of tumor, depending on the primary disease process, determine the scope of resection and whether resection of additional anatomic structures will be necessary, and exclude the presence of regional or distant metastatic disease. As for any other major surgical procedure, patients should undergo a complete physical examination and laboratory studies and have adequate nutritional and performance status to withstand a major operation. Radical cystectomy necessarily will involve reconstruction of the urinary tract, diversion of the urinary stream, or both. As such, patients should undergo preoperative evaluation and counseling regarding the most appropriate choice for urinary diversion: incontinent diversion, continent diversion, or orthotopic neobladder creation. Preoperative consultation with an enterostomal therapist with marking for optimal stoma placement is recommended. With regard to preoperative bowel management, recent data from the colorectal literature showed no difference in complication rates between those who were prepped and those who were not. Of note, surgeons may still elect to prep when using the colon for diversion, because it may have the advantage of technical ease in bowel handling. Prophylactic antibiotics should be administered and thromboembolic prophylaxis methods should be in place prior to surgery.

SURGICAL PROCEDURE

Box 6-2 MASTER SURGEON'S PRINCIPLES

- The retropubic space of Retzius, paravesical spaces, and pararectal spaces should be fully developed to optimize exposure
- Resection of the anterior vaginal wall should be limited to the surface area juxtaposed to the bladder base
- Preservation of the urethra and division of the ureters as distally as possible will maximize options for urinary diversion/reconstruction

The female patient is positioned supine and slightly frog-legged or in low lithotomy in stirrups to facilitate access to the vagina. The abdomen is prepared from the xiphoid to the pubis; the vagina is also prepped. A Foley catheter is inserted on the field.

Initial incision is lower midline from the symphysis pubis to umbilicus; we prefer an infraumbilical incision, which can be superiorly extended, as needed, depending on exposure requirements. Dissection is carried down through the subcutaneous tissues to expose the anterior rectus fascia. The anterior rectus fascia is incised and the rectus muscle bellies are retracted laterally. The transversalis fascia is incised, exposing the preperitoneal space. The bladder is then bluntly dissected anteriorly off the pubis and pelvic sidewalls to expose the retropubic space of Retzius. The retractor is usually placed at this point, and the peritoneum can be opened with sharp incision.

The urachus is identified, ligated, and a clamp is placed for applying traction to the bladder. Most cystectomies for gynecologic malignancy will be performed in the recurrent setting in which patients likely would have undergone previous hysterectomy and bilateral salpingo-oophorectomy. If not, then removal of the uterus and adnexa is included in the scope of resection. Incising the peritoneum lateral to the bladder will expose the round ligaments, which are identified and divided followed by incision of the broad ligaments to expose the ureters. The pelvic sidewall peritoneum is opened and the paravesical and pararectal spaces are developed bilaterally. The ovarian vessels in the infundibulopelvic ligaments are identified and divided. The fallopian tube/utero-ovarian ligament pedicles are clamped and divided, and the adnexa are removed from the field to facilitate exposure. The ureters are isolated

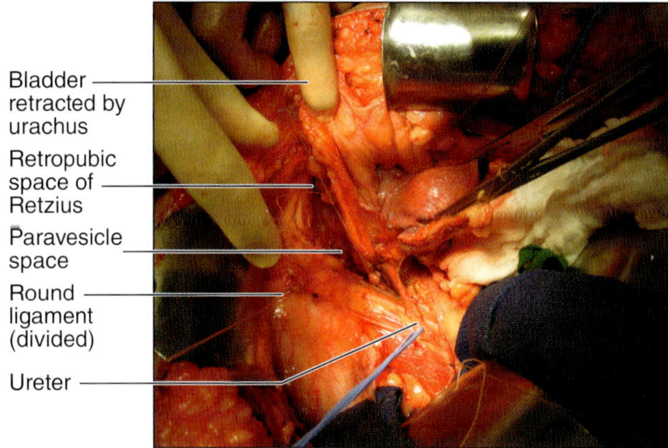

Fig. 6-2. Lateral pelvic wall dissection. The ureter is completely mobilized and the retropubic space of Retzius, paravesical space, and pararectal space are unified.

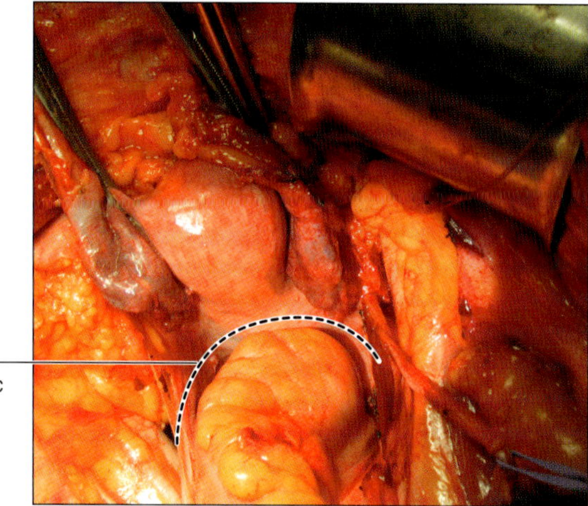

Fig. 6-3. Line of cul-de-sac incision.

with vessel loops and dissected both proximally and distally toward the bladder and divided to provide enough length for later diversion construction (Figure 6-2). We usually ligate the distal ureters before dividing them to allow for distention of the ureters to make subsequent spatulation for diversion easier.

If a previous pelvic lymphadenectomy was not performed, then we usually perform it at this point during the operation. Upon completion of the lymph node dissection, the obliterated medial umbilical ligaments are identified at the take-off from the internal iliac arteries and divided. This allows greater upward mobility on the bladder. The uterus is stitched to the bladder so it does not fall into the posterior dissection. Long Pean clamps can be placed on the uterus to facilitate manipulation of the surgical specimen. Traction is placed on the uterus at this point, pulling the uterus and bladder anteriorly, while a sponge stick is used to place the rectosigmoid colon on stretch posteriorly, exposing the cul-de-sac for incision (Figure 6-3). The rectovaginal space is developed using sharp and blunt dissection, and the vagina is then mobilized off of the rectosigmoid colon. An iodine-soaked sponge stick is then placed in the vagina and directed upward to help identify the cervix, which is easily palpable. The posterior vaginal wall is then incised with electrocautery below the level of the cervix to keep the cervix attached to the uterus. With the surgical specimen placed on medial stretch, the lateral vascular pedicles, which consist of the anterior division of the internal iliac artery and related branches, can be divided between clamps and secured with sutures and clips or controlled with a device such as the LigaSure up to the level of the endopelvic fascia (Figure 6-4). The anterior vaginal wall defect will depend on tumor size and location but preservation of the lateral neural plexus of the vagina is preferred, as it is the location of innervation of the clitoris.

Next the dissection moves anteriorly, exposing and incising the endopelvic fascia. The pubourethral ligaments are identified and divided, then the dorsal venous complex is ligated and divided. This will provide exposure of the urethra. To ensure complete excision of the bladder with urethra, an option is to incise the periurethral tissue sharply around the catheter at the level of the urethral meatus. Traditional pelvic exenteration will include urethrectomy with a small strip of anterior vaginal wall. The vaginal defect is then closed with a running absorbable suture in a clamshell fashion. Occasionally, additional mobilization of the vaginal wall is required to close the vagina without tension. The posterior wall can be sharply dissected off the anterior rectum to provide this mobility prior to closure. If orthotopic diversion is planned, then the bladder neck is occluded with a clamp or Foley balloon and the urethra is transected at the bladder neck junction. It is important to limit the urethral dissection to preserve good function of the urethral sphincter muscle.

At this point, cephalad traction is placed on the Foley/bladder neck clamp to dissect the posterior bladder and resect the associated segment of the anterior vaginal wall. The lateral soft-tissue pedicles are identified at this time and can be controlled and divided with clamps and suture ligation, clips, or hemostatic devices, such as LigaSure (Figure 6-5). The specimen is passed off at this time and if the vaginal wall is thinned or previously incised, an omental flap can be interposed prior to neobladder placement (Figure 6-6). Drain placement and management is specific to the type of diversion performed and is at the discretion of the surgeon.

POSTOPERATIVE CARE

Box 6-3 PERIOPERATIVE MORBIDITY

- The most common complications are ileus, wound infection, and thromboembolic events
- Prior irradiation increases the risk of intestinal anastomotic leak and ureteral stricture

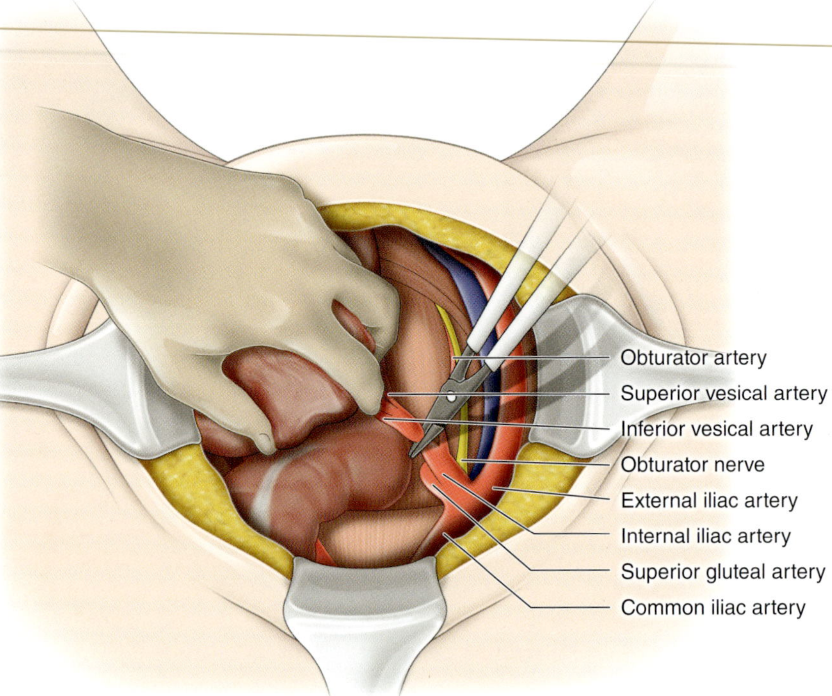

Fig. 6-4. Ligation of the anterior division of the internal iliac artery (lateral vascular pedicle).

Recently more high volume centers have moved toward a set clinical pathway that stream lines the perioperative care for patients undergoing cystectomy. One study showed that outcomes are less dependent on individual surgeon experience and more so on center volume, likely owing to set clinical pathways and coordination with specialized ancillary staff.[9] Prolonged nasogastric tube decompression is unnecessary, and diet can usually be rapidly advanced. Early feeding prior to return of bowel function has also been shown to be safe and may trend toward earlier discharge.[10] Perioperative antibiotics should be discontinued by 24 hours postoperatively in the absence of gross stool spillage.[11] Perioperative pain management varies among individual patients and treatment centers. If possible, utilizing a dedicated pain service, especially with placement of epidural analgesics, will assist in adequate pain control and more expedient recovery. Data have shown

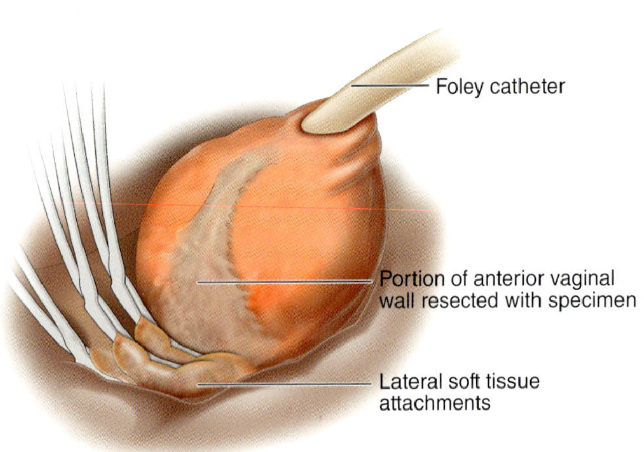

Fig. 6-5. Resection of lateral pelvic wall soft-tissue attachments between clamps.

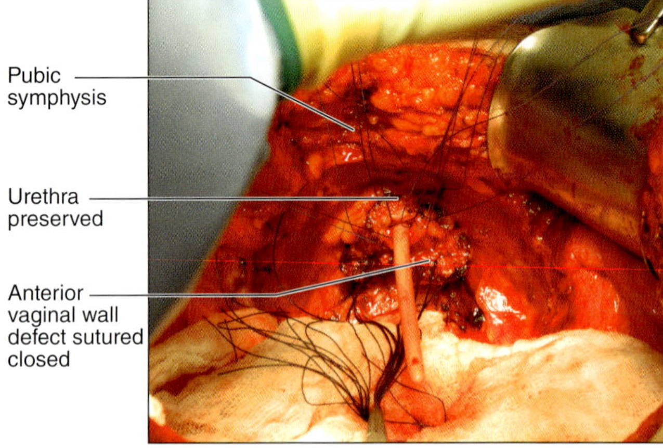

Fig. 6-6. Postradical cystectomy surgical field; the anterior vaginal wall defect has been closed (posterior sutures). The urethra has been preserved and is prepared (anterior sutures) for orthotopic neobladder creation.

decreased narcotic use among patients undergoing laparoscopic and robotic procedures.[12,13] The Jackson-Pratt or other common abdominal drain can be removed around the time of discharge, around days 5 to 7.

With regard to anticoagulation, postoperative mechanical and chemical venous thromboembolic (VTE) prophylaxis should be initiated as soon as possible, taking into account each individual patient's risk of bleeding. VTE prophylaxis should be continued throughout hospitalization. In addition, some studies have shown benefit for a more prolonged course of chemical VTE prophylaxis following discharge; thus, VTE prophylaxis is recommended particularly for patients undergoing major surgery for cancer.[14,15]

Ostomy planning and care are vital to patient quality of life following surgery. It is useful to have the ostomy nursing staff meet with the patient and family to demonstrate appliance application and to provide appropriate supplies prior to discharge.

Despite the improvements in surgical technique and perioperative care, radical cystectomy, with urinary diversion, continues to have one of the highest complication rates among surgical procedures. Ninety-day readmission rates at major treatment centers are as high as 27%, with overall 90-day complication rates as high as 64%. The most common grade 3 complications include ileus (15%–18%), wound dehiscence (3.5%–4.6%), wound infection (2.9%–9.3%), deep venous thrombosis (3.5%–5.3%), acute renal failure (0.9%–3.2%), small bowel obstruction (2.5%–7.2%), and pelvic abscess (2.1%–4.3%). Grade 4 complications include myocardial infarction (1.3%–3.5%), septic shock (2.8%–4.5%), cerebrovascular accident (0.4%–0.7%), and pulmonary embolism (1.8%–3.2%). The 90-day mortality rate ranges from 1.5% to 6.9% in the largest studies.[16-19]

A correlation between higher preoperative ASA score or Charlson comorbidity score and intraoperative blood loss has been noted in some studies. Interestingly, age alone has not been shown to be an independent risk factor for complications in this patient population, prompting surgeons to operate on patients who are elderly but are otherwise healthy.[20,21] Patients who undergo radiotherapy prior to surgery (as is often the case in gynecologic malignancy), are at a higher risk for complications, such as intestinal anastomotic leaks and ureteral anastomotic strictures, which can occur in as many as 11% of cases.

LONG-TERM OUTCOMES

Box 6-4 DELAYED COMPLICATIONS

- Primarily related to the type of urinary diversion
- May include impairment of quality of life and body image

Long-term outcomes in patients undergoing cystectomy will be divergent based on the disease process involved. For example, in cases of urothelial carcinoma of the bladder, the pathologic stage will largely determine outcomes with pT0, pTa, pTis 10-year recurrence-free survival rates at 86%, 89%, and 74% respectively, for lymph node negative disease. Those with more invasive but localized disease (pT2N0/pT3aN0), have 10-year recurrence-free survival rates of 87% and 76%, respectively, while those with lymph node positive disease have a far worse 10-year recurrence-free survival rate of only 34%.[22]

Contrasting with the above data are the long-term results for gynecologic cancer. Most of these cases are performed for recurrent gynecologic cancer, such as cervical cancer, and often have been previously treated with chemotherapy or radiotherapy. A European study assessed survival in a population of patients with gynecologic cancer, of whom one-half had received previous therapy.[23] The study found a disease-specific 5-year survival rate of 36.5% and correlated survival with surgical margin status, a finding common to many such reports.[23] Likewise, recent data on patients undergoing extended pelvic resections for recurrent gynecologic malignancies found an overall 5-year survival rate of 0% versus 48% for patients with positive margins versus those with negative margins at resection.[24] In addition, studies have demonstrated a poor overall survival rate in this population, ranging from 27% to 34% across periods of more than 50 months. Poor prognosis was associated with positive nodal status, cervical squamous cell histology, and positive surgical margins. Of note, endometrial histology had improved survival among patients with gynecologic cancers who underwent removal of the bladder.[25-27]

Radical cystectomy is a surgery with known significant morbidity in the perioperative period and beyond. Much of the extended morbidity is a result of the urinary diversion. The overall effect is one that impacts the health status of the patient on multiple levels, including physical, psychological, sexual, and social levels. There have been extensive research efforts to analyze the health-related quality-of-life in this population. With regard to urinary diversion, urologic experts have recommended orthotopic neobladders, with the assumption that recreating the "normal" voiding mechanism and eliminating external drainage bags will increase patient satisfaction. However, quality-of-life data on urinary diversion have not shown significant improvement in these parameters for patients with orthotopic diversion.[28] Data from validated questionnaires were prospectively collected and analyzed from a gynecologic malignancy population and revealed a significant decline at 3 months for sexual, psychological, and daily activities, with a return to baseline for these parameters at 12 months.[29]

MINIMALLY INVASIVE SURGICAL APPLICATIONS

The first LRC was first described by Parra et al[30] in 1992. Since then, the minimally invasive technique has been compared with open radical cystectomy in oncologic and perioperative outcomes. However, the laparoscopic technique has only shown small benefits with limited follow-up.[5] The largest series of LRC was conducted by Huang et al.[31] A total of 171 patients with urothelial carcinoma were studied; the mean follow-up of the study was 37 months (3–83) and demonstrated similar overall survival (73.7%), cancer-specific survival (81.3%), and recurrence-free survival (72.6%) rates as open radical cystectomy.[32] However, the minimally invasive approach has never gained wide acceptance due to the flat learning curve and skills required for this operation.[33] With the advent of robotics, in 2003 Menon et al[34] demonstrated the feasibility of robotic-assisted radical cystectomy. The clear advantages of the robotic instrumentation over laparoscopy and accumulated experience from robotic prostatectomy have increased surgeon comfort and interest in adopting robotic-assisted radical cystectomy into the minimally invasive armamentarium. Currently, high-volume surgeons have tackled the difficult job of adopting and improving the extirpative portion of the operation, as well as including the reconstructive portion of the operation with the robotic platform.

SUMMARY

Radical cystectomy in the female patient is most often indicated for recurrent gynecologic cancer involving the bladder and internal genitalia (if present). Compared with the classic anterior exenteration, radical cystectomy may allow preservation of a greater extent of vaginal wall and the option of orthotopic neobladder creation. Despite advances in perioperative care, morbidity can be significant; therefore, proper patient selection is critical.

REFERENCES

1. Whitmore WF, Jr., Marshall VF. Radical total cystectomy for cancer of the bladder: 230 consecutive cases five years later. *J Urol.* Jun 1962;87:853-868.
2. Walsh PC, Schlegel PN. Radical pelvic surgery with preservation of sexual function. *Ann Surg.* Oct 1988;208(4):391-400.
3. Parra RO, Andrus CH, Jones JP, Boullier JA. Laparoscopic cystectomy: initial report on a new treatment for the retained bladder. *J Urol.* Oct 1992;148(4):1140-1144.
4. Menon M, Hemal AK, Tewari A, et al. Nerve-sparing robot-assisted radical cystoprostatectomy and urinary diversion. *BJU Int.* Aug 2003;92(3):232-236.
5. Haber GP, Campbell SC, Colombo JR, Jr., et al. Perioperative outcomes with laparoscopic radical cystectomy: "pure laparoscopic" and "open-assisted laparoscopic" approaches. *Urology.* Nov 2007;70(5):910-915.
6. Salem S, Mitchell RE, El-Alim El-Dorey A, Smith JA, Barocas DA. Successful control of schistosomiasis and the changing epidemiology of bladder cancer in Egypt. *BJU Int.* Jan 2011;107(2):206-211.
7. Djaladat H, Bruins HM, Miranda G, Cai J, Skinner EC, Daneshmand S. Reproductive organ involvement in female patients undergoing radical cystectomy for urothelial bladder cancer. *J Urol.* Dec 2012;188(6):2134-2138.
8. Waggoner SE. Cervical cancer. *Lancet.* Jun 28 2003;361(9376):2217-2225.
9. Morgan TM, Barocas DA, Keegan KA, et al. Volume outcomes of cystectomy—is it the surgeon or the setting? *J Urol.* Dec 2012;188(6):2139-2144.
10. Zaid HB, Kaffenberger SD, Chang SS. Improvements in safety and recovery following cystectomy: reassessing the role of pre-operative bowel preparation and interventions to speed return of post-operative bowel function. *Curr Urol Rep.* Feb 10 2013.
11. Nelson RL, Glenny AM, Song F. Antimicrobial prophylaxis for colorectal surgery. *Cochrane Database of Systematic Reviews (Online).* 2009(1): CD001181.
12. Porpiglia F, Renard J, Billia M, et al. Open versus laparoscopy-assisted radical cystectomy: results of a prospective study. *J Endourol.* Mar 2007;21(3):325-329.
13. Basillote JB, Abdelshehid C, Ahlering TE, Shanberg AM. Laparoscopic assisted radical cystectomy with ileal neobladder: a comparison with the open approach. *J Urol.* Aug 2004;172(2):489-493.
14. Bergqvist D, Agnelli G, Cohen AT, et al. Duration of prophylaxis against venous thromboembolism with enoxaparin after surgery for cancer. *N Engl J Med.* Mar 28 2002;346(13):975-980.
15. Guyatt GH, Eikelboom JW, Gould MK, et al. Approach to outcome measurement in the prevention of thrombosis in surgical and medical patients: Antithrombotic Therapy and Prevention of Thrombosis, 9th ed: American College of Chest Physicians Evidence-Based Clinical Practice Guidelines. *Chest.* Feb 2012;141(2 Suppl):e185S-e194S.
16. Stimson CJ, Chang SS, Barocas DA, et al. Early and late perioperative outcomes following radical cystectomy: 90-day readmissions, morbidity and mortality in a contemporary series. *J Urol.* Oct 2010;184(4):1296-1300.
17. Shabsigh A, Korets R, Vora KC, et al. Defining early morbidity of radical cystectomy for patients with bladder cancer using a standardized reporting methodology. *Eur Urol.* Jan 2009;55(1):164-174.
18. Quek ML, Stein JP, Daneshmand S, et al. A critical analysis of perioperative mortality from radical cystectomy. *J Urol.* Mar 2006;175(3 Pt 1):886-889; discussion 889-890.
19. Svatek RS, Fisher MB, Matin SF, et al. Risk factor analysis in a contemporary cystectomy cohort using standardized reporting methodology and adverse event criteria. *J Urol.* Mar 2010;183(3):929-934.
20. Horovitz D, Turker P, Bostrom PJ, et al. Does patient age affect survival after radical cystectomy? *BJU Int.* May 2 2012.
21. Morgan TM, Keegan KA, Barocas DA, et al. Predicting the probability of 90-day survival of elderly patients with bladder cancer treated with radical cystectomy. *J Urol.* Sep 2011;186(3):829-834.
22. Stein JP, Lieskovsky G, Cote R, et al. Radical cystectomy in the treatment of invasive bladder cancer: long-term results in 1,054 patients. *J Clin Oncol: official journal of the Am Soc Clin Oncol.* Feb 1 2001;19(3):666-675.
23. Spahn M, Weiss C, Bader P, Frohneberg D, Studer UE, Burkhard FC. The role of exenterative surgery and urinary diversion in persistent or locally recurrent gynecological malignancy: complications and survival. *Urol Int.* 2010;85(1):16-22.
24. Andikyan V, Khoury-Collado F, Sonoda Y, et al. Extended pelvic resections for recurrent or persistent uterine and cervical malignancies: an update on out of the box surgery. *Gynecol Oncol.* May 2012;125(2):404-408.
25. Benn T, Brooks RA, Zhang Q, et al. Pelvic exenteration in gynecologic oncology: a single institution study over 20 years. *Gynecol Oncol.* Jul 2011;122(1):14-18.
26. Baiocchi G, Guimaraes GC, Rosa Oliveira RA, et al. Prognostic factors in pelvic exenteration for gynecological malignancies. *Eur J Surg Oncol: the journal of the Eur Soc Surg Oncol and the British Association of Surgical Oncology.* Oct 2012;38(10):948-954.
27. Baiocchi G, Guimaraes GC, Faloppa CC, et al. Does histologic type correlate to outcome after pelvic exenteration for cervical and vaginal cancer? *Ann Surg Oncol.* Dec 5 2012.
28. Gerharz EW, Mansson A, Hunt S, Skinner EC, Mansson W. Quality of life after cystectomy and urinary diversion: an evidence based analysis. *J Urol.* Nov 2005;174(5):1729-1736.
29. Rezk YA, Hurley KE, Carter J, et al. A prospective study of quality of life in patients undergoing pelvic exenteration: Interim results. *Gynecol Oncol.* Feb 2013;128(2):191-197.
30. Parra Ro AC, Jones JP. Laparoscopic cystectomy: initial report on a new treatment for the retained bladder. *J Urol.* 1992;148:1140-1144.
31. Huang J, Lin T, Liu H, et al. Laparoscopic radical cystectomy with orthotopic ileal neobladder for bladder cancer: oncologic results of 171 cases with a median 3-year follow-up. *Eur Urol.* Sep 2010;58(3):442-449.

32. Stein JP LG, Cote R. Radical cystectomy in the treatment of invasive bladder cancer: long-term results in 1,054 patients. *J Clin Oncol.* 2001;19:666-675.
33. Aboumarzouk OM, Drewa T, Olejniczak P, Chlosta PL. Laparoscopic radical cystectomy: a 5-year review of a single institute's operative data and complications and a systematic review of the literature. *Int Braz j Urol : official journal of the Brazilian Society of Urology*. May-Jun 2012;38(3):330-340.
34. Menon M, Hermal AK, Tewari A, et al. Nerve-sparing robot-assisted radical cytoprostatectomy and urinary diversion. *BJU Int*. 2003;92:232-236.

Chapter 7. Abdominoperineal Excision of the Rectum

Julio Garcia-Aguilar, MD, PhD

INTRODUCTION

The oncologic removal of the rectum often requires both an abdominal and a perineal approach. During the abdominal portion of the procedure, the superior rectal vessels are controlled, the rectum and mesorectum dissected, and colostomy created. During the perineal portion, the rectum and anus are detached from the ischiorectal fat, the levator muscles, and whatever portion (if any) of the distal portion of the genitourinary organs not planned for removal. The boundary between the abdominal and perineal parts of the procedure is delineated by the levator muscles. The abdominoperineal excision (APE) of the rectum is now much safer than when it was first introduced more than a century ago. However, despite the advances in surgical technique and perioperative care, it remains a surgical challenge due to the complex anatomy of the pelvis.

For many years after its original description, the APE was the only surgical option for patients with rectal cancer. As a result of advances in the understanding of the dissemination of rectal cancer, along with improvements in surgical technique and instrumentation, and the use of neoadjuvant therapy, most rectal cancers are now treated with sphincter-saving procedures (SSPs). APE has been relegated to the treatment of very distal rectal cancers involving the sphincter complex or the levator muscles. Therefore, the division of the levators muscles is a critical step of the operation that determines the oncologic outcomes.

Almost immediately following the initial description of APE, surgeons began introducing minor modifications to the procedure. The number of options has recently expanded with the introduction of minimally invasive techniques. The abdominal part of the operation can be performed as an open, laparoscopic, or robotic procedure; the perineal part can be performed with the patient in lithotomy or in the prone position. In any case, successful APE requires perfect knowledge of the anatomy of the abdomen, pelvis, and ischiorectal fossa, as well as adherence to a few sound surgical principles. The APE operation is very similar to the pelvic exenteration with perineal phase, which is described in Chapter 8. The current chapter will specifically focus on the APE for distal rectal cancers.

BACKGROUND AND HISTORICAL PERSPECTIVE

Surgical treatment of rectal tumors did not become feasible until the introduction of the colostomy by the French surgeon, Jean Amussat, during the Napoleonic wars. Distal proctectomy through the perineum, which reaches within a few centimeters of the promontory, was already being performed by Lisfranc and others in the 1830s. However, it was not until the late nineteenth century that surgeons really began to regularly perform this operation.[1]

The perineal excision of the rectum was performed in 2 stages. The first stage consisted of a minilaparotomy to inspect the peritoneal cavity for signs of tumor dissemination, and to create a loop or double-barrel colostomy. In the second stage, performed several days later, the surgeon removed the anus, the ischiorectal fat, the levators, the rectum, and at least a portion of the mesorectum up to the level of the promontory.[2] This operation had 2 flaws: (1) it did not remove the lymph nodes located along the superior rectal vessels, and (2) it left a portion of colon and mesocolon attached to the distal limb of the stoma, which often resulted in a chronic perineal sinus. Earnest Miles is credited with introducing the modern APE in his seminal article published in 1908.[3] In the years prior to this seminal publication, Miles, like most of his contemporaries, had treated rectal cancer with conventional perineal proctectomy. Of the 57 patients with rectal cancer whom he treated, 54 developed recurrent tumor within 3 years following surgery. Detailed autopsy studies on these patients revealed that most of the recurrences were located in the portion of mesorectum that had been left in place during surgery and along the superior rectal vessels, arising at the pelvic peritoneum, the pelvic mesocolon, or the lymph nodes located at the bifurcation of the left common iliac artery. Miles called these areas "the zone of upward spread." The perineal proctectomy addressed the lateral and distal tumor spread, but not the "upward spread." The operation he devised to address this was performed in one stage, and included the creation of an abdominal colostomy, removal of the entire "pelvic colon because its blood supply was contained in the zone of upward spread," the "whole of the pelvic mesocolon below the point where it crosses the common iliac artery," the "group of lymph nodes situated over the bifurcation of the common iliac artery," and the anus, ischiorectal fat, and levator muscles "as far outward as their origin from the white line as to include the lateral zone of spread." Although this operation was initially associated with a rate of perioperative mortality higher than 40%, it soon became the standard treatment of rectal cancer. Attempts to broaden the scope of the operation by removing the lymph nodes along the internal iliac vessels failed to provide a survival advantage, and increased the risk of perioperative complications and long-term bladder dysfunction.

Miles started the abdominal part of the operation with the patient supine in the Trendelenburg position. He then turned the patient to the right lateral and semiprone position to complete the perineal part. In later years, other surgeons introduced modifications to make it simpler and safer. The synchronous combined abdominal and perineal excision, performed simultaneously by two different teams, was first performed by Kirschner and popularized by Lloyd–Davis, who introduced the leg rests that allowed the patient to be placed in the lithotomy position. The Lloyd–Davis modification has been preferred for more than 100 years.[4]

Recent advances in understanding the mechanisms of recurrence after rectal cancer surgery have re-emphasized 2 aspects of Miles' operation probably ignored by many surgeons for decades: the need to remove the entire mesorectum, and the lateral division of the levator muscle. Although some surgeons had always performed the dissection of the "pelvic mesocolon" (now called mesorectum) in the bloodless areolar space "anterior to the sacral ligaments," as proposed by Miles, many were performing the dissection inside of the mesorectum to avoid the vascular and neural pelvic structures. Incomplete excisions of the mesorectum can leave behind portions of the lymph node–bearing fat surrounding the rectum, and even expose the tumor itself. The need to remove the entire mesorectum in every rectal cancer patient using sharp dissection following the areolar plane outside the fascia propria of the rectum was reintroduced by Heald in 1982.[5] The importance of the presence of tumor at the circumferential resection margin was reported in 1985 by Quirke,[6] who demonstrated a much higher rate of recurrence when tumor reached the circumferential resection margin than when the margin was free of tumor.

The second important development is the renewed emphasis on dividing the levators "as far outwards as their origin from the white line, so as to include the lateral zone of spread." Although in his original description Miles emphasized the importance of dividing the levators laterally,[3] close to their insertion in the pelvic sidewall, many surgeons divide the levators closer to the rectal wall. These changes occurred over time as surgeons extended the abdominal dissection progressively closer to the levator muscles to perform anastomosis in patients with tumors amenable to a sphincter-saving procedure. However, extending the abdominal dissection to the pelvic floor, in a patient with distal rectal cancer that infiltrates the levator or the anal sphincter, leads to the division of the levators close to the rectal wall, increasing the risk of positive circumferential resection margin and local recurrence.[7]

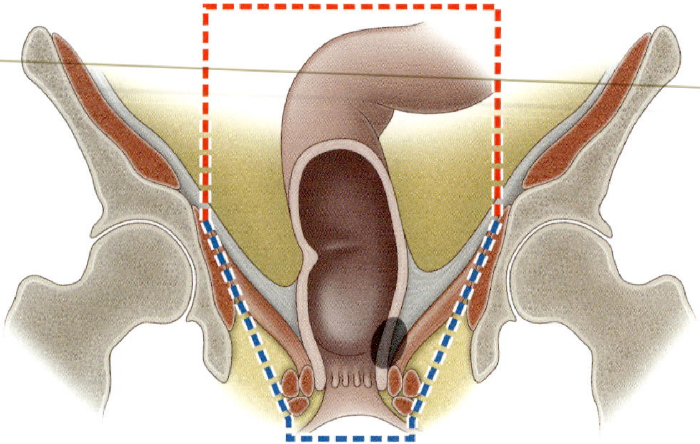

Fig. 7-1. Overview of cylindrical abdominal perineal resection.

These deviations in surgical technique from the original procedure described by Miles are considered, by some, to be the main reason why APE for low rectal cancer is associated with a greater risk of recurrence compared to low anterior resection (LAR) for higher tumors. The newly named "cylindrical," or "extralevator" APE, is an attempt to avoid these shortcomings by emphasizing complete excision of the mesorectum and lateral section of the levator muscles (Figure 7-1).

INDICATIONS AND CLINICAL APPLICATIONS

Adenocarcinoma located in the distal rectum is the most common indication for an APE. Most patients with tumors penetrating the muscularis propria or metastasized to the mesorectal lymph nodes require removal of the rectum and the mesorectal envelope. For most patients with midrectal tumors, the rectum is transected below the end of the mesorectum and intestinal continuity is re-established by double-stapling colorectal anastomosis. For patients with distal rectal tumors, the surgeon must decide whether removal of the tumor with a negative margin is compatible with sphincter preservation, or whether it requires APE. The need to achieve a safe margin of normal rectal wall distal to the tumor, in order to avoid local recurrence, must be balanced against the ability to retain enough rectum attached to the anus so that safe colorectal or coloanal anastomosis (CAA) can be achieved. For decades, 5 cm was the minimum length of normal rectal wall distal to the tumor that was considered oncologically safe. Later studies have shown that cancer cells rarely spread distally along the bowel wall farther than 1 cm from the macroscopic distal end of the tumor. Consequently, the required margin of normal bowel distal to the tumor was reduced to 2 cm.[8] Recent evidence suggests that margins as short as 1 cm do not increase the risk of recurrence, particularly in patients treated with neoadjuvant chemoradiation therapy.[9] Therefore, in most patients, the need for APE, rather than SSP, is due to the inability to obtain a negative circumferential resection margin, rather than a negative distal margin. In general, APE is indicated when distal rectal cancer penetrates beyond the muscularis propria and infiltrates the levator muscle or anal sphincter. A digital examination and an endoscopy provide valuable information about the relationship of the tumor to the anal canal. High-resolution magnetic resonance imaging (MRI) and computed tomography (CT) modalities that provide axial, sagittal, and coronal views can demonstrate the relationship of tumor to the levator muscles and the external anal sphincter with a high degree of accuracy.

In the past, before optimal imaging of the rectum was widely available, many patients with rectal cancer were brought to the operating room with the intention of determining intraoperatively whether the sphincter was salvageable by LAR or CAA, or whether APE and permanent colostomy would be required. The decision to perform an APE was made only after the rectum had been mobilized to the pelvic floor and the tumor was found to be too close to, or to infiltrate, the levator muscle or the anal sphincter. In trying to decide intraoperatively if SSP was feasible, distal dissection was often carried to the levator hiatus, where the rectal wall is not covered by mesorectum and is in direct contact with the levator muscles. If the surgeon found that SSP was not feasible, then the levators were usually divided at the point of their dissection from the pelvis, very close to the rectal wall in the specific area where the tumor was usually located. These "waisted" APE specimens often resulted in exposure of the tumor at the radial resection margin.[10] However, the new high-resolution imaging modalities help surgeons decide preoperatively whether a patient is a candidate for SSP or will require APE.[11] Knowing in advance what procedure is to be performed reduces uncertainty for the patient and improves operative planning and execution.

Abdominoperineal excision of the rectum is also the operation of choice for patients with anal squamous cell carcinoma that persists or recurs after chemotherapy and radiation, because these tumors usually involve the anal canal and levator muscle. Occasionally, APE is required for less common tumors of the anorectal region such as anal melanoma, sarcoma, or gastrointestinal stromal tumors. Extended APE is sometimes required for vulvar, vaginal, or prostate cancers involving the distal rectum or anal sphincter. In addition, APE of the rectum is part of the total proctocolectomy performed for patients with familial adenomatous polyposis or other hereditary polyposis syndromes. Finally, APE is commonly performed in patients with inflammatory bowel disease, either as part of a proctocolectomy for ulcerative or granulomatous colitis, or as a separate procedure in the setting of isolated anorectal Crohn disease.

ANATOMIC CONSIDERATIONS

The key to successful APE is a perfect understanding of the anatomy of the rectum and anus, the vessels and nerves of the pelvis, the pelvic floor musculature, and the ischiorectal fossa. The key structures described in this section are depicted in Chapter 2.

The pelvic floor, also known as the pelvic diaphragm, comprises the levator ani and coccygeus muscles. The levator muscle is a thin, broad layer of muscle that inserts in the inner wall of the pelvis and unites with the muscle of the opposite side to form the greater part of the pelvic diaphragm. The anterior portion inserts in the posterior aspect of the pubic bones lateral to the symphysis and runs posteriorly and obliquely to join the perineal body. These are known as the levator prostate or pubovaginalis. The next muscular fascicle, known as the puborectalis, extends from the posterior aspect of the pubic bone and loops around the back of the rectum, becoming continuous with the muscle of the opposite side. The lower fibers of the puborectalis intermingle with the fibers of the upper portion of the external sphincter. The ileococcygeus and pubococcygeus insert in the pubis and in the tendinous arch of the obturator fascia, extending obliquely downward and backward from/toward the perineal body, the anal sphincter, the anococcygeal ligament, and the coccyx. The levator muscles create a funnel-shaped diaphragm with a central opening delineated by the puborectalis sling and the symphysis of the pubis, which allows passage of the urethra and the rectum in both males and females, and the vagina in females. The puborectalis, pubococcygeus, and ileococcygeus are divided during APE. The coccygeus muscle extends from the spine of the ischium and the sacrospinous ligament and inserts in the coccyx. The coccygeus muscle is in the same plane as the levators but is more posterior, and it is usually not divided during APE.

The rectum corresponds to the distal 15 cm of the large bowel, but neither its beginning nor end is sharply defined by specific anatomical landmarks. Proximally, the sigmoid colon transitions into the rectum at the rectosigmoid junction. This is a poorly defined region where the relatively narrow lumen of the sigmoid colon widens to become the rectum. From the outside, the outer longitudinal muscles forming the taenia coli (characteristic of the sigmoid colon) spread diffusely, becoming the uniform longitudinal muscular layer of the rectum. This occurs approximately at the level of the promontory, but the relationship of the rectosigmoid junction to the promontory depends on the laxity of the mesorectum. Distally, the rectum transitions into the anal canal at the level of the anorectal ring, a palpable anatomical landmark that corresponds to the impromptu of puborectalis on the bowel wall. The anal canal extends from the anorectal ring to the anal verge, the palpable groove between the distal edge of the internal sphincter and the subcutaneous portion of the external sphincter. The rectum contains the 3 valves of Houston, which are occasionally used as reference to locate rectal lesions. However, it is more practical to describe the location of a rectal tumor by measuring the distance of the lesion from the anal verge. This is best accomplished with a rigid proctoscope that permits simultaneous viewing of the tumor, the anal verge, and the measuring marks on the instrument.

The mesorectum is the visceral mesentery of the rectum derived from the dorsal mesentery of the hindgut. It contains the terminal branches of the superior rectal vessels and the lymphatic drainage of the rectum. The upper portion of the rectum is located above the anterior peritoneal reflection; it is covered with peritoneum in the front and on both sides, and has a posterior mesorectum attached to the concavity of the sacrum, which is a continuation of the mesentery of the sigmoid colon. Below the peritoneal reflection, the rectum is completely extraperitoneal and fully surrounded by mesorectum. At that level, the mesorectum is a cushion of loose connective tissue posterolaterally surrounding the rectum, covered by a thin, glistening membrane called the fascia propria of the rectum. It posteriorly extends from the promontory to Waldeyer fascia, a condensation of connective tissue spanning the area from the fourth sacral vertebra to the anorectal ring. Posteriorly, the mesorectum is separated from the presacral fascia by an avascular plane of loose areolar tissue. The plane between the fascia propria of the rectum and the presacral fascia is the natural plane of dissection during radical proctectomy.

The mesorectum is thick posteriorly, where it has a characteristic bilobular appearance. Anteriorly, however, it is either absent (in the upper intraperitoneal portion of the rectum) or reduced to a thin layer of areolar tissue (in the mid and distal rectum). The fascia propria of the rectum is also thinner anteriorly than posteriorly. In the front, the thin mesorectum is separated from the urogenital organs by a remnant of the fusion of two layers of the embryological peritoneal cul-de-sac known as Denonvilliers fascia. The anatomic appearance of Denonvilliers fascia varies, from a barely visible translucent membrane to a distinct, tough, leathery layer of connective tissue separating the seminal vesicles or vagina from the rectal wall. The fascia propria of the rectum and Denonvilliers fascia are important anatomic landmarks in rectal cancer surgery.

The mesorectum distally tapers off as the rectum funnels down toward the anorectal ring, where the longitudinal layer of the muscularis propria of the rectum is in direct contact with the levator muscle. The proximity of the rectal wall to the levator muscle should be taken into consideration when deciding between APE or SSP in the setting of transmural rectal cancers located at or below the level of the anorectal ring.

Below the peritoneal reflection, the mesorectum intermingles on both sides of the pelvis with a condensation of connective tissue surrounding the autonomic nerves that pass from the pelvic plexus to the rectum. These bilateral condensations of the endopelvic fascia are known as lateral ligaments and connect the pelvic sidewall with the mesorectum. In some individuals, the lateral ligaments contain accessory middle rectal vessels; the middle rectal artery usually immediately runs above the levator muscles.

The blood supply of the rectum primarily comes from the superior rectal artery, which is the continuation of the inferior mesenteric artery after it gives off the left colic artery. The superior rectal artery gives several sigmoidal branches before diving into the mesorectum, where it gives multiple branches to the rectum. The superior rectal vein has a parallel course to its homonymous artery, on its way to join the left colic vein to form the inferior mesenteric vein draining into the splenic vein. The lower portion of the rectum also gets blood supply from the internal iliac vessels. The middle rectal artery, an inconsistent branch of the inferior vesical artery, is usually located deep in the pelvis, running over the levator muscle toward the distal wall of the rectum. The inferior rectal artery is a branch of the pudendal artery and provides blood supply to the anal canal and anal sphincter. The middle and inferior rectal vessels anastomose with the upper rectal vessels to supply enough blood to the entire rectum. As in other locations, the middle and inferior rectal veins follow the course of the homonymous arteries and drain into systemic circulation through the internal iliac veins. Anastomosis between the superior and middle rectal vessels represents the potential portosystemic communication that becomes relevant in patients with portal hypertension.

The anatomy of the autonomic pelvic nerve system is particularly relevant when performing APE, because it is close to the plane of dissection during different parts of the operation. Damage to these nerves can result in urinary dysfunction, sexual dysfunction, or both. The hypogastric plexus, located in front of the aorta, contains predominantly preganglionic sympathetic fibers originating from the lumbar sympathetic trunk. The fibers of the hypogastric plexus converge at the level of the aortic bifurcation into well-defined hypogastric nerves, which laterally course across the internal ileal vessels toward the lateral pelvic sidewall. There they join the splanchnic pelvic nerves, containing primarily postganglionic parasympathetic fibers from S3 to S4, to form the pelvic plexus. Branches of the pelvic plexus provide innervation to the distal ureter, the vas deferens, the seminal vesicles, urinary bladder, and prostate. Some branches of the pelvic plexus also provide innervation to the distal rectum, passing though the lateral rectal ligaments, or lateral stalks. Finally, distal to the lateral rectal ligaments, the distal pelvic plexus forms the urogenital neurovascular bundles that pass close to the posterolateral aspect of the seminal vesicles or the vagina, extending toward the apex of the prostate and the neck of the bladder.

The pudendal nerve provides most of the innervation of the perineal region, and must be preserved during the perineal portion of APE. It originates from the inferior aspect of the sacral plexus and contains sensitive, motor, and parasympathetic postganglionic fibers. Passing behind the sciatic spine it enters Alcock canal in the lateral wall of the ischiorectal fossa, and branches into the inferior hemorrhoidal nerve, the perineal nerve, and the dorsal clitoral nerve. Some of these branches are divided during perineal dissection.

PREOPERATIVE PREPARATION

Box 7-1 KEY SURGICAL INSTRUMENTATION

- Long-bladed retractors (Saint Mark or Wylie) for abdominal approach
- Lone Star, Beckman-Adson, Deaver, and Gelpi retractors for perineal approach
- Gastrointestinal anastomosis (GIA) stapling device
- Electrocautery
- 30-degree or flexible-tip camera, vessel-sealing device, and endoscopic staplers (for laparoscopic approach)

Although mortality has dramatically decreased in the last century, APE is still a formidable operation associated with significant morbidity. Patients should undergo cardiac and pulmonary evaluation prior to surgery. Patients should also be marked and counseled for a colostomy. The necessity of full mechanical bowel cleansing is controversial, but, at the very least, patients should receive an enema to cleanse the rectum of fecal matter. In addition, they should receive perioperative antibiotics and deep venous thrombosis prophylaxis. Patients must be informed about the potential risks and complications of the procedure. They should also be counseled about the possible long-term outcomes, particularly sexual and urinary dysfunction. In addition, they should be educated by a stoma therapist regarding the practicalities of living with a permanent stoma.

Although most surgeons prefer a sequential abdominal-perineal approach, a combined synchronous 2-team approach may be advantageous when speed is essential. The synchronous 2-team approach, always performed in lithotomy position, also allows the abdominal and perineal surgeons to simultaneously work in developing the appropriate planes. However, for both surgeons to work simultaneously, patient's positioning is such that neither surgeon can have as optimal visualization of the surgical field as they would working sequentially.

For the lithotomy position, the stirrups should be placed as low as possible on the rail of the operating table so that they do not interfere with the position of the surgeon or assistants during the abdominal part of the procedure. The buttocks should protrude from the end of the operating table to provide adequate access to the perineum, but the sacrum should be supported by a soft gel pad to prevent pressure sores. The hips should be minimally flexed and abducted, and the knees flexed at nearly 90 degrees. When securing the legs to the stirrups, it is essential to avoid pressure over the external fibular nerve as this can result in temporary or permanent foot drop. Appropriate fitting of the leg in the stirrup is particularly important in patients who are obese, because excessive compression can lead to compartment syndrome. The rectum should be irrigated and the anus closed with a double purse-string suture before beginning. When the abdominal part is performed through a laparotomy, self-retaining retractors such as Balfour or Bookwalter, are required. However, a disposable large Alexis retractor also provides adequate exposure while protecting the wound. Long-bladed retractors such as the Saint Mark retractor or a pair of Wylie renal vein retractors are necessary to expose the depths of the pelvis. A long Cooley suction tube is useful not only as a suction device, but also works as a retractor in the depths of the pelvis. A Lone Star retractor is useful during the initial phases of the perineal part, but a deeper self-retained retractor such as a Beckman-Adson, and handheld Deaver retractor or short Wylie, are usually needed to expose the levator muscles. A pair of Gelpi retractors can also be utilized during the perineal dissection, in particular when it is performed in lithotomy. The use of a headlight is strongly recommended to afford sufficient illumination during both parts of the procedure. If the operation is laparoscopically performed, then a 30-degree camera or camera with a flexible tip and high resolution is required, as well as adequate graspers, an energy device to seal the vessels, and endoscopic staplers. If the operation is robotically performed, then we recommend using monopolar scissors, bipolar graspers, a vessel sealer, and an EndoWrist stapler.

SURGICAL TECHNIQUE

Box 7-2 MASTER SURGEON'S PRINCIPLES

- Care should be taken to avoid injuring the superior hypogastric plexus during abdominal approach
- Dissection should be carried in front of Denonvilliers fascia for anterior tumors
- Dissection can be safely performed behind Denonvilliers fascia in the setting of other tumors
- Pudendal nerve must be preserved during perineal approach
- In patients treated with neoadjuvant radiation, and for those who are smokers, obese, and have diabetes, flap reconstruction of the perineum should be considered prior to closure

Abdominal Part: Open Approach

The abdominal part can be performed though a lower midline or low transverse laparotomy. Both incisions provide sufficient exposure to the superior rectal vessels, the sigmoid colon, and the pelvic structures. The transverse incision causes less pain and is cosmetically more appealing. When a rectus muscle flap is required to close the perineal wound, a midline incision is preferable.

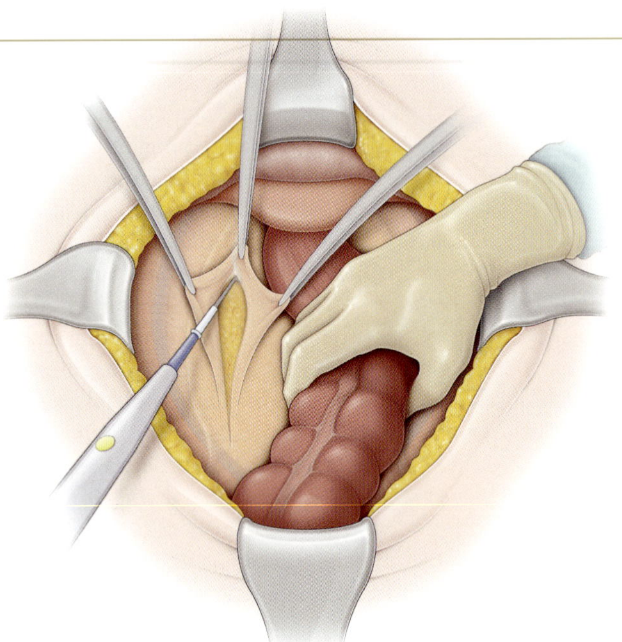

Fig. 7-2. Mobilization of sigmoid colon (left side).

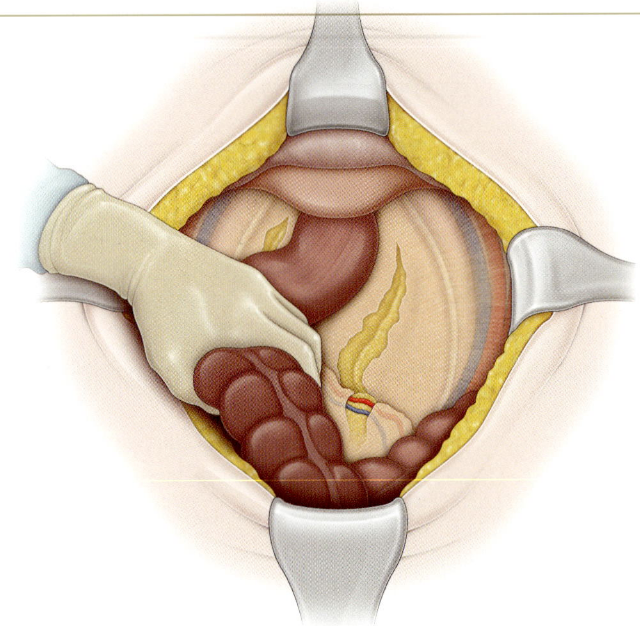

Fig. 7-3. Mobilization of sigmoid colon (right side).

As in any other colorectal cancer procedure, the operation begins with a thorough examination of the abdomen and pelvis. The sigmoid colon is mobilized by dividing the attachments and adhesions to the lateral abdominal and pelvic sidewall. The incision is carried cephalad toward the splenic flexure and distally toward the pelvis (Figure 7-2). The mesentery of the sigmoid and descending colon is lifted from the retroperitoneal attachments, exposing the left gonadal vessels and the left ureter. The sigmoid colon is retracted anteriorly and laterally to expose the root of the sigmoid mesentery. Next, an incision is made in the peritoneum, in the right side of the base of the sigmoid mesocolon, proximal to the promontory (Figure 7-3). A plane is developed underneath the superior rectal vessels, between the origin of the inferior mesenteric artery and the promontory. Care should be taken to avoid injuring the superior hypogastric plexus, situated between the superior rectal vessels and the bifurcation of the aorta.

The superior rectal vessels are isolated between the origin of the left colic vessels and the first sigmoidal vessels, divided between clamps, and ligated. The mesentery of the sigmoid colon is divided toward that point of the sigmoid colon chosen to create the end sigmoid colostomy. The sigmoid colon is finally divided by firing of a linear staple. The proximal end of the divided sigmoid colon and the descending colon should be sufficiently mobilized to ensure a tension-free, well-vascularized colostomy.

The areolar space behind the fascia propria of the rectum is opened by pulling the stump of the superior rectal vessels away from the promontory. The areolar tissue separating the mesorectal fascia from the parietal pelvic fascia is then dissected along the concavity of the sacrum using electrocautery unit (Figure 7-4). The dissection is carried posteriorly as far as the sacrococcygeal junction, and from the midline to the sides. Care should be taken to preserve the hypogastric nerves, which are laterally brushed as they course along the pelvic

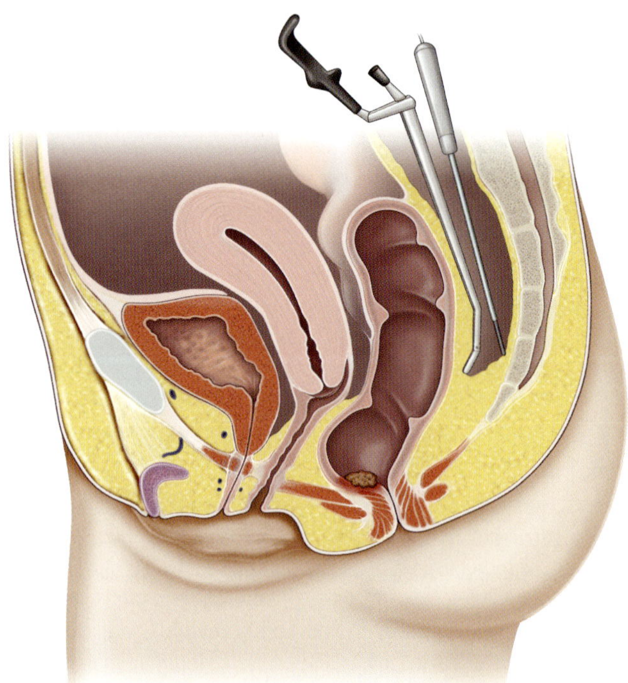

Fig. 7-4. Posterior dissection (sagittal view).

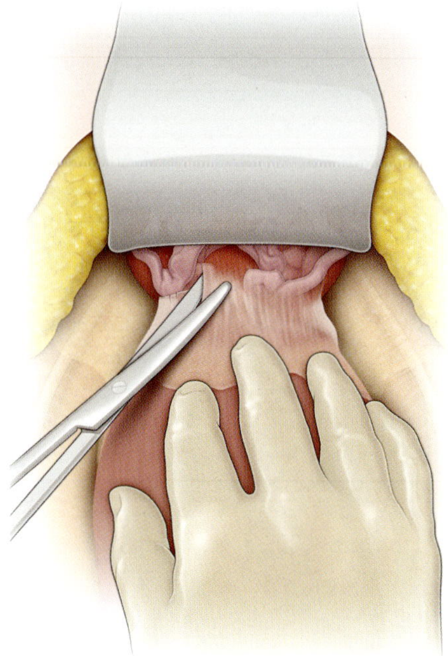

Fig. 7-5. Anterior dissection (sagittal view).

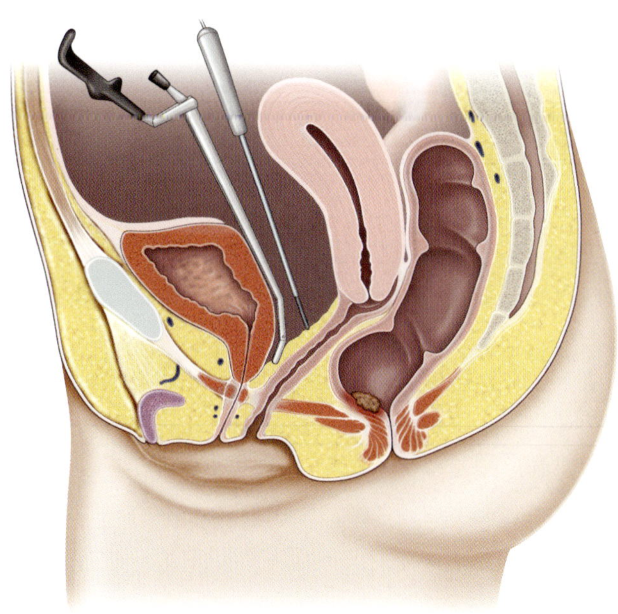

Fig. 7-6. Anterior dissection (surgeon's view).

wall. Distally, the pelvic splanchnic nerves should be preserved as they course from the anterior sacral foramina to join the pelvic plexus. The lateral stalks are then exposed by providing traction of the rectum to the contralateral side of the pelvis, and are divided using electrocautery. A forceful retraction can bring the parietal pelvic fascia and the pelvic plexus within reach of the electrocautery, resulting in inadvertent injury. The dissection is continued until the origin of the levator muscle is reached. Finally, the peritoneum is opened in the cul-de-sac, and dissection carried halfway down the vagina (Figures 7-5 and 7-6). The anterior dissection can be performed in different planes, depending on the location of the tumor in the circumference of the rectum. In the setting of anterior tumors, dissection should be carried in front of Denonvilliers' fascia to avoid dissecting into the tumor. In the setting of other tumors, dissection can be safely performed behind Denonvilliers fascia.

The line formed by the sacrococcygeal junction, the upper portion of the levators, and the upper prostate/mid-vagina, represents the landmark where the perineal dissection will meet the plane dissected from the abdomen.

Perineal Part: Lithotomy Position

A tray with a separate set of instruments is prepared. The rectum is irrigated and aspirated, and the anal orifice closed with a double purse-string suture. A Lone Star retractor is used to expose the perianal area. An elliptical incision is made around the anus (Figure 7-7). The incision is carried through the ischiorectal fossa until the anococcygeal ligaments and levator muscles are exposed (Figure 7-8). The pelvis is entered by dividing the anococcygeal ligament close to the tip of the coccyx. The levator muscles in each side are then hooked with the index finger, the tissue spread apart with the thumb and second finger and divided with electrocautery. The pudendal nerve is protected in Alcock canal in the lateral wall of the ischiorectal fossa, but the branches to the anal sphincter and the levator muscles—the inferior hemorrhoidal nerve and the perineal nerves—must be transected.

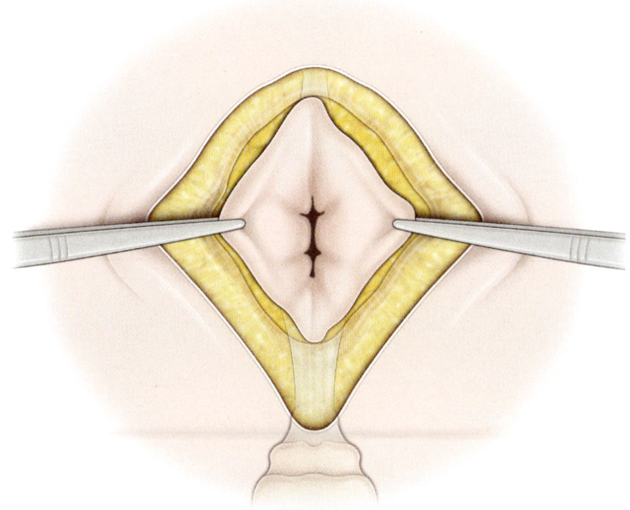

Fig. 7-7. Incision of perineum (prone, with elliptical perineal excision).

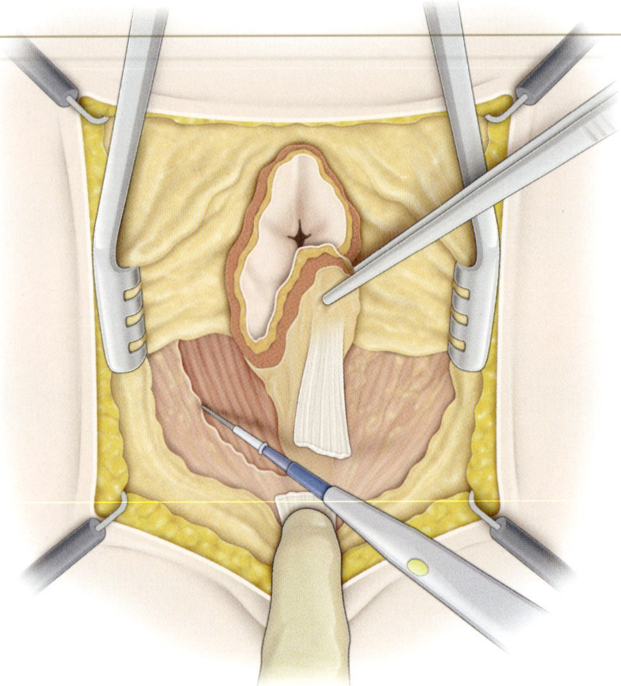

Fig. 7-8. Perineal dissection, taking down levator muscles.

The plane between the anterior aspect of the anal sphincter and the transverse perineal muscle is carefully developed by incising the perineal body. The anterior aspects of both arms of the puborectalis muscles are divided next (Figure 7-9). The anterior-most branches of the pudendal nerve, the dorsal clitoral nerve, run close to the point of transection of the puborectalis muscle. The nerves should be identified and preserved. The central portion of the anterior dissection, between the puborectalis muscles, is the most difficult part of the perineal dissection because there is no clear tissue plane. The perineal body connects the upper portion of the anal sphincter with the transverse perineal muscle, the bulbospongiosus muscle and the distal portion of the membranous urethra. This tissue must be sharply divided with electrocautery. Passing the index finger into the pelvis, between the vagina and the anterior wall of the rectum, helps guide the distal portion of the anterior dissection. Delivering the specimen through the open portion of the wound also helps identify the anterior plane of dissection.

Once the specimen has been removed the field must be extensively irrigated from the pelvis. The perineal defect is closed by approximating the fat of the ischiorectal fossa with interrupted, absolvable stitches. The skin is approximated with interrupted vertical mattress sutures.

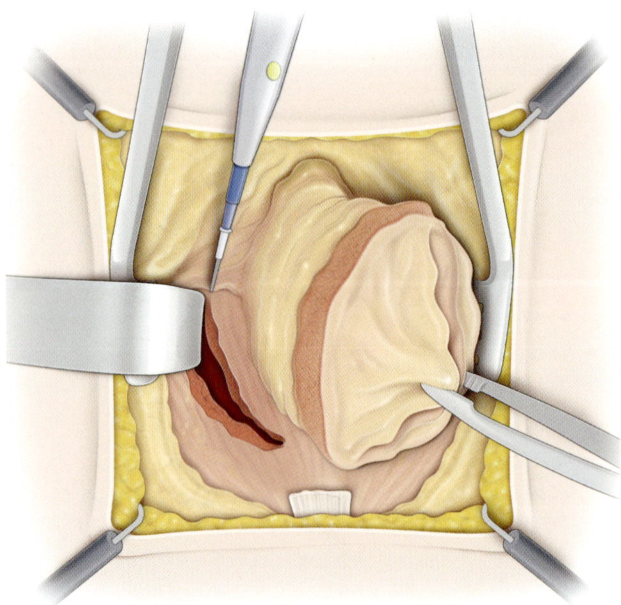

Fig. 7-9. Perineal dissection, mobilizing anus.

COLOSTOMY

A circular incision large enough to accommodate the colon is then made at the marked colostomy site. The incision is carried through the subcutaneous tissue until the anterior sheath of the rectus muscle is reached. The sheath is longitudinally opened, and the fibers of the rectus muscle are longitudinally split. The posterior rectal sheath is also longitudinally opened. In terms of size, the defect should fit 2 fingers. The divided end of the sigmoid colon is exteriorized through the stoma, avoiding any twisting of the colon. When the procedure is performed laparoscopically, the orientation of the mesentery should be inspected after the end of the colon has been brought to the outside, to avoid twisting the stoma. The stoma is not mature until the laparotomy or trocar wounds have been closed. Then the staple line is trimmed, and the stoma is matured with interrupted absorbable sutures.

CLOSURE OF THE PERINEAL WOUND

In most patients undergoing APE, the perineal wound can be primarily closed. If the levators have been divided at or close to their insertion, then the only layers that can be approximated in the midline are the fat of the ischiorectal fossa, the subcutaneous fat, and the skin. However, many perineal wounds that have been closed primarily become infected, dehiscent, or both. The risk is especially high in patients who are obese and have diabetes, those who smoke, and in patients treated with neoadjuvant radiation. A number of flap procedures may be used in these patients to fill the space left after removal of the rectum with well-vascularized tissue, reducing the risk of perineal wound complications. Pelvic floor reconstruction is addressed in Chapters 16 to 18.

POSTOPERATIVE CARE

Box 7-3 PERIOPERATIVE MORBIDITY

- Ureteral or urethral injury
- Perineal wound infection/dehiscence
- Parastomal ischemia or bleeding

Although APE is an extensive surgical procedure, most patients are not postoperatively admitted to the intensive care unit but are instead transferred to a regular surgical floor after recovering in the postanesthesia care unit. The physiologic postoperative ileus tends to be short after APE compared with SSP, and most surgeons do not use postoperative nasogastric suction. A liquid diet is initiated the day following surgery, and it is advanced as tolerated. The Foley catheter is removed once the patient is able to ambulate; however, it may be maintained longer in patients with urinary retention or incontinence, particularly women, to avoid contamination of the perineal wound.

Patients are encouraged to get out of bed the day after surgery but are advised to avoid sitting for several days, particularly if they have undergone a flap reconstruction of the perineum. In these patients, a pneumatic bed may be helpful. If pelvic suction drains have been placed, they are maintained until output is minimal. Thromboembolic prophylaxis is continued until the patient is ambulating. The perineal wound is frequently inspected for signs of infection, as this is the most common postoperative complication. A consultation with a stoma therapist is important so that the patient can become comfortable with stoma care while still in the hospital.

Patients are seen in clinic 2 to 3 weeks after surgery for assessment of the surgical incisions, evaluation of urinary function, and monitoring of the stoma. The nonreabsorbable perineal stitches are usually removed at this time. A new visit with the stoma therapist is necessary in order to reassess the size and type of appliance, once postoperative edema has subsided.

Despite recent advances in surgical technique and perioperative care, APE remains a formidable operation associated with some mortality, significant morbidity, and long-lasting sequelae that permanently impair function and quality of life.[12] The reported perioperative mortality ranges from 0.5% to 3%, and more than 30% of patients develop perioperative complications such as perineal wound infection and dehiscence, abdominal wound infection, pelvic abscess, urinary retention, urinary tract infection, ileus, bowel obstruction, and deep venous thrombosis.[13,14] Intraoperative complications such as pelvic bleeding, ureteral injury, and urethral injury are not uncommon. Acute stoma-related complications such as ischemia, bleeding, mucocutaneous separation, skin irritation, and retraction are also common.

Perineal wound complications are particular common and present a serious clinical problem. They are a common cause of prolonged hospital stay, readmission to the hospital, and increased costs.[15-17] Rates of perineal wound complications as high as 40% have been reported in patients treated with extralevator APE.[18] The risk of perineal infection and dehiscence is higher in patients who are obese, have diabetes, are smokers, and patients treated with neoadjuvant radiation.[14,19] Perineal wound separation often requires prolonged wound care, and may cause indefinite delay in the delivery of adjuvant chemotherapy.[16]

LONG-TERM OUTCOMES

Box 7-4 DELAYED COMPLICATIONS

- Parastomal hernia, necrosis, stenosis, and leakage
- Bowel obstruction
- Perineal hernia
- Sexual and urinary dysfunction

Long-term stoma-related complications are extremely common in patients following APE. These include skin irritation, stenosis, leakage, superficial necrosis, prolapse, bleeding, retraction, odor, and parastomal hernia. Postoperative parastomal complications may not improve with time, and the rate of parastomal hernia increases over time.[20,21] Some patients require hospital readmission and additional surgery for serious complications such as bowel obstruction, incisional hernia, or perineal hernia. Some patients may have persistent perineal pain.[17]

Patients with rectal cancer who are treated with APE often experience sexual and urinary dysfunction related to injury of the autonomic nerves during surgery.[22] The risk of autonomic nerve dysfunction seems to be higher in patients treated with neoadjuvant radiation.[23,24] As a result of these complications and long-term sequela, patients with rectal cancer report severe difficulties in several quality-of-life domains, especially those relating to sexual function and body image.[25,26] However, the overall quality of life for patients after APE does not seem to be worse compared with patients with rectal cancer who have undergone SSP.[27,28]

Historically, patients with rectal cancer treated with APE had higher local recurrence rates and poorer overall survival rates compared with patients treated with SSP.[29] Even introduction of the principles of total mesorectal excision in the last three decades did not change these disparities. A review of the combined experience of 5 European randomized rectal cancer trials investigated whether these differences in outcomes are attributable to the tumor and patient characteristics that led to selection of a specific procedure, or to the procedure itself.[30] The study found that, compared with patients treated with SSP, those with rectal cancer who were treated with APE were more likely to have a positive circumferential resection margin (5% vs 10.6%) and local recurrence (11.4% vs 19.7%).

In addition, patients with APE had a decreased 5-year cancer-specific survival (65.1% vs 76.6%) and 5-year overall survival (59.5% vs 70.1%) rates compared with patients undergoing LAR.[30] A multivariate logistic regression analysis indicated that the differences in positive circumferential resection margin, local recurrence, and 5-year cancer-specific survival rates were independent from the factors typically associated with a decision to perform APE (age, sex, and tumor distance from the anal verge). These data suggest that the surgical procedure itself is partly responsible for the differences in outcomes.[30] The results of other prospective studies, such as the ACCORD trial, have also demonstrated that APE is an independent predictor of a positive circumferential resection margin.[31] However, some retrospective analyses of institutional case series in the United States contradict these results by concluding that APE is not independently associated with a higher rate of positive circumferential resection margins or worse oncologic outcomes.[13]

Numerous studies have investigated the causes of the different outcomes between APE and LAR by performing detailed pathologic examination of APE surgical specimens. A detailed, standardized pathologic examination of surgical specimens in a Dutch rectal cancer trial demonstrated that the high rate of positive circumferential resection margin, tumor perforation, and local recurrence observed in APE compared with patients undergoing SSP might be related to the plane of dissection followed during the perineal portion of the procedure.[32] In 64% of patients, the dissection was carried at the external surface of the external sphincter, while in 36% the dissection was carried within the muscle itself, or in the submucosa. Many patients in this last group had perforated surgical specimens. A more recent study correlating high resolution pretreatment MRI with detailed pathologic examination of the surgical specimen confirmed that the surgical waisting was usually located between 30 and 42 mm from the anal verge, an area corresponding to the puborectalis muscle.[10] These findings have led to a resurgence of the "extralevator" APE, in which the levators are divided "as far outward as their origin from the while line so as to include the lateral zone of spread," as originally described by Miles.[3] The extralevator APE avoids waisting in the surgical specimen, and for that reason is also known as the "cylindrical APE." Compared with conventional APE, the extralevator APE results in a greater distance between the muscularis propria or internal sphincter to the circumferential resection margin, a lower rate of positive circumferential resection margin, and a lower rate of specimen perforation.[33] However, the data comparing the long-term oncologic outcome of patients treated with conventional versus extralevator APE are limited.[18,34] Although surgical technique is a prognostic factor in patients with distal rectal cancer, some studies suggest that differences in outcomes cannot be explained by technical factors alone, and suggest that distal rectal cancers are more aggressive—of higher grade, and with a different pattern of lymphatic spread—compared with more proximal tumors.

MIS APPLICATIONS

The abdominal part of the APE can be performed with minimally invasive surgery. Both traditional laparoscopic and robotic approaches have been used. The abdominal portion of both the laparoscopic and robotic approaches are described in the following sections.

Abdominal Part: Laparoscopic Approach

A Hasson trocar is placed either above or below the umbilicus. A 12-mm trocar is placed in the right lower quadrant, and 5-mm trocars in the right upper quadrant and in the left side of the abdomen, at the stoma site. After the peritoneal cavity is inspected, the patient is placed in the Trendelenburg position with the right side down. The small bowel is moved out of the pelvis. An incision is made in the right side of the root of the mesentery of the sigmoid colon, over the right iliac artery. The areolar space behind the superior rectal vessels is entered, preserving the branches of the superior hypogastric plexus that lie anterior to the bifurcation of the aorta. The left ureter is immediately identified, running toward the left iliac artery. The mesentery of the sigmoid colon is lifted from the retroperitoneal attachments, from medial to lateral. The left gonadal vessels should be identified and should remain in the retroperitoneum. The medial-to-lateral dissection should be continued underneath the mesentery of the sigmoid colon all the way to the line of Toldt. The dissection should be extended cephalad to free the mesentery of the descending colon. The superior rectal vessels should be dissected and divided by firing of an endoscopic stapler, an energy device, or between large clips. The left colic vessels should be preserved.

The attachments of the sigmoid colon to the pelvic sidewall are taken while the colon is pulled medially, until the plane that was opened during the medial-to-lateral dissection is reached. Then the attachments of the remaining sigmoid colon and descending colon are taken down along the left gutter to provide sufficient colonic mobilization for the creation of a tension-free colostomy.

Once the descending and sigmoid colon are completely mobilized, the mesorectal dissection starts by applying traction anteriorly from the stump of the superior rectal vessels in order to open the areolar space behind the fascia propria of the rectum, at the level of the promontory. The hypogastric nerves, clearly identified at this level as they course toward the pelvic sidewalls, should be carefully separated from the fascia propria of the rectum and brushed posteriorly and laterally. The peritoneum is opened on both sides of the rectum all the way to the cul-de-sac, and the rectum is lifted from the concavity of the sacrum by sharply dividing the areolar attachments of the fascia propria of the rectum to the presacral fascia. The lateral ligaments are divided. The anterior dissection to separate the rectum from the urogenital organs is performed last, following the principles outlined in the open procedure. The perineal part is completed next, followed by creation of the end colostomy and placement of any pelvic drains.

Abdominal Part: Robotic Approach

Laparoscopic dissection of the mesorectum is a technically demanding procedure due to 2-dimensional visualization, the use of long and nonarticulating instruments, difficulty handling the rectum and providing traction and countertraction during dissection, and the unnatural position required of the surgeon. The robotic da Vinci platform (Intuitive Surgical, Sunnyvale, California) eliminates some of these difficulties by providing tridimensional visualization, articulating instruments that resemble the human wrist, scale of motion, enhanced surgeon control of camera and instruments, and improved ergonomics. The downside of the robotic approach is that, once the platform is docked, the patient's position cannot be changed to take full advantage of gravity for exposure.

The position of the trocar is similar to the laparoscopic approach, with the camera located around the umbilicus, a 12-mm trocar in the right lower quadrant, a 5-mm trocar in the right upper quadrant, and two 8-mm trocars in the left side. The cart is docked over the left hip at 45% in relation to the axis of the patient. The patient is placed in the Trendelenburg position, right side down, before the robot is docked.

The procedure is conducted following the same steps outlined for the laparoscopic approach: initial vascular control, medial-to-lateral mobilization of the colon, and posterior-to-anterior mesorectal dissection.

The enhanced visualization provided by the da Vinci robotic platform allows lateral division of the levators from the pelvis. Entering the ischiorectal fossa from the pelvis facilitates the perineal dissection.

SUMMARY

APE is a formidable operation. First described by Miles in 1908,[3] for many years it was the only curative option for rectal cancer. With the advent of SSPs, APE is now less frequently performed. It is usually reserved for patients with distal rectal cancers invading the anal sphincter and levator musculature. Over time, changes in APE occurred as surgeons, influenced by the techniques of sphincter-sparing surgery, extended abdominal dissection progressively closer to the levators. These technical deviations from the original procedure described by Miles had unintentionally worse results. A resurgence of strict adherence to the principles of APE, including wider resection of the pelvic floor, has led to clearer resection margins and lower rates of recurrence.

REFERENCES

1. Campos FG, Habr-Gama A, Nahas SC, Perez RO. Abdominoperineal excision: evolution of a centenary operation. *Dis Colon Rectum.* 2012;55(8):844-853.
2. J.P. L-M. The surgical treatment of cancer of the rectum. *Am J Surg.* 1939;46(1):40-44.
3. Miles WE. A method of performing abdomino-perineal excision for carcinoma of the rectum and of the terminal portion of the pelvic colon. *Lancet.* 1908;172(4451):1812-1813.
4. Lloyd-Davis OV. Synchronous combined excision of the rectum: report of 1,638 resections. *Dis Colon Rectum.* 1964;7:440-441.
5. Heald RJ, Husband EM, Ryall RD. The mesorectum in rectal cancer surgery–the clue to pelvic recurrence? *Br J Surg.* 1982;69(10):613-616.
6. Quirke P, Durdey P, Dixon MF, Williams NS. Local recurrence of rectal adenocarcinoma due to inadequate surgical resection. Histopathological study of lateral tumour spread and surgical excision. *Lancet.* 1986;2(8514):996-999.
7. Marr R, Birbeck K, Garvican J, et al. The modern abdominoperineal excision: the next challenge after total mesorectal excision. *Ann Surg.* 2005;242(1):74-82.
8. Williams NS, Dixon MF, Johnston D. Reappraisal of the 5 centimetre rule of distal excision for carcinoma of the rectum: a study of distal intramural spread and of patients' survival. *Br J Surg.* 1983;70(3):150-154.
9. Bujko K, Rutkowski A, Chang GJ, Michalski W, Chmielik E, Kusnierz J. Is the 1-cm rule of distal bowel resection margin in rectal cancer based on clinical evidence? A systematic review. *Ann Surg Oncol.* 2012;19(3):801-808.
10. Salerno G, Chandler I, Wotherspoon A, Thomas K, Moran B, Brown G. Sites of surgical wasting in the abdominoperineal specimen. *Br J Surg.* 2008;95(9):1147-1154.
11. Shihab OC, Heald RJ, Rullier E, et al. Defining the surgical planes on mri improves surgery for cancer of the low rectum. *Lancet Oncol.* 2009;10(12):1207-1211.
12. Rothenberger DA, Wong WD. Abdominoperineal resection for adenocarcinoma of the low rectum. *World J Surg.* 1992;16(3):478-485.
13. Reshef A, Lavery I, Kiran RP. Factors associated with oncologic outcomes after abdominoperineal resection compared with restorative resection for low rectal cancer: Patient- and tumor-related or technical factors only? *Dis Colon Rectum.* 2012;55(1):51-58.
14. Nissan A, Guillem JG, Paty PB, et al. Abdominoperineal resection for rectal cancer at a specialty center. *Dis Colon Rectum.* 2001;44(1):27-35; discussion 35-26.
15. Bullard KM, Trudel JL, Baxter NN, Rothenberger DA. Primary perineal wound closure after preoperative radiotherapy and abdominoperineal resection has a high incidence of wound failure. *Dis Colon Rectum.* 2005;48(3):438-443.
16. Wiatrek RL, Thomas JS, Papaconstantinou HT. Perineal wound complications after abdominoperineal resection. *Clin Colon Rectal Surg.* 2008;21(1):76-85.
17. Welsch T, Mategakis V, Contin P, Kulu Y, Buchler MW, Ulrich A. Results of extralevator abdominoperineal resection for low rectal cancer including quality of life and long-term wound complications. *Int J Colorectal Dis.* 2013;28(4):503-510.
18. West NP, Anderin C, Smith KJ, Holm T, Quirke P. Multicentre experience with extralevator abdominoperineal excision for low rectal cancer. *Br J Surg.* 2010;97(4):588-599.
19. Marijnen CA, Kapiteijn E, van de Velde CJ, et al. Acute side effects and complications after short-term preoperative radiotherapy combined with total mesorectal excision in primary rectal cancer: Report of a multicenter randomized trial. *J Clin Oncol.* 2002;20(3):817-825.
20. Formijne Jonkers HA, Draaisma WA, Roskott AM, van Overbeeke AJ, Broeders IA, Consten EC. Early complications after stoma formation: a prospective cohort study in 100 patients with 1-year follow-up. *Int J Colorectal Dis.* 2012;27(8):1095-1099.
21. Robertson I, Leung E, Hughes D, et al. Prospective analysis of stoma-related complications. *Colorectal Dis.* 2005;7(3):279-285.
22. Hendren SK, O'Connor BI, Liu M, et al. Prevalence of male and female sexual dysfunction is high following surgery for rectal cancer. *Ann Surg.* 2005;242(2):212-223.
23. Marijnen CA, van de Velde CJ, Putter H, et al. Impact of short-term preoperative radiotherapy on health-related quality of life and sexual functioning in primary rectal cancer: Report of a multicenter randomized trial. *J Clin Oncol.* 2005;23(9):1847-1858.
24. Stephens RJ, Thompson LC, Quirke P, et al. Impact of short-course preoperative radiotherapy for rectal cancer on patients' quality of life: data from the Medical Research Council CR07/National Cancer Institute of

Canada Clinical Trials group c016 randomized clinical trial. *J Clin Oncol.* 2010;28(27):4233-4239.

25. Camilleri-Brennan J, Steele RJ. Objective assessment of morbidity and quality of life after surgery for low rectal cancer. *Colorectal Dis.* 2002;4(1):61-66.
26. Ho VP, Lee Y, Stein SL, Temple LK. Sexual function after treatment for rectal cancer: a review. *Dis Colon Rectum.* 2011;54(1):113-125.
27. Pachler J, Wille-Jorgensen P. Quality of life after rectal resection for cancer, with or without permanent colostomy. *Cochrane Database Syst Rev.* 2012;12:CD004323.
28. How P, Stelzner S, Branagan G, et al. Comparative quality of life in patients following abdominoperineal excision and low anterior resection for low rectal cancer. *Dis Colon Rectum.* 2012;55(4):400-406.
29. How P, Shihab O, Tekkis P, et al. A systematic review of cancer related patient outcomes after anterior resection and abdominoperineal excision for rectal cancer in the total mesorectal excision era. *Surg Oncol.* 2011;20(4):e149-e155.
30. den Dulk M, Putter H, Collette L, et al. The abdominoperineal resection itself is associated with an adverse outcome: the European experience based on a pooled analysis of five European randomised clinical trials on rectal cancer. *Eur J Cancer.* 2009;45(7):1175-1183.
31. Rullier A, Gourgou-Bourgade S, Jarlier M, et al. Predictive factors of positive circumferential resection margin after radiochemotherapy for rectal cancer: the French randomised trial accord12/0405 prodige 2. *Eur J Cancer.* 2013;49(1):82-89.
32. Nagtegaal ID, van de Velde CJ, Marijnen CA, van Krieken JH, Quirke P. Low rectal cancer: a call for a change of approach in abdominoperineal resection. *J Clin Oncol.* 2005;23(36):9257-9264.
33. West NP, Finan PJ, Anderin C, Lindholm J, Holm T, Quirke P. Evidence of the oncologic superiority of cylindrical abdominoperineal excision for low rectal cancer. *J Clin Oncol.* 2008;26(21):3517-3522.
34. Han JG, Wang ZJ, Wei GH, Gao ZG, Yang Y, Zhao BC. Randomized clinical trial of conventional versus cylindrical abdominoperineal resection for locally advanced lower rectal cancer. *Am J Surg.* 2012;204(3):274-282.

Chapter 8. Pelvic Exenteration

Javier F. Magrina, MD and
Paul M. Magtibay, MD

BACKGROUND AND EVOLUTION

Exenteration was first reported by Brunchswig in 1948 as a palliative procedure, and, in his subsequent series of 561 patients collected from 1948 to 1964, the operative mortality was 26% and the 5-year survival rate was 20%.[1] Advances in anesthesia, surgical instrumentation, technique, pelvic floor reconstruction, antibiotics, fluid management, blood products, the use of intermediate or intensive care units, and the training of gynecologic oncologists have decreased operative mortality; in addition, improved patient selection preoperatively and intraoperatively have increased survival rates. At the Mayo Clinic from 1950 to 1986, the operative mortality rate decreased from 12% to 6.7%, and the 5-year survival rate increased from 26% to 41%.[2] Patient rehabilitation has also remarkably improved. From loss of vaginal function and 1 or 2 permanent stomas, reconstructive techniques have resulted in no stoma bags (due to low rectosigmoid anastomosis and continent urinary reservoir), and restoration of vaginal function by using different type of pedicle flaps. Other factors to consider for all exenteration candidates are the need for family support due to long rehabilitation, usually 6 months or longer depending on the extent of the operation and whether there were or not postoperative complications, quality of life before and after surgery, and the need for appropriate care if an exenteration cannot be performed or cure is not achieved.

INDICATIONS AND CLINICAL APPLICATIONS

Pelvic exenteration remains a salvage operation when other forms of therapy have been exhausted. Most candidates are patients with cervical cancer postirradiation or those with advanced primary disease. Because of dosimetry improvements and the addition of sensitizing concomitant chemotherapy, the number of exenteration candidates has decreased, with only about 8% of patients with advanced cervical cancer being candidates. Other candidates are patients with recurrent endometrial, vaginal, urethral, vulvar, rectal, bladder, and, even occasionally, ovarian malignancies. Most often, the clinical scenario for consideration of exenterative surgery involves a cervical or endometrial cancer patient presenting with a recurrence after having received pelvic irradiation for a postsurgical recurrence. Occasionally, patients with an advanced primary malignancy of the vulva or vagina, who are not candidates for irradiation, are best treated by primary pelvic exenteration.

Prognostic Factors and Contraindications

Prognostic factors impacting survival and the risk of morbidity include the patient's age, body mass index (BMI), general medical condition, the origin site of the primary lesion, the time interval from primary treatment to recurrence, the volume and location of the recurrent lesion, histological type of tumor, lymphatic invasion, degree of tissue invasion and pelvic viscera involved, parametrial invasion, levator muscle invasion, postresection margins, positive nodes, peritoneal involvement, small bowel involvement, lateral pelvic wall extension or fixation, invasion of other soft tissues or bone, and extrapelvic metastases.[2-6] The combination of several adverse prognostic factors decreases survival rates.[5]

Optimal candidates for pelvic exenteration are young patients in good health with a normal BMI presenting with an isolated central pelvic recurrence from squamous cervical carcinoma postirradiation or chemoirradiation, localized only to the cervix or to the cervix and the upper-most portion of the vagina, with a tumor volume of less than 5 mL, no lymphatic invasion, no parametrial extension, negative nodes, no metastases, and an interval of more than 2 years from completion of irradiation.[5]

Older age is not a contraindication to exenterative surgery; although it is associated with increased morbidity, age does not adversely impact survival.[7] Similarly, obesity is not a contraindication but may affect the likelihood of morbidity. Patients in poor medical condition may simply not survive the operation or its complications. Properly selected patients with endometrial adenocarcinoma recurrence have a similar survival outcome as patients with cervical cancer recurrence.[8] Patients with persistent or recurrent tumor within 6 months from primary treatment have poor survival rates even with complete resection.[5] Factors such as tumor volume, location, degree of invasion, and extension to parametria and levators are important because they may impact the likelihood of obtaining satisfactory surgical margins. In general, large tumors portend decreased survival as compared with small lesions. Tumor volume is a factor in type I exenterations due to the cephalad extension of the lesions with direct peritoneal or small bowel involvement, but is not a factor in type II or III indicating that in these cases complete tumor resection is more important than the lesion volume.[2] Complete resection (negative margins) is associated with increased survival. Incomplete resection (positive margins) has a dismal prognosis,[3,5] with a median survival of only 4 months.[9] A long interval (> 1 year) from primary treatment to recurrence is a favorable prognostic factor.[5] Low rectal anastomosis has been associated with an increased risk of local recurrence.[10,11] Although the cause is unknown, a potential factor could be an increased propensity for narrow margins resulting from attempted preservation of the rectum.

There are a number of both absolute and relative contraindications to exenterative surgery. The presence of extrapelvic metastasis at any site (such as supraclavicular nodes, grossly enlarged aortic nodes, liver, lung, omentum, and peritoneum) and extensive lateral pelvic wall involvement, are contraindications for an exenteration because the disease is not resectable or curable.

Exenterations With Very Low or No Survival: Absolute Contraindications

Absolute contraindications to exenterative surgery are extrapelvic involvement of any organ, grossly positive aortic nodes, peritoneal metastases, or situations in which completely resection cannot be achieved because the disease is not curable. Other adverse factors, such as microscopic aortic node metastases, lateral pelvic wall involvement, positive pelvic nodes, or involvement of bony pelvic structures are not absolute contraindications (see relative contraindications) but they may result in a lower survival. The combination of several adverse factors has an increasingly unfavorable impact on survival.

Contraindications to an exenteration are discovered in about 50% of patients explored for an exenterative procedure. In an early series, reasons for abandoning the procedure were pelvic sidewall involvement, positive aortic nodes, small bowel or cecal involvement, and liver metastases.[12] Patients undergoing an abandoned exenteration attempt have a dismal prognosis. Approximately 75% of such patients die during the first year, 95% have expired by the end of the second year, and only 5% of patients survived for longer than 2 years.[12] Adverse surgical factors are evaluated both preoperatively and at surgical exploration. Minimally invasive surgical exploration 48 to 72 hours prior to a planned exenteration can identify patients with surgical contraindications and avoid a laparotomy (see MIS exploration prior to exenteration in Minimally Invasive Surgery Applications section).

Exenterations With Decreased Survival (15%–20%): Relative Contraindications

The presence of positive pelvic or aortic nodes, involvement of the pelvic peritoneum, sigmoid colon, small bowel, ovaries, tubes, fixation to the pelvic wall fascia, involvement of other soft tissues or bone, even when the lesion is completely resected, have been shown to result in decreased survival rates. Any of these findings reduce the likelihood of cure, and, because there are no other therapeutic alternatives, one may still consider proceeding with exenterative surgery. However, the presence of several adverse prognostic factors may be an indication for not proceeding with the exenteration. In our experience, factors associated with a decreased survival[2,6] were observed in 15% of patients with type I, in 27% of patients with type II, and in 17% of patients with type III exenterations.[2] When analyzing the entire group of patients with adverse factors, the 2- and 5-year survival rates were 47% and 17%, respectively.[6] In a separate series of patients with adverse factors analyzed by the type of exenteration, there were no survivors among patients undergoing a type I or III exenteration, while a 28% 5-year survival rate was obtained for patients with type II.[2] Exenterations with decreased survival have been named palliative, however, this term is misnomer since palliative procedures are directed to improve symptomatology and not survival rates.

1. Positive nodes

There are several issues to consider in the presence of positive nodes prior to deciding to proceed with an exenteration. These factors include lymph node location (pelvic, aortic, sigmoid mesentery, groin, or other), whether the disease is microscopic or macroscopic, the number of involved nodes, whether nodal disease is unilateral or bilateral, extracapsular involvement, and surgical resectability. For instance, 1 or 2 unilateral positive pelvic nodes may not influence survival when other unfavorable factors are not present.[6] In our experience, the survival of patients with positive nodes was 46% at 2 years and 23% at 5 years.[6] In an earlier series of the Mayo Clinic there were no survivors with positive pelvic nodes,[13] probably due to additional negative prognostic factors. A single aortic node with microscopic metastasis may not be a reason to abort an exenteration but multiple microscopic or grossly positive aortic nodes, especially if fixed, are an absolute contraindication. Positive groin nodes, when resectable and treatable with adjuvant groin irradiation, are not a contraindication in the presence of negative pelvic nodes.

2. Peritoneal involvement

Involvement of the peritoneum overlying the recurrent lesion or direct contact of the lesion with the adnexa, sigmoid, small bowel, cecum, or omentum are not absolute contraindications, but these conditions require removal of all the involved tissues.[6] Small bowel resection was the most common additional tissue resected in type I exenterations due to the cephalad growth of the lesion with peritoneal or adjacent bowel involvement. In contrast, there were no bowel resections in patients with a type III exenteration due to the distal location of the lesions.[2]

3. Lateral pelvic wall extension

Extension to the pelvic wall was considered an absolute contraindication in the past when discovered on pelvic examination. However, complete resection has been achieved in

29% of patients with apparent extension to lateral pelvic wall with a 32% 10-year survival rate.[3] In some patients, fixation to the pelvic wall is secondary to radiation fibrosis and the recurrence can be easily resected. Others have lesions invading the pelvic wall muscular fascia of the obturator internus, levators, and coccygeus muscles, and are resectable (see *Extended Radical Parametrectomy*). Others have unresectable disease involving into or past the large sciatic notch or have large fixed recurrences attached to the external iliac vessels, which may be resectable, but these patients are left with subclinical residual disease and are not curable unless intraoperative irradiation is administered. Partial resections should not be attempted because they will not result in cure.

When preoperative evaluation of patients with postirradiation disease with lateral pelvic wall extension appears resectable, we recommend additional external pelvic irradiation (usually 4000 cGy in about 4 weeks), followed by an exenterative procedure 4 weeks later. An effort to achieve complete resection must be made in these instances, because local control is directly related to the size of the residual tumor. Once the resection is completed, intraoperative electron irradiation (Mobetron, IntraOp Medical, Sunnyvale, California) is delivered through a metal cylinder of an appropriate diameter to cover the selected target area (Figure 8-1). A dose of 1250 cGy is delivered in the presence of microscopic disease and may be increased according to the amount of residual visible tumor. Distant metastases and survival rates are directly related to obtaining a complete tumor resection. Tumor bed and local control rates of 81% and 67%, respectively, have been achieved when a complete resection was accomplished in patients with different types of recurrent gynecologic malignancies at different sites and with different surgical procedures.[14] In the absence of intraoperative electron irradiation, immediate postoperative brachytherapy with iridium 192 needles is an alternative, providing a similar local control rate of 68%.[15] Hollow plastic tubules are sutured directly over the tumor bed providing a homogenous dose (Figure 8-2) and are exteriorized through the anterior abdominal wall (Figure 8-3). An omental flap is created and sutured over the tubules to prevent direct bowel contact with them. The tubules are pulled out once the brachytherapy is completed. For intraoperative electron and brachytherapy irradiation, the survival rates were 55% and 44%, respectively, and severe complications were observed in 15% compared with 33% of patients, respectively.[14,15]

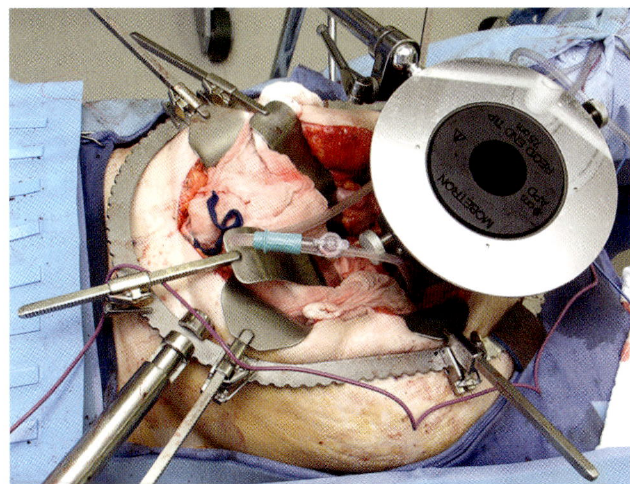

Fig. 8-1. Intraoperative electron irradiation (Mobetron, IntraOp Medical, Sunnyvale, California). A round cylinder is applied directly to the area of previous attachment of the tumor to the pelvic wall. The bowel and ureter are mobilized out of the irradiation field.

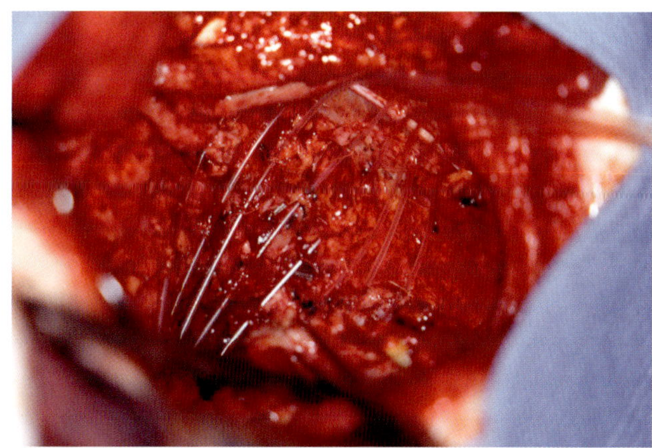

Fig. 8-2. A series of hollow tubules have been sutured on the lateral pelvic wall in the tumor bed of a resected cervical recurrence. The obturator nerve is seen on the upper part of the tumor bed.

4. Bone involvement

Bone involvement is different than periosteal attachment or fixation, which is easier to resect. Factors to consider prior to bone resection are whether complete resection of the entire

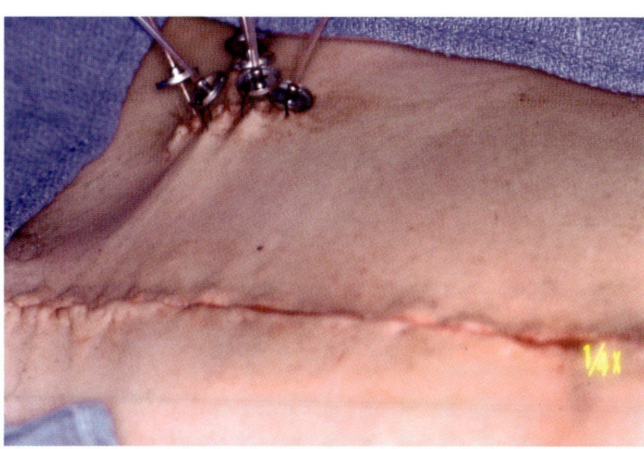

Fig. 8-3. The tubules are exteriorized through the anterior abdominal wall for postoperative insertion of iridium 192 needles, and once the appropriate dose has been delivered they are pulled out.

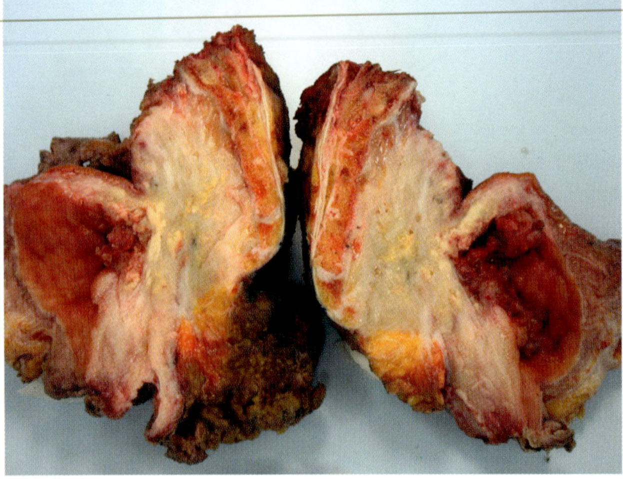

Fig. 8-4. Specimen of an extended total pelvic exenteration type III, including the distal sacrum and coccyx.

lesion is possible, the risk of associated morbidity, long-term sequelae, and any other adverse prognostic factors. Bone invasion is associated with decreased survival rate even when all disease is resected.[6] We recommend a similar approach to patients with lateral pelvic wall extension: preoperative irradiation, followed by tumor and bone resection, and administration of intraoperative irradiation. When the recurrent lesion is fixed to the periosteum, periosteal, or superficial bone resection with an osteotome will achieve complete clearance. The pubic symphysis can be resected without significant disability, as can the ischial tuberosity and a portion of the ischium ramus if necessary to achieve disease clearance. In time, a callus is formed between both ends of the transected bone providing some degree of stability. Most recurrences invading the sacrum are resectable since, as a rule, they tend to be distally located. Sacral involvement below S2 is considered resectable (Figure 8-4) while more proximal disease is generally unresectable. In our institution, preoperative consultation is obtained with an orthopedic oncologist who performs the bone resection.

5. Necrotic tumor recurrence vs irradiation necrosis

Necrotic tissue secondary to irradiation ischemia may appear as necrotic tumor recurrence and may not provide viable tissue for a pathologist to confirm or rule out recurrent malignancy. Infrequently, an exenterative procedure is performed in a patient with necrotic, malodorous tissues, with an annoying vaginal discharge and severe pain only to find no evidence of malignancy on final pathological examination. In a Mayo Clinic series, 4 (3.4%) patients were exenterated with a preoperative clinical suspicion of cancer but without histological confirmation of recurrence.[13] Two (1.2%) patients had actual recurrence on the specimen but no tumor was found in the other 2. These procedures result in a marked improvement of patient's quality of life, especially if they have intractable pain, fistulous tracts, or both.

6. Triad of symptoms

The triad of ipsilateral hydronephrosis, leg swelling, and sciatica has usually been considered a contraindication for an exenteration. Most of these lesions, especially when large, are unresectable. However, the authors have operated in patients with such symptomatology where the symptoms were not directly related to recurrent disease, the lesion was resectable, and the exenteration was curative. In many instances, the final decision of unresectability will be made at the time of surgical exploration.

ANATOMIC CONSIDERATIONS

Types of Exenteration

The classification of exenterations into 3 main categories—anterior, posterior, and total—reflects only the specific viscera removed. This classification fails to address the caudal level of resection of the viscera and the excision of other soft tissues, bone, or both. The Mayo classification of exenterations[16] provides a further understanding of the extent of the operation by taking into consideration the preservation or removal of additional tissues in addition to the pelvic viscera, including:

a. Level of resection of the pelvic viscera (above or below levator muscle),
b. Levator muscles,
c. Perineal membrane,
d. Vulva or vulva-perineum-anus (vulvectomy or vulvoanusectomy),
e. Additional soft tissues, such as small bowel, sigmoid, groin nodes, psoas muscle (Figure 8-5), pelvic wall muscles (Figure 8-6), or bone, such as pubic symphysis, pubic

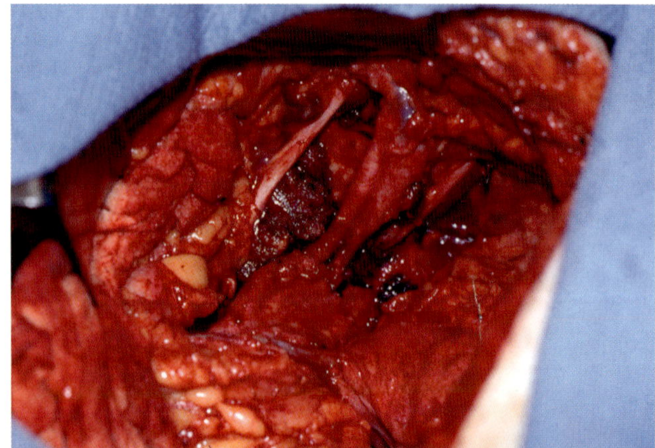

Fig. 8-5. Extended exenteration. Resection of leiomyosarcoma recurrence involving the left external iliac vessels and psoas muscle. The recurrence has been dissected off the external iliac vessels and a segment of the psoas muscle has been resected. The left femoral nerve can be seen lateral to the external iliac vessels exiting the pelvis below the left inguinal ligament. Narrowing of the middle portion of the external iliac vessels secondary to tumor compression is also seen.

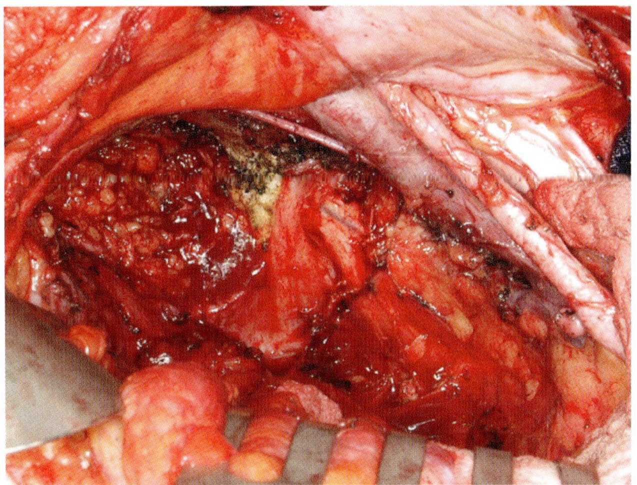

Fig. 8-6. Extended pelvic wall resection. The arterial and venous hypogastric system of the right pelvic wall has been excised as well as the internal obturator and levator muscles for recurrent cervical carcinoma involving the pelvic wall.

ramus, ischial tuberosity, and sacrum (Figure 8-4), or other structures (extended exenteration).

Using the above criteria, there are 3 main categories of exenterations, ie, anterior, posterior, and total, depending on the specific pelvic viscera removed. Each category is divided into 3 types, ie, types I (supralevator), II (infralevator), and III (infralevator with vulvectomy or vulvoanusectomy; Figure 8-7).

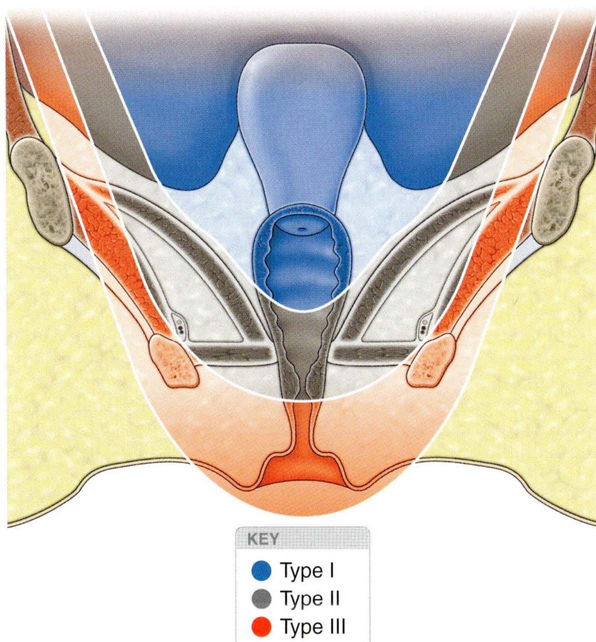

Fig. 8-7. Pelvis diagram showing the three levels of resection in pelvic exenterations: I, II, and III. Type I: supralevator. Type II: infralevator. Type III: infralevator with vulvectomy or vulvoanusectomy.

The tissues removed in each type are summarized in Table 8-1. Type I involves resection of the pelvic viscera above the levator muscle (with preservation of levators, distal vagina, perineal membrane, urethra, vulva, and anus; Figure 8-8). Type II includes resection of the pelvic viscera below the levator muscles as well as the levator muscles (Figure 8-9A). There are 2 levels of visceral resection in type II:

a. Proximal to the urethral meatus, vaginal introitus, and anus, with preservation of the perineal membrane and perineum (Figure 8-9B), or
b. Resection, including the urethral meatus, vaginal introitus, perineum and/or anus, and the medial portion of the perineal membrane (Figures 8-9C and D).

Type III is for distal or vulvovaginal lesions and involves type II b resection with excision of the perineal membrane plus a vulvectomy or vulvoanusectomy (Figures 8-10A to D). The term *extended exenteration* is added to any one of the described types when additional tissues or bone are removed.

PREOPERATIVE EVALUATION

Box 8-1 KEY INSTRUMENTATION

- Long curved clamps, such as Shallcross clamp, long curved scissors, and Russian forceps
- Electrocautery with long tip; vessel-sealing device
- Self-retaining retractor
- Stapling instruments for intestinal and vascular applications
- Clip applier with large and small size clips

Preoperative evaluation is directed to assess the medical condition and the extent of the disease (pelvic and extrapelvic) of potential exenteration candidates. Patients in poor medical condition may simply not survive the operation because of the fluid and metabolic changes experienced during and after surgery and are not appropriate candidates. A medical examination should include palpation of nodal areas, especially the supraclavicular nodes. A detailed pelvic examination is performed to determine the lateral and caudal margins of the lesion, which in the presence of radiation fibrosis may be difficult or impossible to ascertain. In patients with severe pain or a narrow, tender, or irradiated vagina, it is preferable to perform an examination under anesthesia, at which time biopsies can be obtained, and cystoscopy and proctoscopy examinations can also be performed. Smooth parametrial induration may be fibrosis, not tumor, and be resectable. Positron emission tomography/computed tomography scan is the preferred imaging test to evaluate for metastatic disease. The presence of extrapelvic metastatic disease is an absolute contraindication. In the absence of metastases, the magnitude

Table 8-1. Types of exenterations according to tissues resected in addition to pelvic viscera.

Excision	I	II	III
Pelvic viscera	Above levator	Below levator	Below levator
Levator muscles	None	Partial or extensive	Extensive
Perineal membrane	None	(A) None or (B) minimal	Extensive or complete
Urethral meatus-vaginal introitus-anus	None	(A) None or (B) circumscribed resection	Extensive
Vulva	None	None	Extensive
Other soft tissues and/or bone with any type[a]			

[a]Extended exenteration: small bowel, psoas muscle, groin nodes, ischial tuberosity, pubic bone, sacrum, other.

of involvement of the viscera, soft tissues, and bones of the pelvis must be carefully evaluated.

Patient counseling about the proposed operation and the resulting permanent life style changes related to urinary, intestinal, and vaginal functions require time and compassion. A strong family support is necessary for the long postoperative recovery, usually 6 months or longer when facing complications, which, unfortunately, are common. Consultation with a stoma nurse is necessary to assess for potential stomal sites and patient and family education of stoma care and potential complications.

On the day prior to the exenteration, the stoma site is marked in the standing position, the patient should remain on clear liquids after lunch and until midnight, have a bowel preparation at home, and take an evening shower with a chlorhexidine brush for the abdominal and vulvoperineal skin, which is repeated in the morning of the surgery day. All patients are typed and screened, and depending on the planned type of exenteration, with 2 or more units of blood crossmatched. Stockings and intermittent pneumatic devices are used in all patients and placed prior to the operation. Prophylactic antibiotics are administered 1 hour before the operation and repeated at 3 hours. It is advisable to have an anesthesia team familiar with the intraoperative management of the serious potential complication that can accompany exenterative surgery.

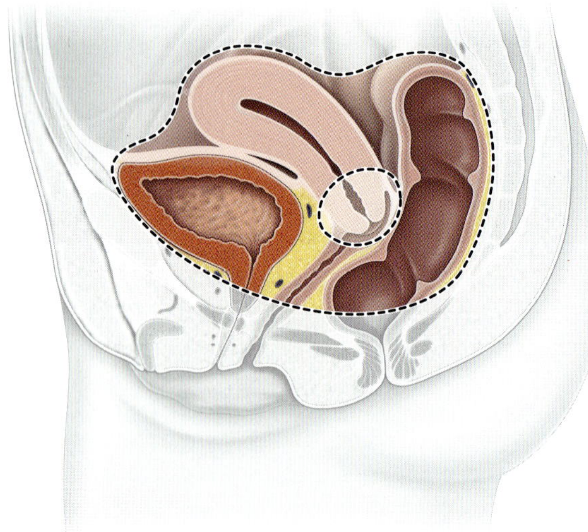

Fig. 8-8. Diagram showing the level of resection in type I total pelvic exenteration.

SURGICAL PROCEDURE

Box 8-2 MASTER SURGEON'S PRINCIPLES

- Adequate exposure with an adequate size incision and a self-retaining retractor are a must for every exenteration
- Sharp dissection of pelvic spaces is usually the rule for previously irradiated patients
- Be prepared for unexpected bleeding at any time
- Division of the ureters, rectum, or both is not performed until there is assurance of no contraindications
- The omentum must be preserved for layering the denuded pelvic floor, an important part of the operation
- Inferior epigastric arteries must be preserved when vaginal reconstruction involves the rectus muscle

General Considerations

Because prolonged anesthesia time is associated with increased morbidity and mortality, the surgeon must be prepared to proceed expeditiously and have an extensive knowledge of the pelvic anatomy and surgical techniques for the management of ureters, bladder, vagina, rectum, small bowel, pelvic and

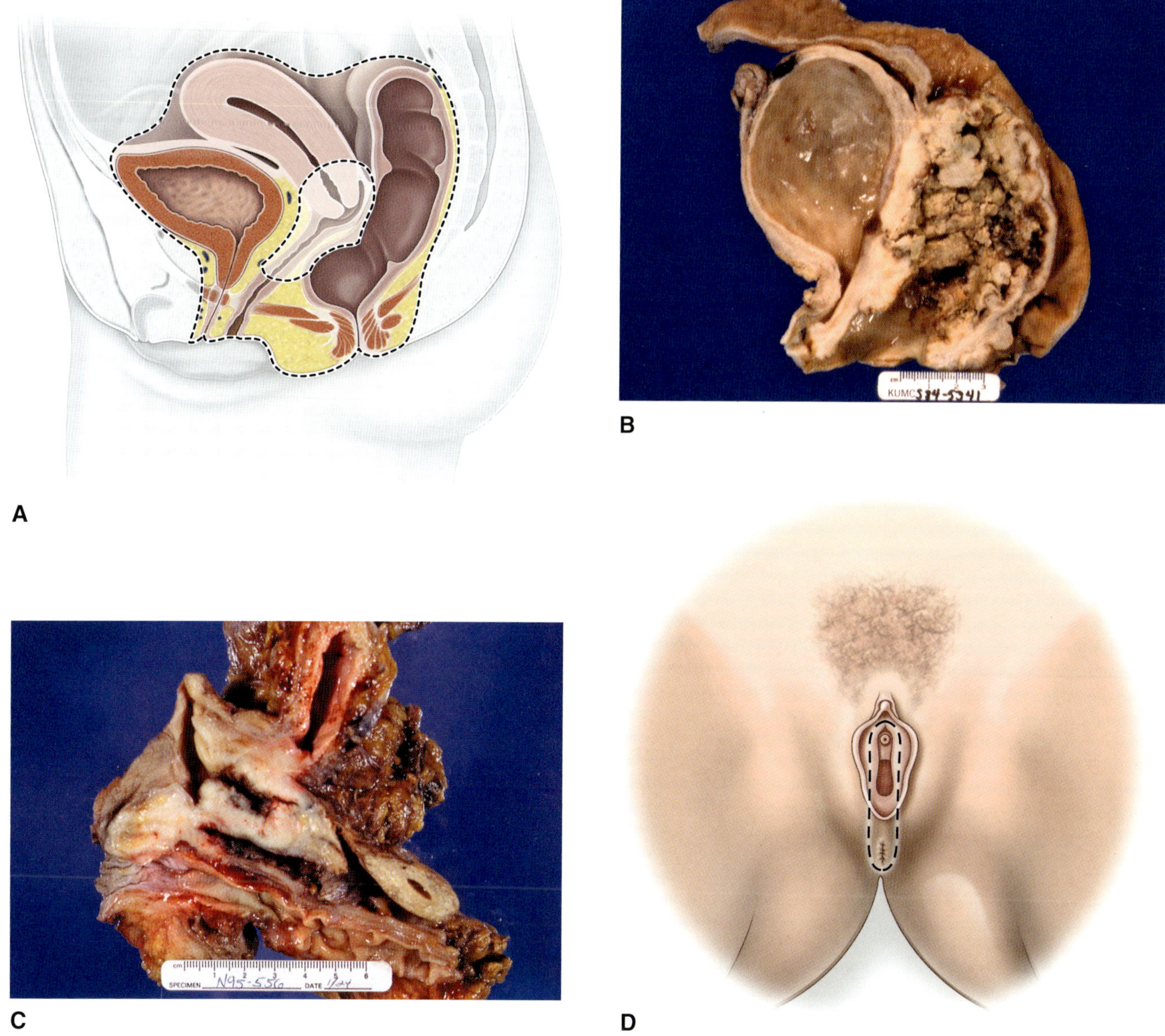

Fig. 8-9. (A) Total pelvic exenteration type II. Level of resection of pelvic organs. (B) Total pelvic exenteration type IIA. Specimen of large recurrent cervical carcinoma with preservation of urethral meatus, vaginal introitus, perineum, and anus. (C) Total pelvic exenteration type IIB. Specimen of recurrent cervical carcinoma with resection of urethral meatus, vaginal introitus, perineum, and anus.(D) Total exenteration type IIB showing the limited resection of urethral meatus, vaginal introitus, perineum, and anus as in the specimen of Figure 8-9C.

aortic nodes, and vulva, as well as being versed in reconstructive techniques for the urinary, vaginal, and intestinal tracts. Equally important is preparation for the management of severe hemorrhage, which can occur even with the best technique. The addition of other surgical teams in the operation room may not be in the best interest of the patient due to difficulty with coordination of schedules, different approaches, difference in level of experience of the surgeons, and the need for different operating room personnel, resulting in a "cluttered" operating room. We prefer a single surgeon for the exploration, exenterative, and reconstructive abdominal phases and a second surgeon for the reconstructive vulvovaginal phase simultaneously with the reconstructive abdominal phase.

The surgeon must exercise creativity and surgical judgment, and possess physical endurance and mental strength to determine and carry out the type of resection best suited for each patient. When the resection is tailored to the patient's disease and anatomy, each operation is different. For instance, a fixed, right parametrial recurrence may require complete resection of the right hypogastric vessel system while on the contralateral side these vessels can be preserved. A lesion extending into the right lower vaginal third near the introitus, will require ipsilateral levator, perineal membrane, and vulvar

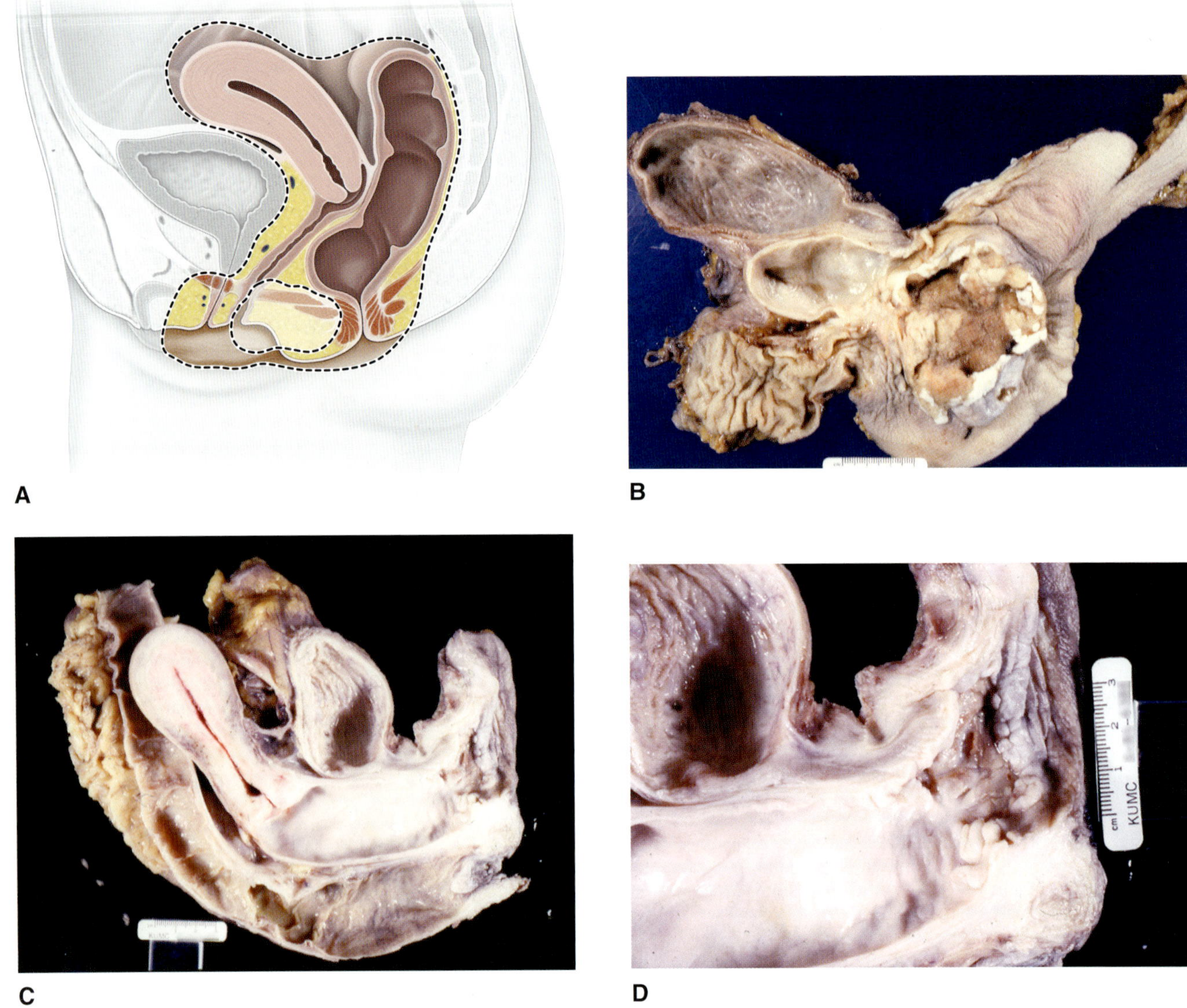

Fig. 8-10. (A) Total exenteration type III. The vulva, including the labia majora, the perineum and perianal tissues are excised in addition to the pelvic viscera, levator muscles, and perineal membrane. (B) Total exenteration type III. Surgical specimen of type III total pelvic exenteration showing large ulcerated vulvar carcinoma (on the right) and bladder, vagina (opened), and rectum on the left. (C) Surgical specimen of total exenteration type III for recurrent vaginal carcinoma postirradiation involving the distal left lateral vaginal wall, vaginal introitus, urethra, and posterior vaginal wall (ulcerated lesion). (D) Higher magnification of the left vaginal ulcerated lesion seen in Figure 8-10C.

resection, while the symmetrical contralateral tissues may be spared. Radiation fibrosis, which increases with the passage of years, may obliterate the usual pelvic spaces the surgeon is familiar with, requiring a more extensive resection than one may have planned originally. Alternatively, a small central recurrence in a patient with preservation of the spaces and planes of dissection may result in a radical or extended radical hysterectomy, instead of an exenteration. Obliteration of the vesicovaginal or rectovaginal spaces may require a total exenteration instead of the planned anterior or posterior exenteration, which would have been adequate to obtain clear margins. We have observed that patient survival is not affected by the type of exenteration, assuming complete tumor resection is accomplished.[2]

The type of instrumentation used for the division of vascular pedicles and soft tissues is a personal preference. Our preference is to use electrocautery for transection of soft tissues and a vessel-sealing device for vascular pedicles, unless it appears unsafe in which case the standard clamp-cut-suture technique is used. Soft rubber rugs are placed on the floor of both sides of the operating table for the surgeon and assistants to stand on.

Patient Position

The patient is placed in a low semilithotomy position using Allen stirrups with heel but not calf pressure. Leg position is intermittently checked during the operation by a circulating nurse. The full abdomen, vulva, perineum, anus, buttocks, and upper thighs are prepped and draped to provide immediate access when needed. A small degree of Trendelenburg facilitates bowel retraction in the upper abdomen, improves venous flow, and allows direct lighting to the deep aspects of the pelvis. One operating room light is positioned perpendicular to the surgical field and focused on the upper pelvis and lower abdomen while a second light is positioned over the patient's head at an angle and directed to the deepest part of the pelvis. The small bowel and sigmoid are placed in the upper abdomen and packed with a long gauze pack or blue towels depending on the weight of the patient, and held in place with malleable self-retracting blades attached to the retractor's ring.

Surgical Technique

Exenterative surgery follows a series of segments or phases:

a. Exploratory phase: surgical exploration to determine resectability and absence of contraindications
b. Exenterative phase: removal of pelvic viscera and other tissues
c. Vulvo-vaginal-anal phase: completion of the exenterative phase with removal of additional vulvo-vaginal-anal tissues
d. Hemostasis phase: meticulous hemostasis after the exenterative phase is completed
e. Reconstructive phase: there is an abdominal reconstructive phase and a vulvo-vaginal-anal reconstructive phase. They consist of the reconstruction of the urinary and intestinal tracts and restoring vaginal function. In our opinion, this is when 2 surgical teams may be working concurrently to shorten the operating time.

1. Exploration phase: evaluation of resectability and contraindications

Patients with no obvious preoperative contraindications are submitted to an examination under anesthesia, cystoscopy, proctoscopy, and surgical exploration prior to proceeding with an exenteration because almost half of the patients are found to have contraindications or unresectable disease during this evaluation.[12] Both examinations can be performed by laparoscopy or robotics 48 to 72 hours prior to the planned exenteration to avoid an unnecessary laparotomy in case of adverse findings (see MIS exploration prior to exenteration in Minimally Invasive Surgery Applications section).

Examination under anesthesia, cystoscopy, and proctoscopy are usually performed prior to surgical exploration with particular attention to the caudal and lateral extension of the lesion. Should there be any obvious contraindications, the surgical exploration is abandoned. In the absence of an obvious contraindication, surgical exploration is warranted, as pelvic examination alone can be inaccurate for predicting surgical resectability. In one series, central lesions on pelvic examination were found to be unresectable after exploration in 35% of patients, while 28% of lateral pelvic wall lesions were able to be completely resected.[17]

There are 2 main objectives and 4 major areas of assessment during the surgical exploration. The 2 objectives are:

a. Evaluation of resectability: Is it possible to obtain a complete resection?
b. Evaluation of contraindications: Are there any contraindications?

The 4 major areas of assessment are:

a. Peritoneal metastases, direct peritoneal involvement, and involvement of attached bowel, adnexa, or other structures to the lesion
b. Aortic nodal metastases, including the infrarenal nodes
c. Fixation/extension of the recurrent lesion to the lateral pelvic wall
d. Pelvic node metastases

The order of performance varies according to the findings on preoperative evaluation and not all elements may be necessary if a contraindication is quickly noted (eg, peritoneal metastases). During the exploration phase the surgeon must avoid cutting any structures (ureters, bowel) to allow for an easy retreat in the case of adverse findings. In the absence of contraindications and after complete resectability has been assured, the procedure can be performed at the same surgical setting or 2 or 3 days later once the negative findings at laparoscopy have been discussed with the patient and her family.

A midline laparotomy incision is made. Intestinal and omental adhesions are sharply removed and efforts are made to preserve the omentum for ensuing pelvic floor covering. Pelvic peritoneal cytology is obtained. A thorough visual exploration of the peritoneal surfaces of abdomen and pelvis and of the omentum is carried out. Palpation is an added benefit of laparotomy. Aortic lymphadenectomy, including the infrarenal nodes, is then performed. Intraoperative frozen section is requested of the nodes and of any peritoneal lesion, suspicious or not. In the pelvis, most patients will have variable degrees of retroperitoneal fibrosis from previous irradiation and/or surgery, and palpation of the pelvic walls without retroperitoneal dissection will not provide valuable information as to resectability. The degree of fibrosis is directly related to the amount of time that has elapsed since completion of irradiation, and sharp dissection of the pelvic spaces will be necessary. The dissection is performed first on the side with the more lateral extension of the disease. The peritoneum over the psoas muscle is incised from the round ligament, which is transected, to above the pelvic brim. The external iliac vessels are exposed up to the common iliac artery bifurcation. Any enlarged nodes are removed for frozen section. The dissection is continued over the internal iliac artery until its anterior division. The superior vesical artery is followed caudally to the lateral aspect of the bladder. Sometimes, it may be easier to identify the superior vesicle artery by pulling it with a clamp or Russian forceps lateral to the bladder and tracing it in a retrograde fashion to its origin at the internal iliac artery. Mobilizing the superior vesical artery and the bladder medially while holding the external iliac vessels laterally, the paravesical space is developed. This dissection can be more or less tedious depending on the degree of fibrosis. Medial to the internal iliac artery and lateral to the ureter and in the direction of the coccyx, the pararectal space is developed. Significant effort must be made sometimes to open these spaces compared with a nonirradiated pelvis. Between both spaces one can palpate the parametrial web extending inferiorly to the levator muscle. Biopsies of the parametrium must be performed if there is a question of involvement. Pelvic lymphadenectomy is performed if there is any remaining nodal tissue.

In the absence of contraindications, the operation continues to evaluate the resectability of the lesion, the type of pelvic viscera involved, the caudal level of resection, and the excision of other tissues (types I, II, or III; Table 8-1). To determine the type of visceral involvement, the vesicovaginal or rectovaginal spaces may have to be dissected, and biopsies obtained of the bladder or rectal wall if there is a question about the potential for conservation of one of them. In the case of small central recurrences or clearly anterior or posterior lesions, this dissection is not necessary. We have encountered situations in which both organs could be preserved and radical hysterectomy with radical vaginectomy accomplished a complete resection of the lesion. In other instances, extended radical hysterectomy with segmental resection of bladder, ureter, and/or rectum avoided an exenteration on a permanent or temporary basis.[18] These alternative operations, although they may result in a cure, they are associated with a high risk of fistula formation. The caudal level of visceral resection may be determined in the office, such as is the case for vulvar or distal vaginal lesions, or during the examination under anesthesia, but sometimes it cannot be determined until the operation has progressed enough as to clearly determine the full extent of the tumor.

2. Exenterative phase

Once resectability and absence of contraindications have been established, the operation continues to the exenterative phase, tailoring the resection in all directions, ie, lateral, anterior, posterior, and caudally, to obtain negative margins of adequate size.

a. The exenterative phase usually follows an orderly process consisting of:
b. radical or extended radical parametrial resection, and
c. resection of pelvic viscera above or below levators, with or without resection of levators, perineal membrane, and vulva or vulva-perineum-anus.

Because the uterus and vagina are radically removed in all patients, the exenterative phase is started with a radical parametrial and paravaginal resection on the side of more extensive involvement which, depending on the degree of fibrosis and the size, fixation, and extension of the recurrent lesion, may be the most demanding part of the operation. Exceptional situations may be rectal recurrences fixed to the sacrum, especially if occurring after previous rectosigmoid resection with anastomosis, or vulvovaginal lesions fixed to the pubic bone. All exenterative phases are completed abdominally in type I exenterations, about one-half of the type II operations are completed abdominally, and none of the type III operations are completed abdominally.[2] In the latter 2 instances, the exenterative phase is completed through a vulvar approach. Once the lateral parametria have been divided, the operation continues according to the visceral involvement.

Parametrial Resection. The parametrial resection is one of the most important parts of the operation. There are 2 types of parametrial resection, radical and extended radical. The surgeon must recognize the importance of obtaining clear margins, and tailor the resection to the lesion. A tumor extending only to the right requires a complete excision of the right parametrium while being more conservative on the left. A recurrent lesion fixed to the pelvic wall will require an extended radical parametrial resection on that side (see below) while being less radical on the contralateral side. Once the parametrial resection is completed, the caudal extent of the lesion is ascertained again, confirming the level of transection of the pelvic viscera and aiming for wide (about 2 cm) margins.

Radical parametrial resection. The extent of parametrial resection is similar to that of a radical hysterectomy and radical vaginectomy combined, reaching the level of the levator muscles.

The lateral pelvic spaces will have been developed during the exploration phase. With a Deaver retractor in the paravesical space and another in the pararectal space, the parametria are clearly delineated. The parametria are divided at their origin from the hypogastric artery and vein with successive applications of a vessel-sealing device to the level of the levator muscle or between 2 long curved clamps (Shallcross clamps) applied to the entire length of the parametrium. In the latter case, the parametrium is then cut and the pedicle is secured with a running suture, the clamp removed, and then the pedicle is oversewn with the same running suture in the opposite direction and tied. Another option consists in applying a loose continuous running suture from one to the other end of the pedicle, including the clamp in the suture. Hemostasis is obtained by removing the clamp and tightening both ends of the suture. The pedicle is then resutured in the opposite direction (using the same suture) in a continuous-locking fashion and tied at the same end where the suture was started.

With limited mobility, there may be space for only 1 parametrial clamp; once the parametrium is cut, hemostasis can be achieved on the specimen side by applying direct pressure over a laparotomy pad. Sometimes the parametria are markedly thickened from fibrosis or the space so reduced that division by vessel sealing or clamping is not possible and cutting with scissors is the only option, surprisingly with minimal or no bleeding. Any bleeding vessels are secured independently with sutures, clips, or vessel-sealing applications or with pressure over a laparotomy pad.

Extended radical parametrial resection. Resection of the internal iliac arterial and venous system, preferably below the origin of the superior gluteal artery, is sometimes necessary, including the fascia or the pelvic wall muscles with their fascia to obtain a complete tumor resection (Figure 8-6). The lateral extent of the tumor may be secondary to direct extension of the recurrent lesion or due to grossly enlarged, matted, and fixed pelvic nodes. Typically, these nodes are found surrounding the obturator nerve, attached to the obturator internus muscle and pelvic brim, lying atop the lumbosacral trunk and first sacral root. The superior gluteal artery is found exiting the pelvis between the lumbosacral trunk and first sacral root and it is preserved if not involved by tumor. There are usually no major vessels lateral to these lesions that can be separated from the muscular fascia and nerve roots with sharp and blunt dissection. The muscular fascia can be removed to eliminate subclinical disease. Vascular stapling devices provide an expeditious and usually safe division of confluent veins deep on the lateral wall, which may be otherwise difficult to control by suturing, especially if the sutures are not hemostatic. Surgical clips may also be effective.

In exceptional situations in the presence of a long-standing single, isolated, lateral pelvic wall recurrence involving bone, sciatic nerve, and external iliac vessels, and in a patient with intractable pain, the situation can be approached by hind quarter leg amputation (Figure 8-11).

Visceral Resection. The extent of visceral resection, as for parametrial resection, is tailored to the lesion and is defined by the viscera removed (bladder, rectum, or both), and the caudal extent of resection as type I, II, or III. Rarely, 2 operations will be performed identically due to fibrosis, location, size, fixation, and extent of visceral invasion of the recurrent lesions. The rates of the different types of exenterations[2] are indicated below. The 3 most common types of exenterations by order of frequency are total type II, anterior type II, and total type I.[2] Extended exenterations make up approximately 10% of our exenterations and occur more commonly in association with type III exenterations.[2] A detailed technique is provided under total exenteration and further detailed by category and type. In our experience, the exenterative phase is completed abdominally in all patients with type I, in about one-half of the patients with type II, and in none of the patients with type III exenteration.[2]

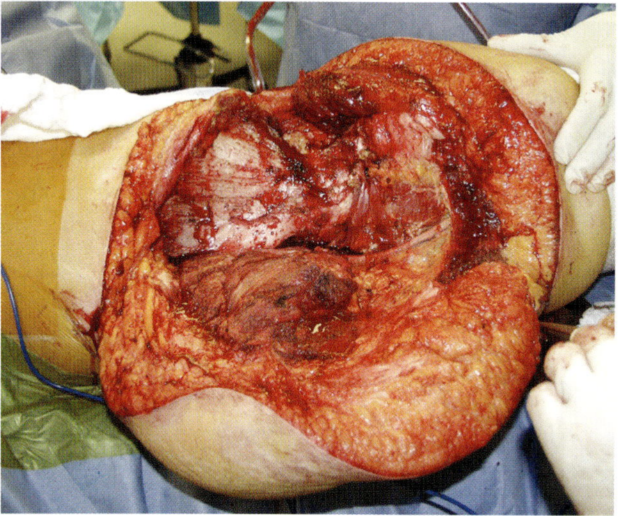

Fig. 8-11. Hindquarter amputation of the right extremity. This patient presented with an isolated pelvic wall recurrence involving external iliac vessels, bone, and sciatic nerve and no metastatic disease. The lesion was unresponsive to previous chemotherapy and had remained stable for 3 years in the absence of any treatment.

Total Exenteration. A radical parametrial resection is performed first (see *Parametrial Resection*) followed by division of the attachments of the bladder and rectum, which are described here. Total type II is the most common type of exenteration in our experience.[2]

Division of the bladder attachments. There are 4 bladder attachments which need to be divided: (1) the peritoneum ventral and lateral to the bladder, (2) the loose areolar connective tissue of the retropubic (Retzius) space, (3) the vascular pedicle of the superior vesical artery, and (4) the bladder attachments to the levator muscle. The peritoneum over the superior aspect of the bladder is incised transversely at the midline and extended toward the round ligament pedicles, following the lateral walls of the bladder, to join the already divided pelvic peritoneum. The bladder is mobilized from the pubic bone by blunt dissection through the retropubic space, communicating the retropubic space with the paravesical spaces, exposing the urethra piercing the levator muscles, and the internal obturator, pubococcygeus, and ileococcygeus muscles. The superior vesical arteries (lateral umbilical ligaments) are divided at each side of the bladder. The attachments of the bladder to the levator muscle are divided from lateral to medial. Distending the bladder with 300 mL of water prior to its mobilization facilitates the identification of the bladder margins, particularly if performed by laparoscopy or robotics.

Division of the rectosigmoid attachments. There are 7 attachments of the rectosigmoid that need to be divided: the pelvic peritoneum at the base (right and left) of the sigmoid mesentery, the loose areolar connective tissue of the presacral space, the sigmoid mesentery (including the vascular pedicles of the superior hemorrhoidal vessels), the sigmoid colon, the vascular pedicles of the middle hemorrhoidal vessels (not always present), Waldeyer's fascia, and the lateral ligaments of the rectum.

With ventral and left lateral traction on the sigmoid, a peritoneal incision is made at the base of the right mesosigmoid starting at the level of the aortic bifurcation and reaching the already incised right pelvic peritoneum in the depths of the pelvis below the right ureter (this preserves the peritoneum attached to the ureter). A symmetrical peritoneal incision is carried out on the left side of the mesosigmoid. By increasing sigmoid traction the air will penetrate the areolar presacral tissue and facilitate the presacral dissection. Using the index and middle fingers, pointing to the rectum, the presacral space is carefully dissected between the mesorectal fascia (on the rectum) and Waldeyer's fascia (on the sacrum) to the level of the levators. There is a typical "swooshing" sound when lifting up the rectum from the sacrum in the correct plane of dissection. The avascular areolar plane of dissection between both of these fascias is known as the "holy plane," because it facilitates a bloodless separation of the rectum from the sacrum. Resistance will be felt at above the level of the levators where the Waldeyer's fascia extends anterolaterally and fuses with the mesorectal fascia, accounting for the feeling of resistance. Waldeyer's fascia must be separated from the mesorectal fascia at this point of attachment with careful blunt dissection or preferably using a cautery with a long tip. Making the mistake of ripping it off from the anterior aspect of the sacrum or dissecting between Waldeyer's fascia and the sacrum may result in severe bleeding from the vertebrobasilar veins. These veins end on small openings on the surface of the sacral bone, draining into a lacunar space inside the sacrum. When disrupted or detached from the sacrum, a rapid and large amount of blood loss will occur. Management of presacral bleeding from these veins is discussed below.

The mesosigmoid should be now free from the sacral promontory and sacrum. The superior hemorrhoidal vessels are selectively sealed and divided, followed by division of the sigmoid mesentery to the point of proximal transection of the sigmoid, avoiding the left ureter. The sigmoid is transected with a stapling device. By ventral and caudal traction on the transected sigmoid further presacral dissection is carried out to the level of the anococcygeal ligament (formed by the retrorectal fusion of both pubococcygeus muscles and inserting to both sides of the coccyx). The vascular pedicles of the middle hemorrhoidal arteries (not always present) are fine structures located in the lateral ligaments of the rectum. The lateral ligaments of the rectum become apparent at its mid-level running posterolaterally and ending caudally into the base of the lower rectum. By advancing the tip of a Shallcross clamp through the distal portion of the lateral ligaments of the rectum and then opening the clamp wide, an avascular space is developed to allow the application of a vessel-sealing device or Shallcross clamp for their division at the levator level. The rectum is ready for transection; however, the level is dependent on the location of the lesion.

Division of the ureters. The ureters are transected above the pelvic brim preserving the peritoneum attached to them and preferably dividing them at a level that is out of the irradiation field.

With division of the parametria, the attachments of the bladder and rectum and ureters, the pelvic viscera are free for distal transection, the level depending on type I, II, and III exenteration, which are described next.

In type I total exenterations, (10% of all exenterations; Figures 8-7 and 8-8),[2] the levator muscles are preserved and the pelvic viscera are transected at or above the levators (Figures 8–12A and B). Using electrocautery, the urethra is transected (and the lumen recognized by the indwelling Foley catheter) followed by the vagina, at or close to the levators. The rectum is cut, using a long scalpel, between a stapling device applied at the point of transection and a Foss clamp is applied proximally. It is not necessary to divide the rectum at the same level as the bladder or vagina as long as the rectal margins are adequate. Preservation of the distal rectum may allow a rectosigmoid anastomosis. The infralevator portions of the urethra, vagina, and rectum and the levator muscles are

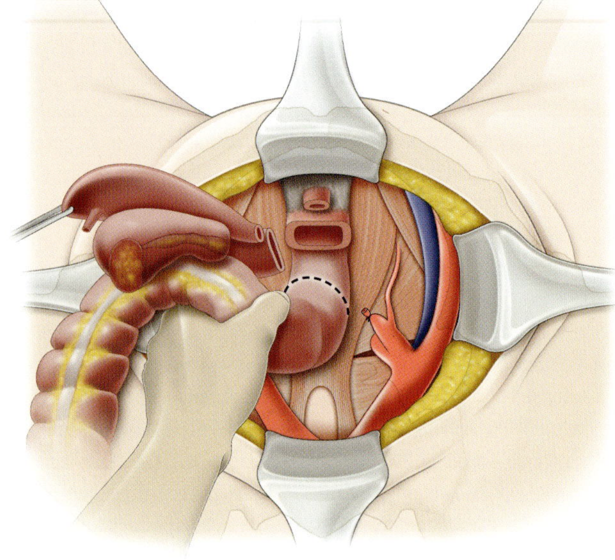

A

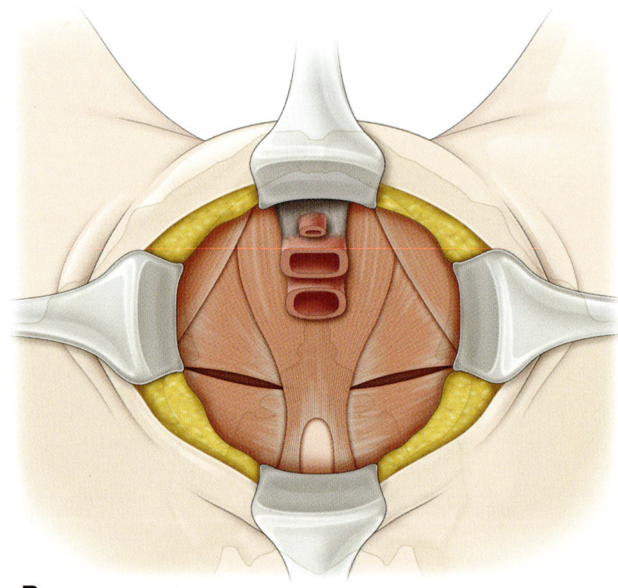

B

Fig. 8-12. (A) Total exenteration type I. The pelvic viscera are transected above the level of the levator muscles. (B) Total exenteration type I. The levator muscles are preserved as well as all infralevator structures.

preserved. Small bleeding is tolerated during the operation until the specimen is removed, followed by meticulous hemostasis. The urethra and vagina are closed with delayed absorbable sutures; alternatively, the vagina is left open at this juncture if a neovagina reconstruction is planned.

Rectosigmoid anastomosis. The proximal sigmoid is brought up to the left lower quadrant as an end colostomy or a rectosigmoid anastomosis is performed in the presence of adequate blood supply to the rectum, an adequate diameter of the sigmoid lumen, and enough length of remaining rectum (preferably ≥ 6 cm above the anorectal junction). Either a hand-sewn or stapled colorectal anastomosis can be performed, according to surgeon preference. If a stapled anastomosis is selected, then a stapling device of the maximum lumenal diameter possible should be utilized. It may be necessary to mobilize the left colon. With contralateral traction on the left colon, an incision is carried out along the white line (of Toldt) up to the splenic flexure. With careful blunt dissection, an avascular plane is developed dorsal to the mesentery of the left colon and ventral to the left ureter and the left kidney, exposing the aorta and abdominal retroperitoneum. If the entire irradiated sigmoid is removed, as it is our preference, then it may be necessary to mobilize the splenic flexure by an orderly transection of the following ligaments: the splenocolic (or colicosplenic) ligament (a double fold of the peritoneum extending from the spleen to the left colon); the phrenocolic (or phrenicocolic) ligament (extending from the left diaphragm to the left colon and attached to the lower pole of the spleen); and, if necessary, the gastrocolic ligament (a portion of the supracolic omentum which consists of attachments of the transverse colon to the stomach). Once these ligaments are divided, using blunt dissection in the same plane of dissection for mobilization of the left colon, the splenic flexure and the transverse colon are mobilized medially, allowing the descending colon to drop into the pelvis for a tension-free anastomosis. An omental J-flap is sutured to the pelvic brim, obturator internus muscle, and pubic bone to cover the entire pelvis. A chest tube No. 26, connected to continuous suction, is left in the pelvis exiting through the anterior abdominal wall. A chest tube is our preferred method of closed-suction drainage, as it will not become clogged with blood clot or debris.

In type II total exenterations (36% of our exenterations; Figures 8-9A to D)[2] the levator muscles are excised to a greater or lesser degree, and the urethra, vagina, and rectum are transected distal to the levator level (Figure 8-13). There are 2 levels of visceral transection in type II exenterations, and are dependent on the caudal margin of the lesion:

a. At or above the urethral meatus, vaginal introitus, and anus (with preservation of the perineum) (Figure 8-9B), or
b. With resection of the urethral meatus, vaginal introitus, perineum, and anus (Figures 8-9C and D).

In the first case, the perineal membrane is preserved and the exenteration is performed abdominally, while in the second case (Figure 8-9D) the medial portion of the perineal membrane (which contains the bulbocavernosus muscles) is

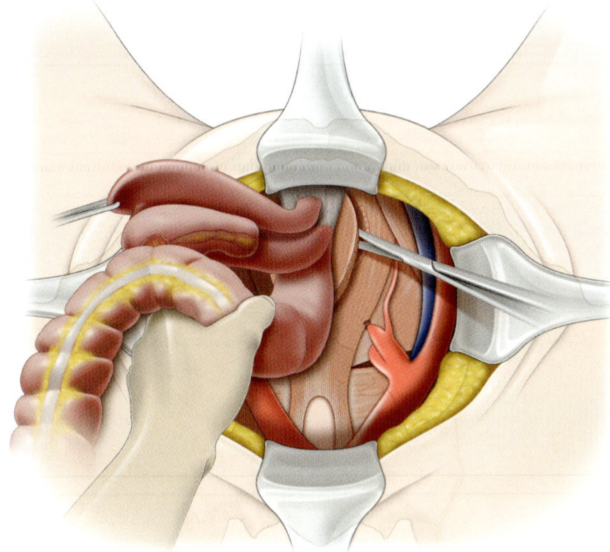

Fig. 8-13 Total exenteration type II. At a difference than type I, the levator muscles are removed with the pelvic viscera and the pelvic viscera transected at a level below the levator muscles.

resected and the resection is completed by an abdominal or vulvar approach, depending on exposure. An almost bloodless exenterative phase will become bloody during transection of the levator muscles and may remain as such until the specimen is removed and there is adequate exposure for meticulous hemostasis.

After the attachments of the bladder and rectum are divided (as described above), the levators are exposed by ventral traction on the viscera. The resection of the levator muscles is carried from ventral to dorsal and the extent of resection is tailored to obtain adequate margins (Figure 8-13A). One will be surprised to see how narrow the levator muscular margins become once they are transected, even if the transection is at their junction with the internal obturator muscle (fascial white line). The pubourethral ligaments, now considered simple extensions of the perineal membrane to the pubic bone, are divided above the urethra, allowing the introduction of the index finger to bluntly detach the urethra from the pubic bone. The levator incision is continued bilaterally detaching the pubococcygeus muscles from the pubic bone and entering the ischiorectal fossa. The levator incision is continued posteriorly following the fascial white line to the ischial spines and from this point the dissection is carried to the anococcygeal ligament or raphe.

a. When the urethral meatus, vaginal introitus, and anus are preserved, the urethra, vagina, and rectum are transected proximally to their external openings and subsequently closed abdominally with delayed absorbable sutures (except the vagina if a vaginal reconstruction is to be performed). The perineal membrane is also preserved. The urethra and vagina are preferably divided with electrocautery.

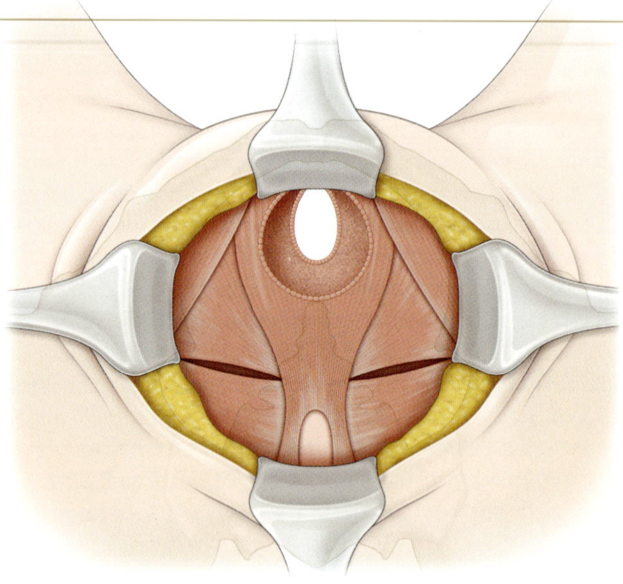

Fig. 8-14. Total exenteration type IIB, including the medial portion of the perineal membrane, urethra, vaginal introitus, perineum, and anus.

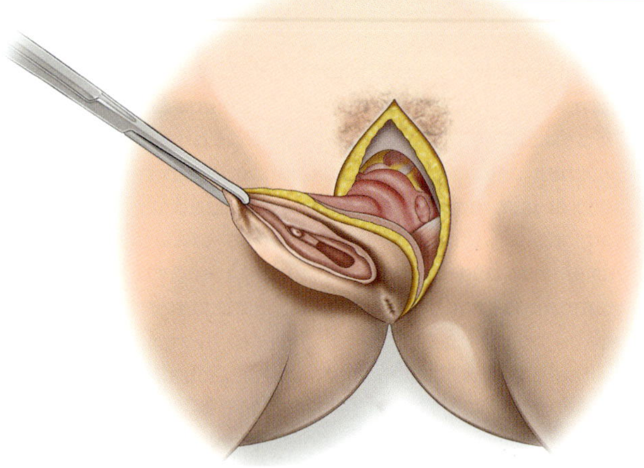

Fig. 8-15. Total exenteration type III. Vulvar phase, including vulvoanusectomy.

A stapling device can be used for the rectal transection, or it can be divided between clamps. It is important to perform the resection below the anorectal junction to avoid mucus formation from residual rectal mucosa.

b. When the entire urethra, vagina, perineum, and anal openings are resected (Figure 8-14), the viscera are pulled cephalad and with the index finger the urethra is further separated from the pubic symphysis by downward pressure until the urethral meatus is reached. Using long curved scissors the mucosa above the urethra is transected outside of the pelvis. By further downward pressure on the urethra with the index finger, the mucosa lateral to the urethral meatus is cut toward the vaginal introitus, and by pulling on the specimen one can excise the entire vaginal introitus (and if not careful the labia minora), the bulbocavernosus muscles (medial portion of the perineal membrane), the perineum and the anus abdominally. After removal of the specimen, a laparotomy pad is placed in the deepest part of the pelvis and the surgeon proceeds to secure hemostasis from the upper part to the deepest part of the pelvis (blood flow follows gravity). Closure may be performed through an abdominal or vulvar approach, depending on the planned reconstruction, exposure (limited in patients who are obese), and extent of resection.

An omental J-flap is created to cover the raw pelvis and is sutured to the pelvic brim, internal obturator muscle, and pubic bone. Two drains are always used. A chest tube No. 26, connected to continuous suction, is left in the pelvis below the omental flap and exiting through the right lower anterior abdominal wall. The large bore of the chest tube will prevent clogging during the postoperative course. A Jackson-Pratt drain is left in the ischiorectal fossa connected to a closed vacuum system and brought out through the anterior vulva, in a site where it will not interfere with sitting.

In type III total exenterations, which account for 5% in our experience[2] (Figures 8-11A to C), a vulvar phase is always required (Figure 8-15). We prefer the vulvo-perineal-anal resection associated with a total type III exenteration to be performed by the operating surgeon while the vulvo-anal closure and/or vulvovaginal reconstruction performed by a second surgeon while the operating surgeon is proceeding to the abdominal reconstruction.

The operation follows the technique of a type IIB exenteration. However, once the parametria and the attachments of the bladder and rectum are divided, the levator muscles may be divided or it may be preferable to leave the levator transection through a vulvo-anal approach, because this part of the operation may be associated with increased blood loss and there is a large surgical field created by the resection of the entire vulva, perineum, and anus. (Figures 8-16A to C). Laparotomy pads are placed and packed tight in the pelvis around the specimen, the self-retracting blades are removed and the abdominal incision is covered with wet blue towels. The patient is placed in a high semilithotomy position. A vulvo-anal incision is centered on the lesion including at least 2 cm of grossly free margins (Figure 8-16B). The incision is continued cephalad to the clitoris and dorsal to the anus, including the labia majora. The vagina and urethra are freed by the division of the perineal membrane (consisting of the ischiocavernosus, bulbocavernosus, and superficial perineal transverse muscles sandwiched between the superficial and inferior fascia of the perineal membrane) along the pubic symphysis, pubic rami, and extending to each ischial tuberosity if needed. The transection will meet the point where the urethra has already been dissected from above and the

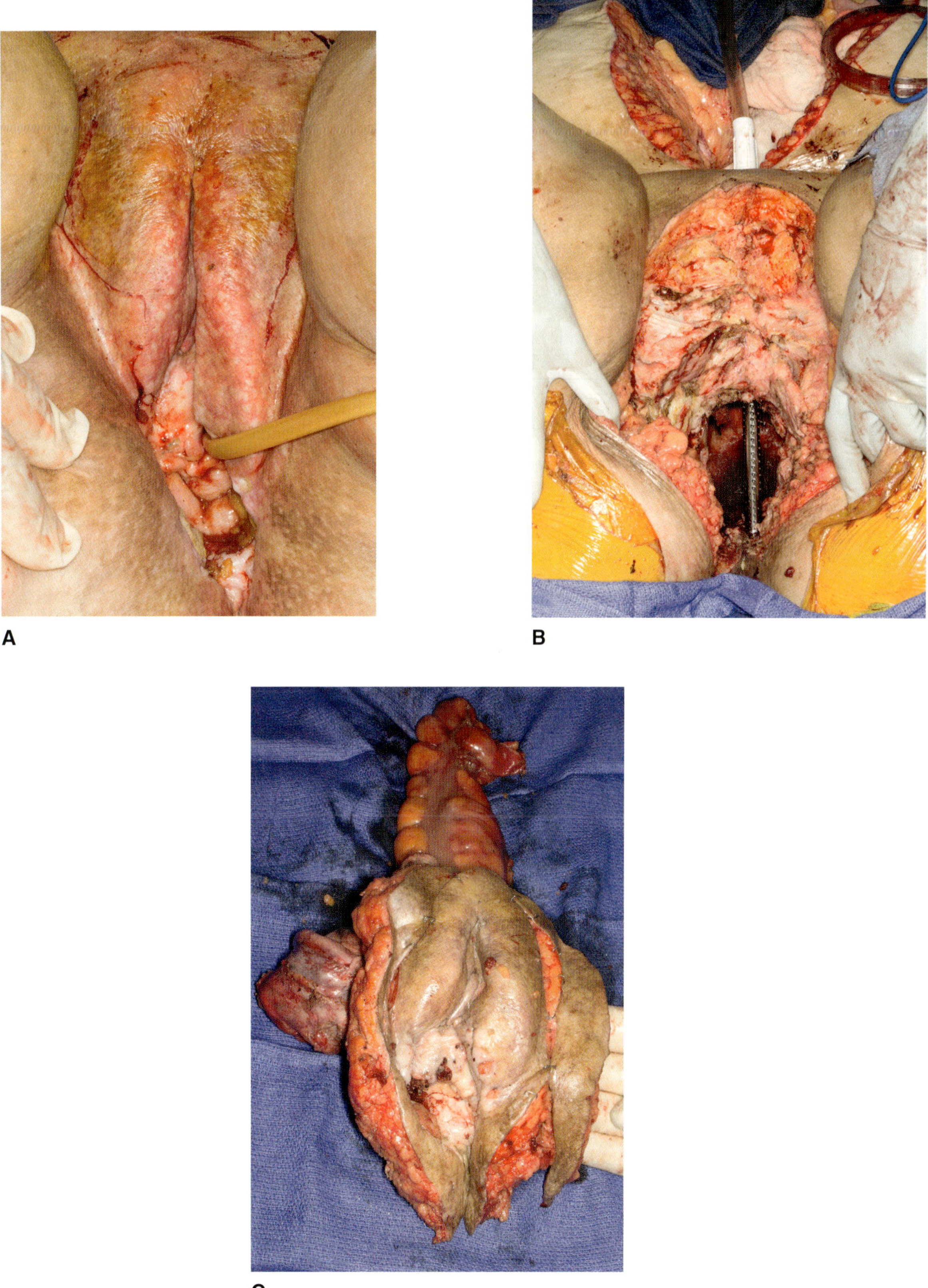

Fig. 8-16. Total exenteration type III. (A) Vulvar recurrence postirradiation and previous excision. (B) Vulvar defect post vulvo-perineal-anal excision. (C) Surgical specimen.

specimen becomes free anteriorly. The next step is to free the specimen posteriorly. There are 3 rectal attachments that need to be divided: the anococcygeal ligament or raphe, the levator muscles, and the inferior hemorrhoidal vascular pedicles. The incision dorsal to the anus is carried into the deep soft tissue, transecting the anococcygeal ligament in the midline (unless already performed abdominally) until the laparotomy pads left in the pelvis are identified. By sliding the index finger in the midline of the presacral space, the remaining levator muscles or attachments of the rectum to the levator muscles are identified and divided with a cautery over a finger, first on the right, leaving a laparotomy pad for hemostasis, and then on the left side. The inferior hemorrhoidal pedicles are divided bilaterally at about the 4 and 8 o'clock positions, as well as any remaining attachments of the rectum or vagina. Once the specimen is free, it is pulled through the large vulvo-perineal-anal defect. Meticulous hemostasis is performed reaching as cephalad as possible, because it may be easier than through an abdominal approach.

There are 3 options for the management of the vulvo-perineal-anal wound: primary closure, closure with a large pedicle flap, or closure with vaginal reconstruction. The latter 2 methods are described in the *Vulvovaginal and Pelvic Floor Reconstruction* section. For primary closure, the levator muscles are sutured first to each other in the midline if possible with interrupted delayed absorbable sutures, and then the fat tissue of the ischiorectal fossa is sutured to the midline to eliminate dead space. The vulvar incision is closed with interrupted nonabsorbable monofilament sutures and a Jackson-Pratt drain connected to a closed vacuum system is left in the ischiorectal fossa and brought out through the anterior vulva, in a site where it will allow for comfortable sitting. The patient is repositioned in a low semilithotomy position, the wet towels are removed, the self-retracting blades reinserted, and the laparotomy pads are removed. Meticulous hemostasis is performed. An omental J-flap is created to cover the raw pelvis and is sutured to the pelvic brim, internal obturator muscle, and pubic bone. A chest tube No. 26, connected to continuous suction, is left in the pelvis below the omental flap and exiting through the right lower anterior abdominal wall.

Anterior Exenteration. Radical parametrial resection is performed first followed by separation of the rectum from the vagina, transection of the uterosacral ligaments, and division of the bladder attachments.

Separation of vagina from rectum. Once the parametria are resected, the peritoneum of the cul-de-sac is incised transversely at its deepest portion and extended laterally to the already transected pelvic peritoneum. The rectovaginal space is bluntly or sharply dissected, depending on the degree of fibrosis, to the level of the levator muscles. The lateral rectal walls, which creep up on the medial aspect of the uterosacral ligaments, are bluntly reflected dorsally, thus exposing the dorsal aspect of the uterosacral ligaments that are divided at the level of the lateral rectal wall. With ventral and lateral traction on the specimen, any distal paravaginal tissues are divided. The specimen is free of its rectal and lateral attachments.

Division of the bladder attachments. There are 4 bladder attachments which need to be divided: the peritoneum ventral and lateral to the bladder, the loose areolar connective tissue of the retropubic space (of Retzius), the vascular pedicle of the superior vesical artery, and the bladder attachments to the levator muscle. The peritoneum over the superior aspect of the bladder is transversely incised at the midline and extended toward the round ligament pedicles, following the lateral walls of the bladder, to join the already divided pelvic peritoneum. The bladder is mobilized from the pubic bone by blunt dissection through the retropubic space, communicating the retropubic space with the paravesical spaces, exposing the urethra piercing the levator muscles, and the obturator internus, pubococcygeus and ileococcygeus muscles. The superior vesical arteries (lateral umbilical ligaments) are divided at each side of the bladder. The attachments of the bladder to the levator muscle are divided from lateral to medial. Distending the bladder with 300 mL of water prior to its mobilization facilitates the identification of the bladder margins, particularly if performed by laparoscopic or robotic surgery.

Type I Anterior Exenterations. Type I anterior exenterations account for 8% of exenterations in our experience,[2] the levator muscles are preserved, and the urethra and vagina are transected at or above the levators. Using electrocautery, the urethra is transected (and its lumen recognized by the indwelling Foley catheter) followed by the division of the vagina, and any remaining attachments to the levators, at or close to the levator muscles. The specimen is removed. The urethra, distal vagina, rectum, anus, and the entire levator muscles are preserved. Some small bleeding is tolerated until the specimen is removed to accomplish an expeditious operation but meticulous hemostasis should be achieved once the specimen is removed. The urethra and vagina (if no reconstruction is planned) are closed with delayed absorbable sutures. An omental J-flap is used to cover the entire pelvis and is sutured to the lateral rectal walls, pelvic brim, internal obturator muscle, and pubic bone. A closed suction drain is placed in the pelvis, as previously described.

Type II Anterior Exenterations. These are the second most common type of exenterations in our experience (16%),[2] and in this type of resection the bladder and vagina are transected below the level of the levators, including the ventral aspect of the levator muscles. There are 2 levels of distal transection of the pelvic viscera in type II anterior exenterations depending on the caudal extent of the lesion:

a. At or above the level of the urethral meatus and vaginal introitus, or
b. With resection of the urethral meatus and vaginal introitus.

When the transection is above the vaginal introitus, the perineal membrane is preserved and the exenteration is performed abdominally. On the other hand, when the urethral meatus and vaginal introitus are resected, the medial portion of the perineal membrane (which contains the bulbocavernosus muscles) is also excised and the exenteration is completed either through an abdominal or vulvar approach.

With ventral traction on the viscera, the levator muscles are exposed. The resection of the levators is carried from ventral to dorsal and the extent of their resection is tailored to obtain adequate margins. The pubourethral ligaments, now considered simple extensions of the perineal membrane to the pubic bone, are divided with electrocautery above the urethra, allowing the introduction of the index finger to bluntly detach the urethra from the pubic bone. The levator incision is started adjacent to the urethra and pubic bone using electrocautery and continued bilaterally following the pubic bone toward the fascial white line, detaching the pubococcygeus muscles from the pubic bone and exposing the ischiorectal fossa. The levator incision is continued posteriorly over the fascial white line to the ischial spines and toward the lateral rectal wall, preserving the dorsal levator muscles and anococcygeal ligament.

With the use of electrocautery, the urethra is transected above or including the urethral meatus. Similarly, the vagina is resected at the level of the introitus or slightly above. By pulling on the specimen one can excise the entire urethral meatus and vaginal introitus, avoiding a vulvar phase for resection. The specimen is removed. A laparotomy pad is left in the depth of the pelvis and hemostasis is obtained from the pelvic brim to the deep aspects of the pelvis. Closure of the vulvar incision may be performed through and abdominal or vulvar approach, depending on exposure and the planned reconstruction. Two drains are always used. A Jackson-Pratt drain is left in the ischiorectal fossa connected to a closed vacuum system and brought out through the anterior vulva at a site where it will allow for comfortable sitting. A chest tube No. 26, connected to continuous suction, is left in the pelvis exiting through the right lower anterior abdominal wall. A chest tube will not become clogged.

Type III Anterior Exenterations. Type III anterior exenterations account for 5% of all exenteration[2] and are similar in scope to the type IIb operation; however, in the type III variant the extent of resection includes the entire perineal membrane and vulva. After the parametria, the paravaginal tissues and the bladder attachments are divided and the vagina is separated from the rectum; the levator muscles are transected abdominally, which is a difference from a type III total exenteration in which they may be divided through a vulvar approach. The extensions of the perineal membrane to the pubic bone (previously known as pubourethral ligaments) are divided above the urethra, allowing the introduction of the index finger to bluntly detach the urethra from the pubic bone. The levator incision is started adjacent to the urethra and pubic bone and continued laterally toward the fascial white line and ischial spine, exposing the ischiorectal fossa. From the ischial spine, the excision is directed toward the level of transection of the uterosacral ligaments, preserving the dorsal levator muscles and anococcygeal ligament. Laparotomy pads are packed tight in the pelvis around the specimen, the self-retracting blades are removed and the abdominal incision is covered with wet towels. The patient is placed in a high semilithotomy position.

A circumscribing vulvar incision is made and centered on the recurrent lesion to obtain at least 2 cm of gross free margins. The incision is continued ventrally to include the clitoris and a portion of the mons pubis if needed, laterally to include the labia majora, and extended dorsally toward the perineum just below the posterior vaginal wall, as one would do for a rectocele repair, to meet the contralateral incision. The perineal membrane (including the superficial and inferior fascia and the ischiocavernosus, bulbocavernosus, and superficial perineal transverse muscles) is excised from the pubic symphysis to each ischial tuberosity; while deepening the perineal membrane incision, the pelvic laparotomy pads are identified. The rectovaginal space is dissected through the transverse perineal incision until it meets the level of dissection accomplished abdominally. Any remaining attachments to the levator muscles are divided.

Meticulous hemostasis is performed reaching as cephalad as possible, although exposure will be reduced as compared with type III total exenteration.

There are 3 options for the management of the vulvar wound, ie, primary closure, closure with a large pedicle flap, or closure with vaginal reconstruction. The latter 2 methods are described in the *Vulvovaginal and Pelvic Floor Reconstruction* section. For primary closure, any remaining levator muscles are sutured to the midline with absorbable interrupted sutures, as well as the fat tissue of the ischiorectal fossa, to eliminate dead space. The vulvar skin is closed with interrupted nonabsorbable monofilament sutures. A Jackson-Pratt drain is left in the ischiorectal fossa connected to a closed vacuum system and brought out through the anterior vulva, at a site where it will allow for comfortable sitting. The patient is then repositioned in a low semilithotomy position, the wet towels are removed, the self-retracting blades reinserted, and the laparotomy pads are removed. An omental J-flap is used to cover the raw pelvis and sutured to the rectum, pelvic brim, obturator internus muscle, and pubic bone. A chest tube No. 26, connected to continuous suction, is left in the pelvis below the omental J-flap and exteriorized through the right lower anterior abdominal wall.

Posterior Exenteration. Posterior exenteration is the least frequently performed procedure for several reasons. The cervix is not in direct contact with the rectum (although the bladder is) due to the interposition of the cul-de-sac peritoneum. For this reason, cervical cancer recurrences will usually invade the bladder first. The dissection of the vesicovaginal space and the ureters may be difficult or impossible due to radiation fibrosis and is associated with a high risk of vesical or ureteral fistula. For this reason, and not uncommonly, a planned posterior exenteration will evolve into a total exenteration when the bladder dissection is not possible or carries a high risk for fistula formation.

A radical parametrial resection is performed first, followed by separation of the bladder from the vagina, parametrial ureteral dissection, and rectosigmoid resection.

Separation of the vagina from the bladder and parametrial ureteral dissection. Separation of the vagina from the bladder and parametrial ureteral dissection requires 3 steps: dissection of the vesicovaginal space, division of the vesicouterine ligaments (ventral and sometimes dorsal), and division of the paravaginal tissues. It is preferable to preserve as much of the anterior vaginal wall as possible, even if only in its distal part, to prevent fistula formation and maintain some degree of vesical neck and bladder support.

Once the parametrial resection is accomplished, the vesicovaginal space is sharply dissected for a satisfactory distance to obtain an adequate anterior margin of surgical resection, and preferably with the bladder distended with 200 to 300 mL of water to facilitate the identification of the correct dissecting plane in the presence of fibrosis. The ureters are left attached to the lateral pelvic peritoneum until the point at which they cross under the uterine arteries, where they are separated from the pelvic peritoneum. With the bladder retracted with a manual or self-retaining retractor, the tip of a Shallcross clamp is advanced into the parametrial tunnel at the 12 o'clock position along the ureteral adventitia, and carefully advanced until it exits the tunnel near the anterior vaginal wall, separating the ventral vesicouterine ligament from the ureter. The ventral vesicouterine ligament is divided, exposing (or "unroofing") the ureter, which is mobilized laterally with short touches of an electrocautery or scissors until it is lifted from the vaginal wall, exposing the dorsal vesicouterine ligament, which is then divided if necessary. This allows the division of the lower paravaginal tissues and the attachments of the vagina and rectum to the levator muscles.

Division of the rectosigmoid attachments. There are 7 attachments of the rectosigmoid that need to be divided: the pelvic peritoneum at the base (right and left) of the sigmoid mesentery, the loose areolar connective tissue of the presacral space, the sigmoid mesentery (including the vascular pedicles of the superior hemorrhoidal vessels), the sigmoid colon, the vascular pedicles of the middle hemorrhoidal vessels (not always present), Waldeyer's fascia, and the lateral ligaments of the rectum.

With ventral and left lateral traction on the sigmoid colon, a peritoneal incision is made at the base of the right mesosigmoid starting at the level of the aortic bifurcation and connected to the already incised right pelvic peritoneum in the depths of the pelvis below the right ureter (this preserves the peritoneum attached to the ureter). A symmetrical peritoneal incision is carried out on the left side of the mesosigmoid. By increasing sigmoid traction, the air will penetrate the areolar presacral tissue and facilitate the presacral dissection. Using the index and middle fingers, pointing to the rectum, the presacral space is carefully dissected between the mesorectal fascia (on the rectum) and Waldeyer's fascia (on the sacrum) to the level of the levators. There is a typical "swooshing" sound when lifting up the rectum from the sacrum in the correct plane of dissection. The avascular areolar plane of dissection between both of these fascias is known as the "holy plane," because it facilitates a bloodless separation of the rectum from the sacrum. Resistance will be felt at or above the level of the levators where the Waldeyer's fascia extends anterolaterally and fuses with the mesorectal fascia, therefore the feeling of resistance. Waldeyer's fascia must be separated from the mesorectal fascia at this point of attachment with careful blunt dissection or preferably using a cautery with a long tip. Making the mistake of avulsing it off from the anterior aspect of the sacrum or dissecting between Waldeyer's fascia and the sacrum may result in severe bleeding from the vertebrobasilar veins. These veins end on small openings on the surface of the sacral bone, draining into a lacunar space inside the sacrum. When disrupted or detached from the sacrum, a rapid and large amount of blood loss will occur. Management of presacral bleeding from these veins is discussed below (section on Presacral Bleeding).

The mesosigmoid should be now free from the sacral promontory and sacrum. The superior hemorrhoidal vessels are selectively sealed and divided, followed by division of the sigmoid mesentery to the point of proximal transection of the sigmoid, avoiding the left ureter. The sigmoid is transected with a stapling device. By ventral and caudal traction on the transected sigmoid colon, further presacral dissection is carried out to the level of the anococcygeal ligament (formed by the retrorectal fusion of both pubococcygeus muscles and inserting to both sides of the coccyx). The vascular pedicles of the middle hemorrhoidal arteries (not always present) are fine structures located in the lateral ligaments of the rectum. The lateral ligaments of the rectum become apparent at its midlevel running posterolaterally and ending caudally into the base of the lower rectum. By advancing the tip of a Shallcross clamp through the distal portion of the lateral ligaments of the rectum and then widely opening the clamp, an avascular space is developed, wide enough to allow the application of a vessel-sealing device or Shallcross clamp for their division of the lateral ligaments at the levator level. The rectum is ready for transection, the level depending on the location of the lesion. The resection is continued as described for a type I, II, or III procedure, depending on the location of the tumor.

Type I Posterior Exenteration. In our experience, type I posterior exenteration is the most uncommonly performed exenteration (1%).[2] In the presence of a rectal stump of sufficient length (measuring ≥ 6 cm from the anorectal junction), adequate blood supply to the rectum, and an adequate size of the lumen of the sigmoid and rectum, this type of exenteration allows for a rectosigmoid anastomosis. Mobilization of the left colon and splenic flexure may be necessary for a tension-free anastomosis.

The anterior vagina is transected at the previously selected level, preserving as much length as possible but without compromising margins. The posterior vaginal wall may be transected more distally if needed. A stapling device is applied at the point of transection of the rectum and a Foss clamp is applied proximally and the rectum cut in between with a scalpel. The specimen is removed and the vagina is closed with delayed absorbable suture, unless a vaginal reconstruction is planned. The proximal sigmoid colon is anastomosed to the rectal stump or is brought up to the left lower quadrant as an end colostomy.

Rectosigmoid anastomosis. In the presence of adequate blood supply to the rectum, an adequate diameter of the sigmoid lumen, and sufficient length of the remaining rectum (preferably ≥ 6 cm above the anorectal junction), rectosigmoid anastomosis may be performed. The technical procedure for colorectal anastomosis is the same as described above for a type I total exenteration.

Type II Posterior Exenteration. In the type II posterior exenteration, which accounts for 5% of exenterations,[2] the uterus, vagina, rectosigmoid, and the dorsal aspect of the levator muscles and perineal membrane are resected. Once the radical parametrial resection, the separation of the bladder from the vagina, the parametrial ureteral dissection, and the division of the rectal attachments are completed, the bladder is held with a wide Deaver manually or with a wide self-retracting bladder blade. This maneuver enhances the exposure of the rectovaginal space and prevents unintentional bladder or ureteral injury. The levator muscle is transected with an electrocautery starting at the level of the lateral walls of the vagina and proceeding posteriorly to the anococcygeal ligament or raphe, which is also transected, entering the ischiorectal fossa posteriorly. A transverse incision is made on the upper vagina and continued along the lateral walls of the vagina to the appropriate level of transection. The posterior vaginal wall may be transected at a lower level than the anterior one, if possible, to preserve as much as of the anterior vaginal wall as possible. The posterior vaginal wall is left attached to the rectum.

There are 2 options for the distal transection of the posterior vagina and rectum:

a. above the vaginal introitus and anus, or
b. with resection of the vaginal introitus, perineum, and anus.

By pulling on the specimen, the vagina is transected above the vaginal introitus, the perineum is preserved, and the rectum is cut at the level of the anorectal junction. This is a type IIa exenteration. When the transection includes the vaginal introitus, the perineum, and the anus, the dorsal and medial portion of the perineal membrane is also excised (including the superficial perineal muscle and the posterior aspect of the bulbocavernosus muscle). This is a type IIb exenteration and is usually completed through a vulvar approach.

There are 3 options for the management of the vulvo-anal wound: primary closure, closure with a large pedicle flap, or closure with vaginal reconstruction. The latter 2 methods are described in the *Vulvovaginal and Pelvic Floor Reconstruction* section. For primary closure, the levator muscles are sutured to each other in the midline, if possible, with interrupted absorbable sutures followed by closure of the fat tissue of the ischiorectal fossa to eliminate dead space. The vulvar and perianal skin are sutured to the midline with interrupted nonabsorbable monofilament sutures and a Jackson-Pratt drain connected to a closed vacuum system is left in the ischiorectal fossa and brought out through the anterior vulva, at a site where it will allow for comfortable sitting. The patient is then placed in a low semilithotomy position, the self-retracting blades replaced, and the wet towels and laparotomy pads are removed.

An omental J-flap is used to cover the entire pelvis and is sutured to the lateral rectal walls, pelvic brim, obturator internus muscle, and bladder peritoneum. A chest tube No. 26 connected to continuous suction is left in the pelvis below the omental flap, exiting through the right lower anterior abdominal wall.

Type III Posterior Exenteration. Type III posterior exenterations account for 3% of exenterations[2] and are usually performed for vulvar, anorectal or distal, vaginal lesions involving the posterior vaginal wall. Occasionally this operation is performed for primary tumors of the same locations not amenable to chemoirradiation. In addition to the uterus, vagina and rectum, levator muscles, and perineal membrane, the vulva, perineum, and perianal tissues are extensively resected, leaving a much larger defect than in a type IIB posterior exenteration (Figures 8-17A to C). Recurrent rectal malignancy following previous surgery, irradiation, or both is usually densely attached to the sacrum and difficult to excise.

The abdominal portion of the exenterative phase is carried out as a type IIB posterior exenteration; however, the resection of the levator muscles may be left for a vulvo-anal approach. Laparotomy pads are placed and packed tight in the pelvis around the specimen, the retracting blades are removed, and the abdominal incision is covered with wet towels. The patient is placed in a high semilithotomy position. A perianal incision is started dorsal to the anus and continued toward the anterior vaginal wall, including the perianal tissues and the posterior aspect of the labia majora. The dorsal aspect of the perineal membrane is resected as lateral as the pubic bone and ischial tuberosity if needed. The specimen needs to be mobilized posteriorly from its 3 attachments, ie, anococcygeal ligament or raphe, levator muscles, and inferior hemorrhoidal vascular pedicles. The incision dorsal to the anus is carried deeper into the soft tissues, transecting the anococcygeal raphe or ligament with electrocautery (unless already performed abdominally) and continuing until the laparotomy pads left at the completion of the abdominal part are identified. By sliding a couple of fingers in the midline of the lower presacral space, the remaining levator muscles or attachment of the rectum to the levator muscles are identified and divided with a cautery over the fingers, first on the right, leaving a laparotomy pad for hemostasis, and then on the left side. The inferior hemorrhoidal pedicles are ligated bilaterally at about the 4 and 8 o'clock positions, and the remaining connective tissue attachments of the rectum and posterior vagina are divided. The specimen is pulled through the vulvo-anal defect. Meticulous hemostasis is performed reaching as cephalad as possible since it may be easier than through an abdominal approach.

As previously described, there are 3 options for the management of the vulvo-anal wound, ie, primary closure, closure with a large pedicle flap, or closure with vaginal reconstruction.

Extended Exenterations. Extended exenterations account for 11% of exenterations.[2] In circumstances where

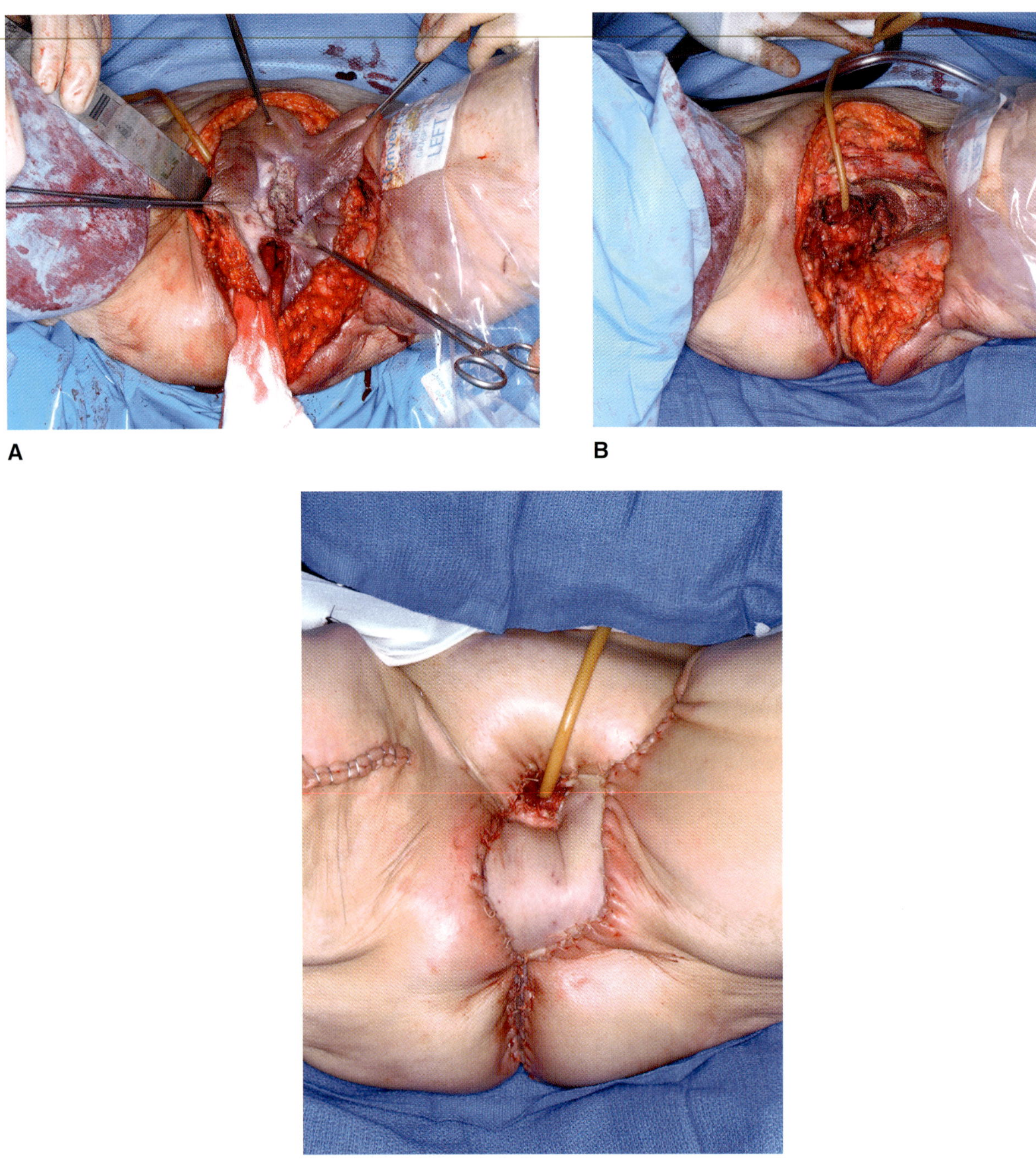

Fig. 8-17. Extended posterior exenteration type III. (A) Vulvar-perineal-anal excision. (B) Vulvar defect including partial resection of left pubic ramus and adductor muscles. (C) Closure with gracilis muscle pedicle flap.

localized, recurrent pelvic cancer is fixed to or is invading other soft tissues or bone, the surgeon must decide during the exploration phase whether it is resectable, whether a complete resection can be achieved, and the value of such resection in regard to the associated morbidity, long-term sequelae, and cure rate. About 1 in 10 of patients in our series underwent an extended exenteration, which was necessary in 2% of anterior, 5% of posterior, and 5% of total exenterations and they were more commonly associated with type III resection. The type of additional tissues resected is dependent on the type of exenteration, which is dictated by the size and location of the lesion. For instance, the small bowel was the most commonly resected additional tissue in type I, followed by type II (33%; due to the cephalad growth of the recurrent lesions), while there were no bowel resections in type III procedures (performed for distal lesions). For the same reasons, groin node dissection was performed in 86% of patients with type III exenterations while there were none in the other 2 types. Lateral recurrences fixed to the external iliac vessels and invading the psoas muscle may require segmental resection of the psoas muscle (Figure 8-5). Lateral recurrences fixed to pelvic wall fascia may require an extended radical parametrectomy with resection of pelvic wall fascia and muscles (Figure 8-6). In lower vaginal lesions requiring a type II or III exenteration, the lesion may be attached or invade portions of the pubic bone (Figure 8-17B), which is resectable.

Rectal recurrences, especially when resulting from a primary cancer of the rectum, commonly will attach or invade the sacrum. Resection of the sacrum can be accomplished whenever the involvement is below the S2 level (Figure 8-4). Lesions involving the sacrum proximal to S2 are considered unresectable. Through a vulvar approach, the coccyx and lower sacrum are dissected from the subcutaneous tissue up to the level of sacral transection. The sacrospinal and sacrotuberal ligaments, and the coccygeal muscles are transected first followed by sacral transection. Vulvovaginal or vulvar recurrences may require bilateral groin node dissection and, depending on their location, may require segmental resection of the pubic bone, ischial tuberosity, or coccyx. In rare and highly selected situations, a lower extremity may be removed in association with an exenteration (Figure 8-11).

3. Hemostasis phase

Once the viscera are removed and surgical exposure has been optimized, meticulous hemostasis must be obtained by the use of electrocautery, sutures, clips, or temporary pressure. Hemostatic substances may occasional be of use and the surgeon must ensure they are available and learn their applications and risks prior to the procedure. The surgical field will continue to ooze for several days from all deperitonealized surfaces. For that reason, a suction drain is always left in the depths of the pelvis exiting through the lower anterior abdominal wall, and a second one exiting through the vulva in types II and III exenterations. Our preference is to use a chest tube No. 26 connected to continuous wall suction because it will not become clogged. It is removed when the drainage is about 50 mL or less in 24 hours.

When facing a bleeding site that cannot be completely controlled by any of the common hemostatic measures available, the pelvis may be heavily packed with long gauzes or multiple laparotomy pads attached to each other, laying over a chest tube placed near the bleeding site (see Lateral Pelvic Wall Bleeding).

Management of Intraoperative Bleeding. Every surgeon who has performed enough of these operations has been surprised by how quickly the entire pelvis can be filled with blood when a parametrial suture has failed or pelvic veins have retracted behind a suture. The following are suggestions for management of a few bleeding situations which they usually occur when least expected and will tax the skills of any surgeon.

Lateral Pelvic Wall Bleeding. Severe lateral pelvic wall bleeding is usually from transected confluent veins and it is sometimes difficult to visualize the bleeding vessels. Pressure with a gauze pack and lifting up gingerly one edge at a time, with the assistant handling preferably two suction devices, will be helpful to visualize the bleeding site. Strong irrigation will wipe out any residual blood and allow the bleeding source to be localized, which then can be clamped, clipped, or controlled with finger pressure. Clips are most useful in deep areas since there is no need for tying. The surgeon must have a straight and a right-angle clip applier available for a perpendicular placement of the clips to the bleeding vessel. Sewing below the fingertip as the finger pressure is slightly released using a fine needle and suture (4-0 Prolene, eg, precut to 5 cm and with a LAPRA-TY [Ethicon, Somerville, New Jersey] at its end), and taking wide and deep bites may catch any retracted veins or occlude them by tension of the overlying tissues. Once the bleeding is controlled, the suture is secured with another LAPRA-TY (Ethicon, Somerville, New Jersey), eliminating the need to tying in a deep area and the associated the risk of avulsing the veins. If there are any nerve roots (lumbosacral trunk, sacral roots) near the bleeding site, they must be exposed to ensure they are excluded from the hemostatic sutures. In spite of precise, hemostatic sutures the bleeding may be decreased but not completely controlled. Applying a hemostatic substance over the oozing site or on the surface of a laparotomy pack and leaving the pack in place with pressure by a malleable blade attached to the retractor ring or by a Harrington retractor held by the second assistant may provide hemostasis while the operation continues in the opposite site. If by the end there is still persistent bleeding or oozing, then leaving a long gauze tightly packed for 3 days with an end exiting through the perineal wound or a small incision in the lower abdomen will likely control the oozing site. If bleeding persists in spite of packing, as noted by drain suction and decreasing hemoglobin (Hgb) values in spite of blood transfusions, then a MAST (Military Anti-Shock Trousers) suit for 48 hours will probably be effective.[19] In desperate situations, the surgeon may leave a hemostatic clamp in situ, close the abdomen, and return to the operating room for removal 2 to 3 days later.

Arterial bleeding is easier to see and, thus, to manage. However, major injuries to the aorta, common iliac, or external iliac vessels require an expert vascular surgeon and the use of selective techniques.

Presacral Bleeding. Bleeding from the sacrum above Waldeyer's fascia is easy to control with pressure, fine sutures or clips. These bleeding veins are laying on the surface of the upper sacrum and are easy to identify and control. Dangerous and rapid bleeding occurs with disruption of the vertebro-basilar veins below Waldeyer's fascia. These veins end on the surface of the sacral bone, draining their blood directed into a lacunar space inside the sacrum. If disrupted and detached from the sacrum, a rapid and large amount of blood loss will occur. Packing and pressure will control the bleeding temporarily. Because there are only small venous openings on the sacral surface with no vein endings to suture, the only effective hemostatic measure is to plug the bleeding openings by muscle coagulation. A 1 × 1 × 1 cm segment of rectus (or any other muscle) is cut and held against the bleeding hole by the tip of a long clamp (without grasping the muscle). The tip of an electrocautery (at 100 watts) is applied to the long clamp until the muscle is desiccated, becoming fixed to the bone, and plugging the bleeding hole. Bone wax is difficult to use because it will stick to your fingers or instrument used to apply it and will not effectively plug the bleeding site.

Levator Muscles Bleeding. In infralevator exenterations it is advisable to leave the transection of the levators until all other attachments are divided and to proceed expeditiously during that part of the operation. Transection of the levators may be the first major blood loss of the operation. The edges of the transected levator muscles, even when using an electrocautery connected to a coagulating current, may result in continuous blood loss until the specimen is removed and there is improved visualization for hemostasis. Continuous cautery application to the bleeding muscle may not be effective due to tissue or blood carbonization, and lifting up a sticky cautery tip may restart the bleeding. To prevent this, continuous suction is applied at the bleeding site while a long DeBakey forceps with closed ends is applied directly over the bleeding muscle and the tip of an electrocautery (at 80 watts) is applied to the DeBakey forceps.

4. Reconstructive phase

There are 2 reconstructive phases:

a. Abdominal, which includes the urinary and intestinal tracts and pelvic floor management, and
b. Vulvovaginal, which addresses vaginal reconstruction, vulvo-anal wound, and pelvic floor management.

Reconstruction is discussed in the sections on *Gastrointestinal Tract, Urinary Tract,* and *Vulvovaginal and Pelvic Floor Reconstruction.*

POSTOPERATIVE CARE

Box 8-3 PERIOPERATIVE MORBIDITY

- The most common immediate stoma complications are ischemia/ necrosis and retraction
- The most common delayed stoma problems are parastomal hernias and stenosis
- Bowel obstruction and intestinal fistulas are the most common intestinal complications
- Metabolic acidosis may be an early and/or delayed complication and is dependent on the type of urinary reconstruction
- Ureteral leaks generally occur in the immediate postoperative period, while ureteral strictures are delayed problems

Care in the immediate postoperative period following exenterative surgery should be individualized according to the specific medical condition of the patient and the extent of the procedure performed. In most cases of exenterative surgery, a period of observation in an intensive care unit setting for 24 to 72 hours is advisable. Routine nasogastric tube decompression is unnecessary. In general, oral feeding can be resumed once the patient is extubated and bowel sounds are present; however, some surgeons prefer to wait for advance diet until passage of flatus per rectum or colostomy. Parenteral nutrition should be considered if there is evidence of malnutrition (serum albumin < 3.0 g/dL) preoperatively or a prolonged period (> 7 days) of bowel rest is anticipated. Prophylactic antibiotics should be re-dosed during or immediately after the operation, depending on the duration of the procedure. In instances of gross fecal contamination, antibiotic coverage should be extended 72 hours following surgery. Incisions, flaps, and stomas should be inspected daily for integrity and evidence of vascular perfusion. Mechanical and pharmacologic thromboembolic prophylaxis should be continued at least until the patient is fully ambulatory.

Postoperative Complications

Postoperative complications are common, occurring in about 1 in 2 patients,[2,4,20-22] and, although varying in type, they occur with an overall similar frequency among the 3 types of exenterations.[2] The risk of complications is related to multiple factors, including the medical condition and nutritional status of the patient, history of previous surgery, prior irradiation, the extent of pelvic viscera removed, the type of exenteration, the length of the operation, the amount of blood loss, the techniques of reconstruction of the urinary and intestinal tracts and the vagina, and the method of reconstructing the pelvic floor. For instance, reconstruction of the pelvic floor with an omental flap or vaginal reconstruction with pedicle grafts, which brings a new blood supply to the empty pelvis, is associated with a decreased complication rate, especially of intestinal origin (48% vs 82%).[20] Bringing a new blood supply to the pelvis reduces the rates of intestinal obstruction (12% vs 28%)[20] and/or enteric fistulae (3.4% vs 20%)[17] as well as pelvic abscess formation (6.9% vs 20%).[10,17] However, the risk of urinary complications, such as infection, fistula, or ureteral stricture, remains unchanged.[20] Anastomotic leaks occur usually only in patients with rectosigmoid anastomosis, and higher leak rates are observed in patients with previous irradiation (67% vs 26%),[20] and the risk is higher as the anastomosis approaches the anal verge (< 5 cm).[10,11] A protective colostomy is indicated with the combination of previous irradiation and an anastomosis less than 5 cm from the anal verge, because it is associated with a high leak rate.[11] The reported leak rate from a literature review in patients with previous irradiation was 93% as compared with 29% without irradiation.[11] Vulvar wound complications only occur with type II and III exenterations.

Early Complications

Early complications (< 30 days) are usually related to cardiovascular, pulmonary, and metabolic derangements, sepsis,

Table 8-2. Perioperative morbidity, reoperation, mortality, and survival for pelvic exenteration in series with more than 100 patients.

	Year	N	Morbidity	Mortality	5-year survival	Reoperation due to complications
Schmidt et al[4]	2012	282	51	5	41	8
Magrina et al[2]	1997	133	44	5	41	12[a]
Maggioni et al[21]	2009	106	66	0	47[b]	13[c]
Rossi et al[22]	2011	205	40	4.6		
Goldberg et al[10]	2006	103	25	1	48	
Crozier et al[32]	1995	105	40	10	38	
Jakowatz et al[20]	1985	104	51	12	27	
Rodriguez Cuevas et al[24]	1988	252	45	10	49[d]	

[a]Additional 11% for vaginal reconstruction completion or reoperation.
[b]52% cervical, 35% endometrial, 19% vaginal, 16% vulvar.
[c]10.3 reoperation for late complications (> 30 days).
[d]3 years, only cervical cancer.

pelvic abscess, ureteral or rectosigmoid anastomotic leaks, bowel obstruction, fistulas, and wound and stoma problems. Ureteral leaks (14%) are a common problem and seem to occur with equal frequency with continent or incontinent conduits.[10] Bowel obstructions and/or intestinal fistulas are reported in 10% to 15% of patients. Although bowel obstruction and fistulas can occur at any time during the postoperative period, 78% of bowel obstructions but only 56% of intestinal fistulas occur during the first 30 days after surgery.[23] The development of intestinal fistula is associated with a much higher postoperative mortality as compared to bowel obstruction.[23] Pulmonary embolism has been reported in 3.5% of patients.[4]

Early Reoperations

Early reoperation (< 30 days) for the correction of postoperative complications is necessary in about 1 in 10 patients (8%–13%).[2,4,21] In one study reoperations for ureteral leaks were noted in 28% of patients.[10] Reasons for reoperation may include ureteral leaks, wound (abdominal and vulvar) complications, necrotic pedicle flaps, intestinal anastomosis leaks, intestinal fistulas, rectosigmoid anastomotic leaks, stoma retraction or necrosis, and others.[11] A rule of thumb is that any patient requiring more than 2 operations for the correction of major complications will die during the postoperative course. Therefore, utmost attention has to be made to prevent complications and to provide successful correction of any major complication.

Operative Mortality Rates

The operative mortality of more recent series including more than 100 patients is shown in Table 8-2. The operative mortality has decreased throughout the years[2,4,24] from an early operative mortality rate around 20%[1,24] to a more recent mortality rate ranging from 0% to 5%. Patient selection is an important factor in minimizing the operative mortality rate, since in the hands of the same surgeons the operative mortality rate during the years 1960 to 1965 was 9.8%, while for the years 1963 to 1965 it was 2.3%.[13] Anterior exenterations have decreased morbidity and mortality as compared with total pelvic exenterations.[4,13,24]

LONG-TERM OUTCOMES

Box 8-4 DELAYED COMPLICATIONS

- The most common delayed stoma complications are stricture and parastomal hernia
- The most common urinary conduit complications are recurrent urinary infections and stricture of the ureteral anastomosis

Delayed Complications

Delayed complications (> 30 days) are related to the exenteration type, the viscera removed, and the techniques used for reconstruction of the urinary and intestinal tracts and vagina. For instance, perineal hernias only occur with type IIb and III exenterations. Delayed complications, although they may be different, occurred with equal frequency in each type of exenteration.[2] Complications include bowel obstruction, intestinal fistulas, revision of continent urinary pouch, recurrent urinary tract infections, parastomal hernias, stoma stenosis, ureteral or intestinal anastomotic strictures, perineal hernias, and problems associated with vaginal reconstruction (strictures, prolapse).

Late Reoperations

Late reoperations (> 30 days) are necessary due to either complications or as a secondary operation for completion of vaginal reconstruction in about 1 in 10 patients (10.3%–11%).[2,21] In our experience 11% of patients had reoperations related to vaginal reconstruction, and all were on patients with type II or III exenterations. Late reoperations are more commonly performed for intestinal fistulas, rectosigmoid anastomosis leaks, vaginal stenosis/revision, perineal hernia, stomal stenosis, parastomal hernia, ureteral strictures, revision of a continent pouch, repair of prolapse of a sigmoid colon neovagina, and others.

Survival

Comparison of the survival, morbidity, and mortality rates from exenteration series is difficult due to many factors influencing the results. Among these factors are the time period of the study, the primary site of the malignancy (cervix, uterus, urethra, rectum, ovary, vulva, vagina), the histologic type of the tumor (squamous, adenocarcinoma, sarcomas, melanomas), whether the tumor is primary, persistent, or recurrent disease, and whether exenteration is performed postsurgery, postirradiation, or both (healing is gravely affected by irradiation; previous surgery and irradiation are a combination for increased morbidity). Intraoperative adverse prognostic factors associated with low survival include the patient's general medical condition, the time interval from original diagnosis to recurrence, lesion size, and others are also important. Large differences in survival have been noted when analyzing 3 prognostic factors: the time interval to recurrence, tumor size, and pelvic wall fixation on pelvic examination, with survival rates ranging from 0% to 82%.[5]

In general, series including all types of patients with different origins and types of tumors and variable prognostic factors and patient conditions have reported a survival rate around 40%. In the series by Maggioni et al,[21] the survival rate by tumor origin was 51% for cervical lesions, 35% for endometrial, 19% for vaginal, and 16% for vulvar lesions. In another series of 31 patients with recurrent endometrial adenocarcinoma, the 5-year survival rate was 45%.[8] Patients with primary vulvar lesions have increased survival (70%) as compared with patients with recurrent vulvar cancer (38%).[25]

MINIMALLY INVASIVE SURGERY APPLICATIONS

Minimally Invasive Surgery Exploration Prior To Exenteration

About 50% of exenterations are abandoned during surgical exploration. Because a number of factors that would be contraindications to an exenteration can be identified by minimally invasive surgery (MIS), we prefer to perform a laparoscopic or robotic exploration 48 to 72 hours prior to a planned exenteration. The use of laparoscopy or robotics assessment preceding an exenteration has several advantages over an open exploration at the time of a planned exenteration.

a. Patients are counseled for a pre-exenteration exploration. Once completed and the surgeon is confident of no surgical contraindications, the patient is then counseled for an exenteration
b. If contraindications for an exenteration are discovered at laparoscopic or robotic exploration, then the patient can avoid the full counseling for an exenteration (marking stoma sites, discussing reconstructive techniques, postoperative care, vaginal function, complications, and other information) and a laparotomy is avoided.
c. At the exenteration, the operating time is reduced because there is no exploration phase and the resectability of the lesion has already been determined allowing the surgeon to proceed directly to the exenterative phase of the operation.
d. There is improved utilization of operating room time since the blocked time for the planned exenteration will be used.
e. The examination under anesthesia, cystoscopy and proctoscopy are performed at same setting of the laparoscopic or robotic exploration.

In a report of 13 patients, the operating time for pre-exenteration assessment was 150 minutes and the blood loss was 50 mL. Contraindications to an exenteration were discovered in 75% of patients. The laparoscopic findings were corroborated at the time of the exenteration in those patients who were found to have no contraindications.[26]

Minimally Invasive Surgery For Exenteration

There are only a few reports describing the role of laparoscopy and robotics for pelvic exenteration. The first report of the use of laparoscopy for anterior pelvic exenteration with Miami pouch urinary reconstruction was in 2004.[27] There are 2 other reports of laparoscopic pelvic exenteration. In one of them,[27] 5 patients underwent type I, II, and III exenterations, including anterior, total, and posterior. The mean operating time was 6 hours (range: 4.5–9), the mean blood loss was less than 500 mL, and the mean length of hospitalization was 27 days. The hospital stay was not reduced by the MIS approach. Another series[28] included 7 patients undergoing palliative exenterations for improvement of quality of life. The mean operating time was 3.8 hours, mean blood loss was 250 mL, and the mean hospital stay was 8 days (range: 7–21).

The first report of a robotic exenteration was in 2009 with 1 patient.[29] In 2010, there were 2 reports, one with 2 patients undergoing an anterior supralevator exenteration[30] with a hospital stay of 8 days, and another with 3 patients.[31] In the latter report the range of the operating times was 6 to 10 hours, blood loss 200 to 500 mL, and hospital stay of 25 to 53 days. All 3 patients required a 10-cm laparotomy incision for the urinary reconstruction. At the present, there does not appear to be a major benefit of MIS technologies for pelvic exenteration.

SUMMARY

Pelvic exenteration is an operation reserved for patients with recurrent or advanced pelvic malignancies in the absence of contraindications, the availability of other treatment modalities, and in the presence of complete tumor resectability. It is associated with a complication rate of 25% to 66%, a reoperation rate of 8% to 13%, a recent operative mortality of 0% to 5% and a 5-year survival rate of 41% to 48%. Patient selection and surgical technique are important factors for survival and morbidity.

REFERENCES

1. Brunschwig A. What are the indications and results of pelvic exenteration? *JAMA*. 1965;194(3):274.
2. Magrina JF, Stanhope CR, Weaver AL. Pelvic exenterations: Supralevator, infralevator, and with vulvectomy. *Gynecol Oncol*. 1997;64(1):130-135.
3. Jurado M, Alcazar JL, Martinez-Monge R. Resectability rates of previously irradiated recurrent cervical cancer (pircc) treated with pelvic exenteration: Is still the clinical involvement of the pelvis wall a real contraindication? A twenty-year experience. *Gynecol Oncol*. 2010;116(1):38-43.
4. Schmidt AM, Imesch P, Fink D, Egger H. Indications and long-term clinical outcomes in 282 patients with pelvic exenteration for advanced or recurrent cervical cancer. *Gynecol Oncol*. 2012;125(3):604-609.
5. Shingleton HM, Soong SJ, Gelder MS, Hatch KD, Baker VV, Austin JM , Jr. Clinical and histopathologic factors predicting recurrence and survival after pelvic exenteration for cancer of the cervix. *Obstet Gynecol*. 1989;73(6):1027-1034.
6. Stanhope CR, Symmonds RE. Palliative exenteration–what, when, and why? *Am J Obstet Gynecol*. 1985;152(1):12-16.
7. Matthews CM, Morris M, Burke TW, Gershenson DM, Wharton JT, Rutledge FN. Pelvic exenteration in the elderly patient. *Obstet Gynecol*. 1992;79(5 (Pt 1)):773-777.
8. Morris M, Alvarez RD, Kinney WK, Wilson TO. Treatment of recurrent adenocarcinoma of the endometrium with pelvic exenteration. *Gynecol Oncol*. 1996;60(2):288-291.
9. Fotopoulou C, Neumann U, Kraetschell R, et al. Long-term clinical outcome of pelvic exenteration in patients with advanced gynecological malignancies. *J Surg Oncol*. 2010;101(6):507-512.
10. Goldberg GL, Sukumvanich P, Einstein MH, Smith HO, Anderson PS, Fields AL. Total pelvic exenteration: The albert einstein college of medicine/montefiore medical center experience (1987 to 2003). *Gynecol Oncol*. 2006;101(2):261-268.
11. Jurado M, Alcazar JL, Baixauli J, Hernandez-Lizoain JL. Low colorectal anastomosis after pelvic exenteration for gynecologic malignancies: Risk factors analysis for leakage. *Int J Gynecol Cancer*. 2011;21(2):397-402.
12. Haas T, Buchsbaum HJ, Lifshitz S. Nonresectable recurrent pelvic neoplasm. Outcome in patients explored for pelvic exenteration. *Gynecol Oncol*. 1980;9(2):177-181.
13. Symmonds RE, Pratt JH, Welch JS. Exenterative operations. Experience with 118 patients. *Am J Obstet Gynecol*. 1968;101(1):66-77.
14. Garton GR, Gunderson LL, Webb MJ, Wilson TO, Cha SS, Podratz KC. Intraoperative radiation therapy in gynecologic cancer: Update of the experience at a single institution. *Int J Radiat Oncol Biol Phys*. 1997;37(4):839-843.
15. Hockel M, Sclenger K, Hamm H, Knapstein PG, Hohenfellner R, Rosler HP. Five-year experience with combined operative and radiotherapeutic treatment of recurrent gynecologic tumors infiltrating the pelvic wall. *Cancer*. 1996;77(9):1918-1933.
16. Magrina JF. Types of pelvic exenterations: a reappraisal. *Gynecol Oncol*. 1990;37(3):363-366.
17. Jurado M, Bazan A, Alcazar JL, Garcia-Tutor E. Primary vaginal reconstruction at the time of pelvic exenteration for gynecologic cancer: morbidity revisited. *Ann Surg Oncol*. 2009;16(1):121-127.
18. Peregrin-Alvarez I, Akl MN, Morrow CP, Magrina JF. Metastatic and recurrent adenocarcinoma of the uterine cervix: a long-term survival of 16 years. *Eur J Gynaecol Oncol*. 2010;31(3):333-335.
19. Pearse CS, Magrina JF, Finley BE. Use of mast suit in obstetrics and gynecology. *Obstet Gynecol Surv*. 1984;39(7):416-422.
20. Jakowatz JG, Porudominsky D, Riihimaki DU, et al. Complications of pelvic exenteration. *Arch Surg*. 1985;120(11):1261-1265.
21. Maggioni A, Roviglione G, Landoni F, et al. Pelvic exenteration: Ten-year experience at the european institute of oncology in milan. *Gynecol Oncol*. 2009;114(1):64-68.
22. Rossi M, Chiantera V, De Iaco P, et al. Morbidity and outcomes after pelvic exenteration for gynecological malignancies: a retrospective multicentric study of 205 patients. *Eur Soc Gynaecol Oncol*. 2011;21:S429.
23. Webb MJ, Symmonds RE. Management of the pelvic floor after pelvic exenteration. *Obstet Gynecol*. 1977;50(2):166-171.
24. Rodriguez Cuevas H, Torres A, de la Garza M, Hernandez D, Herrera L. Pelvic exenteration for carcinoma of the cervix: Analysis of 252 cases. *J Surg Oncol*. 1988;38(2):121-125.
25. Miller B, Morris M, Levenback C, Burke TW, Gershenson DM. Pelvic exenteration for primary and recurrent vulvar cancer. *Gynecol Oncol*. 1995;58(2):202-205.
26. Plante M, Roy M. Operative laparoscopy prior to a pelvic exenteration in patients with recurrent cervical cancer. *Gynecol Oncol*. 1998;69(2):94-99.
27. Ferron G, Querleu D, Martel P, Letourneur B, Soulie M. Laparoscopy-assisted vaginal pelvic exenteration. *Gynecol Oncol*. 2006;100(3):551-555.
28. Puntambekar SP, Agarwal GA, Puntambekar SS, Sathe RM, Patil AM. Stretching the limits of laparoscopy in gynecological oncology: technical feasibility of doing a laparoscopic total pelvic exenteration for palliation in advanced cervical cancer. *Int J Biomed Sci*. 2009;5(1):17-22.
29. Lim PC. Robotic assisted total pelvic exenteration: a case report. *Gynecol Oncol*. 2009;115(2):310-311.
30. Davis MA, Adams S, Eun D, Lee D, Randall TC. Robotic-assisted laparoscopic exenteration in recurrent cervical cancer robotics improved the surgical experience for 2 women with recurrent cervical cancer. *Am J Obstet Gynecol*. 2010;202(6):663-e661.
31. Lambaudie E, Narducci F, Leblanc E, Bannier M, Houvenaeghel G. Robotically-assisted laparoscopic anterior pelvic exenteration for recurrent cervical cancer: report of three first cases. *Gynecol Oncol*. 2010;116(3):582-583.
32. Crozier M, Morris M, Levenback C, Lucas KR, Atkinson EN, Wharton JT. Pelvic exenteration for adenocarcinoma of the uterine cervix. *Gynecol Oncol*. 1995;58(1):74-78.

Chapter 9. (Laterally) Extended Endopelvic Resection

Michael Höckel, MD, PhD

BACKGROUND

Insights in the topology of locoregional tumor spread from developmental biology call for redefining the principles of cancer surgery.[1] Surgical procedures translating these concepts into practice have achieved excellent locoregional tumor control at low rates of treatment-related morbidity.[2-5] The corresponding surgical techniques for the therapy of locally advanced and recurrent cancer of the lower female genital tract are termed (laterally) extended endopelvic resection ([L]EER).[6] (L)EER enables R0 resection and locoregional tumor control not only in patients who are regarded as suitable candidates for conventional pelvic exenteration but also in patients with tumors fixed to the pelvic sidewall who are currently excluded from exenteration candidacy either pre- or intraoperatively.[7]

INDICATIONS AND CLINICAL APPLICATIONS

Pelvic sidewall recurrences or locally advanced cancer of the lower female genital tract have traditionally been considered inoperable. If patients with this clinical presentation have not been irradiated, then radiotherapy or combined chemoradiotherapy can lead to remission. However, in the majority of cases, pelvic sidewall disease is diagnosed following primary or adjuvant pelvic irradiation or has not been controlled by radiotherapy. Consequently, patients with persistent and recurrent cervicovaginal cancer following radiotherapy and patients with advanced primary disease with fistulae between the genital and urinary tracts and/or anorectum are candidates for (L)EER if the following conditions are met preoperatively:

a. Exclusion of distant metastases,
b. No tumor involvement at the site of the sciatic foramen, and
c. Physical status and mental fitness adequate for the megaoperation.

Patients with locally advanced disease without fistulae and patients with postsurgical pelvic recurrence in an non-irradiated pelvis are primarily considered for chemoradiation. However, they may be evaluated for (L)EER if the radiotherapist votes for or the patient requests surgical treatment.

ANATOMIC CONSIDERATIONS

A prerequisite for the performance of (L)EER is a working knowledge of the *ontogenetic anatomy* of the pelvis in the human female, which will be briefly outlined here, supplemented by Figures 9-1 to 9-3. For further details, the reader is referred to textbooks and monographs.[8-12]

The pelvic ground plan is laid down in the fourth developmental week through migration, proliferation, and specific interaction of cell lineages from the 3 germ layers (endoderm, mesoderm, ectoderm) that establish 3 *pelvic building blocks:* primitive pelvic wall, terminal gut, and urogenital ridges. Focal interactions of the building blocks lead to the formation of *early metacompartments* such as the mesonephric ducts-cloaca complex and the cloacal folds and membrane complex. During the embryonic period, *late metacompartments* are established within the domains of the early metacompartments. These include the mesonephro-urogenital sinus complex and the genital tubercle-cloacal eminence and plate complex. The late metacompartments provide the territory for the *definitive compartments,* which represent developmental domains independent from each other, thus acting as modules of morphogenesis during the fetal period and thereafter.

Synchronous with the formation of the developmental domains, 3 networks for their support are established from the central primordia: the vascular system from the dorsal aorta, the lymphatic system from the posterior cardinal veins, the nervous system from the spinal neural tube, the spinal neural crest, and the neural cord derived from the caudal eminence. The distal parts of the support system, eg, the lymph capillaries, interact with their recipient compartments and adopt positional information specific for that particular tissue. The proximal parts are conduction structures that transit other compartments within defined *corridors.*

Differentiation of the pelvic compartments during the fetal period is sex specific. The female *endopelvic compartments,* hindgut, bladder primordium, and internal urogenital sinus (UGS) develop into the rectum with its mesorectum, the bladder, and the internal UGS compartment. The latter forms the urethra, distal vagina, and distal rectovaginal septum.[3] Dorsally, the internal UGS compartment is attached to the

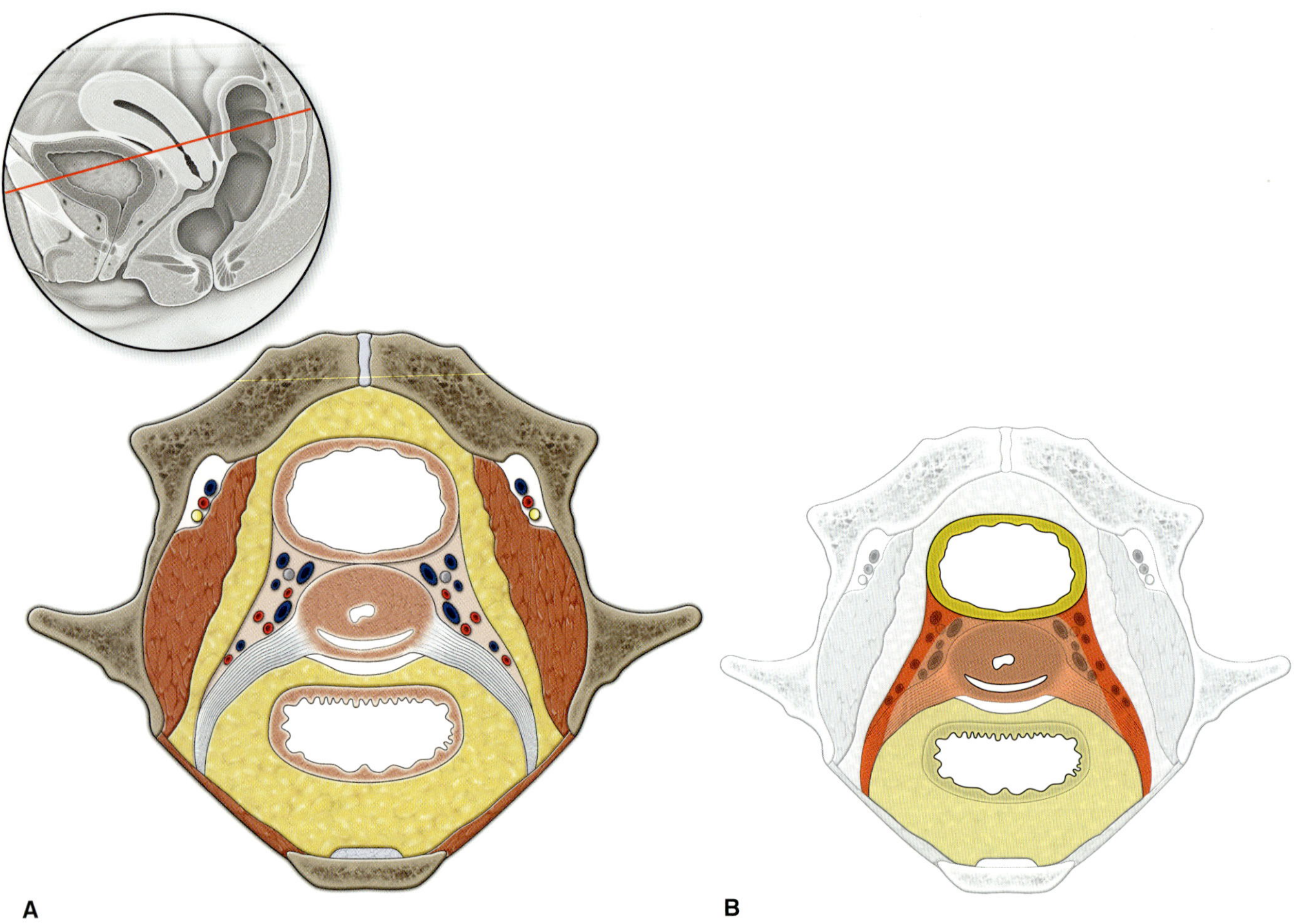

Fig. 9-1. Anatomic drawings of a transverse section of the female pelvis. (A) Illustrates ontogenetic mapping. (B) The sectioning level is indicated by the inset. Dark yellow, bladder; light yellow, hindgut compartment; dark red, urogenital mesentery; light red, Müllerian compartment; orange, ureters.

anterior rectum and mesorectum (see Figure 9-1). Caudally, it merges with the external UGS compartment (see below).

The *mesopelvic compartments* include the gonadal primordia, paramesonephric-mesonephric complex, primordial ureter, and primitive urogenital mesentery. These primordia differentiate in the female pelvis into the ovaries with mesovarium, Müllerian compartment, pelvic ureters, and the definitive pelvic urogenital mesentery. Anatomic details of the Müllerian compartment are described elsewhere.[2,13] The mature *pelvic urogenital mesentery* derived from its primitive precursor consists of fibrofatty tissue providing the corridors for the ureter, the pelvic autonomic nerves, the visceral branches of the internal iliac vessel system, the lymph collectors, and, eventually, the intercalated lymph nodes from the Müllerian, bladder, and UGS compartments. The urogenital mesentery also fixes these compartments to the pelvic wall with a structurally complex "mesopelvic suspensorium," which is fused to the pubo- and iliococcygeus muscles by the arcus tendineus fasciae pelvis anteriorly and to the ischial spine and coccygeus muscles posteriorly (see Figure 9-2). Using the ureter as landmark, the cranial pelvic urogenital mesentery can be formally divided into a supraureteral peritoneal part corresponding to the distal broad ligament and an infraureteral retroperitoneal part loosely attached to the lateral mesorectum. The caudal pelvic urogenital mesentery is located subperitoneally below the level of the obliterated umbilical artery. Laterally, the subperitoneal urogenital mesentery adheres to the perivisceral fat pad and abuts the internal iliac vessel system, proximal sciatic nerve, and sacral plexus. Medially, the subperitoneal urogenital mesentery is continuous with the bladder and the Müllerian parts of the mesometria/mesocolpos (see Figure 9-3).

The *ectopelvic compartments* are represented by the pelvic epidermis, dermis, hypodermis, fasciomusculoskeletal structures, perivisceral and presacral fat pads,[14] as well as the parietal peritoneum. The external UGS compartment matures into all morphologic structures of the vulva except the labia majora, into the gynecologic perineum, and the ventral anal segment.[4]

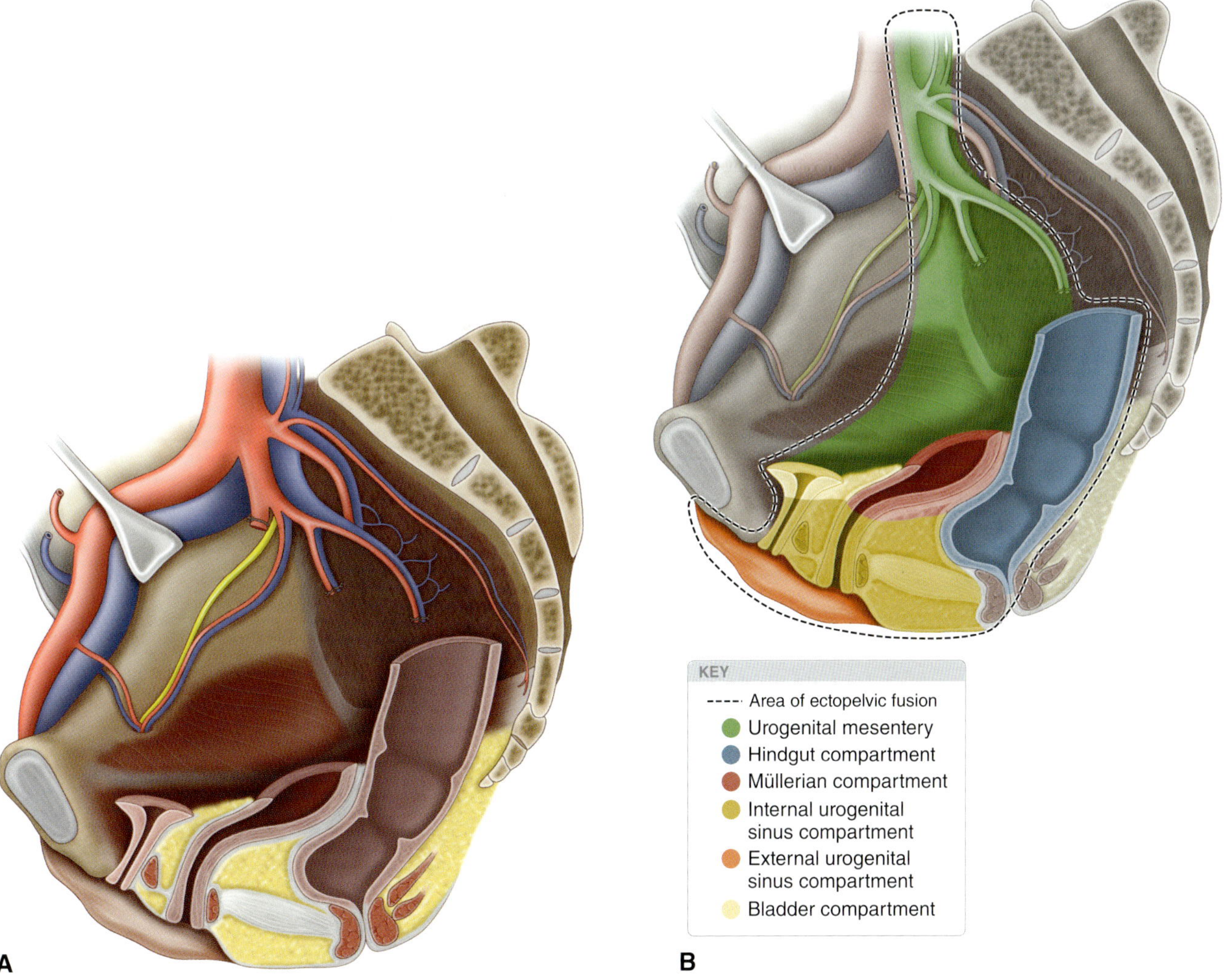

Fig. 9-2. Anatomic drawings of a midsagittal section of the female pelvis. (A) Illustrates ontogenetic mapping. (B) The urogenital mesentery with all transit structures has been omitted. However, its area of ectopelvic fusion is shown by the sickle-shaped shadow. Likewise, the central pelvic organs except their most distal parts are cut off. Dark yellow, internal urogenital sinus compartment; light yellow, bladder compartment; blue, hindgut compartment; dark red, Müllerian compartment; green, urogenital mesentery; light red, external urogenital sinus compartment.

PREOPERATIVE PREPARATION

Box 9-1 KEY SURGICAL INSTRUMENTATION

In addition to a standard laparotomy set and electrosurgical cutting and coagulation devices, the following equipment is useful to perform (L)EER:

- Table-fixed retractor system (eg, Bookwalter, Codman and Shurtleff, Inc., Raynham, Massachusetts) with rings and blades of various sizes
- Vessel-sealing system (eg, LigaSure, Valleylab, Boulder, Colorado) of various sizes
- Cobb periosteal dissectors of various sizes

The locoregional extent of the neoplastic disease is assessed from the clinical examination of the patient under anesthesia during which T2-weighted axial and sagittal high-resolution magnetic resonance imaging (MRI) scans of the pelvis are displayed. Multiple site-directed biopsies are taken and their histopathologic results are awaited. If the pelvic disease is considered treatable with (L)EER by applying the criteria outlined above, positron emission tomography/computed tomography (CT) is ordered to screen for distant metastases. Rarely, diagnostic laparoscopy is necessary to rule out peritoneal carcinomatosis. When distant spread is not obvious, the patient's comorbidity is checked by the anesthesiologist with regard to fitness for the megaoperation. If all prerequisites are met, then the patient is informed about the putative resective and reconstructive aspects of her treatment.

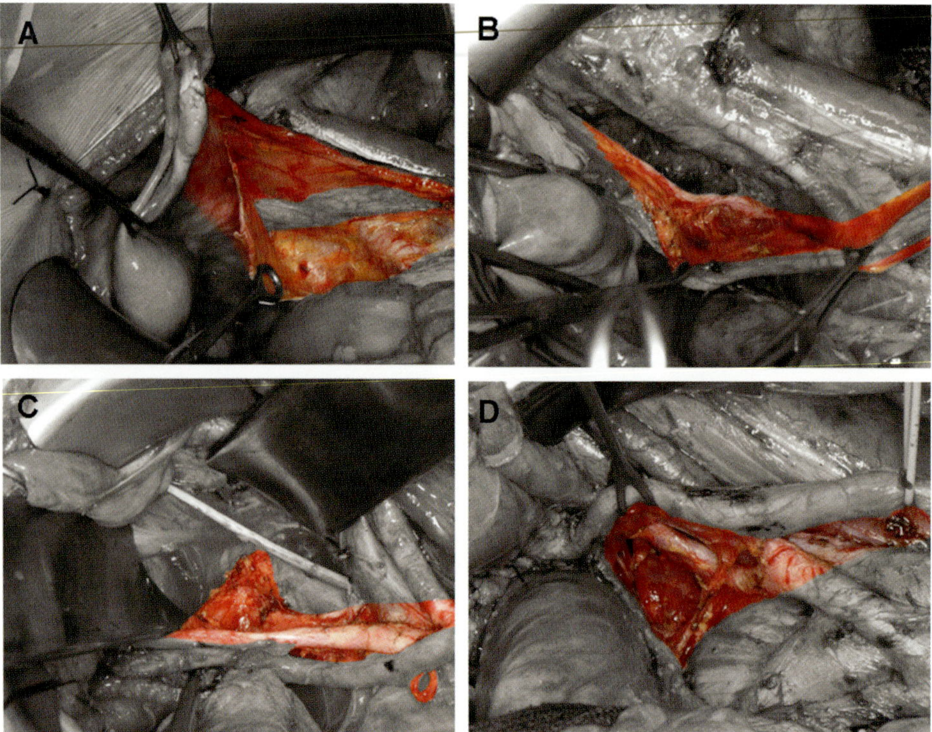

Fig. 9-3. Topographic anatomy of the pelvic urogenital mesentery. The complex structure of the right pelvic urogenital mesentery at successive states of dissection is highlighted red. (A) Exposure of the posterior peritoneal part above the ureter. Below the ureter the medial surface of the retroperitoneal part is partly visible. (B) Removal of the peritoneal part demonstrates the anterior aspect of the retroperitoneal part. (C) Removal of the perivisceral fat body exposes the anterior aspect of the subperitoneal part. (D) Posterior aspect of the subperitoneal part below the internal iliac artery. (Reproduced with permission from Michael Höckel, MD)

To prepare the patient for (L)EER, she receives mechanical bowel cleansing the day prior to surgery. Perioperative antibiotic and anticoagulation medication is administered the evening before surgery.

SURGICAL PROCEDURE

Box 9-2 MASTER SURGEON'S PRINCIPLES

- The surgeon performing (L)EER should read the patient's MRI scans herself/himself, optimally in parallel to physically examining the patient
- The surgeon should be familiar with the ontogenetic anatomy of the female pelvis. She or he should understand the topology of locoregional spread of gynecologic cancer based on embryonic development
- The surgeon should know the biology of wound healing and the pathophysiology of its disturbance from previous radiotherapy, scarring, and obesity

Principles

The aim of *Extended Endopelvic Resection* based on ontogenetic anatomy is to resect multiple pelvic developmental compartments instead of tissues related to functions, ie, multiple pelvic viscera. The Müllerian compartment is resected en bloc with the bladder compartment and eventually with the hindgut compartment. Integrated into these multi-compartment resections is the *proximal* part of the pelvic urogenital mesentery (Figure 9-4). The resection can be caudally expanded by including the internal and external UGS compartments. In these cases, the procedure must be performed both from the abdominal and perineal routes, whereas otherwise solely the abdominal approach is adequate (Figure 9-5).

(L)EER includes the *distal* part of the urogenital mesentery. To ensure the completeness of its caudal resection, the pubo-, ilio-, and coccygeus muscles together with the mesopelvic suspensorium are included in the specimen. Cranial resection of the distal subperitoneal urogenital mesentery necessitates the inclusion of the internal iliac vessel system. Whereas the merging area of the caudal subperitoneal urogenital mesentery with the pelvic wall is

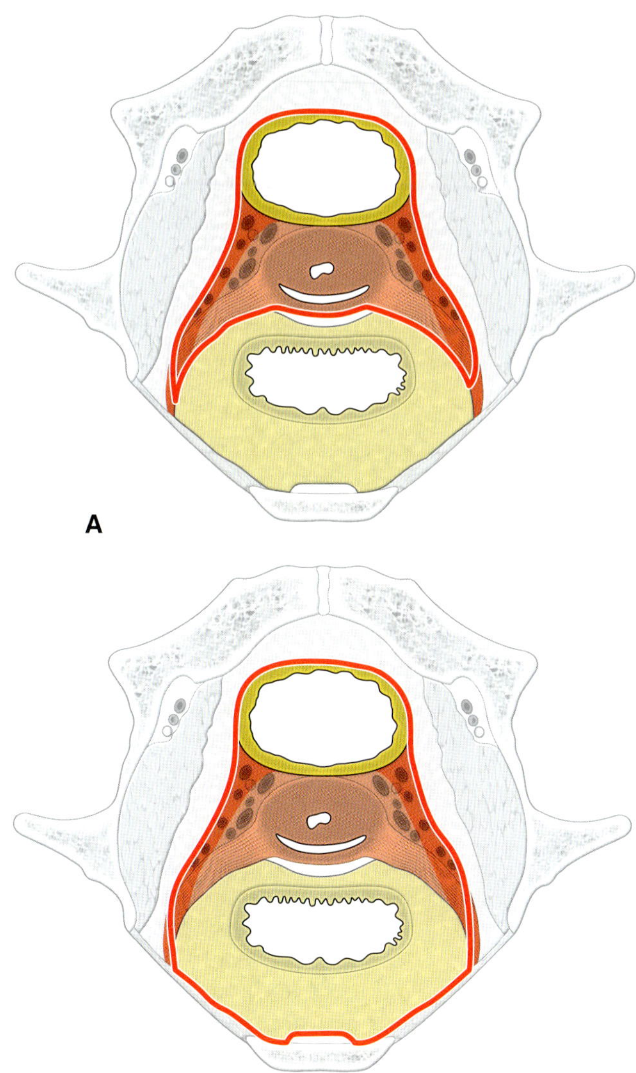

Fig. 9-4. Schematic representation of the major types of extended endopelvic resection. (A) Anterior endopelvic resection (transverse plane, circumferential resection line highlighted). (B) Total endopelvic resection (transverse plane, circumferential resection line highlighted).

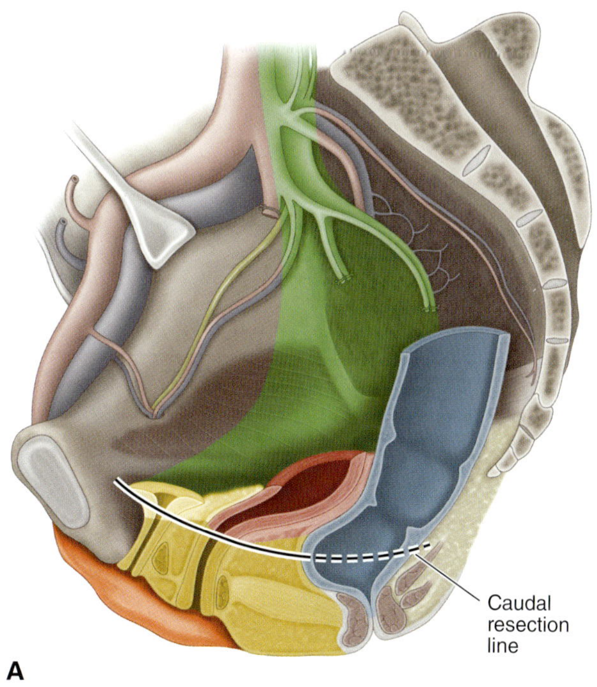

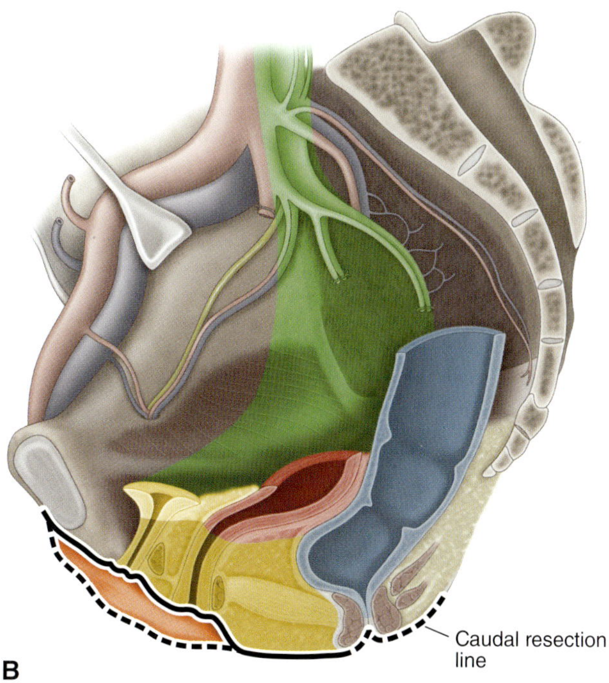

Fig. 9-5. Schematic representation of the major types of extended endopelvic resection. (A) Abdominal total endopelvic resection (sagittal plane, caudal resection line highlighted). (B) Abdominoperineal total endopelvic resection (sagittal plane, caudal resection line highlighted).

defined by the smooth surface of the striated pelvic muscles, the transition of the cranial subperitoneal urogenital mesentery to the internal iliac vessel system and the sacral plexus is complex (Figure 9-6). Consequently, cervicovaginal tumors fixed to the pelvic wall below the sciatic notch level can be reliably resected by the inclusion of these pelvic floor and wall muscles into the en bloc specimen. However, if clinical symptoms or imaging indicate tumor involvement of the pelvic wall at the sciatic foramen, then tumor control can no longer be accomplished with LEER.

A uniform nomenclature describes the specific procedure within the spectrum of (L)EER. Total endopelvic resection designates the inclusion of the bladder compartment and

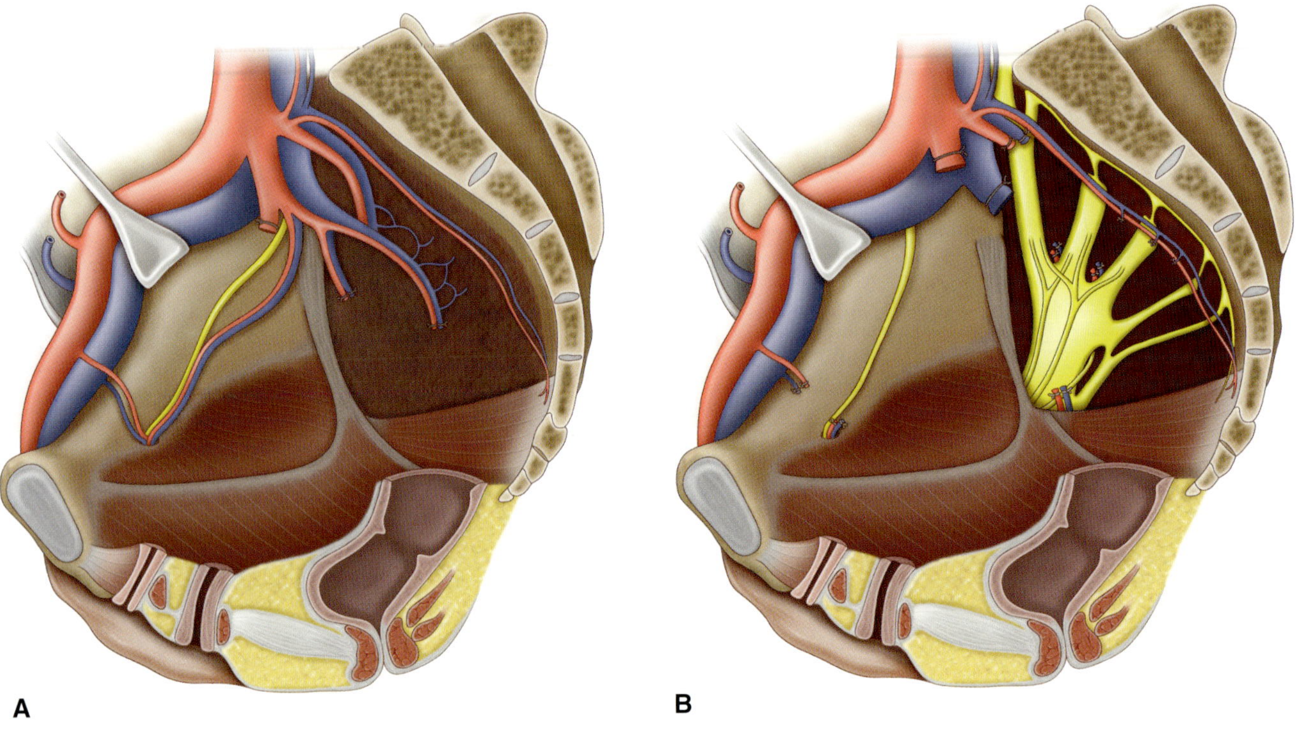

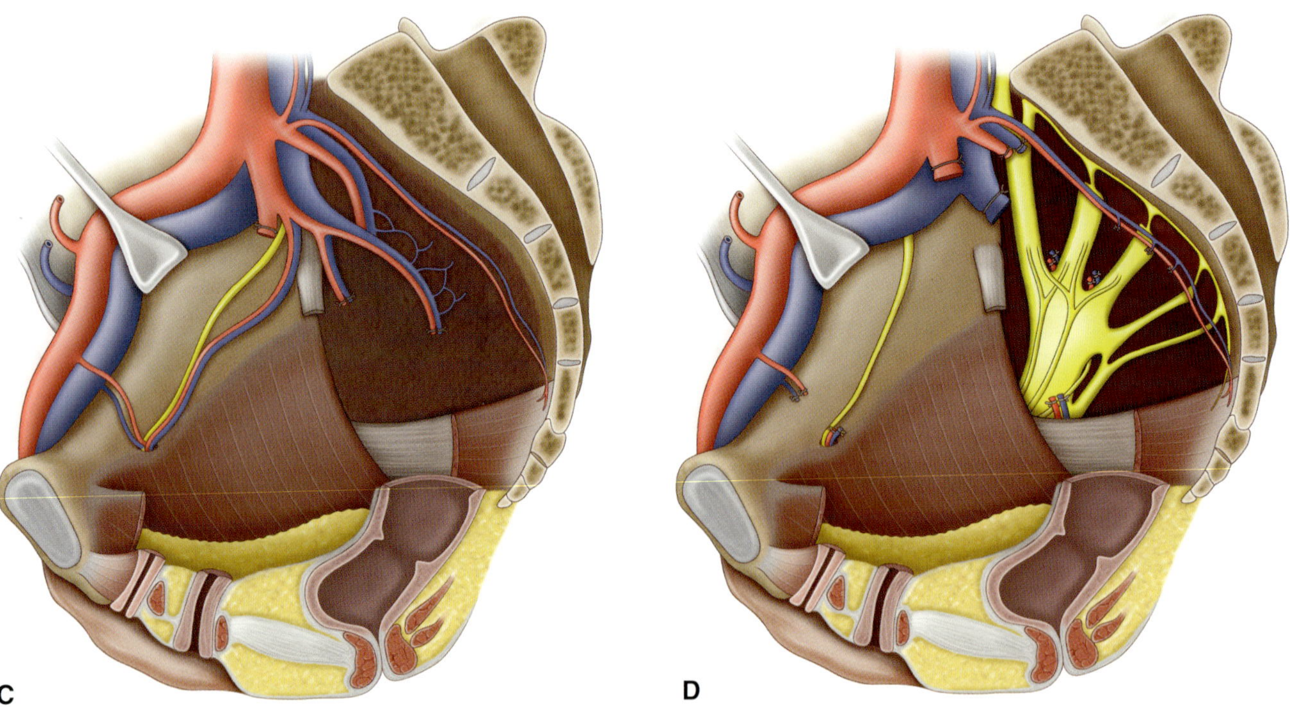

Fig. 9-6. Surgical anatomy of the right pelvic side wall for (L)EER. (A) The urogenital mesentery with all transit structures is removed and the central pelvic organs are cut. (B) Dissection of the caudal part of the distal urogenital mesentery including the pubo-, ilio-, and coccygeus muscles into the (L)EER specimen. (C) Dissection of the rostral part of the urogenital mesentery including the internal iliac vessels into the (L)EER specimen. (D) Dissection of the complete urogenital mesentery including the pubo-, ilio-, and coccygeus muscles and the internal iliac vessels into the (L)EER specimen.

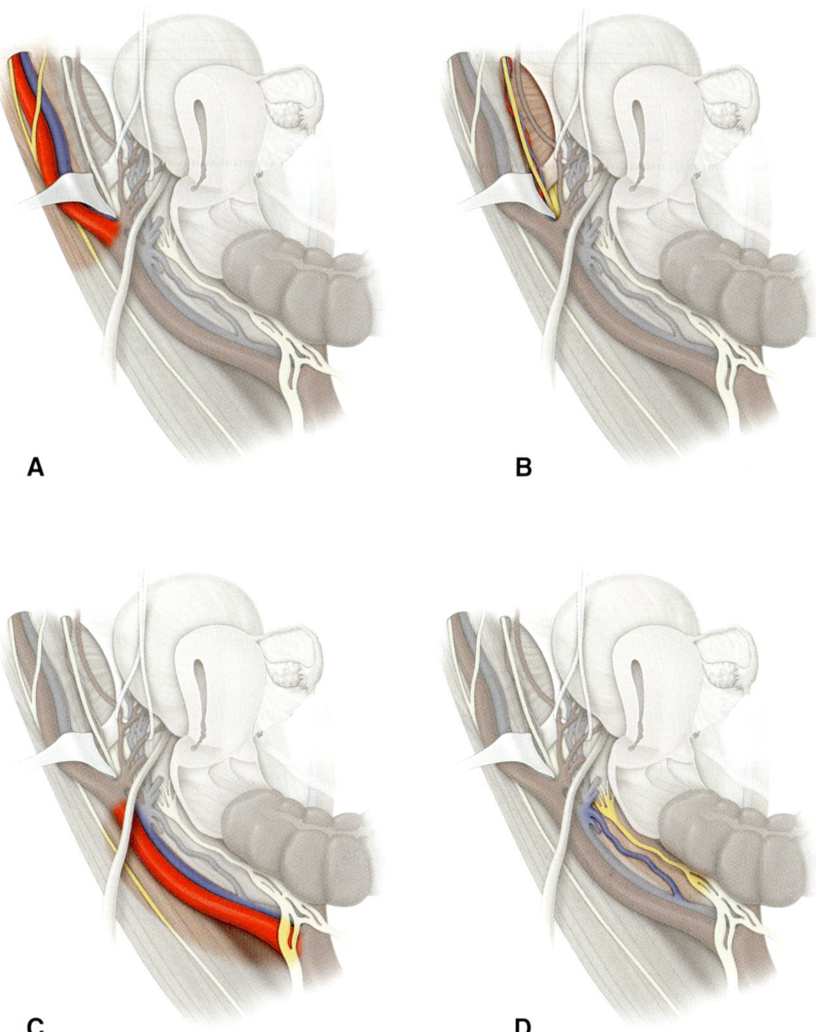

Fig. 9-7. Anatomic drawings of the pelvic lymphatic sub-basins. (A) External iliac. (B) Perivisceral. (C) Common iliac. (D) Presacral. All sub-basins belong to the iliac lymph compartment.

the hindgut compartment; anterior endopelvic resection and posterior endopelvic resection indicate the inclusion of solely the bladder compartments or the hindgut compartment. The abdominal procedure contains the complete Müllerian compartment or its remains in case of prior surgery. The abdominoperineal procedure includes both the Müllerian and the internal UGS compartments and may also integrate the external UGS compartment.

The lateral extension is specified by adding supplementary information, ie, right, left, caudal, and rostral part of the distal subperitoneal urogenital mesentery.

Therapeutic lymph node dissection (tLND) based on ontogenetic anatomy supplements (L)EER for regional tumor control (Figures 9-7 and 9-8). Pelvic tLND is performed in all patients who have not undergone surgical and/or radiation therapy of the lymph node regions before and in those whose previous treatment for lymph node metastases has been incomplete.

Para-aortic lymph node dissection is carried out first to the level of the inferior mesenteric artery, and the surgical specimen is histopathologically examined using frozen sections. If no metastases are detected, then the procedure is terminated. Otherwise, dissection proceeds further cranially in the same manner up to the level of the left renal vein. In case of tumor involvement of the uterine corpus the infra renal para-aortic lymph node region is a first-line basin. High para-aortic tLND is carried out irrespective of the pelvic nodal state (Figures 9-9 and 9-10).

Pelvic reconstruction for vital organ functions lost by the resective procedure should adhere to the following principles:

a. Choosing the optimal procedure from several reconstructive options considering the patient's preference,
b. Setting surgical safety over patient comfort in case of doubt, and
c. Strictly avoiding irradiated tissue for reconstruction.

This topic is dealt with in depth in Chapters 11 through 18.

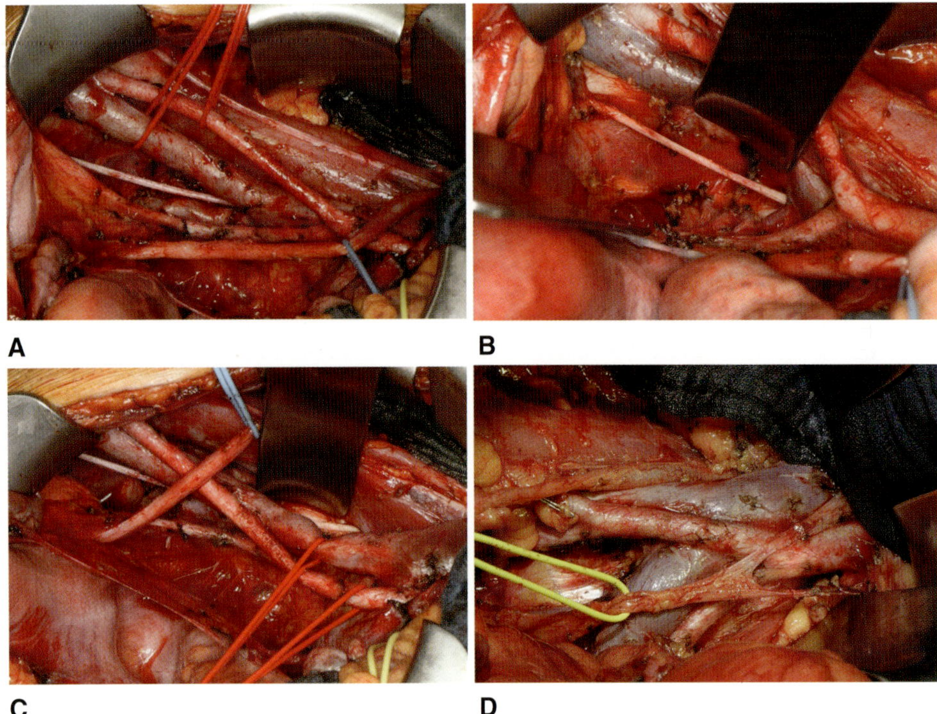

Fig. 9-8. Intraoperative situs following therapeutic pelvic lymph node dissection. The following regions have been completely cleared from lymphatic fatty tissue. (A) External iliac. (B) Perivisceral. (C) Common iliac. (D) Presacral. (Reproduced with permission from Höckel M, Horn L-C, Tetsch E, Einenkel J. Pattern analysis of regional spread and therapeutic lymph node dissection in cervical cancer based on ontogenetic anatomy. *Gynecol Oncol.* 2012;125:168.)

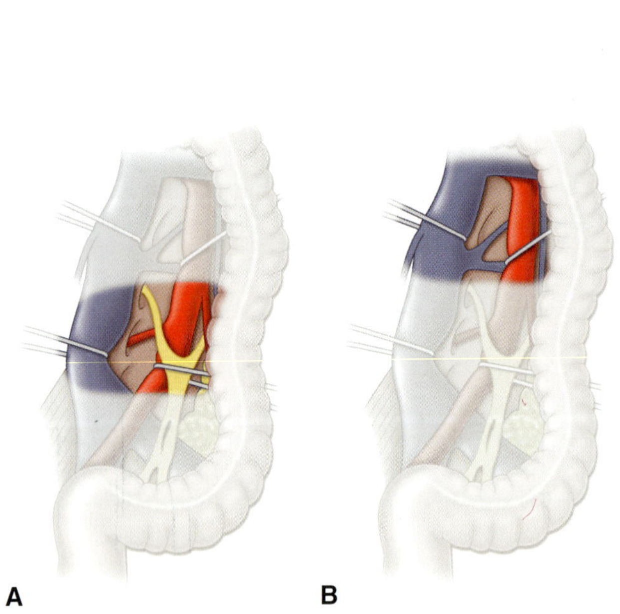

Fig. 9-9. Anatomic drawings of the para-aortic lymphatic sub-basins. (A) Infra mesenteric. (B) Infrarenal. Both sub-basins belong to the lumbar and mesenteric lymph compartments. (Adapted with permission from Höckel M, Horn L-C, Tetsch E, Einenkel J. Pattern analysis of regional spread and therapeutic lymph node dissection in cervical cancer based on ontogenetic anatomy. *Gynecol Oncol.* 2012;125:168.)

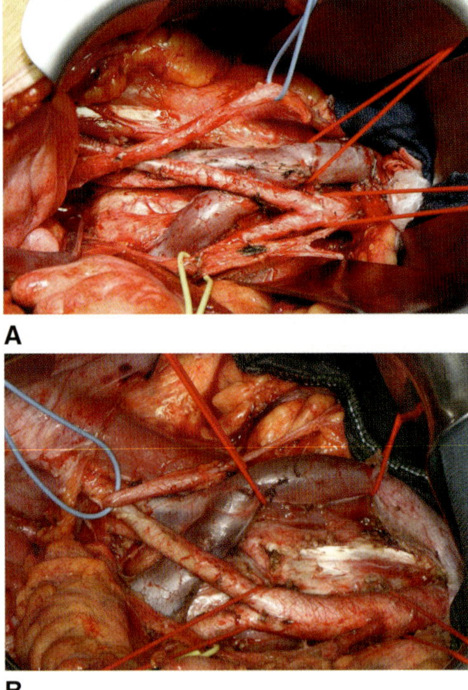

Fig. 9-10. Intraoperative situs following therapeutic para-aortic lymph node dissection. The following regions have been completely cleared from lymphatic fatty tissue. (A) Inframesenteric. (B) Infrarenal. (Reproduced with permission from Höckel M, Horn L-C, Tetsch E, Einenkel J. Pattern analysis of regional spread and therapeutic lymph node dissection in cervical cancer based on ontogenetic anatomy. *Gynecol Oncol.* 2012;125:168.)

Practice

1. Laparotomy and retroperitoneal access

A midline hypo- and epigastric laparotomy is performed. Postoperative, postinflammatory, and connatal peritoneal adhesions are lysed. The peritoneal surfaces and the extent of the pelvic disease are explored. Access to the retroperitoneum is gained through peritoneal incisions at the pelvic sites of the psoas muscles, the paracolic gutters, and along the radix mesenterii. The infundibulopelvic ligaments, ureters, and superior hypogastric plexus are exposed. By mobilizing the cecum and ascending colon, the duodenum, and the sigmoid colon cranial-ward the inferior vena cava and the abdominal aorta with the para-aortic lymph nodes and the nervi splanchnici lumbales are exposed. A sling around the sigmoid colon facilitates the surgical step-specific positional changes and the traction of this bowel part. The site of the connatal sigmoid adhesions is marked by a suture for the exact refixation at the end of the procedure.

2. Para-aortic lymph node dissection

For para-aortic tLND the ascending colon, the duodenum and descending colon and sigmoid colon are mobilized further cranial-ward above the level of the left renal vein. The ovarian vessels and the major lumbar splanchnic nerves are exposed. Both proximal ureters mark the lateral sites of the dissection fields. The ovarian vessels are sealed at their origin and cut. If not encased by lymph node metastases or retroperitoneal fibrosis, then the lumbar splanchnic nerves are preserved. By adventitia stripping the superficial para-caval, inter-aortocaval, and para-aortic lymph node chains are removed from the origin of the inferior mesenteric artery to the aortic bifurcation. Thereafter, the caval vein and the abdominal aorta at that site are undermined and elevated with elastic slings. If necessary for the lifting of the large vessels, lumbar arteries and veins are sealed and cut. The retro-caval and retro-aortic lymph tissue is then completely removed exposing the anterior spine. The sympathetic trunk is preserved bilaterally.

Infrarenal para-aortic tLND is performed in the same manner from the level of the left renal vein to the origin of the inferior mesenteric artery (inframesenteric tLND). Para-caval, inter-aortocaval, para-aortic, retro-caval, and retro-aortic lymph tissue are completely removed.

3. Pelvic lymph node dissection

Pelvic tLND is prepared by incision of the peritoneum at the anterior and posterior base of the broad ligament, dissection of the round ligament and caudal-ward mobilization of the "infundibulopelvic ligament," with the ovarian vessels sealed and cut at their origins. The adnexa may be sealed and cut for a better view of the surgical field. The ureters along with their mesoureters are mobilized within the urogenital mesenteries caudal-ward down to their intersection with the vascular mesometria. Laterally, the fine vascular connections of the mesoureter with the internal/common iliac vessels should be preserved. Dorsally to the ureters, the hypogastric nerves and the inferior hypogastric plexus are identified and exposed. The parietal peritoneum is further incised caudally to the inguinal canal bilaterally, and the obliterated umbilical arteries are exposed to their origin from the internal iliac arteries. The para-visceral spaces are now developed by shifting the urogenital mesentery from the fat pads exposing the arcus tendineus and the pubo- and iliococcygeus muscles caudally.

Pelvic tLND is started by adventitia stripping of the external iliac vessels. Both artery and vein are completely freed of all lymphatic tissue. tLND is continued by the removal of the perivisceral fat pads containing the supra- and infraobturator, internal iliac, and inferior gluteal lymph node regions. To complete this step, the parietal branches of the internal iliac lymph node system must be sealed and cut, and the proximal sciatic nerve is then fully exposed. The obturator vessels may be included in the specimen, but the obturator nerve is spared unless encased by lymph node metastases. At the end of this step the endopelvic part of the internal obturator muscle, the pubo- and iliococcygeus muscles and the fascial connections of the endopelvic suspensorium to the sciatic spine are exposed. Pelvic tLND is continued by adventitia stripping of the common iliac vessels. To complete this step, again parietal branches have to be sealed and cut exposing the lumbar and first sacral branches of the lumbosacral trunk. This maneuver also allows the clearance of the superior gluteal lymph node region. The pelvic tLND is completed with the removal of the presacral fat pad down to the S2 level.

4. Laterally extended endopelvic resection

For locally advanced primary and postirradiation locally recurrent tumors of the cervix uteri and vagina, representing the major indication, surgical treatment necessitates *abdominoperineal anterior endopelvic resection* with or without lateral extension. Technical aspects of these procedures will be demonstrated in some detail first. The other variants of (L) EER are compiled in brief thereafter.

The *abdominal part* of the anterior endopelvic resection with or without lateral extension is initiated with the mobilization of the bladder compartment toward the symphysis and the ascending pubic bones (Figure 9-11). The ureters are cut before they intersect with the vascular mesometrium (Figure 9-12). The dissection sites are sent to frozen section histopathological examination to rule out microscopical tumor involvement. The ureters are temporarily splinted by soft catheters that direct the urine into bags. The peritoneum of the rectouterine pouch is incised as a "u" opening dorsally, and the rectum is pushed cranial-ward to separate the ligamentous mesometria of the Müllerian compartment from the hindgut compartment. These structures are sealed and cut at the level of the anterior rectum bilaterally (Figures 9-13 and 9-14). The hypogastric artery and veins are also dissected. The hypogastric artery is mobilized from its surrounding attachments and sealed and cut or divided between clamps and suture ligated (Figures 9-15 and 9-16). All parietal branches have to be sealed

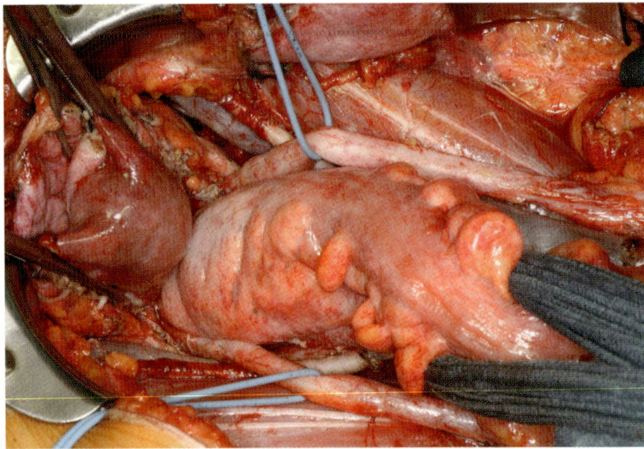

Fig. 9-11. Intraoperative situs of anterior endopelvic resection after therapeutic pelvic lymph node dissection.

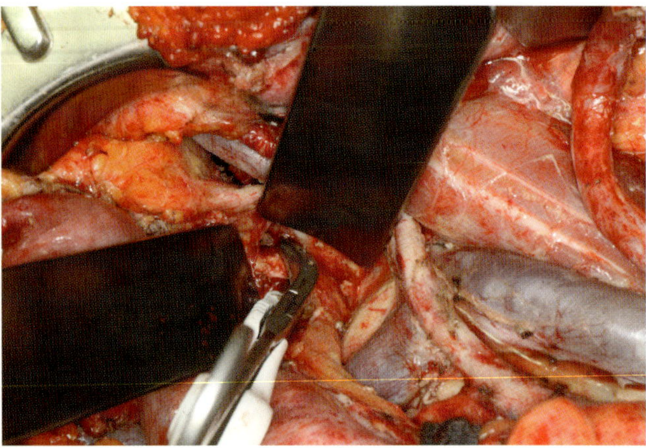

Fig. 9-13. Intraoperative abdominal situs of anterior endopelvic resection. Sealing and dissection of the right ligamentous mesometrium together with anterior branches of the inferior hypogastric plexus at the lateral mesorectum.

and cut before the internal iliac vessels can be completely detached from the common iliac vessels in case of lateral extension ([L]EER). The hypogastric artery is retracted, exposing the parietal branches of the hypogastric vein, which are divided individually and ligated (Figure 9-17). Once all parietal arterial and venous branches have been secured, the hypogastric vein is also divided (Figure 9-18). Parallel to the stepwise vascular dissection the ligamentous mesometrium, the major elements of the endopelvic suspensorium, are sealed and cut at the level of the lateral mesorectum (Figure 9-19). The anterior branches of the inferior hypogastric plexus are included in the (L)EER specimen. Once the fibers of the endopelvic suspensorium attached to the ischial spine are cut, the endopelvic fascia covering the pelvic floor muscles are reached (Figure 9-20). The ilio- and pubococcygeus muscles are incised at the tendineus arc of the pelvic fascia and mobilized medially against the surface of the ischioanal fossa

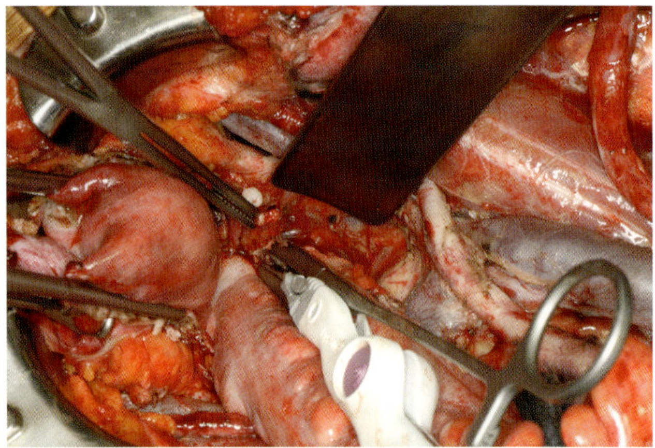

Fig. 9-14. Intraoperative abdominal situs of anterior endopelvic resection. Sealing and dissection of the right mesocolpos together with anterior branches of the inferior hypogastric plexus at the lateral mesorectum.

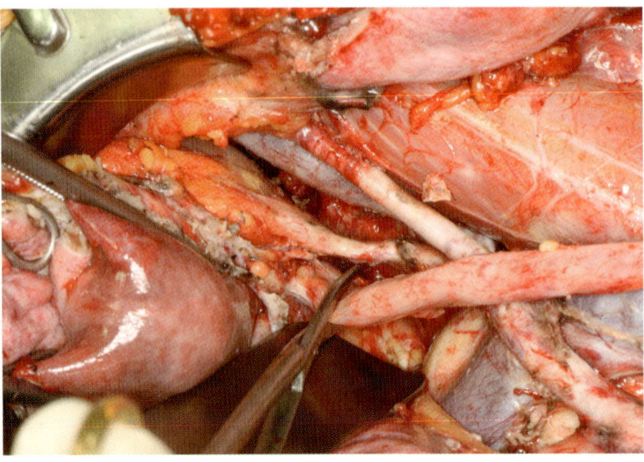

Fig. 9-12. Intraoperative abdominal situs of anterior endopelvic resection. Transection of the right ureter 2-cm proximal to its intersection with the vascular mesometrium.

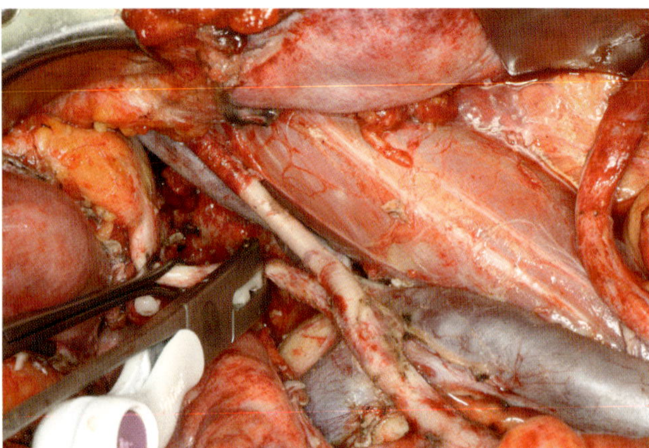

Fig. 9-15. Intraoperative abdominal situs of anterior endopelvic resection. Sealing, ligating, and dissection of the right hypogastric artery at its origin.

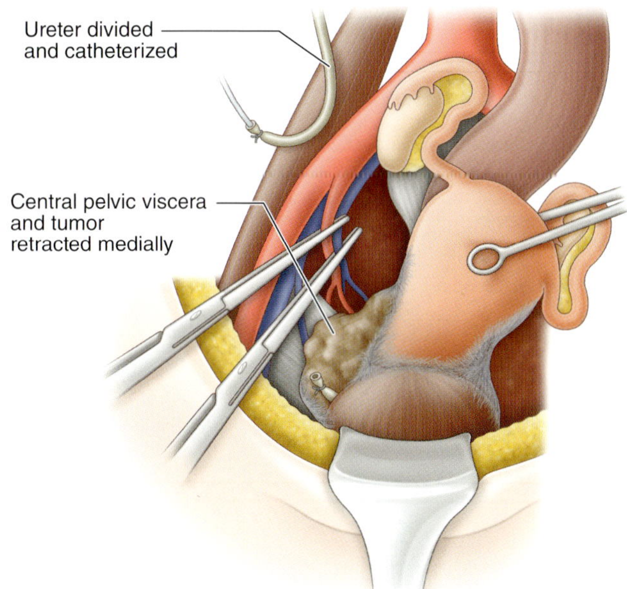

Fig. 9-16. The pelvic viscera and tumor specimen are retracted medially, exposing the hypogastric artery for clamping, division, and suture ligation.

(Figure 9-21). The internal pudendal vessels are identified as they course into the pubococcygeus muscle and sealed and cut (Figure 9-22) or divided between clamps. Depending on the extent of the tumor, the muscular dissection can also be laterally extended, including the complete levator ani muscle

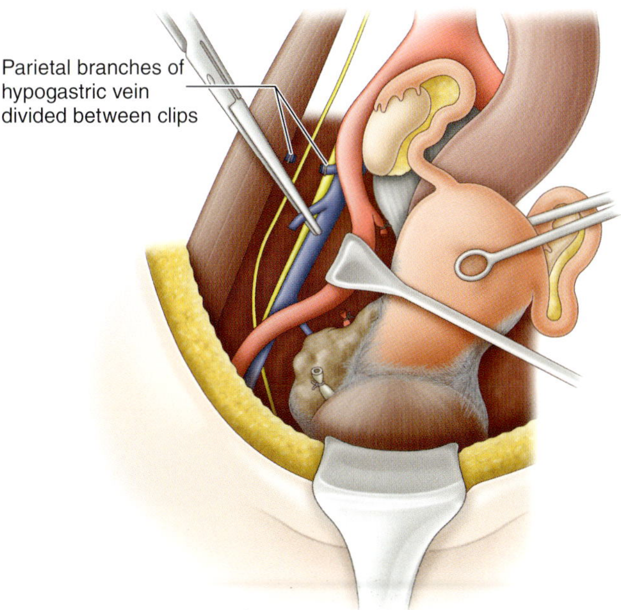

Fig. 9-17. The parietal branches of the hypogastric vein are isolated individually, clamped, divided, and suture ligated before dividing the hypogastric vein.

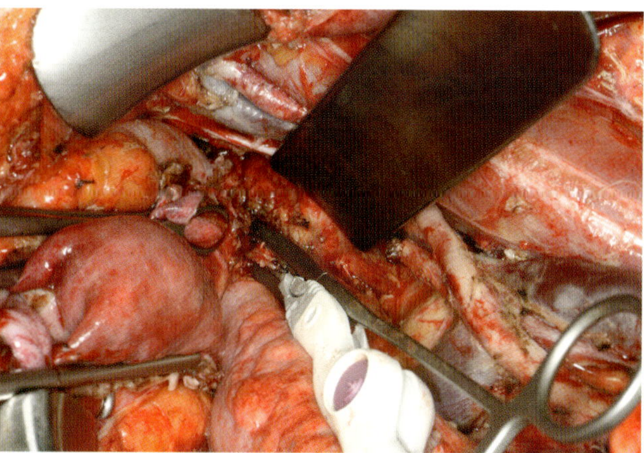

Fig. 9-18. Intraoperative abdominal situs of anterior endopelvic resection. Sealing and dissection of the right hypogastric veins at their insertion.

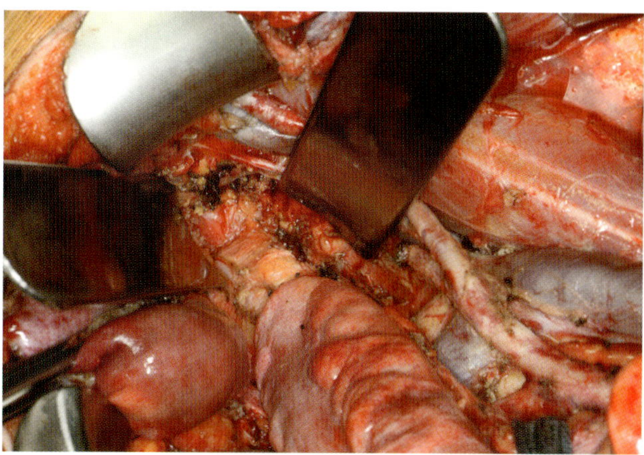

Fig. 9-19. Intraoperative abdominal situs of anterior endopelvic resection after sealing and dissection of the attachments of the mesopelvic suspensorium to the right sciatic spine.

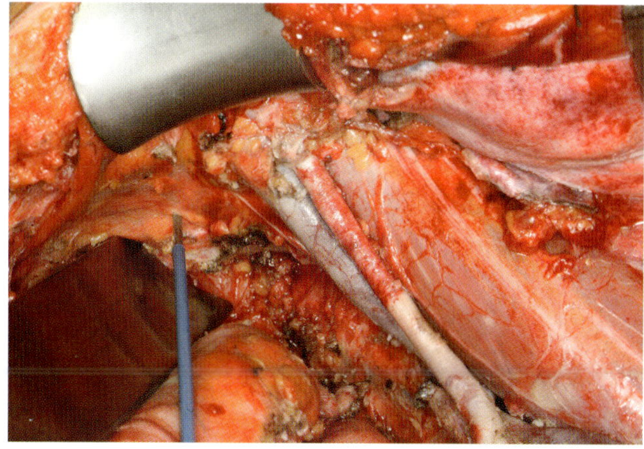

Fig. 9-20. Intraoperative abdominal situs of laterally extended anterior endopelvic resection. Muscular incision at right tendineus arc.

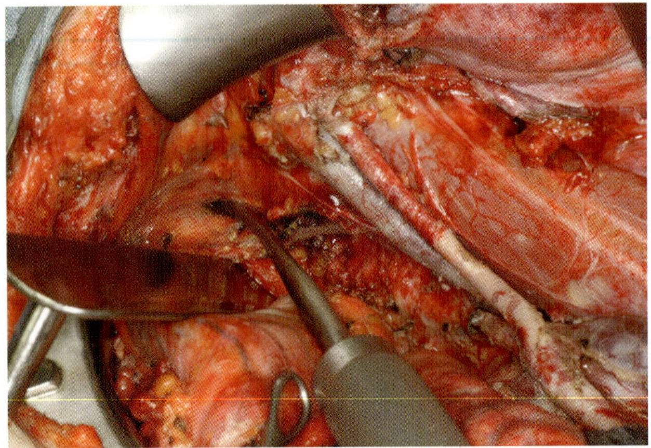

Fig. 9-21. Intraoperative abdominal situs of laterally extended anterior endopelvic resection. Mobilization of the right iliococcygeus muscle medially by use of a Cobb periosteal dissector.

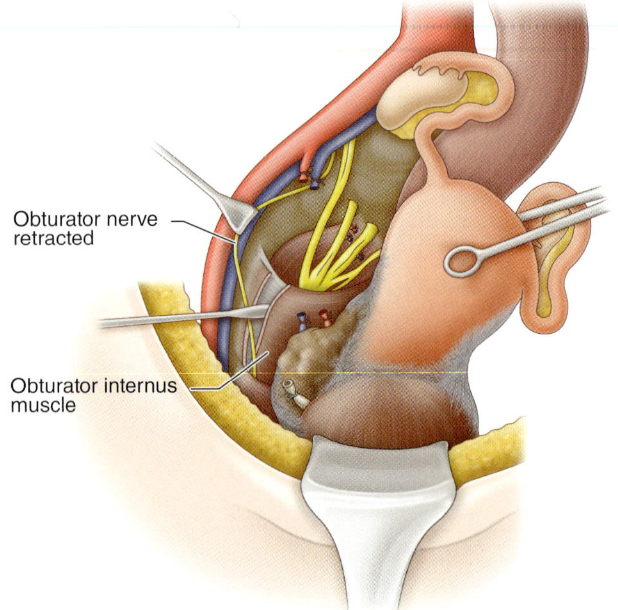

Fig. 9-23. The obturator internus muscle is incised ventrally and separated from the obturator membrane and acetabulum using a Cobb periosteal dissector.

and the endopelvic part of the internal obturator muscle. In this case, the obturator internus muscle is incised ventrally at the site of the obturator nerve, which is either elevated or divided if it is incorporated in the tumor. The obturator internus muscle is separated from the obturator membrane and acetabulum by use of a Cobb periosteal dissector (Figure 9-23). Completion of the muscular resection at the sidewall exposes the fatty tissue within the ischiorectal fossa (Figure 9-24). Dorsally, the distal ligamentous mesometrium forming the proximal rectovaginal septum are separated from the anterior rectal wall reaching the level below the levator ani plate (Figure 9-25). Ventrally, the periurethral vessels are sealed and cut (Figure 9-26).

The patient is then turned into the lithotomy position for the *perineal part* of (L)EER. The perineal skin incision is made at the Hart's line of the minor labia and at the anterior and posterior commissure of the vulva, including the complete vestibulum (Figure 9-27). The anal sphincter and anal canal are separated from the posterior distal part of the internal UGS compartment (Figure 9-28). Laterally, the internal UGS compartment is separated from the deep vulvar structures (bulbi vestibulares, vestibular glands). Anteriorly, the pubourethral ligaments are sealed and cut allowing to pull the complete (L)EER specimen through the genital hiatus (Figures 9-29 and 9-30). The completed resection results in a generous pelvic defect that may be prone to herniation or fistula formation (Figures 9-31 and 9-32). For the prevention of hiatus genitalis

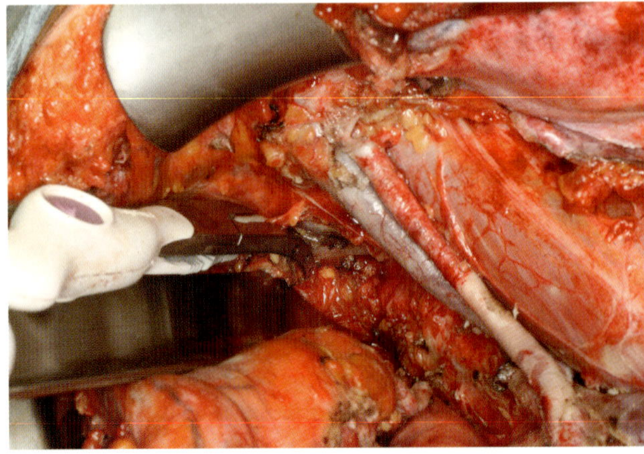

Fig. 9-22. Intraoperative abdominal situs of laterally extended anterior endopelvic resection. Sealing of branches of the right internal pudendal vessels to the pubococcygeus muscle.

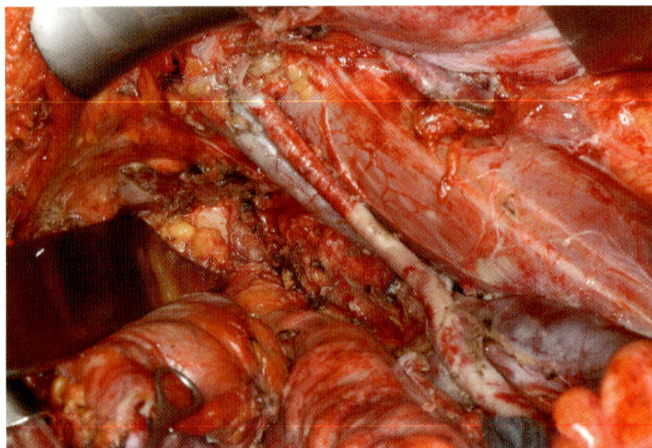

Fig. 9-24. Intraoperative abdominal situs of laterally extended anterior endopelvic resection after completing the muscular dissection exposing the fatty tissue of the ischiorectal fossa.

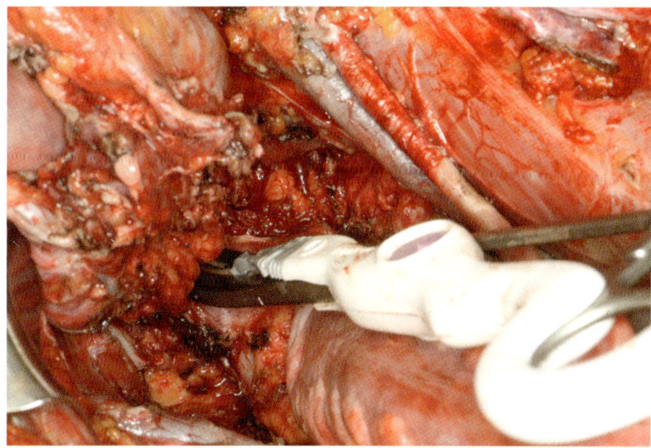

Fig. 9-25. Intraoperative abdominal situs of laterally extended anterior endopelvic resection. Sealing and dissection of the distal mesocolpos.

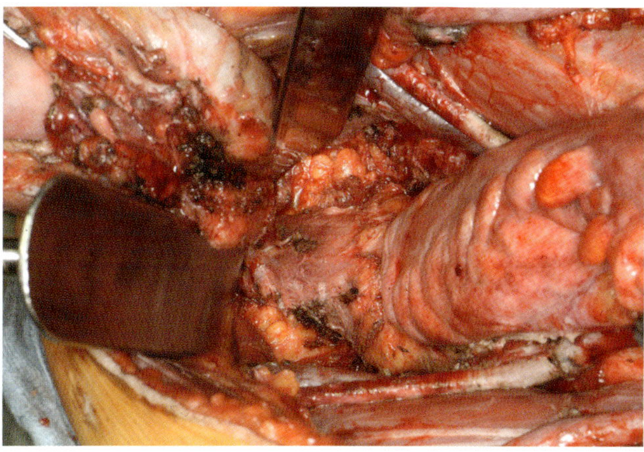

Fig. 9-26. Intraoperative abdominal situs of laterally extended anterior endopelvic resection after completion of the abdominal part.

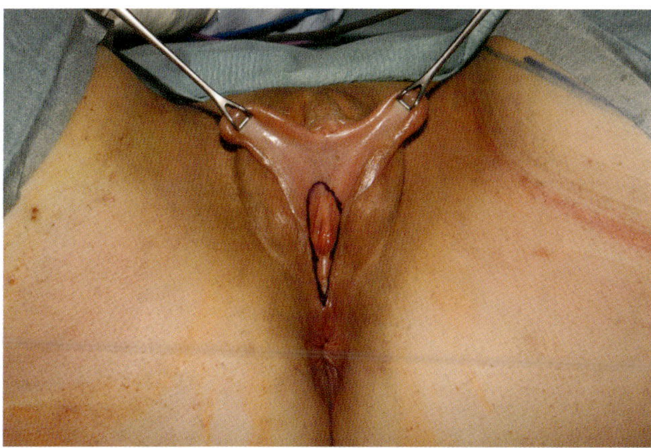

Fig. 9-27. Intraoperative perineal situs of abdominoperineal anterior endopelvic resection. Perineal incision line.

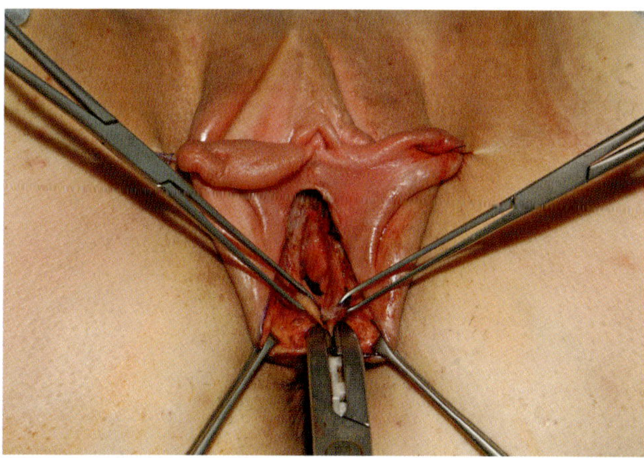

Fig. 9-28. Intraoperative perineal situs of abdominoperineal anterior endopelvic resection. Sealing and dissection of the attachments of the rectovaginal septum to the anorectum.

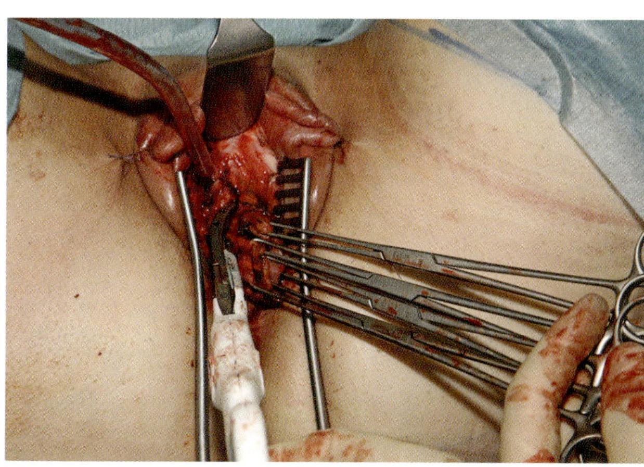

Fig. 9-29. Intraoperative perineal situs of abdominoperineal anterior endopelvic resection. Sealing and dissection of the right pubourethral ligament.

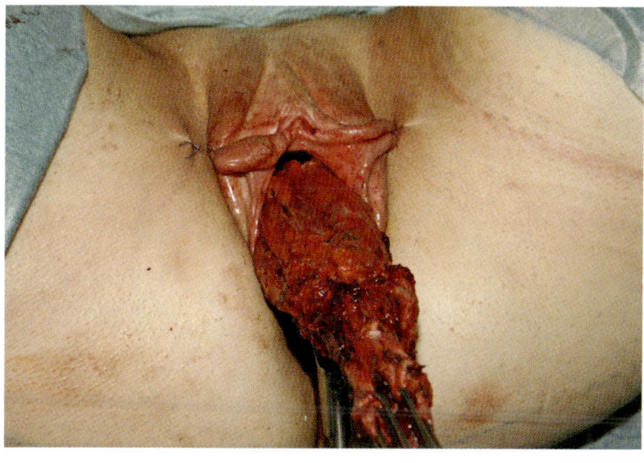

Fig. 9-30. Intraoperative perineal situs of abdominoperineal anterior endopelvic resection. Pulling of the specimen through the genital hiatus.

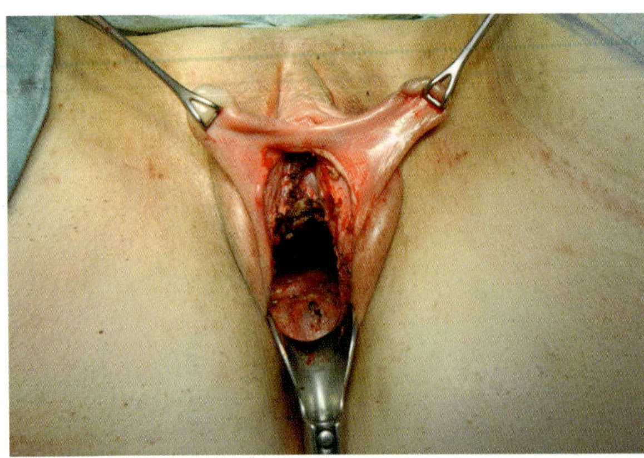

Fig. 9-31. Intraoperative perineal situs of abdominoperineal anterior endopelvic resection after completion of the resective phase demonstrating the open genital hiatus.

herniation and for the formation of a neovestibulum, a pudendal thigh flap elevated from the genitocrural region is useful.

After returning the patient to the supine position, supravesical urinary reconstruction is performed. An omentum majus flap is raised and transposed to the denuded pelvis. Sewn to the rim of the parietal peritoneum, symphysis, and rectum, it should completely cover and vascularize the sub- and retroperitoneal surgical field of the pelvis. After abdominopelvic lavage a closed-suction indicator drain is placed and the laparotomy is closed.

If the tumor involves the hindgut compartment, *total* (L)EER is indicated. The bowel continuity is interrupted at the retrosigmoidal transition or a lower more appropriate site. In the abdominal part of the procedure the posterior dissection plane is set to the dorsal mesorectum. The inferior hypogastric plexus are resected along with the complete endopelvic suspensorium. The coccygeus muscles

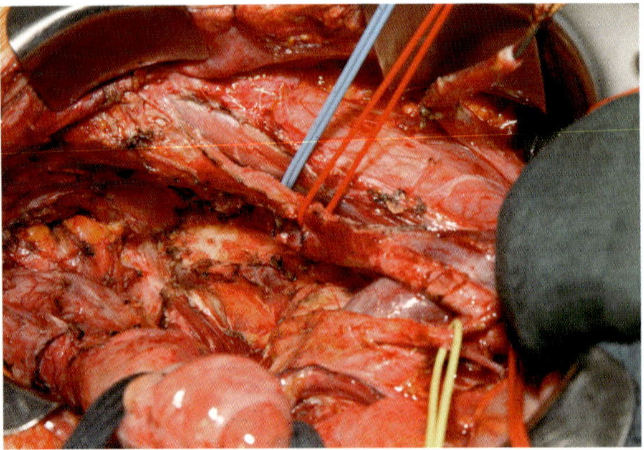

Fig. 9-32. Intraoperative abdominal situs of laterally extended anterior endopelvic resection after completion of the abdominal resection phase exposing the right iliolumbar trunk and proximal sciatic nerve and the iliorectal fat separated by the sacrospinous ligament and coccygeus muscle.

and sacrospinous ligaments can be included in the muscular dissection step if needed. The perineal incision is extended perianally, and the anus and anal canal are included in the (L)EER specimen.

POSTOPERATIVE CARE

Box 9-3 PERIOPERATIVE MORBIDITY

- Infective wound breakdown is causal for most of the early postoperative morbidity. Therapeutic secondary healing should be considered in the irradiated and morbidly obese patient.
- Sectional imaging (CT) should be requested early in case of suspected intra-abdominal morbidity.
- Skillful interventional radiologic techniques can prevent re-operation particularly in case of urologic complications.

Patients treated with (L)EER should receive intensive care surveillance during the early postoperative period. Most patients can be transferred to intermediate or low care facilities after 1 to 2 days. Treatment-related mortality rates can be kept below 2%; in our series, it has been 0 since 1999. However, moderate and severe complications of up to 50% must be taken into consideration when counseling the patient. Treatment-related morbidity is mainly due to pretreatment tissue alterations and significantly increases with the complexity of the reconstructive procedures. The complications following (L)EER treatment are compiled in Table 9-1. Most moderate and severe complications are related to infection and to reconstruction failures.

LONG-TERM OUTCOMES

Box 9-4 DELAYED COMPLICATIONS

- Late morbidity refers mainly to the reconstruction of the bladder function. Regular urologic check-ups should ensure early intervention to prevent damage of the upper urinary tract.
- As lymph edemas are aggravated by erysipelas, early antibiotic therapy should be administered in case of even small skin lesions at the lower extremities.
- Perineal and abdominal herniation is pronounced with postoperative weight gain. The patient should be advised to watch her weight.

(L)EER has been evaluated by a prospective clinical trial at the University of Leipzig School of Radical Pelvic Surgery

Table 9-1. Moderate and severe complications of (L)EER treatment.

	Early			Late		
Complications	**G2**	**G3**	**G4**	**G2**	**G3**	**G4**
Cardiopulmonary[a]	2%					
Cutaneous[b]	1%			3%		
Gastrointestinal[c]	7%	3%		4%		
Neurologic[d]	2%					
Urinary[e]	7%	1%	1%	1%	1%	
Vascular[f]	9%			3%		

Data from 91 patients treated during March 1999 to March 2012.[6]
[a]Pneumonia, pulmonary edema (early).
[b]Laparotomy dehiscence, partial flap necrosis, donor site dehiscence (early); perineal hernia, abdominal wall hernia (late).
[c]Bowel obstruction, anastomosis insufficiency, bowel fistula, generalized peritonitis, rectum stump dehiscence, pelvic abscess (early); parastomal hernia (late).
[d]Temporary paresis of femoral and sciatic nerve.
[e]Bleeding, anastomotic insufficiency, ischemic necrosis of conduit, pouch neobladder, hydronephrosis (early); stenosis of urostoma, pouch incontinence (late).
[f]Postoperative bleeding, deep venous thrombosis, pulmonary embolia (early); infected lymphocyst, leg edema (late).

since 1998. (L)EER achieved a 100% R0 resection rate without abortion of any procedure during the resective phase.[6] R0 resection has been proven to be the most important factor for pelvic tumor control and cure.[7] Locoregional tumor control of 90% and overall survival rates of 60% have been obtained in the treatment of locally advanced and recurrent cancer, the majority of them being tumors fixed to the pelvic side wall, which are usually not considered for surgical treatment at all. Late complications are listed in table 9-1. Lymph edema and long-term failure of surgical reconstruction represent late morbidity related to (L)EER and tLND.

SUMMARY

Procedures termed (L)EER have been developed for the treatment of locally advanced and recurrent uterovaginal cancer translating new insights of locoregional tumor spread into surgical practice. Extended endopelvic resection extirpates the mature tissue derived from multiple ontogenetic developmental domains such as the Müllerian, bladder, urogenital sinus compartments, as well as the proximal urogenital mesentery. If indicated, the hindgut compartment can be included into the abdominal resection. To integrate the urogenital sinus compartments, the procedure has to be performed abdominoperineally. Resection of the distal urogenital mesentery—necessary for the surgical treatment of disease fixed to the pelvic wall—mandates the inclusion of the internal iliac vessel system and/or pelvic wall and floor muscles. These procedures are termed (L)EER, which reliably achieve R0 resection in patients with locally advanced and recurrent uterovaginal cancer if tumor fixation at the region of the sciatic foramen and peritoneal spread can be excluded.

REFERENCES

1. Höckel M. Cancer permeates locally within ontogenetic compartments: clinical evidence and implications for cancer surgery. *Future Oncol.* 2012;8(1):29-36.
2. Höckel M, Horn L-C, Manthey N, et al. Resection of the embryologically defined uterovaginal (Müllerian) compartment and pelvic control in patients with cervical cancer: a prospective analysis. *Lancet Oncol.* 2009;10(7):683-692.
3. Höckel M, Horn L-C, Illig R, Dornhöfer N, Fritsch H. Ontogenetic anatomy of the distal vagina: Relevance for local tumor spread and implications for cancer surgery. *Gynecol Oncol.* 2011;122(2):313-318.
4. Höckel M, Schmidt K, Bornmann K, Horn L-C, Dornhöfer N. Vulvar field resection: novel approach to the surgical treatment of vulvar cancer based on ontogenetic anatomy. *Gynecol Oncol.* 2010;119(1):106-113.
5. Höckel M, Horn L-C, Tetsch E, Einenkel J. Pattern analysis of regional spread and therapeutic lymph node dissection in cervical cancer based on ontogenetic anatomy. *Gynecol Oncol.* 2012;125(1):168-174.
6. Höckel M, Horn L-C, Einenkel J. (Laterally) extended endopelvic resection: surgical treatment of locally advanced and recurrent cancer of the uterine cervix and vagina based on ontogenetic anatomy. *Gynecol Oncol.* 2012;127(2):297-302.
7. Höckel M, Dornhöfer N. Pelvic exenteration for gynaecologic tumours: achievements and unanswered questions. *Lancet Oncol.* 2006;7(10):837-847.
8. Sadler TW. *Langman's Medical Embryology.* 9th ed. Philadelphia, PA: Lippincott, Williams & Wilkins; 2004.
9. Larsen WJ. *Human Embryology.* 3rd ed. Philadelphia, PA: Churchill Livingstone; 2001.
10. O'Rahilly R, Müller F. *Human Embryology and Teratology.* 3rd ed. New York, NY: Wiley-Liss; 2001.
11. Keibel F. Zur Entwicklungsgeschichte des menschlichen Urogenitalapparates. In: *Archiv für Anatomie und Physiologie.* Leipzig:1896:55-156.
12. Van der Putte SCJ. The development of the perineum in the human. In: *Advances in Anatomy, Embryology and Cell Biology.* Vol. 177. New York, NY: Springer; 1975.
13. Höckel M, Horn L-C, Fritsch H. Association between the mesenchymal compartment of uterovaginal organogenesis and local tumour spread in stage IB-IIB cervical carcinoma: a prospective study. *Lancet Oncol.* 2005;6(10):751-756.
14. Fritsch H, Kühnel W. Development and distribution of adipose tissue in the human pelvis. *Early Hum Dev.* 1992;28(1):79-88.

Chapter 10. Bone and Extended Pelvic Resections

Rudy S. Suidan, MD,
David G. McKeown, MD, and
Patrick J. Boland, MD

BACKGROUND

Most recurrent and locally advanced gynecologic malignancies carry a poor prognosis. Advances in multimodality management have improved local control and overall survival (OS).[1-3] Historically, tumors invading the pelvic sidewall or involving the major vessels or nerves were considered inoperable. Early reports of central pelvic exenteration were discouraging and associated with high perioperative mortality (28%) and major complications (100%).[4] Advances in several medical disciplines have resulted in greatly improved outcome and reduced morbidity and mortality in the management of these complex tumors. Increasingly effective chemotherapy and refinement in methods of radiation administration have rendered these large tumors, most of which had previous radiation therapy, amenable to wide surgical resection.

The use of modern imaging technology has improved our ability to accurately outline the anatomy of the tumors preoperatively and rule out distant metastases. Several studies have shown that obtaining negative surgical margins of resection is essential to local tumor control and improvement of OS.[1] Preoperative medical assessment and management, expert anesthesia, and postoperative intensive care have reduced perioperative mortality to less than 5%.[1-3] The majority of patients undergoing radical pelvic surgery including those with recurrent endometrial and cervical tumors have already had surgery and radiation therapy. Patients with locally advanced primary carcinomas and a minority with advanced primary or recurrent sarcomas may also be candidates for the type of radical pelvic surgery described in this chapter.

INDICATIONS AND CLINICAL APPLICATIONS

This chapter describes the surgical management of a small group of tumors, which, due to their proximity to or invasion of bone, require bony pelvic resections in order to achieve a wide surgical margin. We also discuss management of tumors involving major vessels and nerves. Major sidewall soft tissue resections are discussed in Chapter 9.

Bony involvement occurs from extension of tumor growth into the periosteum by direct invasion or by spread through local vessels into the bone (local metastasis). In some cases, the tumors do not actually involve bone but are inseparable from it, such that a wide resection can only be accomplished by resecting the adjacent bone. Better understanding of the functional anatomy of the pelvis and our ability to reconstruct following major bony resections has made these procedures possible. Resection of the periacetabular area or the hip usually requires extensive reconstruction, while resection of the area above and below the hip may not.[5] It should be emphasized that the number of patients who are suitable candidates following full local and systemic staging are few and that a multidisciplinary approach is essential to ensure a satisfactory outcome.

ANATOMIC CONSIDERATIONS

A thorough knowledge of the topographic and functional anatomy of the pelvis is essential for surgeons embarking on these operations. Knowledge of the topographic anatomy ensures that the surgeon is familiar with important landmarks and relationships of various structures to each other, enabling safe and effective resections. Familiarity with functional anatomy allows the surgeon to decide whether surgery is feasible, if it would result in an acceptable quality of life, and whether soft tissue and bony reconstruction are necessary. This knowledge is also important when counseling patients preoperatively.

The true pelvis is tilted 60° anterior to the long axis of the body, so that on digital examination per rectum or vagina, the pubic bone, ischial spine, and tip of coccyx are in the same horizontal plane (Figure 10-1). These are landmarks that are also helpful intraoperatively. The lumbosacral nerve and sympathetic trunks will be found deep to the common iliac vessels anterior to the sacral ala (Figure 10-2). The ureter, adherent to the peritoneum, crosses the bifurcation of the common iliac arteries. The piriformis muscle is a key anatomic structure in

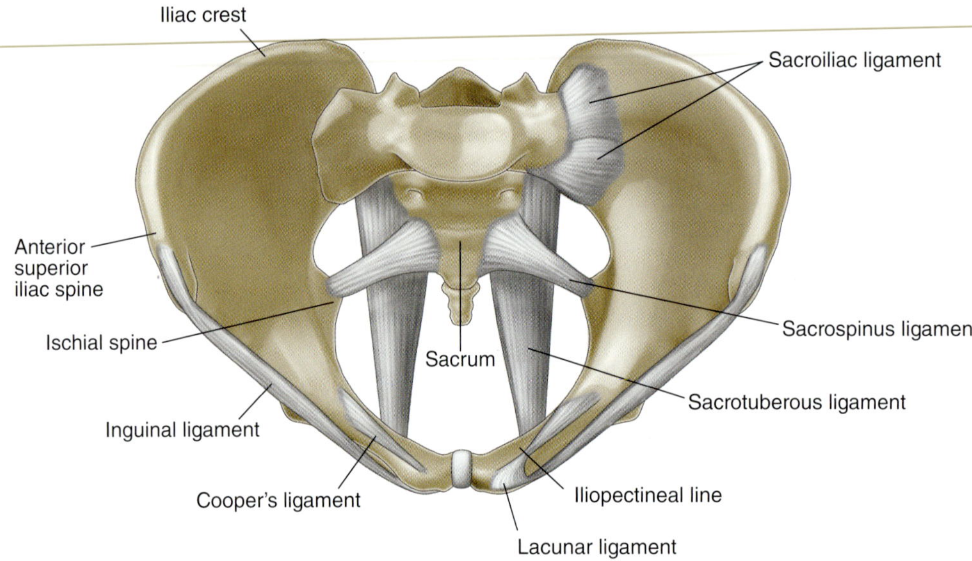

Fig. 10-1. Bony pelvis with ligaments.

the pelvis and can be readily identified (Figure 10-3). It lies above the palpable ischial spine and sacrospinous ligament, and it runs through the greater sciatic notch. The superior gluteal vessels and nerves pass above the piriformis to exit the pelvis and supply the abductor muscles of the hip. The sciatic nerve, inferior gluteal, and pudendal neurovascular structures lie anterior to the piriformis and pass posteriorly out of the pelvis above the sacrospinous ligament. The pudendal nerve and vessels curve over the ischial spine and enter the ischiorectal fossa. The anterior sacral foramina can be easily identified and their emerging sacral roots visualized. The obturator nerve lies on the sidewall of the pelvis lateral to the iliac vessels. It passes through the obturator foramen with the obturator vessels anteriorly and inferiorly.

The functions of the bony pelvis include supporting and protecting its contained viscera and neurovascular structures, and transmission of body weight to the lower limbs. It is a semirigid ring composed of the innominate bone (the entire fused ilium, ischium, and pubis) laterally and the sacrum posteriorly (see Figure 10-1). Anteriorly, the pubic bones join at the symphysis pubis, a relatively weak cartilaginous joint. Posteriorly, the innominate bone, often referred to as the hip bone, articulates with the sacrum through bilateral strong sacroiliac joints. This articulation extends from the S1 to the S3 segments. The sacroiliac joint is a complex one, consisting of a small synovial joint anteriorly, which allows minimal gliding motion. However, most of the articulation is composed of very strong ligaments that are both intra-articular and extra-articular. The posterior spinal pelvic ligaments are some of the strongest in the body. The articular surfaces of the joints are irregular and afford some stability, but overall stability is dependent on the strong sacroiliac ligaments. Removal of the inferior two-thirds of the sacroiliac joint requires surgical stabilization. The anterior symphysis pubis and posterolateral sacrospinous and sacrotuberous ligaments afford minor stability, and their removal usually causes little disability. Major resection of the innominate bone, which disrupts the transmission of weight from the spine to the lower limb, usually requires reconstruction.

The sidewall of the true pelvis is largely lined by the obturator internus, which is covered by the dense pelvic fascia. A tendinous fascial arch extending from the ischial spine posteriorly to the pubis anteriorly along this muscle forms the origin of the pelvic floor muscles. These muscles support the pelvic and abdominal viscera, especially during periods of increased intraabdominal pressure. They also surround the vagina, bladder neck, and rectum, acting as an adjuvant sphincter. When resecting the pelvic floor muscles, surgical reconstruction using muscle flaps from the abdomen and thigh help restore these important functions.

Ligation of the internal iliac (hypogastric) vessels is well tolerated (see Figure 10-3). Resection of the common or external iliac arteries requires reconstruction. Ligation or resection of the common or external iliac veins usually results in lower limb edema. Venous reconstruction is typically not successful, but early postoperative pressure bandaging can control subsequent lower limb swelling.

The autonomic nerves lie in the pelvic plexus adjacent to the internal iliac arteries and their branches (see Figure 10-3). They are composed of the parasympathetic fibers from the second, third, and fourth sacral nerves, and the sympathetic fibers from the sympathetic trunks entering the pelvis from the lower thoracic and upper lumbar spine. These nerves supply the bladder, rectum, and reproductive organs. Parasympathetic fibers are motor to rectal and bladder detrusor muscles and relax their sphincters. Sympathetic fibers contract sphincters and constrict vessels. These nerves can be destroyed with sacral and posterior pelvic resections, resulting in bowel incontinence, bladder obstruction, and loss of sexual function.

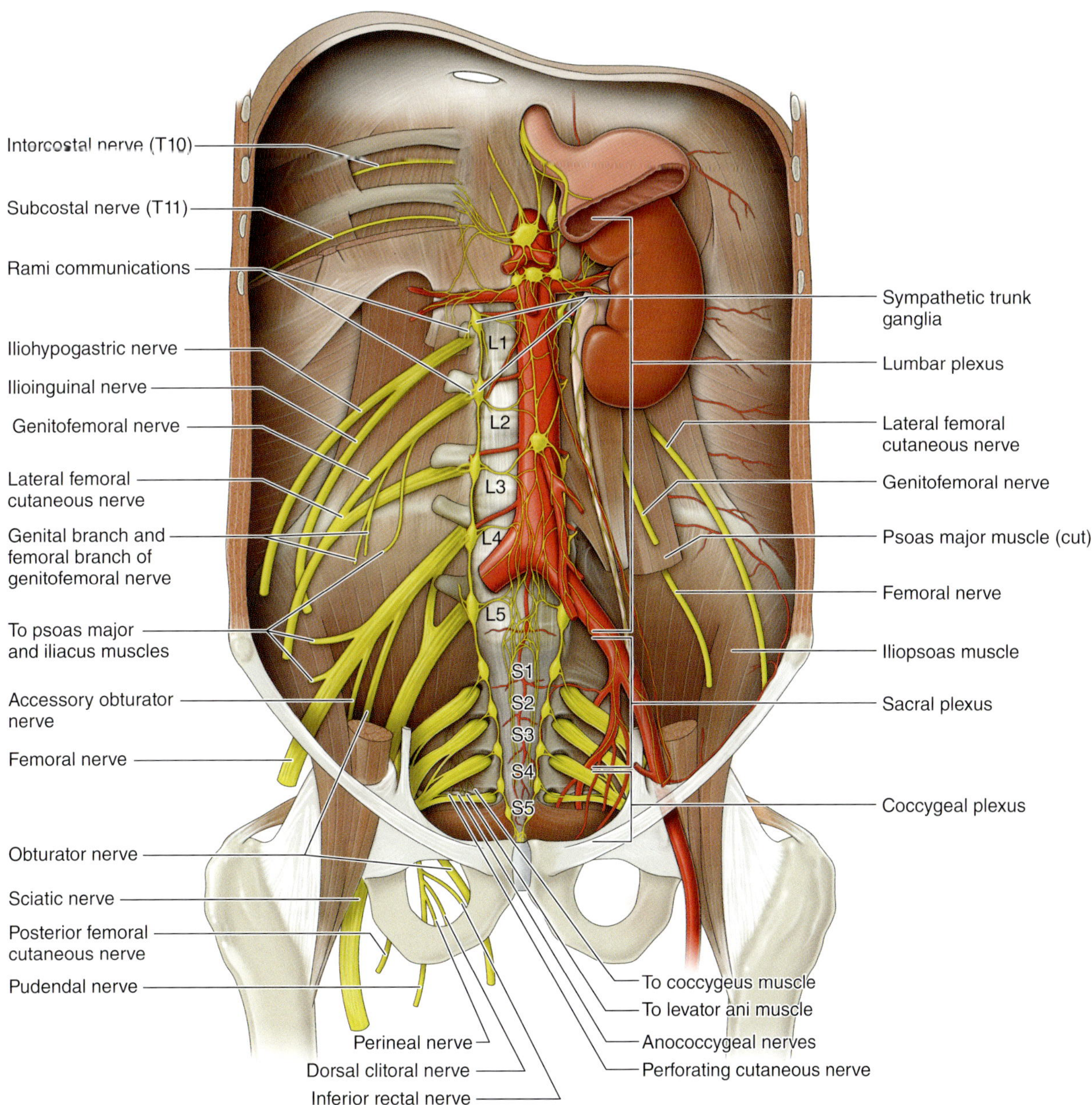

Fig. 10-2. Anterior view of pelvic inlet showing major neurovascular structures entering the pelvis.

The femoral, sciatic, and obturator nerves are the major spinal nerves supplying the lower limbs (see Figure 10-2). The obturator nerve adducts the thigh and its sacrifice results in only mild disability. Resection of the sciatic or femoral nerves does result in significant disability. The sciatic nerve supplies the hamstring muscle, all the muscles of ankle and toe flexion, and sensation to the leg below the knee and foot, with the exception of a small pretibial area which is supplied by the saphenous branch of the femoral nerve. The femoral nerve supplies the quadriceps muscles, which extend the knee and stabilize the leg when walking. It also supplies sensation to the anterior and medial thigh and pretibial areas. Patients can walk when either nerve is excised; however, removal of both nerves results in such disability that limb salvage is usually contraindicated.

Resection of the sacral plexus above the piriformis muscle results in significantly more ambulatory disability than resections below this muscle, as the gluteal nerves that supply the abductor muscles of the hip will be sacrificed (see Figure 10-2). This results in loss of lateral hip stabilization, in addition to the loss of ankle and foot motion. The pudendal nerve exits the pelvis lateral to sciatic and gluteal nerves at the top of the ischial spine. It immediately enters the ischiorectal fossa supplying motor function to the pelvic floor, lower vagina, anal canal, and urethra. Every effort should be taken to preserve this nerve.

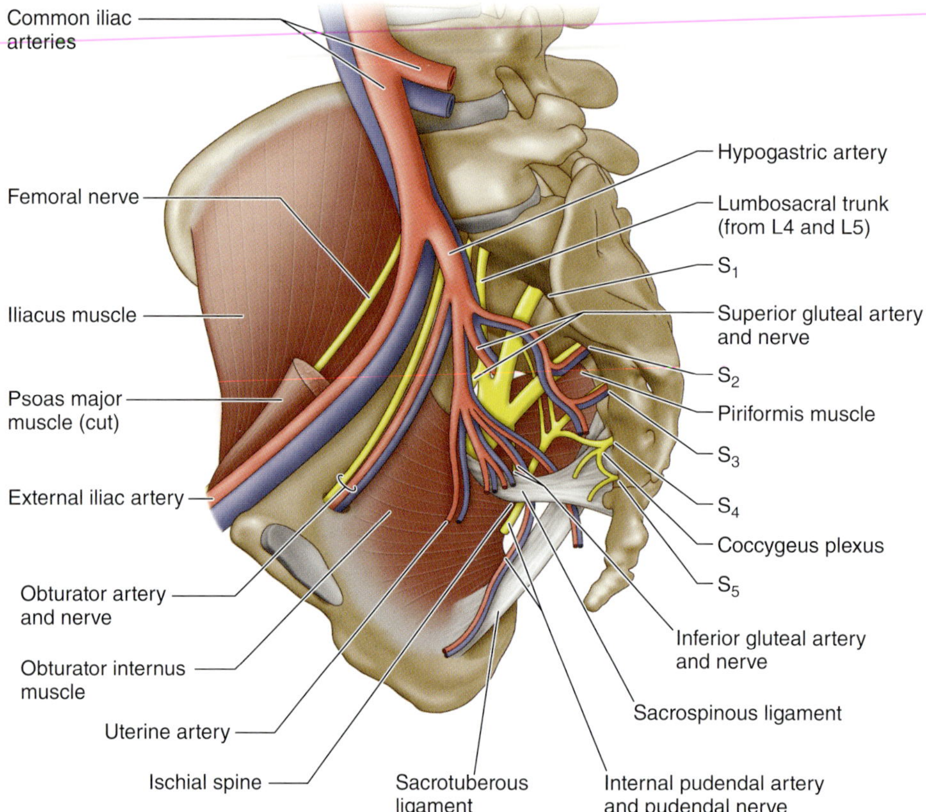

Fig. 10-3. Pelvic sidewall showing sacral plexus and major vessels.

PREOPERATIVE PREPARATION

Box 10-1 KEY SURGICAL INSTRUMENTATION

- Osteotome and oscillating saw
- Self-retaining retractor
- Long pelvic instruments
- Electrocautery with long tip
- Peripheral nerve stimulator

A detailed preoperative history and physical examination must be carried out by all involved surgeons. Patients with poor performance status and significant comorbidity should not be subjected to these procedures until the status is satisfactorily upgraded. Objective neurologic findings in the lower limbs such as loss of peripheral nerve function or loss of bowel and/or bladder function usually indicate invasion of nerve, which will necessitate their removal en bloc with the tumor. In selected patients at high risk of prolonged postoperative bleeding, which may constitute a contraindication to anticoagulation, preoperative insertion of an inferior vena caval filter may be prudent.

Imaging of the pelvis including plain radiographs, computed tomography (CT), and magnetic resonance imaging (MRI) scans are essential to study the extent of the tumor and plan surgery. It is also necessary to rule out systemic extrapelvic metastases in these patients using positron emission tomography (PET)/CT scans before considering surgery. Recent data have shown that PET/MRI had greater diagnostic confidence and inter-reader agreement than either MRI or PET/CT in patients with recurrent gynecologic cancers.[6]

SURGICAL PROCEDURE

Box 10-2 MASTER SURGEON'S PRINCIPLES

- Obturator nerve may be excised with little disability
- Unilateral resection of either the femoral or sciatic nerve is possible with satisfactory postoperative ambulatory function
- Resection of the sacral plexus above the piriformis muscle results in significantly greater ambulatory disability than resection below it
- Pudendal nerve preservation is important if resection not indicated
- Resection of the common or external iliac artery requires reconstruction
- Disruption of the hip and periacetabular pelvis should be reconstructed

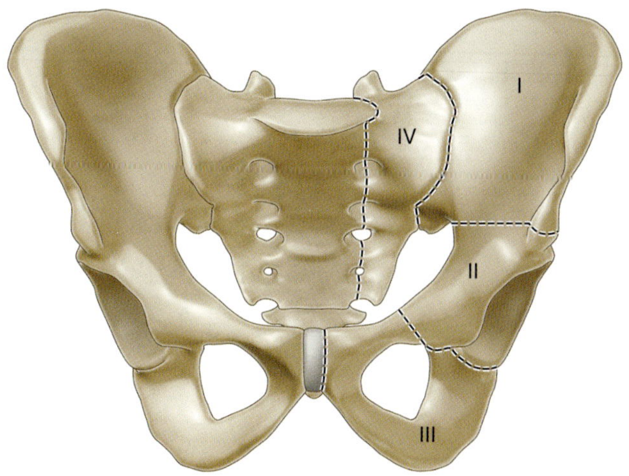

Fig. 10-4. Types of pelvic resections: Type I (ilium), Type II (periacetabular), Type III (ischium and pubis), Type IV (sacra ala).

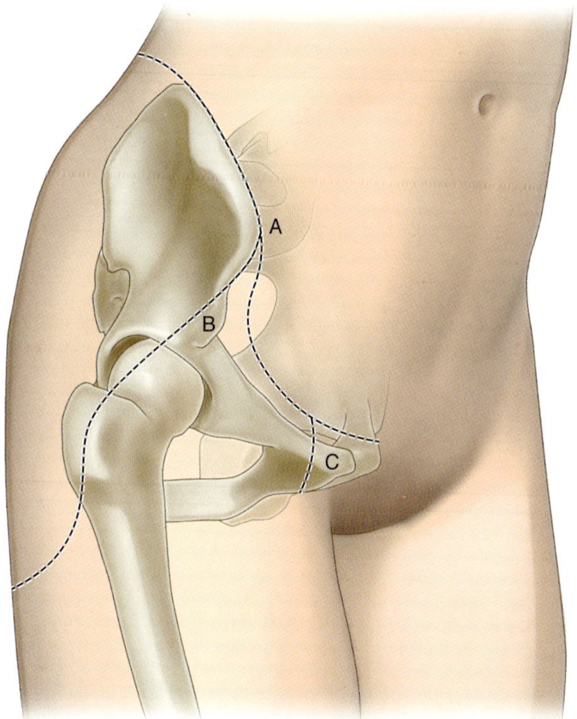

Fig. 10-5. Surgical exposures for pelvic resections. (A) Ileo-inguinal. (B) Ileo-femoral. (C) Perineal.

Pelvic Bone Resections

Curative surgery for localized pelvic tumors can only be accomplished with a wide resection with negative pathologic margins (R0 resection). In suitable cases, all or parts of the hemipelvis (innominate bone) and surrounding soft tissue can be resected while preserving a functional lower limb below.

Pelvic bone resections have been classified into four types based on the structures removed (Figure 10-4)[7,8]:

a. Type I: ilium
b. Type II: periacetabular
c. Type III: ischium and pubis
d. Type IV: sacral ala

Each type can be extended to include adjacent areas. Complete resection of the innominate bone with sacral ala is classified as a Type I, II, III, and IV resection. This is also known as an extended internal hemipelvectomy.

Technique

The surgical approach to the pelvis is done through an iliofemoral incision with an ilioinguinal and perineal extension (Figure 10-5).[9] Any part or all of this incision is used depending on the area being resected. Resection Types I and II can be carried out through the iliofemoral portion alone while exposure of the pubic body and rami require the ilioinguinal portion.

With the patient lying in a floppy lateral position, the incision is made starting posteriorly between the 12th rib and iliac crest. This extends parallel to the iliac crest and curves inferiorly at the anterior superior iliac spine to a point below the greater trochanter where it curves posteriorly below the gluteal crease. Quadratus lumborum and abdominal wall muscles attached to the ilium are divided allowing access to the extraperitoneal structures. Anterior to this, the iliac fossa is visualized, exposing the iliopsoas and pelvic sidewall structures. The ureter and vessels are separated from the muscles. The sciatic notches are exposed. The internal iliac vessels may be divided and ligated at this time, if necessary.

Exposure of the outer portion of the pelvis is accomplished by creating a flap consisting of the skin and gluteus maximus. The lateral hip (greater trochanter) is exposed and further dissection posteriorly exposes the sciatic notch and its contents below and the sacroiliac joint above. If the superior and inferior iliac vessels have been preserved anteriorly, care is taken to prevent damaging them since they provide an important blood supply to this large flap. The deep gluteal muscles (medius and minimus) can be detached from the iliac bone either by subperiosteal resection or trochanteric osteotomy. In cases where tumor involves the muscles, these muscles would be resected en-bloc with the bone.

In a Type I resection, the iliac bone is divided through the supra-acetabular bone starting at the sciatic notch and extending anteriorly above the hip joint (see Figure 10-4). The posterior iliac division passes through the sacroiliac joint or sacral ala. If the sacroiliac joint and sacral ala is involved with tumor (Figure 10-6), the resection is carried out through the sacral ala medial to the tumor (Types I and IV). Stabilization following this resection can be achieved by instrumentation extending from the lower spine to the remaining pelvic bone (Figure 10-7).[10] The herniation created by the removal of the pelvic sidewall can be repaired with a mesh.

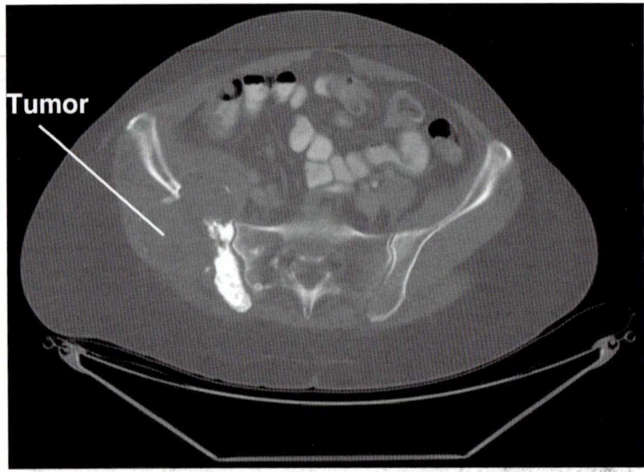

Fig. 10-6. Computed tomography (CT) scan of a patient with recurrent endometrial sidewall carcinoma involving the iliac bone.

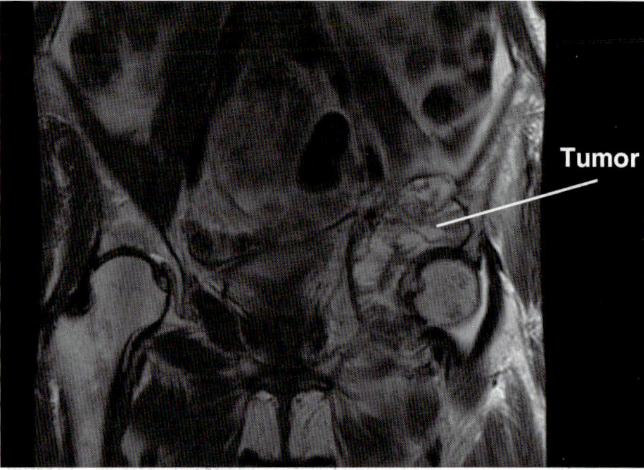

Fig. 10-8. Magnetic resonance imaging of a patient with recurrent endometrial carcinoma invading the acetabulum.

In a Type II resection, the femoral neck is divided and the iliac bone is cut above and below the acetabulum depending on the extent of the tumor (see Figure 10-4). If periacetabular tumors extend high into the iliac bone, then a combined Type I and II resection will be required. In patients with tumor involving the muscles on the inner or outer aspects of the pelvis, these muscles must be resected with the bone. Reconstruction of the hip joint should be performed, if possible, because this type of resection results in significant instability and difficulty weight bearing. In Type II resections reconstruction can be accomplished using a structural periacetabular allograft (transplanted bone harvested from a cadaver) combined with a total hip replacement (Figures 10-8 to 10-10).[11,12]

In combined Type I and II resections (Figures 10-11 and 10-12), alloprosthesis (Figures 10-13 and 10-14) extending from sacrum above to the ischium and pubis below can be used for reconstruction, or a metal cement bridge into which a total hip prosthesis is inserted can also be satisfactory (Figure 10-15).[11] Some surgeons favor no reconstruction, leaving a flail hip (Figure 10-16).

Type III resections of the pelvis below the acetabulum are best performed in lithotomy position using an ilioinguinal

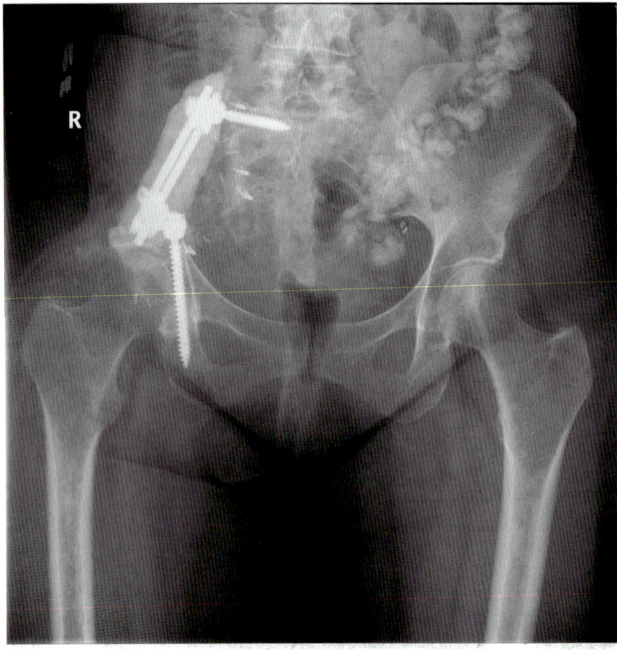

Fig. 10-7. Radiograph of a Type I pelvic resection with spinopelvic reconstruction.

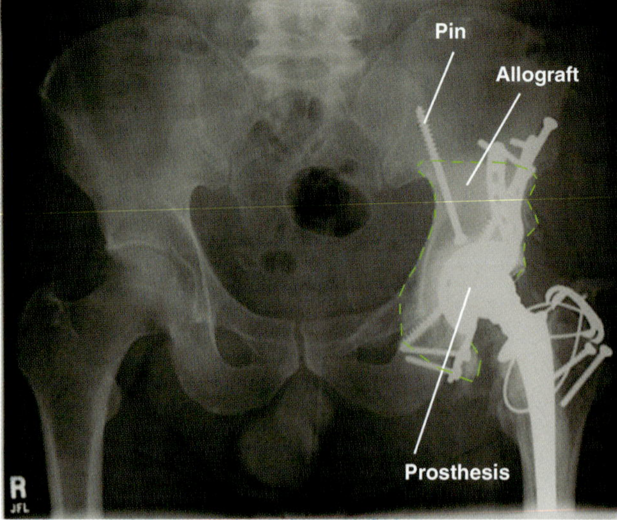

Fig. 10-9. Radiograph of a Type II pelvic resection with reconstruction. Acetabulum and surrounding bone were replaced with an allograft and a total hip joint was inserted into the allograft and femur.

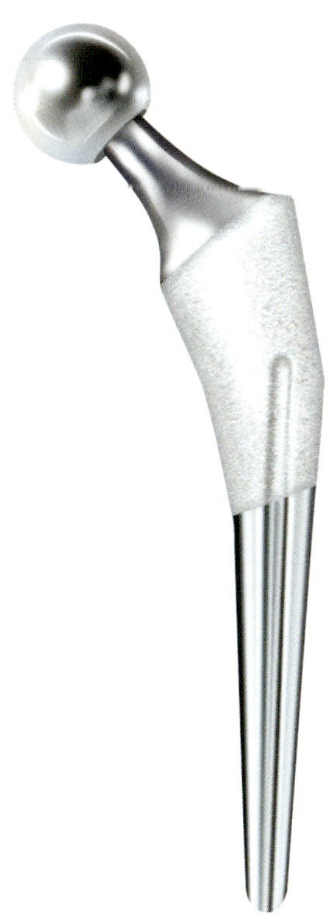

Fig. 10-10. Total hip prosthesis.

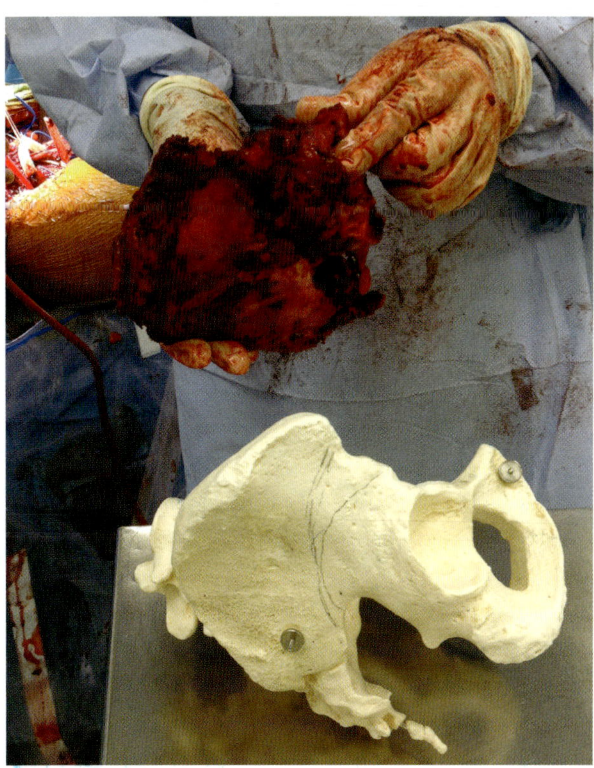

Fig. 10-12. Combined Type I and II resection specimen with model.

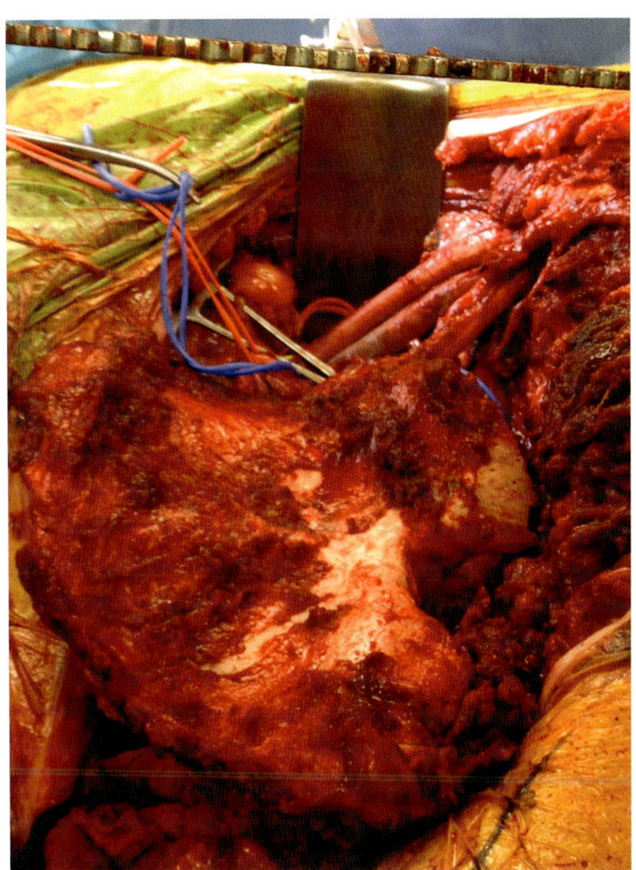

Fig. 10-11. Combined Type I and II resection specimen.

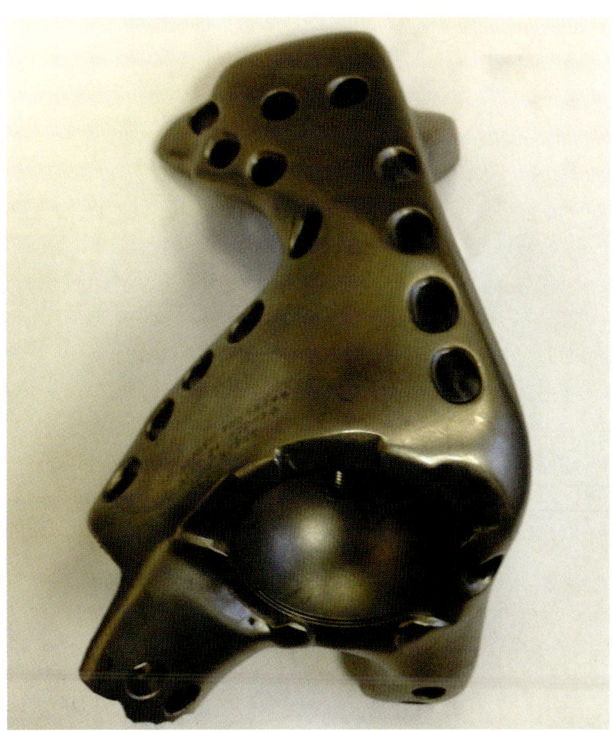

Fig. 10-13. Custom-made metallic prosthesis for reconstruction following Type I and II resection (seen from a lateral angle).

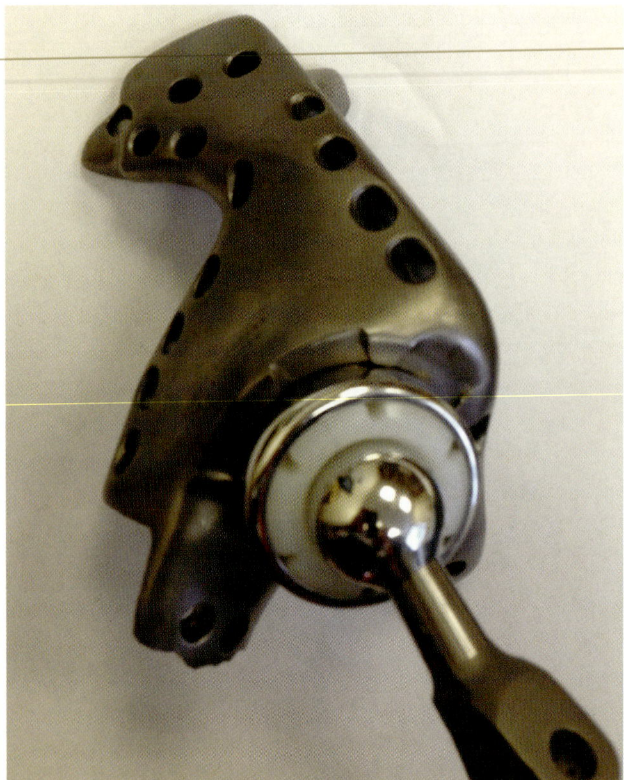

Fig. 10-14. Pelvic metallic prosthesis with a total hip prosthesis inserted.

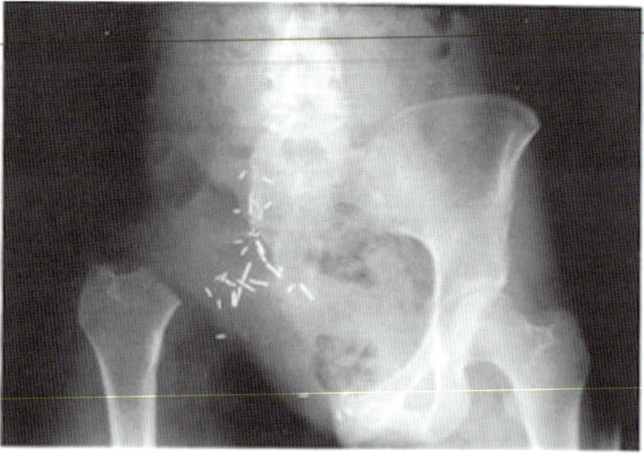

Fig. 10-16. Radiograph of a combined Type I, II, III, and IV resection without reconstruction.

incision with a perineal extension extending to the ischium (Figure 10-17). No reconstruction is necessary for these resections.

Type IV resections usually involve resection of the sacroiliac joint (see Figure 10-4). This is carried out through an inverted U-type incision with the patient lying in a lateral position. Posteriorly, the incision starts at the level of the lower sacroiliac joint. It extends superiorly, over and parallel to the iliac crest. An ileo-inguinal extension can be performed if necessary to increase intraabdominal exposure (see Figure 10-5).[8] Through this incision, the posterior joint can be visualized, and adjacent iliac bone and sacrum are exposed. The anterior sacroiliac joint is approached in a retroperitoneal fashion, elevating the peritoneum and pelvic structures medially. Osteotomes are used to divide the sacrum and iliac bone (Figure 10-18). Reconstruction using sacral pelvic instrumentation and grafting is favored by the authors (Figure 10-19). Patients can ambulate without reconstruction, but this is usually painful and requires the use of crutches.

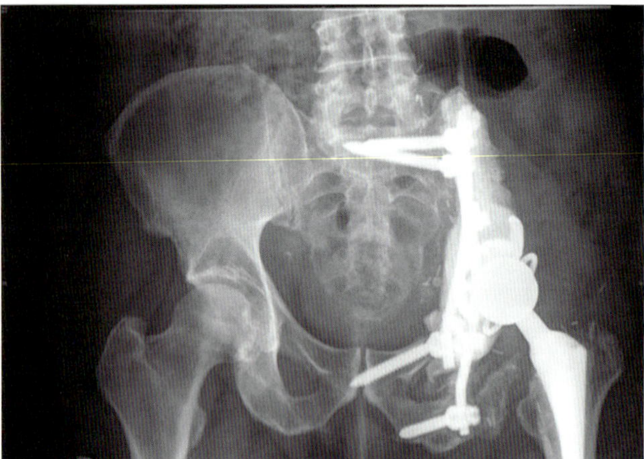

Fig. 10-15. Radiograph of a sacropelvic reconstruction following a combined Type I, II, and IV resection using screws and connecting bars. A constrained total hip replacement was cemented into this metal construct.

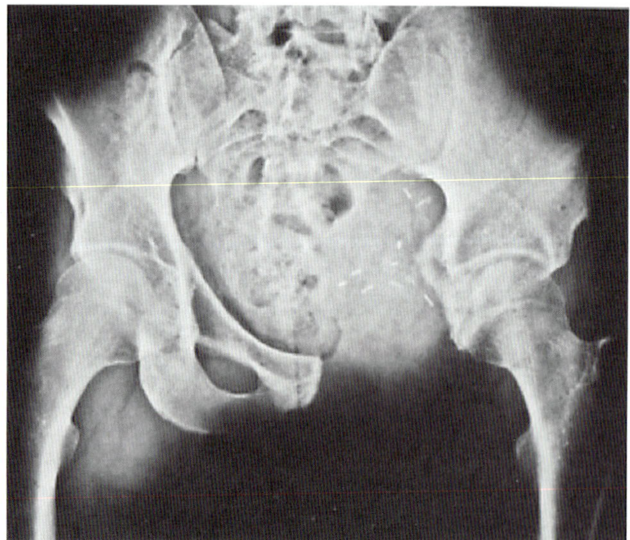

Fig. 10-17. Radiograph of a Type III resection without reconstruction.

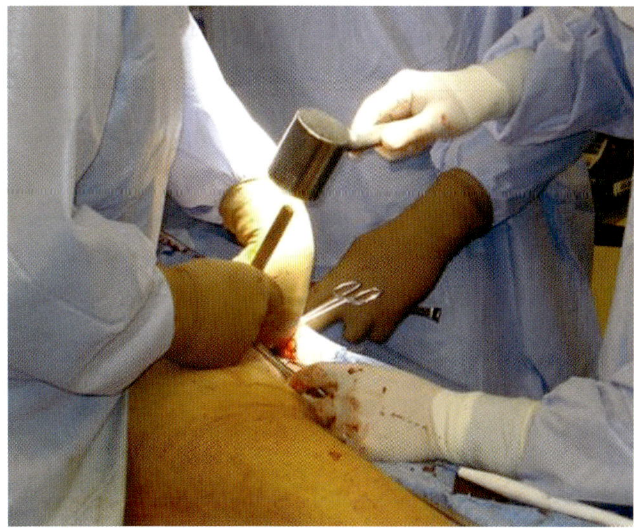

Fig. 10-18. Use of an osteotome to divide the sacrum and iliac bone.

Sacrum

Tumors which involve the sacrum can be dealt by sacral resections. Division of the sacrum preserving at least one S3 root preserves bowel, bladder, and sexual function. Hemisacrectomy preserving all nerves on the contralateral side will also result in normal bowel bladder function, but do require stabilization. High sacral resections through S1 usually require lumbo-sacral stabilization (Figure 10-19).

Major Nerves

Repair of major pelvic nerves in older patients who have had radiation therapy is not successful. Excision of the obturator nerve results in little disability. Patients can function satisfactorily following unilateral resection of either the femoral or sciatic nerves. However, the necessity for resection of both the femoral and sciatic nerves on the same side is usually a contraindication to limb salvage surgery. In a minority of these patients, amputation in the form of a hemipelvectomy should be considered (Figure 10-20).

Femoral Nerve Resection

Tumors involving the psoas muscle and sometimes the pelvic sidewall may surround the femoral nerve, necessitating resection of this nerve. Resection is done through an anterior or retroperitoneal approach (Figure 10-21 and 10-22). Excision results in the inability to extend the knee. Postoperatively these patients are managed with an extensive knee brace, but

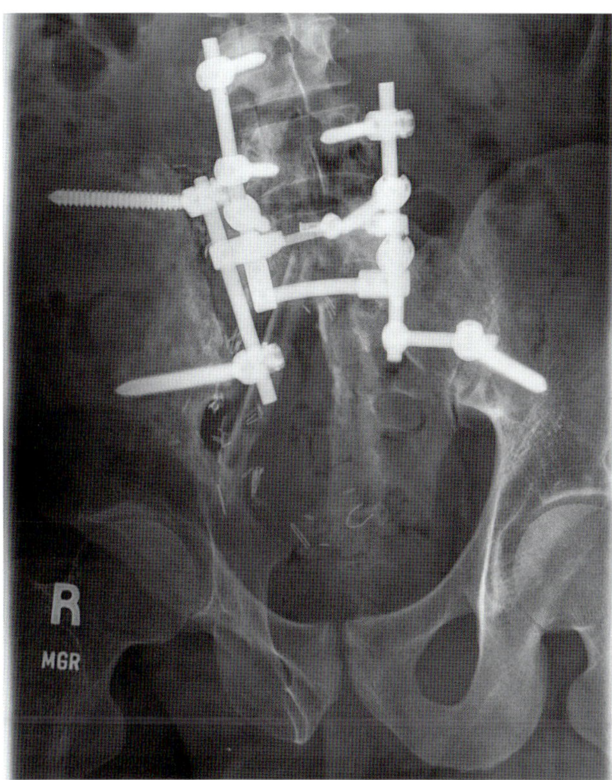

Fig. 10-19. Radiograph of a hemisacrectomy with resection of adjacent iliac bone followed by reconstruction.

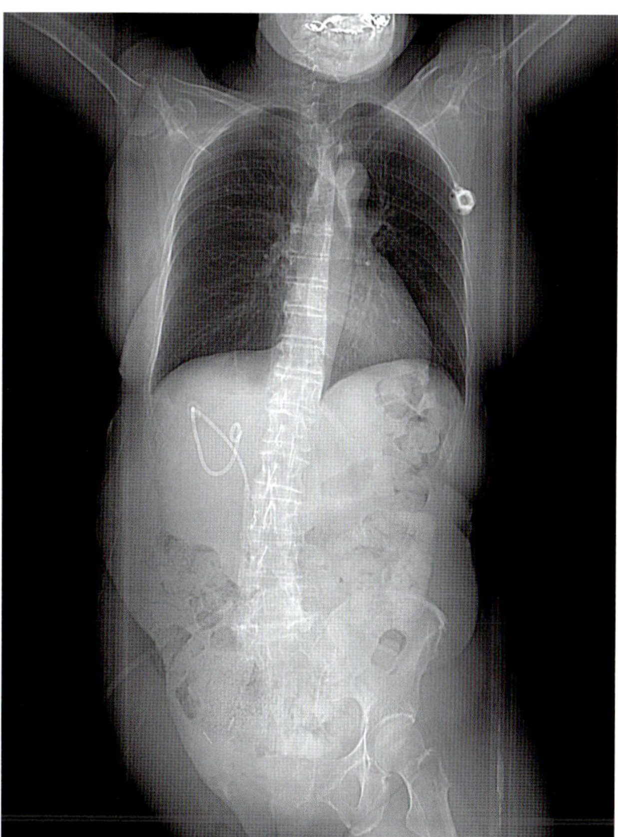

Fig. 10-20. Radiograph of a patient with recurrent endometrial carcinoma who underwent a hemipelvectomy. Part of the sacrum was also resected.

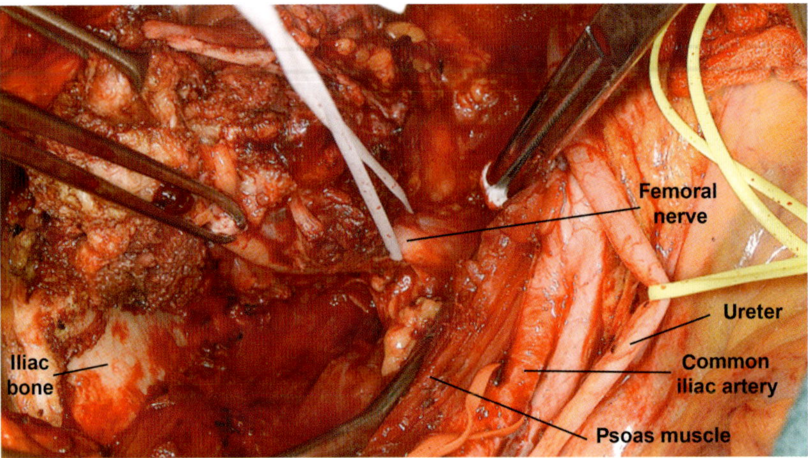

Fig. 10-21. Patient with recurrent endometrial carcinoma involving the psoas muscle and femoral nerve who underwent femoral nerve resection. *(Reproduced with permission from Memorial Sloan-Kettering Cancer Center.)*

with rehabilitation they can learn to walk without a support in most cases.[13]

Sciatic Nerve Resection

Tumors may invade the sacral plexus in the lateral presacral portion of the posterior pelvis or may involve the formed sciatic nerve lying on the piriformis and/or in the sciatic notch. Resection of the plexus alone can be done through a trans-abdominal or retroperitoneal approach. If the lumbosacral nerve trunk (L4-5) is free, then it should be saved maintaining full ankle extension. Excision of the sacral roots proximal to the origin of the formed sciatic nerve will result in greater lower limb dysfunction as already mentioned under functional anatomy. Loss of motor and sensory function to the foot and ankle alone will occur when the sciatic nerve is severed, preserving the gluteal nerves.

Resection of large tumors involving the sciatic nerve extending into the sciatic foramen is best performed using anterior abdominopelvic and posterior buttock incisions (Figure 10-23 and 10-24). The patient is positioned in a floppy lateral decubitus position with the ability to rotate the body anteriorly and posteriorly. Through the anterior approach, the intrapelvic portion is isolated and the nerve or nerve roots are divided above the tumor. The nerve is found lying on the piriformis muscle, which passes laterally through the greater sciatic notch into the buttock. The sacral origin of this muscle is detached. The posterior branches of the internal iliac vessels are divided and ligated (Figure 10-25). If possible, the gluteal and pudendal nerves are spared. The nerve and tumor are then exposed posteriorly through a vertical incision made lateral to the posterior iliac crest and sacrum. The medial origin of the gluteus maximus is severed and the muscle reflected laterally

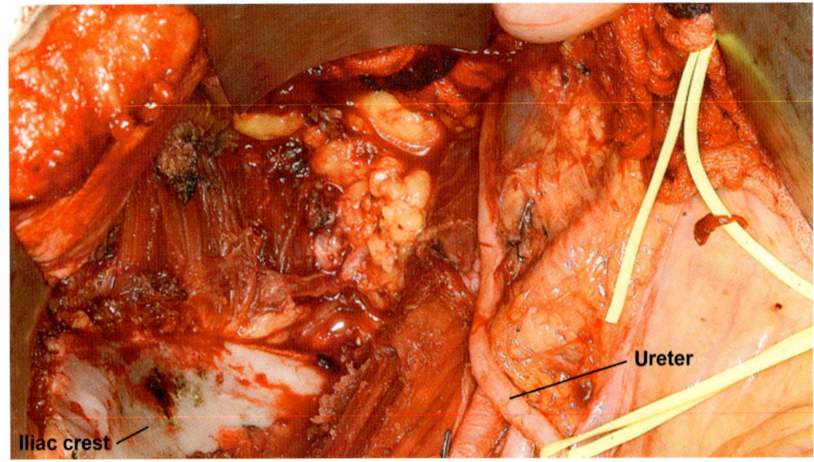

Fig. 10-22. Resection of femoral nerve, psoas muscle, and iliac crest. *(Reproduced with permission from Memorial Sloan-Kettering Cancer Center.)*

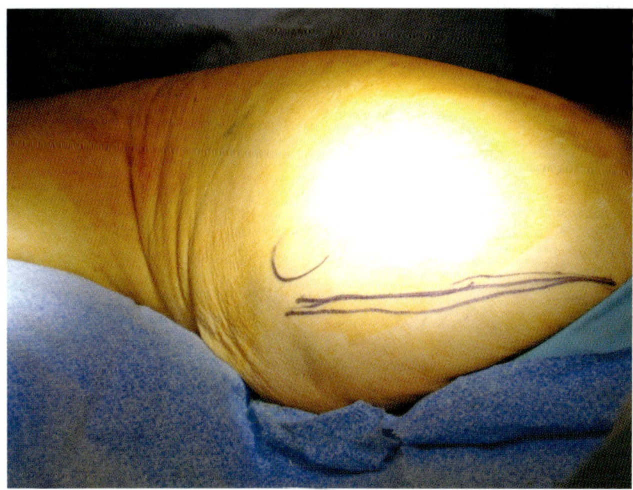

Fig. 10-23. Posterior buttock incision.

exposing the sciatic notch with the sciatic nerve, tumor, and extrapelvic piriformis muscle (Figure 10-26). Exposure is facilitated further by cutting the sacrotuberous and sacrospinous ligaments, which lie deep to the gluteus maximus muscle (Figure 10-27). The superior or inferior gluteal vessels above and below the piriformis are again cut and ligated. The piriformis muscle is sectioned laterally. If the gluteal and pudendal nerves were saved anteriorly, care should be taken to preserve them. If further exposure is necessary, then the bone of the sciatic notch can be excised with a burr or osteotome. Postoperatively, the patient will require a foot-drop brace with crutches initially and later a cane.

Major Vessels

As mentioned earlier, resection of the internal iliac and obturator vessels does not require reconstruction; however, reconstruction is necessary upon resection of the common or external iliac artery (Figure 10-28). Reconstruction can be accomplished with either a vascular graft to replace the resected artery or as a fem-fem bypass graft (Figure 10-29). Resection of the common or external iliac vein will result in lower leg edema, especially in patients who have been irradiated and already have impaired lymphatic drainage. Placement of a venous graft is associated with thrombosis and is not recommended. For these cases, postoperative care involves elevation of the leg and application of lower limb compression hose.

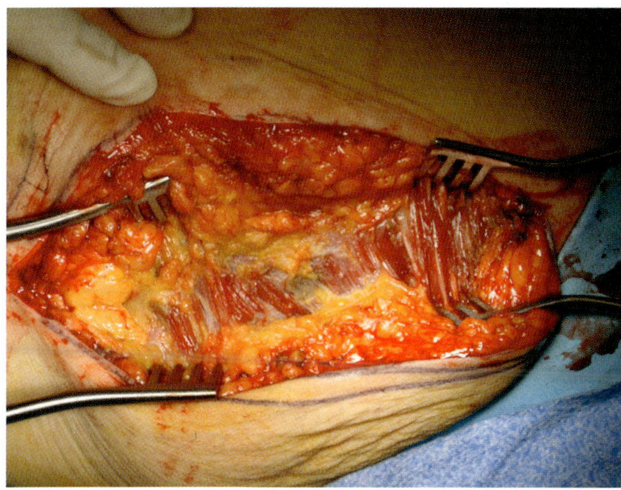

Fig. 10-24. Exposure of gluteus muscles through buttock incision.

POSTOPERATIVE CARE

Box 10-3 PERIOPERATIVE MORBIDITY

- Pelvic abscess
- Neuropathy
- Vascular graft thrombosis

Extended pelvic resections are prolonged extensive procedures at significant risk for blood loss and metabolic acidosis. Intensive care unit (ICU) admission should be considered depending on the extent of the procedure, duration, patient comorbidities, and necessity for ventilatory support. Published literature shows a reported average operative time of 11.4 to 14.4 hours with median blood loss of 1775 to 3700 cc and average transfusion of 5 units of packed red blood cells. Average postoperative length of hospital stay was 15 to 28 days with 36% being admitted to the ICU.[1,2] Patients who undergo sciatic nerve resection require frequent inspection and care of their limbs to prevent decubitus ulceration. The ankle should be splinted in a neutral position. Single-dose antibiotic prophylaxis is used in all cases, except when allografts or prosthesis are used, where antibiotics are continued until drains are removed. Some surgeons will use prophylactic antibiotics for 3 months following insertion of large allografts. For thromboembolic prophylaxis, sequential compression devices are continued postoperatively, and low-molecular weight heparin should be started when the risk of bleeding has diminished, even in cases in which an inferior vena cava (IVC) filter was placed preoperatively. Venodyne boots should not be placed on an extremity in which major vascular resection was carried out. Patients should be mobilized as soon as possible. All these patients will require long-term physical rehabilitation consisting of ambulation training, protected weight bearing when appropriate, and use of orthosis and walking devices as indicated. Prevention of lower limb joint contractures is especially important when nerves have been sacrificed.

Early Complications

Major complications are common, and range overall from 39% to 64%.[1-3] In one series, early major complications (≤ 1 month postoperatively) were reported to occur in 45% of the patients. Eighteen percent had infectious morbidity (pelvic abscess, urosepsis), 14% had neurologic impairment (neuropathy),

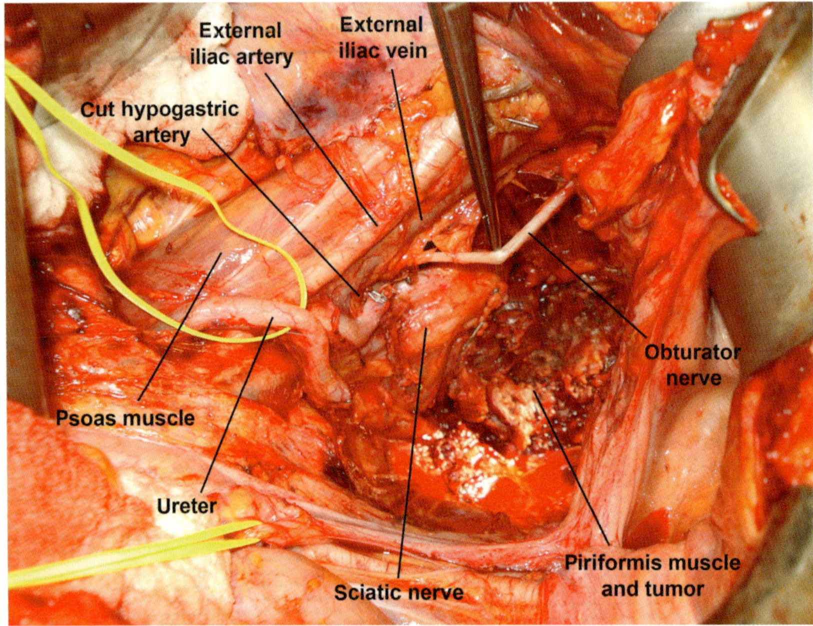

Fig. 10-25. Exposure of sciatic nerve and piriformis muscle through abdominal transperitoneal incision.

and 14% had urinary complications (disruption of appendiceal stroma, neobladder perforation, hydronephrosis). Other complications included hemorrhage and vascular graft thrombosis.[1] Pelvic abscesses are usually successfully treated via drain insertion by interventional radiology and intravenous antibiotics. Patients who have had major nerve resections or amputations frequently develop phantom pain for which anticonvulsants such as gabapentin or pregabalin may be used.[14] Patients with prosthesis who develop early infections should have thorough open debridements performed frequently to prevent prosthetic infection.

LONG-TERM OUTCOMES

Box 10-4 DELAYED COMPLICATIONS

- Fistulas
- Pelvic abscess/sepsis
- Wound infection
- Ureteral obstruction

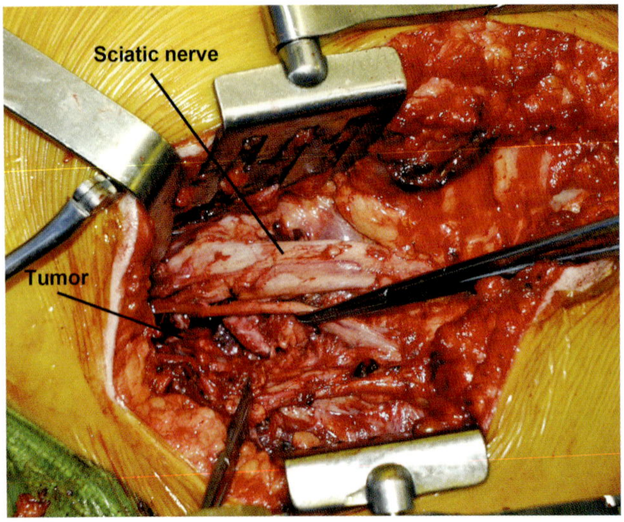

Fig. 10-26. Exposure of sciatic nerve and tumor through buttock incision.

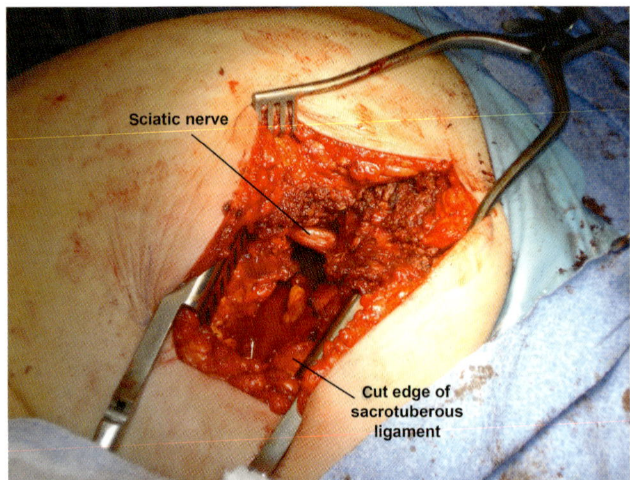

Fig. 10-27. Exposure of sciatic nerve after transection of sacrotuberous ligament. *(Reproduced with permission from Memorial Sloan-Kettering Cancer Center.)*

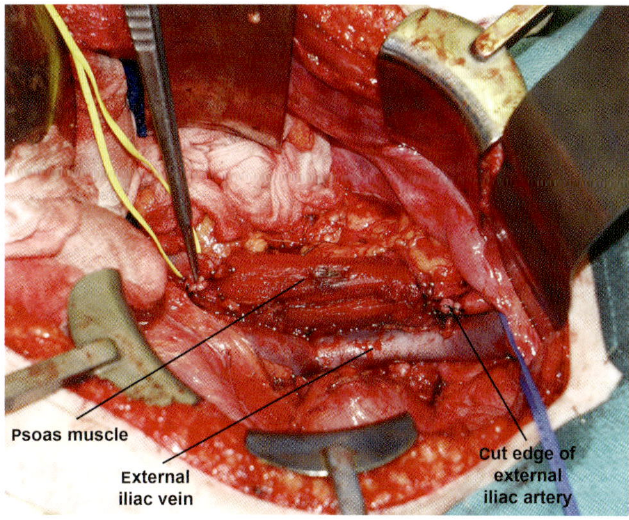

Fig. 10-28. Resection of common and external iliac arteries.

Late Complications

Long-term complications (1–6 months postoperatively) are related to the extent of the procedure, and whether intraoperative radiation therapy was administered. Complications include pelvic abscesses, wound infection, urosepsis, functional ureteral obstruction, fistula, small bowel obstruction, hematoma, neuropathy, and significant lower extremity edema interfering with ambulation.[1-3] Major late complications occur at a rate of 36%. Fistulas occur at a rate of 14% to 16%, involving both the bowel and bladder. Fistulas include enterovaginal, enteroneovaginal, enterocutaneous, enteroarterial, and vesicovaginal.[1,2] Late hardware infections may require removal of prosthesis and allografts.

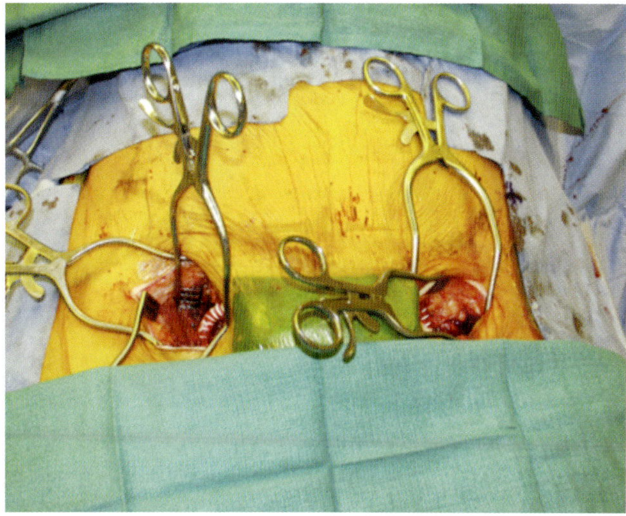

Fig. 10-29. Fem-fem bypass graft after resection of the external iliac artery.

Reoperation

The rate of reoperation is 22% to 27% with a reported readmission rate of 55% at least once during the 6 months following surgery.[1,3] Indications for reoperation include GI (stomal revision, enteral diversion for colovaginal fistula, small bowel obstruction), urinary (neocystoscopy for hematuria, urinary stenting, urinary diversion), and vascular (thrombectomy of vascular bypass graft, iliac artery stenting secondary to pseudoaneurysm formation).

Survival

Five-year OS rates range from 34% to 47%.[1-3] In the Memorial Sloan-Kettering Cancer Center experience (22 patients, 5-year OS 34%),[1] patients who had an R0 resection (microscopically negative margins, n = 17) had a 5-year OS of 48% with a median OS of 44 months. The other 5 patients in whom microscopically negative margins could not be obtained had a 5-year OS of 0%, with a median OS of 27 months. Patients who did not have resection of the common and/or external iliac vessels (n = 17) had a 5-year OS of 49% with a median OS of 44 months, while patients whose surgery did include a major vascular resection (n = 5), had a 5-year OS of 0% and median OS of 27 months. However, only 1 of the 5 patients who underwent a major vascular resection had negative microscopic margins.[1] These findings suggest that negative surgicopathologic margins are critical in achieving long-term survival.

SUMMARY

Extended pelvic resection in patients with recurrent or persistent gynecologic cancer can lead to long-term survival in carefully selected patients. If negative microscopic margins can be obtained, then radical surgical resection of bone, muscle, nerve, and vessels can provide adequate local control in patients who have failed prior surgery and/or definitive radiation therapy. Treatment must be individualized after a comprehensive radiologic evaluation and extensive preoperative assessment and counseling. Major complications remain a hallmark; however, these procedures provide a reasonable option with acceptable morbidity in adequately selected patients in whom surgery is the only potential means of a cure.

REFERENCES

1. Andikyan V, Khoury-Collado F, Sonoda Y, et al. Extended pelvic resections for recurrent or persistent uterine and cervical malignancies: an update on out of the box surgery. *Gynecol Oncol*. 2012;125(2):404-408.
2. Hoeckel M. Laterally extended endopelvic resection. Novel surgical treatment of locally recurrent cervical carcinoma involving the pelvic side wall. *Gynecol Oncol*. 2003;91(2):369-377.
3. Dowdy SC, Mariani A, Cliby WA, et al. Radical pelvic resection and intraoperative radiation therapy for recurrent endometrial cancer: technique and analysis of outcomes. *Gynecol Oncol*. 2006;101(2):280-286.
4. Brunschwig A, Barber H. Pelvic exenteration combined with resection of segments of bony pelvis. *Surgery* 1969;65(3):417-420.

5. Harrington KD. The use of hemipelvic allografts or autoclaved grafts for reconstruction after wide resections of malignant tumors of the pelvis. *J Bone Joint Surg Am*. 1992;74(3):331-341.
6. Vargas HA, Burger IA, Donati OF, et al. MRI/PET provides a roadmap for surgical planning and serves as a predictive biomarker in patients with recurrent gynecological cancers undergoing pelvic exenteration. *Int J Gynecol Cancer*. 2013;23(8):1512-1519.
7. Enneking WF, Dunham WK. Resection and reconstruction for primary neoplasms involving the innominate bone. *J Bone Joint Surg Am*. 1978;60(6):731-746.
8. Yuen A, Ek ET, Choong PF. Research: Is resection of tumours involving the pelvic ring justified? : A review of 49 consecutive cases. *Int Semin Surg Oncol*. 2005;2(1):9.
9. Karakousis CP. Abdominoinguinal incision and other incisions in the resection of pelvic tumors. *Surg Oncol*. 2000;9(2):83-90.
10. Delloye C, Banse X, Brichard B, Docquier PL, Cornu O. Pelvic reconstruction with a structural pelvic allograft after resection of a malignant bone tumor. *J Bone Joint Surg Am*. 2007;89(3):579-587.
11. Abudu A, Grimer RJ, Cannon SR, Carter SR, Sneath RS. Reconstruction of the hemipelvis after the excision of malignant tumours. Complications and functional outcome of prostheses. *J Bone Joint Surg Br*. 1997;79(5):773-779.
12. Uchida A, Myoui A, Araki N, Yoshikawa H, Ueda T, Aoki Y. Prosthetic reconstruction for periacetabular malignant tumors. *Clin Orthop Relat Res*. 1996;(326):238-245.
13. Mavrogenis AF, Soultanis K, Patapis P, et al. Pelvic resections. *Orthopedics*. 2012;35(2):e232-e243.
14. Abbass K. Efficacy of gabapentin for treatment of adults with phantom limb pain. *Ann Pharmacother*. 2012;46(12):1707-1711.

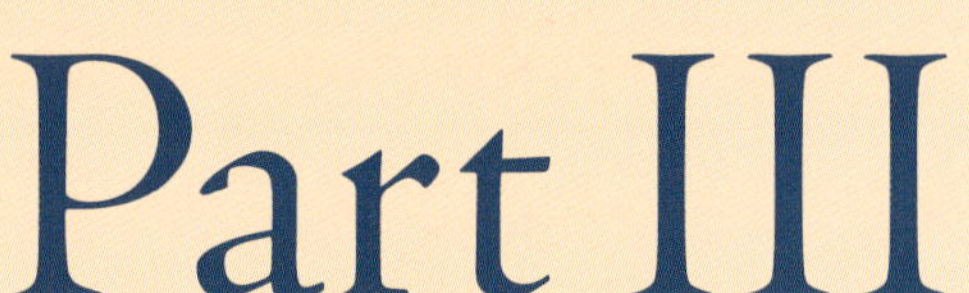

Part III

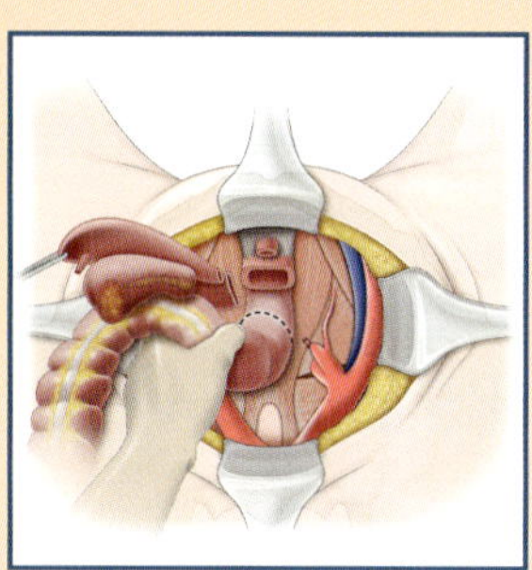

Reconstructive Operations

Section A — Urinary Tract

Section B — Gastrointestinal Tract

Section C — Vulvovaginal and Pelvic Floor Reconstruction

Section D — Management of Complex Abdominal Wall Defects

Section E — Supportive Care

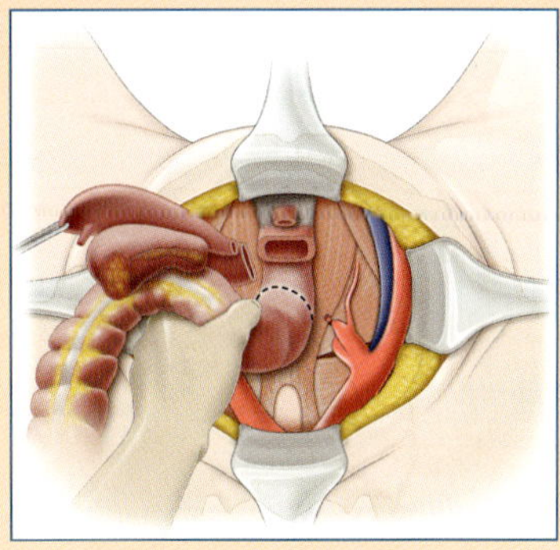

SECTION A URINARY TRACT

Chapter 11. Incontinent Urinary Diversions

Donghua Xie, MD and
Jaspreet S. Sandhu, MD

BACKGROUND

Urinary diversion, defined as rerouting of urine from a normal intact urinary tract, can be classified as either incontinent or continent. Incontinent diversion allows for the free flow of urine outside of the body, which can be collected into an external ostomy appliance.[1,2] Incontinent urinary diversions are performed much more often than continent ones, particularly in patients with complex medical or surgical histories and/or those that have a history of previous radiotherapy.[3,4]

Ureterosigmoidostomy, first performed in 1851 by John Simon, was the first widely used surgical technique for urinary diversion, providing an effective diversion that relied on the anal sphincter for continence. However, its usefulness is limited by deterioration of renal function over time, metabolic complications, and the increased risk for the development of secondary malignancies. Subsequently, substantial progress has been made by incorporating innovative techniques that use isolated bowel segments as either urinary conduits or continent reservoirs and effectively separates the fecal and urinary streams. In the 1950s Bricker used a segment of ileum to which the ureters were anastomosed and a stoma created in the right lower abdomen. The ileal conduit (IC) has subsequently become the gold standard for incontinent urinary diversion.[1,2] Cutaneous ureterostomy, which has been used sparingly in adults due to surgeon concern for ureteral obstruction,[5] is the simplest method of all permanent urinary diversions. However, there are risks of stomal stenosis requiring intubation and pyelonephritis.[6,7]

In this chapter, the most commonly used reconstructive options of incontinent urinary diversion will be discussed, as well as indications and clinical applications, anatomic considerations, surgical procedures, postoperative care, and long-term outcomes.

INDICATIONS AND CLINICAL APPLICATIONS

There are a variety of choices for incontinent urinary diversions (IC, colon conduit [CC], and cutaneous ureterostomy). The choice is determined by patient and medical criteria. Important patient criteria are patient preference, age, comorbidities, body mass index (BMI), and the ability and motivation to perform intermittent self-catheterization. Further considerations are the condition of the segment of bowel to be used, kidney function/upper urinary tract status, and the overall medical condition of the patient. The choice of urinary diversion still remains a very personal decision to be made between the patient, family members, and the physician.[8]

Ileal Conduit

IC urinary diversion remains the gold standard for incontinent urinary reconstruction. Although the introduction of continent urinary diversions has decreased the proportion of these procedures performed, they remain the most common form of urinary diversion.[4] It is a procedure that is obligated for patients with a short life expectancy, reduced kidney function, and for those who cannot manage a continent diversion. Due to the relative ease of formation and shorter operative time, an IC is often used in patients with significant medical comorbidities in an attempt to minimize postoperative complications and the risk of reoperation.[9]

Cutaneous Ureterostomy

Although the IC is the accepted standard due to its safe, well-proven, and low-risk performance, nevertheless it does involve a small bowel resection and ureteroenteric anastomosis, which can lead to increased complications. The uretero-cutaneostomy, consisting of direct routing of the ureters to the skin, is an easier alternative, which was initially shown to have a high rate of stomal stenosis. However, new data suggest that the stomal stenosis rate, measured by need for stent, is comparable to the IC. In addition, quality of life analyses show comparable results. Therefore, cutaneous ureterostomy should be considered as an option for urinary diversion in patients who are critically ill, those with significant previous intestinal surgery, or those with end-stage urinary obstruction, in whom neither cystectomy nor intestinal surgery may be advisable.[7,10-12] It can also be used as a temporary diversion in situations when gastrointestinal diversion is not possible or whenever the bladder needs to be diverted because of fistula or hemorrhage.[13] In cases of failed IC urinary diversion, transureteroureterostomy with cutaneous ureterostomy can be used as a salvage measure.[14] In those patients in whom intestine may not be available for reconstruction (eg, those with short bowel syndrome or Crohn disease), cutaneous ureterostomy remains an option to enable permanent diversion with or without cystectomy.[11]

Colonic Conduit

Although controversial, some believe that the use of ileal segments or the ileocecal reservoir in patients who have been exposed to pelvic radiation may be associated with increased risk of early and late complications.[15] In this circumstance, a colonic conduit, a loop of transverse colon with ureterocolonic anastomosis, is an option. The superior outcome of this urinary diversion is due to the use of nonirradiated segments of the colon and ureter in the radiated population.[16] The transverse colon segment is also an option for salvage of problems related to ICs.[17]

Reconfigured colon segments can be used successfully to replace long ureteral defects. The advantages are use in patients with impaired renal function and lack of small intestine, proximity of the colon to the ureter, optimal cross-sectional diameter of the graft and less intraperitoneal surgical trauma than with ileal substitutes.[21]

ANATOMIC CONSIDERATIONS

Ureter

Complications due to ischemia of the distal ureter, ureteroenteric or stomal (in the case of cutaneous ureterostomy), are a recognized complication of any urinary diversion. Ischemia of the distal ureter is preventable, by taking note of its vascular supply with its common variations and preserving the periureteral adventitial tissue. This reduces the risks of urinary extravasation and ureteral strictures. Special care must be taken when translocating the left ureter across the retroperitoneum to the right; this should be done below the posterior peritoneum overlying the sigmoid colon *above* the level of the inferior mesenteric artery in order to maximize length and avoid kinking. Approximately 5 to 10 cm of well-vascularized ureter is usually left freely mobile for ureterointestinal anastomosis.

For cutaneous ureterostomy, the ureters are tunneled in an extraperitoneal fashion to bilateral abdominal or flank stomas. If a single stoma is required, then translocation of 1 ureter to the other side in a similar manner to translocating the left ureter to the right (as described above) with a subsequent transureteroureterostomy can be performed.

Bowel

As a general principle, any segment of bowel can be used to form a urinary diversion. However, there are metabolic consequences associated with the utilization of each segment based upon the absorptive function of bowel.[18-20] In addition, the length and location of bowel segment used can affect the patient's postoperative bowel function. Conduits should be long enough to warrant an everted stoma and to allow a tension-free ureterointestinal anastomosis. The two types of bowel segment most commonly used for noncontinent urinary diversion are distal ileum and transverse colon.

For IC urinary diversion, the terminal 10 to 15 cm of ileum is typically preserved to maintain adequate absorption of bile salts, vitamin B12, and fat-soluble vitamins. Before deciding on the final limits of the segment, the associated vascular arcades are routinely inspected with translumination through the mesentery to ensure that at least 2 vascular arcades are present. The isolated loop is always left caudal and below the continuous small intestine after performing enteroenteric anastomosis.

Anastomosis

It is important to perform tension-free ureteroileal anastomoses and reduce manipulation of the conduit after completion of the ureteroileal anastomoses. There are multiple ureteroileal anastomotic variants. The Nesbit ureteral implantation technique, adopted and more commonly attributed to Bricker leaves the proximal end of the IC closed. The ureteral ends are spatulated and anastomosed directly via a refluxing technique and separated by about 1 to 3 cm from each other along the antimesenteric side of the conduit. The Wallace variant consists of anastomosing both spatulated ureters together—oriented "head to head" (Wallace I); or oriented in the opposite, "head to tail" direction (Wallace II)—and then directly anastomosing the combined complex to the proximal end of the IC segment.[22] Although a Wallace type of anastomosis is technically simpler due to the creation of only one ureteroenteric anastomosis, complications at this anastomosis put both kidneys at risk for damage. Therefore, the Bricker anastomosis is currently the one more commonly performed.

Stoma

The preferred location of the ileal stoma is the right abdominal quadrant between the umbilicus and the anterior-superior iliac spine. The location should be above or below the waistband and not too close to the umbilicus, the edge of the rectus muscle, a bony prominence or a scar, and must be tested with the patient and preoperatively marked.[7,13,22]

The presence of a stoma and appliance affects a patient's body image. Typically, the ileal or transverse conduit stoma is a standard end ostomy. In patients who are obese, where a short bowel mesentery and thick abdominal wall may prevent the creation of an end-on stoma without undue tension, a loop type of stoma (Turnbull) is commonly advocated.[20]

PREOPERATIVE PREPARATION

Box 11-1 KEY SURGICAL INSTRUMENTATION

- GIA stapler 60 3.8 + 2 reloads
- TA stapler 60 3.5
- LigaSure 20 cm
- Groove director/suture guide
- Surgical clips
- 2-0, 4-0, Vicryl sutures
- 3-0 silk sutures

General

A complete preoperative anesthesiologic assessment, including cardiac testing, renal, and hepatic function, and correction of modifiable medical diseases, such as hypertension, cardiac arrhythmias, and anemia, should be completed in all candidates. Imaging studies of the ureters and kidneys to confirm presence of both kidneys is also required.

Limited bowel preparation has been recognized by many clinical studies as a promising approach in radical cystectomy, which require use of intestinal segments.[23,24] Despite this, the use of complete bowel preparation (polyethylene glycol or sodium phosphate oral solution) has long been advocated to reduce the incidence of postoperative ileus, wound infections, and anastomotic dehiscence.[25] However, recent reports show that preoperative mechanical bowel preparation prior to radical cystectomy with urinary diversion or colorectal surgery does not demonstrate any significant advantage in perioperative outcomes, including gastrointestinal complications.[24,26]

The stoma site is usually marked on the skin by the urologist or stoma therapist. Patients should be fully informed about the risks and benefits of the urinary diversion procedure planned including possible surgical alternatives and sufficient time should be given to patients to understand the impact of everyday aspects related to the selected urinary diversion prior to obtaining informed consent. Patient or family counseling, with the aid of psychologists, oncology nurse specialists, or patients who have previously undergone the chosen procedure, is also helpful.[23]

SURGICAL TECHNIQUE

Box 11-2 MASTER SURGEON'S PRINCIPLES

- Initially divide the ureter as distally as possible as it can always be trimmed back later
- Avoid grasping the ureters with forceps and preserve as much blood supply as possible by preserving periureteral adventitial tissue
- For ileal and sigmoid conduits, tunnel the left ureter under or through the sigmoid mesentery and try to use nonirradiated ureteral segments for the ureterointestinal anastomoses
- The terminal 10 to 15 cm of ileum at the ileocecal junction should be preserved to maintain adequate absorption of bile salts, vitamin B12, and fat-soluble vitamins
- Ensure that ≥ 2 vascular arcades are present in the mesentery supplying the isolated segment
- Restore intestinal continuity before performing ureterointestinal anastomoses
- Perform a standard end-to-side ureteroileal or ureterocolonic anastomosis (Bricker) after appropriately spatulating the ureter
- Ureteral stents should be placed before completing the ureterointestinal anastomosis
- The stoma location should be above or below the waistband and not too close to the umbilicus, the edge of the rectus muscle, a bony prominence or a scar, and must be tested with the patient and preoperatively marked
- The ileal or colonic conduit should be long enough to allow an everted stoma that allows proper placement of stoma appliance

Ileal conduit

After entering the abdomen, a self-retaining retractor is positioned. The ureters are identified and ligated as distally as possible. Temporarily obstructing the ureter with a tie or clip allows for dilatation until it is time for the ureteroileal anastomosis. The ureters are dissected superiorly to the pelvic brim while preserving the adventitia.

Approximately 15 cm from the ileocecal valve, the distal margin of the proposed ileal segment is marked with a silk suture. The length required should be sufficient to span the distance from the stoma site to the sacral promontory. In some cases, a longer span may be needed to bridge the gap between ureter and skin. Mesenteric windows are formed by dividing the peritoneum, fat, and intervening blood vessels. This division can be performed using mosquito hemostats and ties, a stapler, or the monopolar cautery combined with the LigaSure device.[7] A small bowel resection is then performed essentially by using a gastrointestinal anastomosis (GIA) 60/80 stapler. The bowel is put back in contiguity cephalad to the ileal loop using standard technique, specifically a GIA 60/80 stapler for a side-to-side ileal anastomosis and a thoracoabdominal (TA) 60/90 stapler to complete the anastomosis. The staple line is then oversewn using imbricating Lembert sutures of 3-0 silk. The rent in the mesentery is closed using 3-0 silk as well.

The left ureter is passed under the posterior peritoneum under the sigmoid colon mesentery, caudal to the inferior mesenteric artery toward the right side. Alternatively, the left ureter is brought through the sigmoid colon mesentery. With the proximal end of the loop positioned at the level of the sacral promontory, the ureteroileal anastomosis is performed in a standard end-to-side fashion after sharply debriding the distal ureter. A traction suture is placed at the apex of the spatulated ureter (Figure 11-1) to allow manipulation of the ureter during the anastomosis. A 1-cm enterotomy is next created (Figure 11-2), and ureteroileal anastomosis is commenced with absorbable 4-0 or 5-0 sutures in an interrupted fashion (Figures 11-3 and 11-4).[7,13,22,27] Prior to completing each anastomosis, a single J stent should be placed (Figure 11-5). The suture line can be reinforced with interrupted and ventitial sutures if desired (Figure 11-6). Confirmation of the closure is performed at this point by injecting saline using

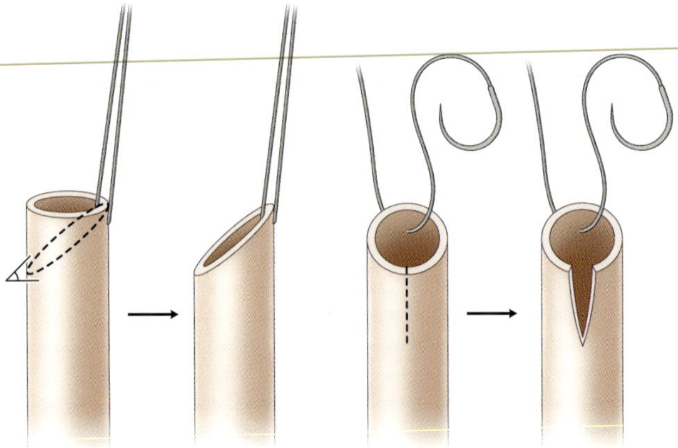

Fig. 11-1. (A) Sharply cut away devitalized end of ureter at a 45-degree angle. (B) Place traction suture through the apex of the spatulated ureter and spatulate the other end.

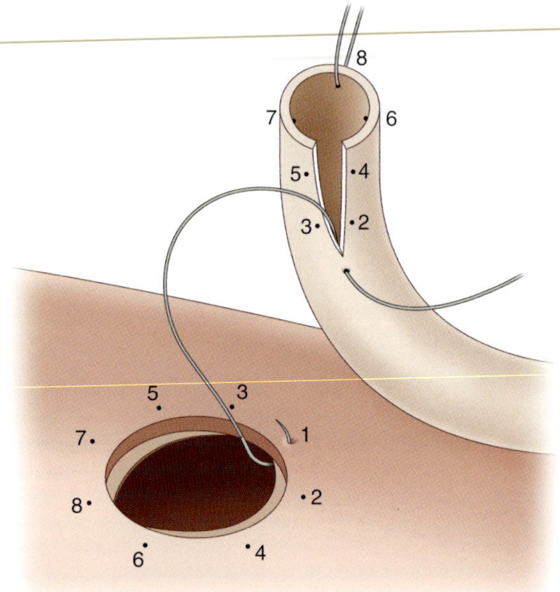

Fig. 11-3. Place a suture at the base of the spatulated ureter (outside in on ureter, inside-out on ileum).

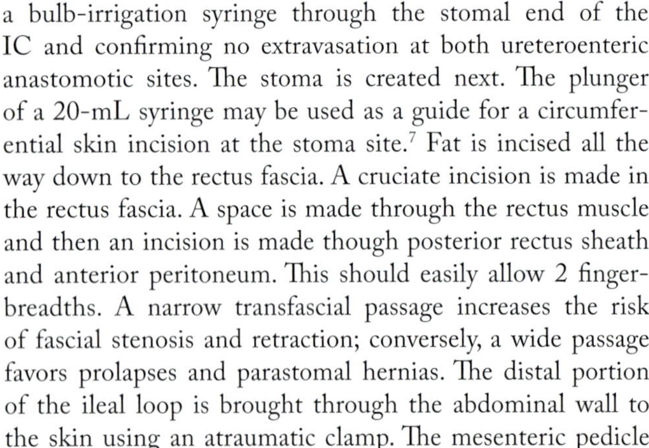

a bulb-irrigation syringe through the stomal end of the IC and confirming no extravasation at both ureteroenteric anastomotic sites. The stoma is created next. The plunger of a 20-mL syringe may be used as a guide for a circumferential skin incision at the stoma site.[7] Fat is incised all the way down to the rectus fascia. A cruciate incision is made in the rectus fascia. A space is made through the rectus muscle and then an incision is made though posterior rectus sheath and anterior peritoneum. This should easily allow 2 fingerbreadths. A narrow transfascial passage increases the risk of fascial stenosis and retraction; conversely, a wide passage favors prolapses and parastomal hernias. The distal portion of the ileal loop is brought through the abdominal wall to the skin using an atraumatic clamp. The mesenteric pedicle should be inspected to make sure it is not twisted, as this can cause severe ischemic damage. The stoma is next matured by first placing 3 fascial sutures, followed by 4 quadrant sutures to rosebud the stoma, both of these are using 2-0 Vicryl sutures. The stoma is then matured by suturing the mucosa to the skin with multiple interrupted 3-0 Vicryl sutures. The ureteral stents are secured with a silk suture to the skin, and an external urine collection device is placed. A 22-French multi-eyed catheter may be placed in the ileal loop for extra drainage.

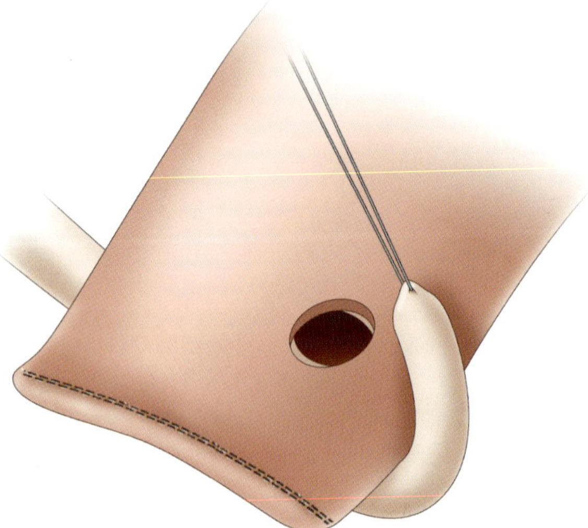

Fig. 11-2. Make 1-cm enterotomy at the butt end of the ileal conduit and bring the ureter around.

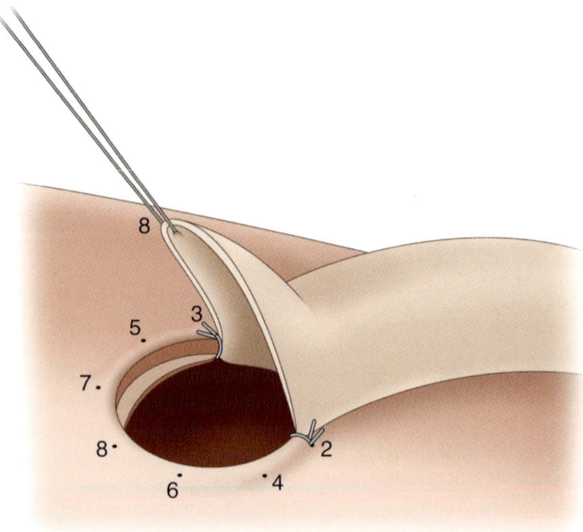

Fig. 11-4. Place 2 more on either side of ureter and tie down for a portion of the ureteroenterostomy.

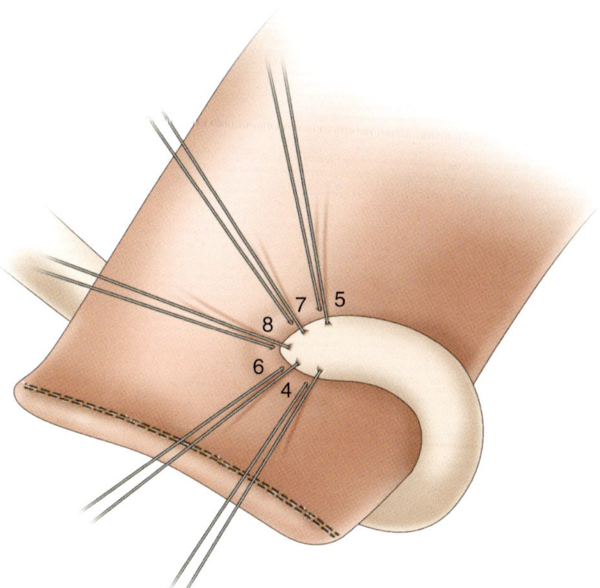

Fig. 11-5. Place 5 additional anastomotic sutures and leave clamped (untied), then place the single-J stent followed by completion of the anastomosis.

The surgeon should verify that the ileocutaneous anastomosis is tension free; otherwise, he or she should not hesitate to redo it. Ureteroileal anastomosis is generally dropped back into the retroperitoneum by suturing the sutured end of the ileal loop to the cut end of the posterior peritoneum, effectively placing the proximal end of the IC and ureteroileal anastomoses in the retroperitoneum. The omentum, when available, is used to wrap the area. One suction drain should be placed in the pelvis. Irrigation of the abdominal cavity with normal saline solution is suggested.[7,13,22] Figure 11-7 shows a representative IC urinary diversion.

Cutaneous Ureterostomy

There are 4 common types of ureterostomies: single ureterostomy, bilateral ureterostomy, double-barrel ureterostomy, and transureteroureterostomy (TUU).

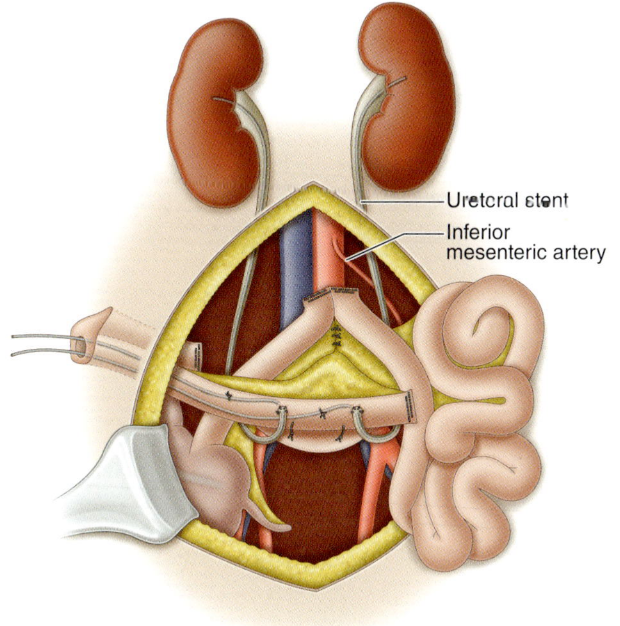

Fig. 11-7. Ileal cutaneous urinary diversion. The completed ileal conduit. (1) The bowel anastomosis is anterior to the conduit and the mesenteric defect closed. (2) The butt is fixed to the sacral promontory and adjacent tissue. (3) The ureters are not kinked, the ureteral anastomoses are dry, and the stents are secured into place. (4) The end of the blind loop of the Turnbull stoma is secured to the peritoneum and posterior rectus sheath.

Generally, the left ureter is mobilized extensively, preserving its adventitia. It is then transposed to the right hemiabdomen above the inferior mesenteric artery. The right ureter is mobilized up to the upper abdomen. After creating an abdominal wall hiatus the latter is stitched with 4 angle polyglactin 2-zero sutures to facilitate mobilization of the 2 ureters to the skin and avoid ureteral compression by large muscle contractility. A skin stoma is created with a double V skin flap and lateral spatulation of the 2 ureters. Ureterostomy is performed through a direct, spatulated end-to-side ureterocutaneous anastomosis. Each ureteral reimplant is intubated with a Double-J stent fixed to the skin with 3-zero nylon sutures. Ostomy is performed at the same site as for classic IC,

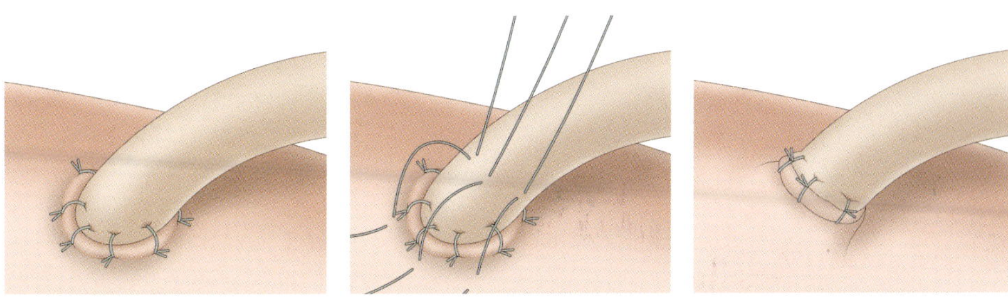

Fig. 11-6. Place 3-4 silk suture through the adventitia of the ileum and ureter and cover the previous suture line.

usually on the right side for bilateral cutaneous ureterostomies or a single right cutaneous ureterostomy, and on the left side for a single left cutaneous ureterostomy.[5,28]

TUU is used in some circumstances. The ureters are carefully mobilized to the bladder, with minimal disruption to their blood supply, then ligated and divided. After creating a retroperitoneal tunnel cranial to the inferior mesenteric artery, the less dilated left or right ureter is transposed to the contralateral side. A V- or U-shaped skin incision is made in the skin, and a track is developed through the abdominal wall in the most direct line. The ureter with the largest diameter is pulled through the track without tension and angulations and spatulated. A 4/0 or 5/0 absorbable suture is placed through the apex of the skin flap into the apex of the ureteral spatulation. The dilated ureter is then incised longitudinally for approximately 2 cm and anastomosed to the other ureter without any tension, using and end-to-side configuration to complete the transureteroureterostomy. An omental flap can be used to secure both anastomoses and the abdominal tunnel. If any doubt existed regarding the integrity of the anastomosis, then 20-mL isotonic solution is injected to the ureters to confirm a watertight anastomosis. If leakage is observed, then additional interrupted sutures are placed or the anastomosis is taken down and redone. At least 2 closed suction drains are left behind; one is placed near the ureteroureteral anastomosis and another in the pelvis.[13,29]

Colonic Conduit

The principle for colonic conduit is similar to that of the IC.[30-32] After entering the peritoneum, the colon is dissected medially; the ureters are identified and transected above the iliac vessels, above the usually irradiated pelvis. Each ureteral dissection is then performed. The left ureter is then passed through a small incision in the mesosigmoid. An approximately 15-cm colonic conduit is then made. The omentum is dissected away from the superior aspect of the transverse colon. The colon is divided with staplers and colon–colon anastomosis is performed. The conduit end chosen to be the stoma is opened and the ureterocolonic anastomoses are performed at the other end with the stoma created and matured in the assigned quadrant similar to an IC.[30-32]

POSTOPERATIVE CARE

Box 11-3 PERIOPERATIVE MORBIDITY

- Ileus
- Bowel obstruction
- Acute pyelonephritis
- Ureteroenteric anastomotic leak
- Ureteral obstruction
- Metabolic disturbance
- Bowel anastomotic leak

During the last decade, enhanced recovery protocols with standardized perioperative plans of care or "fast-track" schedules have emerged as tools to assist patients. Fast-track protocols, incorporating innovative aspects such as non-narcotic analgesics, early institution of oral diet, and drain management have been recognized as a promising approach after radical cystectomy followed by the use of intestinal segments.[23,24]

Mandatory surgical intensive care unit admission is no longer the norm, particularly with the availability of adequate recovery room observation, blood pressure monitoring, and tailored fluid replacement. Nasogastric tube can usually be removed at the end of surgery or the day after. The early administration of oral fluids (day 1) and, if successful, the early restoration of oral feeding is part of most standard postoperative management strategies.[29] The abdominal drains are removed when they stop draining or if drain creatinine is consistent with serum creatinine, whereas the ureteral stents are generally removed 5 to 12 days postoperatively. The role of the stoma therapist is recognized as essential for long-term stoma reliability. Patients should be educated about the most adequate kind of stoma to wear, how and when to replace it, and how to avoid complications related to incorrect handling of the cutaneous device, and skin care.[29,33,34]

The most common short-term complications after urinary diversion are ileus, acute pyelonephritis, bowel obstruction, urine leak, and ureteral obstruction (see Box 3). In addition to the proliferation of fast-track pathways, major strides are being made in reducing intestinal complications, typically the most common cause of short-term morbidity. Vora et al[35] showed that, alvimopan, a drug which behaves as a peripherally acting μ-opioid antagonist, improves gastrointestinal recovery without nasogastric tube decompression after radical cystectomy and urinary diversion. It is important to note that most intestinal segments, which are used to fashion the conduit, are normally colonized with bacteria.[36] The use of perioperative antibiotics and careful postoperative monitoring are important ways that infectious complications, which can contribute to acute morbidity and chronic renal insufficiency, are being reduced.

Teixeira et al[37] evaluated 232 patients who underwent a pelvic exenteration, 74 (32%) of whom had a urinary conduit created. Of these, 47 (64%) had an IC compared with 27 (36%) who had a colonic conduit. Twelve (16%) patients developed a urine leak, of which 9 occurred within the first month. Factors associated with a conduit leak included involvement of R2 surgical margins (43%), the magnitude of the exenteration and a current cardiovascular medical history (27%). Interestingly, urine leaks were not found to be associated with either radiotherapy or chemotherapy. The 30-day leak rate for ICs was 17% (8/47) and 4% (1/27) for colonic conduits, with enterocutaneous fistula only occurring in the IC group (2/47). Fistula, drained collections, and sepsis occurred in 40% of ileal and 19% of colonic conduits ($P < .01$). Of note, patients with a conduit leak had a longer length of stay (59 vs 23 days, $P < .001$).

Metabolic effects of urinary diversion are predictable. Hyperchloremic acidosis is related to the form of urinary diversion, being higher in continent forms than in incontinent diversions. Acute complications of metabolic acidosis may encompass hyperventilation as well as severe changes of serum electrolytes and acid base balance leading to cardiac arrhythmias necessitating immediate hospital treatment with intravenous alkalinizing. It is best detected by arterial blood gas analysis. Chronic acidosis, meanwhile, may lead to osteopenia through hypocalcemia and stimulation of osteoclastic activity. To prevent these complications, prophylactic administration of alkalinizing agents (eg, potassium citrate) should be readily performed.[38]

LONG-TERM OUTCOMES

Box 11-4 DELAYED COMPLICATIONS

- Stoma problems (eg, stenosis, parastomal hernia, bleeding, skin irritation)
- Bowel complications (obstruction, enterocutaneous fistulas)
- Urinary tract infection (due to anastomotic stricture, stomal stenosis, reflux, or stones)
- Ureteral conduit junction stenosis
- Deterioration of renal function
- Urolithiasis
- Ureteral obstruction
- Severe acidosis
- Development of secondary cancers

Multiple reports exist evaluating perioperative complications and long-term outcomes. Pycha et al[40] prospectively evaluated early, short-term, and long-term complications in three different forms of incontinent urinary diversion in 130 high-risk patients undergoing radical cystectomy and incontinent urinary diversion. The patients were divided into 3 groups: IC, CC, and ureteroureterocutaneostomy (UUCS). All patients underwent radical cystectomy (73%) or anterior pelvic exenteration (27%) and 1 form of incontinent diversion. IC was performed in 55, CC in 34, and UUCS in 41 patients, respectively. High comorbidity, mainly diabetes, arteriosclerosis, pulmonary insufficiency, and borderline renal function (creatinine > 1.5 mg %) were present in 12.7% of patients who underwent IC, in 35.2% of those who underwent CC, and in 48.9% of those who underwent UUCS. Overall median follow-up was 16 months (range 5-84) with perioperative mortality occurring in 1.5% of patients. The overall perioperative diversion-unrelated complication rate was 23.6%. IC showed the lowest rate with 18.1%, followed by CC with 26.4%, and UUCS with 32%, respectively. By contrast, major diversion-related complications occurred in 18.1% of IC, in 5.8% of CC, and 0% in UUCS. The same was true for late surgical reinterventions, with 20% for IC, 5.8% for CC, and 2.4% for UUCS. Complications appear to be closely related to the method selected. IC had the highest rate of severe complications as well as surgical reinterventions and late complications in the intestinal tract.[40]

Patients with urinary conduits of all types (particularly those utilizing colon rather than ileum) are at high risk of developing a second primary intestinal adenocarcinoma in the conduit. This population is likely to benefit from surveillance measures aimed at detecting such cancers. The primary form of therapy remains adequate surgical resection. General surgeons should be aware of such patients as they may be involved in the diagnosis of, and surgery for, the cancer in the conduit.[4,41-43] Patients undergoing ureterosigmoidostomy should be given information concerning this risk and should undergo regular colonoscopic surveillance beginning 5 years postoperatively.[44]

Ileal or Colonic Conduit

The primary long-term complications of IC diversion are centered on stomal/peristomal problems (stomal/peristomal lesions, stomal stenosis, stomal retraction), parastomal hernia, conduit stenosis, and renal deterioration.[45,46] Overall, complications occur in roughly 60% of patients, and the number of complications increases with the duration of follow-up, making continued surveillance of these patients mandatory.[9]

Doležel et al[47] studied 131 patients who underwent IC reconstruction and survived at least five years and reported an overall complication rate of 66%. Many patients experienced more than one complication during the first 5 years, and complications continued to develop throughout the study period (beyond 15 years), and 24% developed problems with the stoma (eg, stenosis, parastomal hernia, bleeding, and skin irritation). Bowel complications occurred in 24%, predominantly obstruction, although enterocutaneous fistulas were also observed. Urinary tract infection requiring hospitalization occurred in 23% and was usually associated with postrenal obstruction due to anastomotic stricture, stomal stenosis, or stones. Urolithiasis developed in 9%. A total of 14% developed stenosis requiring open or endoscopic surgical correction at the ureteral conduit junction. Deterioration of renal function was observed in 27%, while hyperchloremic acidosis developed in only 2%.[47] A similar rate of deterioration of renal function was observed, in another series of 178 patients, all of whom had at least 4 years of follow-up.[48]

A study from the Mayo Clinic included 1057 patients who underwent radical cystectomy with conduit urinary diversion using ileum or colon from 1980 to 1998 with complete follow-up information.[49] Patients were followed for long-term clinical outcomes and analyzed for the incidence of diversion-specific complications. Bowel complications were the most common, occurring in 215 patients (20.3%), followed by renal complications in 213 (20.2%), infectious complications in 174 (16.5%), stomal complications in 163 (15.4%) and urolithiasis in 162 (15.3%). The least common were metabolic abnormalities, which occurred in 135 patients

(12.8%); and structural complications, which occurred in 122 (11.5%). Increasing age at cystectomy (hazard ratio [HR] 1.21, $P < .001$), increasing Eastern Cooperative Oncology Group performance status (HR 1.23, $P = .02$) and recent era of surgery (HR 1.68, $P < .001$) were significantly associated with a higher incidence of complications. The authors concluded that conduit urinary diversion is associated with a high overall complication rate but a low reoperation rate.[49] Box 4 lists common delayed complications in patients undergoing incontinent urinary diversions.

Cutaneous Ureterostomy

As with other types of urinary diversion, left ureteral obstruction is a common complication of bilateral cutaneous ureterostomies. Long-term stenting for this particular operation for more than 3 months has been reported to decrease this complication and improved the clinical outcomes of this type of urinary diversion.[5]

MINIMALLY INVASIVE APPROACHES

The outcomes of laparoscopic/robotic-assisted urinary diversion come primarily from retrospective case series with small case numbers, which have shown these approaches to be feasible and safe for IC, cutaneous ureterostomy, and ureterosigmoidostomy.[50-55] Lee et al[56] showed that robot-assisted radical cystectomy can be more cost effective than open surgery in the treatment of bladder cancer at a high-volume, tertiary care referral center, particularly with IC as the urinary diversion choice.

Others have shown a lower rate of perioperative complications with "hybrid" open-laparoscopic-assisted techniques compared to a totally laparoscopic technique. Major complications associated with a totally laparoscopic approach appear to be bowel leak and/or urine extravasation and sepsis.[57] Hybrid laparoscopic-assisted approaches or robot-assisted laparoscopic approaches have shown better operative and short-term clinical outcomes comparable with those of previously reported extracorporeal techniques.[53-55,57] However, larger numbers of patients and longer follow-up will be needed to establish therapeutic equivalence.[57]

SUMMARY

Incontinent urinary diversion techniques are an important part of management of patients after radical pelvic extirpative procedures. There are several options, including IC, cutaneous ureterostomy, and colonic conduit, each with different indications and applications. The IC remains the gold standard. Most patients who undergo this procedure can expect minimal morbidity and mortality and an enhanced quality of life. Significant advances in surgical techniques, a better understanding of isolated bowel segment physiology, and improvements in preoperative and postoperative care have revolutionized the field of urinary diversion. Efforts to refine surgical techniques for incontinent urinary diversions, including the incorporation of newer minimally invasive techniques, are ongoing.

REFERENCES

1. Goodwin WE, Scardino PT. Ureterosigmoidostomy. *J Urol.* 1997;118 (1 pt 2):169-174.
2. Williams O, Vereb MJ, Libertino JA. Noncontinent urinary diversion. *Urol Clin North Am.* 1997;24(4):735-744.
3. Silberstein JL, Poon SA, Maschino AC, et al. Urinary diversion practice patterns among certifying American urologists. *J Urol.* 2013; 189(3):1042-1047.
4. Evans B, Montie JE, Gilbert SM. Incontinent or continent urinary diversion: how to make the right choice. *Curr Opin Urol.* 2010;20(5):421-425.
5. Rodriguez AR, Lockhart A, King J, Wiegand L, Carrion R, Ordorica R, Lockhart J. Cutaneous ureterostomy technique for adults and effects of ureteral stenting: an alternative to the ileal conduit. *J Urol.* 2011;186(5): 1939-1943.
6. Kim CJ, Wakabayashi Y, Sakano Y, Johnin K, Yoshiki T, Okada Y. Simple technique for improving tubeless cutaneous ureterostomy. *Urology.* 2005;65(6):1221-1225.
7. Westney OL. The neurogenic bladder and incontinent urinary diversion. *Urol Clin North Am.* 2010;37(4):581-592.
8. Parekh DJ, Donat SM. Urinary diversion: options, patient selection, and outcomes. *Semin Oncol.* 2007;34(2):98-109.
9. Madersbacher S, Schmidt J, Eberle JM, et al. Long-term outcome of ileal conduit diversion. *J Urol.* 2003;169:985.
10. Rosen MA, Roth DR, Gonzales ET Jr. Current indications for cutaneous ureterostomy. *Urology.* 1994;43(1):92-96.
11. Kaiho Y, Ito A, Numahata K, Ishidoya S, Arai Y. Retroperitoneoscopic transureteroureterostomy with cutaneous ureterostomy to salvage failed ileal conduit urinary diversion. *Eur Urol.* 2011;59(5):875-878.
12. Nogueira L, Reis RB, Machado RD, et al. Cutaneous ureterostomy with definitive ureteral stent as urinary diversion option in unfit patients after radical cystectomy. *Acta Cir Bras.* 2013;28(suppl 1):43-47.
13. Nagele U, Sievert KD, Merseburger AS, Anastasiadis AG, Stenz A. Urinary diversion following cystectomy. *EAU Update Series.* 2005;3: 129-137.
14. Ubrig B, Lazica M, Waldner M, Roth S. Extraperitoneal bilateral cutaneous ureterostomy with midline stoma for palliation of pelvic cancer. *Urology.* 2004;63(5):973-975.
15. Chang SS, Alberts GL, Smith JA Jr, Cookson MS. Ileal conduit urinary diversion in patients with previous history of abdominal/pelvic irradiation. *World J Urol.* 2004;22(4):272-276.
16. Estape R, Mendez LE, Angioli R, Penalver M. Urinary diversion in gynecologic oncology. *Surg.* 2001;81(4):781-797.
17. Schmidt JD, Buchsbaum HJ, Nachtsheim DA. Long-term follow-up, further experience with and modifications of the transverse colon conduit in urinary tract diversion. *Br J Urol.* 1985;57(3):284-288.
18. Mills RD, Studer UE. Metabolic consequences of continent urinary diversion. *J Urol.* 1999;161:1057.
19. Stampfer DS, McDougal WS, McGovern FJ. The use of in bowel urology. Metabolic and nutritional complications. *Urol Clin North Am.* 1997;24:715.
20. Turbull Rb Jr. Intestinal stomas. *Surg Clin North Am.* 1958;38:1361.
21. Lazica DA, Ubrig B, Brandt AS, von Rundstedt FC, Roth S. Ureteral substitution with reconfigured colon: long-term followup. *J Urol.* 2012; 187(2):542-548.
22. Maffezzini M, Gerbi G, Campodonico F, Parodi D. Multimodal perioperative plan for radical cystectomy and intestinal urinary diversion. I. Effect on recovery of intestinal function and occurrence of complications. *Urology.* 2007;69(6):1107-1111.
23. Güenaga KF, Matos D, Wille-Jørgensen P. Mechanical bowel preparation for elective colorectal surgery. *Cochrane Database Syst Rev.* 2011; (9):CD001544.

24. American Society of Anesthesiologist Task Force on Preoperative Fasting. Practice guidelines for preoperative fasting and the use of pharmacologic agents to reduce the risk of pulmonary aspiration: application to healthy patients undergoing elective procedures: a report by the American Society of Anesthesiologist Task Force on Preoperative Fasting. *Anesthesiology.* 1999;90(3):896-905.
25. Raynor MC, Lavien G, Nielsen M, Wallen EM, Pruthi RS. Elimination of preoperative mechanical bowel preparation in patients undergoing cystectomy and urinary diversion. *Urol Oncol.* 2013;31(1):32-35.
26. Colombo R, Naspro R. Ileal conduit as the Standard for urinary diversion after radical cystectomy for bladder cancer. *Eur Urol.* 2010;9(suppl): 736-744.
27. Winter WE III, Krivak TC, Maxwell GL, Elkas JC, Rose GS, Carlson JW. Modified technique for urinary diversion with incontinent conduits. *Gynecol Oncol.* 2002;86(3):351-353.
28. Nogueira L, Reis RB, Machado RD, et al. Cutaneous ureterostomy with definitive ureteral stent as urinary diversion option in unfit patients after radical cystectomy. *Acta Cir Bras.* 2013;28(suppl 1):43-47.
29. Kilciler M, Bedir S, Erdemir F, Zeybek N, Erten K, Ozgok Y. Comparison of ileal conduit and transureteroureterostomy with ureterocutaneostomy urinary diversion. *Urol Int.* 2006;77(3):245-250.
30. Ravi R, Dewan AK, Pandey KK. Transverse colon conduit urinary diversion in patients treated with very high dose pelvic irradiation. *Br J Urol.* 1994;73(1):51-54.
31. Schmidt JD, HJ. Transverse colon conduit diversion. *Urol Clin North Am.* 1986;13(2):233-239.
32. Tobias-Machado M, Starling ES, Korkes F, da Silva MN, Appolonio PR, Wroclawski ER. Video-assisted colonic conduit: a new minimally invasive urinary diversion to patients after pelvic radiotherapy. *Surg Laparosc Endosc Percutan Tech.* 2009;19(4):e119-e122.
33. Haugen V, Bliss DZ, Savik K. Perioperative factors that affect long-term adjustment to an incontinent ostomy. *J Wound Ostomy Continence Nurs.* 2006;33(5):525-535.
34. Gemmill R, Sun V, Ferrell B, Krouse RS, Grant M. Going with the flow: quality-of-life outcomes of cancer survivors with urinary diversion. *J Wound Ostomy Continence Nurs.* 2010;37(1):65-72.
35. Vora AA, Harbin A, Rayson R, et al. Alvimopan provides rapid gastrointestinal recovery without nasogastric tube decompression after radical cystectomy and urinary diversion. *Can J Urol.* 2012;19(3):6293-6298.
36. Wullt B, Holst E, Steven K, et al. Microbial flora in ileal and colonic neobladders. *Eur Urol.* 2004;45:233.
37. Teixeira SC, Ferenschild FT, Solomon MJ, et al. Urological leaks after pelvic exenterations comparing formation of colonic and ileal conduits. *Eur J Surg Oncol.* 2012;38(4):361-366.
38. Fichtner J. Follow-up after urinary diversion. *Urol.* 1999;63(1):40-45.
39. Pycha A, Comploj E, Martini T, et al. Comparison of complications in three incontinent urinary diversions. *Eur Urol.* 2008;54(4):825-832.
40. Salemis NS, Gakis C, Zografidis A, Gourgiotis S. Cutaneous metastasis of transitional cell bladder carcinoma: a rare presentation and literature review. *J Cancer Res Ther.* 2011;7(2):217-219.
41. Jian PY, Godoy G, Coburn M, et al. Adenocarcinoma following urinary diversion. *Can Urol Assoc J.* 2012;6(2):E77-E80.
42. Kälble T, Hofmann I, Riedmiller H, Vergho D. Tumor growth in urinary diversion: a multicenter analysis. *Eur Urol.* 2011;60(5):1081-1086.
43. Azimuddin K, Khubchandani IT, Stasik JJ, Rosen L, Riether RD. Neoplasia after ureterosigmoidostomy. *Dis Colon Rectum.* 1999;42(12): 1632-1638.
44. Wood DN, Allen SE, Hussain M, Greenwell TJ, Shah PJ. Stomal complications of ileal conduits are significantly higher when formed in women with intractable urinary incontinence. *J Urol.* 2004;172(6 Pt 1): 2300-2303.
45. Hautmann RE, Abol-Enein H, Hafez K, et al; World Health Organization (WHO) Consensus Conference on Bladder Cancer. Urinary diversion. *Urology.* 2007;69(1 suppl):17-49.
46. Samuel JD, Bhatt RI, Montague RJ, et al. The natural history of postoperative renal function in patients undergoing ileal conduit diversion for cancer measured using serial isotopic glomerular filtration rate and 99m technetium-mercaptoacetyltriglycine renography. *J Urol.* 2006;176:2518-2522.
47. Doležel J, Capak I, Valik D, et al. Effect of ureterointestinal anastomosis on renal function and morbidity in intestinal urinary diversion. *Scand J Urol.* 2013;47:225-229.
48. Shimko MS, Tollefson MK, Umbreit EC, Farmer SA, Blute ML, Frank I. Long-term complications of conduit urinary diversion. *J Urol.* 2011;185(2):562-567.
49. Turedi S, Incealtin O, Hos G. Complications associated with ureterosigmoidostomy—colon carcinoma and ascendens infection resulting in nephrectomy: a case report. *Acta Chir Belg.* 2009;109(4):531-533.
50. Ma LL, Bi H, Hou XF, Huang Y, Wang GL, Zhao L, Zhang SD. Laparoendoscopic single-site radical cystectomy and urinary diversion: initial experience in China using a homemade single-port device. *J Endourol.* 2012;26(4):355-359.
51. Canda AE, Atmaca AF, Altinova S, Akbulut Z, Balbay MD. Robot-assisted nerve-sparing radical cystectomy with bilateral extended pelvic lymph node dissection (PLND) and intracorporeal urinary diversion for bladder cancer: initial experience in 27 cases. *BJU Int.* 2012;110(3): 434-444.
52. Horstmann M, Kugler M, Anastasiadis AG, Walcher U, Herrmann T, Nagele U. Laparoscopic radical cystectomy: initial experience using the single-incision triangulated umbilical surgery (SITUS) technique. *World J Urol.* 2012;30(5):619-624.
53. Johnson D, Castle E, Pruthi RS, ME. Robotic intracorporeal urinary diversion: ileal conduit. *J Endourol.* 2012;26(12):1566-1569.
54. Pruthi RS, Nix J, McRackan D, et al. Robotic-assisted laparoscopic intracorporeal urinary diversion. *Eur Urol.* 2010;57(6):1013-1021.
55. Azzouni FS, Din R, Rehman S, et al. The first 100 consecutive, robot-assisted, intracorporeal ileal conduits: evolution of technique and 90-day outcomes. *Eur Urol.* 2013;63(4):637-643.
56. Lee R, Ng CK, Shariat SF, et al. The economics of robotic cystectomy: cost comparison of open versus robotic cystectomy. *BJU Int.* 2011;108(11):1886-1892.
57. Haber GP, Campbell SC, Colombo JR Jr, et al. Perioperative outcomes with laparoscopic radical cystectomy: "pure laparoscopic" and "open-assisted laparoscopic" approaches. *Urology.* 2007;70:910.

Chapter 12. Continent Diversions

Timothy Donahue, MD and
Bernard H. Bochner, MD

BACKGROUND

Urinary diversion following cystectomy remains one of the great challenges of radical pelvic surgery because an equivalent replacement for the native bladder has yet to be developed. The bladder is ideally a low-pressure, highly compliant reservoir for the storage of urine with its own intrinsic continence mechanism, sensation, and coordinated, volitional emptying by muscular contraction. In addition, the bladder is generally impermeable, stores sterile urine, and possesses antirefluxing ureters to protect the kidneys and upper tracts from sustained increases in bladder pressure. Recapitulating many of the intrinsic properties of the native bladder and understanding the impact of the choice of bowel segments are paramount to successfully reconstructing the urinary tract. Urinary diversions are broadly divided into 2 main categories: continent and incontinent diversions. In this chapter, we will review the principles, surgical technique, perioperative management, and long-term issues associated with continent cutaneous reservoirs. The other major type of continent diversion, orthotopic urinary diversion is described in Chapter 13.

A continent catheterizable diversion was first described by Gilchrest et al[1] in 1950, but it was not until more than 30 years later when continent cutaneous diversions were routinely performed. Although many different techniques have been described, all are based upon 2 underlying principles: a detubularized, spherical bowel reservoir for storage and a continent, catheterizable stoma for emptying. A variety of continent stomas have been described. The terminal ileum can be tailored and used as a catheterizable limb to take advantage of the nonrefluxing ileocecal valve. The appendix or a tailored segment of bowel can be submucosally tunneled to form a stoma utilizing the principles described by Mitrofanoff.[2] With the Kock or Mainz pouch, a nipple or flap valve is constructed to provide a new continence mechanism. Continent cutaneous reservoirs are an outstanding option for patients in whom an orthotopic urinary diversion is contraindicated.

The Indiana Pouch, a continent cutaneous diversion based upon the terminal ileum and right colon, was first described in 1985 and uses the nonrefluxing ileocecal valve as the continence mechanism. The right hemicolon is detubularized, folded, and is used to fashion a spherical reservoir. The tapered terminal ileum is matured into a stoma either in the right lower quadrant or umbilicus for catheterization of the pouch. Long-term data from multiple institutions have shown this to be a safe and reliable form of urinary diversion, with continence rates that range from 94% to 98%,[3] reoperation rates of 15%, and long-term complications, such as pouch calculi, stomal hernia, stomal stenosis, bowel obstruction, and renal insufficiency, in 17%.[4] Bochner et al[5] described a modification to the ileocecal reservoir whereby the ureters are anastomosed into the terminal ileum as a ureteral substitution segment and a flap valve is developed with the in situ appendix as the catheterizable stoma. This technique is especially useful in patients who have undergone preoperative radiation therapy where excessive manipulation of the ureters can result in devascularization and a higher rate of ureterointestinal anastomotic strictures. In addition, this modification can be used in patients that require resection of ureter for tumor factors. Both techniques will be described in detail.[3,5]

SURGICAL PRINCIPLES

Development of a Low-Pressure System

One of the fundamental principles behind any form of continent urinary diversion is the creation of a low-pressure reservoir. Detubularization of the bowel segment and cross-folding into a sphere forms the maximum capacity reservoir for a given bowel segment and limits the ability of the bowel segment to develop a coordinated and synchronous peristalsis.[6] The spherical configuration maximizes the radius of the reservoir, which according to Laplace law (pressure = tension/radius) will translate into lower filling and storage pressures. Reconfiguration maximizes capacity, therefore, the overall length of bowel required is more limited and this minimizes the surface area available for reabsorption which may reduce metabolic complications. Overall, the spherical reservoir most closely approximates the native bladder by creating a high-capacity, highly compliant reservoir, while minimizing the surface area available for reabsorption of urine and electrolytes during storage. Reconfiguration interferes with the bowel's ability to coordinate a contraction thereby minimizing high-pressure peaks. This may not only be important in upper tract preservation but facilitates continence as well.

Refluxing vs Antirefluxing Systems

The principle behind constructing nonrefluxing anastomoses is to protect the kidneys and upper tracts from sustained high pressures and to prevent ascending bacteriuria. In its normal state, the ureter creates a dynamic, unidirectional flow of urine from the kidney to the bladder by means of peristalsis with the ureter eventually passing at an oblique angle through the bladder wall to its lumen. The intramural portion of the ureter must be of sufficient length (ureteral length to ureteral diameter ratio of 5:1) to allow for passive compression during bladder filling otherwise vesicoureteral reflux (VUR) can occur.[7] Numerous investigators have observed a link between vesicoureteral reflux, upper urinary tract infections or pyelonephritis, and renal scarring. Hutch[8] described increased rates of pyelonephritis in paraplegic patients with VUR, while other investigators noted higher rates of renal scarring and urinary tract infections (UTIs) in children with a history of reflux.[9]

There is significant debate regarding whether the ureterointestinal anastomoses should be constructed in a nonrefluxing or refluxing manner. This was particularly relevant for patients undergoing ureterosigmoidostomy, which diverts the urine into a high-pressure chronically infected system, but has become less of a concern with the development of lower pressure, high-capacity continent reservoirs. With detubularization of the bowel, peristaltic contractions and pressure transmission to the upper tracts is minimized. Berglund and Kock[10] described the volume and pressure characteristics of various intestinal reservoirs and noted that sustained pressures above 25 to 30 cm of water can lead to renal deterioration. Continent cutaneous reservoirs will typically only have sustained pressures above 25 cm of water for approximately 2 minutes per hour during the day, assuming stored volumes below 500 cc or no more than 60% of reservoir capacity.[10]

More recent observations suggest that vesicoureteral reflux is not itself a cause of urinary tract infections. Reflux may deliver colonized urine to the renal pelvis, but it is the sustained stasis of bacteriuria within the upper tracts that is the greater risk factor for pyelonephritis. In children who have reflux and are dysfunctional eliminators, the risk of febrile UTIs or pyelonephritis is significantly higher. Correcting the dysfunctional elimination was one of the most modifiable risk factors for reducing the risk of future infections.[11] As a corollary, stasis of colonized urine within the upper tracts, either secondary to an ureterointestinal anastomotic stricture or from poor emptying of the urinary reservoir, may predispose patients with continent diversions to upper tract infections, pyelonephritis, and increase the risk of long-term scarring.

There appears to be a greater risk of gradual renal deterioration from ureterointestinal anastomotic strictures than from reflux of urine into the upper tracts. Nonrefluxing anastomoses are associated with twice the rate of strictures than refluxing anastomoses, irrespective of the type of bowel segment used. Rates of ureterointestinal strictures with a refluxing anastomotic repair range from 1.7% to 3.6% compared with the 13% to 29% described with the LeDuc nonrefluxing anastomosis technique.[12] Approximately one-half of patients with strictures will require surgical intervention, leading some surgeons to conclude that the greater risk to the upper tracts is ureterointestinal anastomotic stricture rather than reflux. In a group of 126 patients followed for more than 25 years with Kock reservoirs, Jonnson et al[13] concluded that the type of diversion does not significantly impact long-term kidney function as long as any potential strictures are recognized and treated. Refluxing anastomoses are technically simpler to complete and have not been associated with significant rates of upper tract deterioration, thus making them the procedure of choice for ureterointestinal anastomoses.[3,14-17]

Development of Continence Mechanism

There are 4 basic continence mechanisms that may be utilized in the construction of a continent reservoir. Mitrofanoff described tunneling the appendix beneath the tenia of the adjacent cecum to create a continent, catheterizable limb that is brought to the skin surface. This technique may not be feasible if the caliber and/or length of the appendix are inadequate.[2] In the Kock pouch, a nipple valve is constructed by intussuscepting a portion of the small bowel into the lumen of the low-pressure reservoir to serve as the continence mechanism.[18] Due to the complexity of this reconstruction and the relatively high rate of complications with the nipple valve, this technique has not been widely adopted.[19] Expanding upon the flap valve mechanism described by Ghoneim,[20] Skinner[21] adapted the technique to construct a double-T pouch for continent cutaneous diversions which utilizes a serous-lined extramural tunnel instead of intussuscepted small bowel as the flap-valve continence mechanism. The complexity of construction and longer operative times has also limited its widespread adoption. The hydraulic ileal valve, as seen in the Indiana pouch, incorporates the native ileocecal valve, a tapered limb of ileum, and plication sutures at their junction to form the basis of the continence mechanism.[3]

INDICATIONS AND CLINICAL APPLICATIONS

Selection Criteria for Continent Diversions

When considering the creation of a continent diversion, it is of paramount importance to have a motivated patient with realistic expectations regarding the functional outcomes and limitations of the reconstruction. Patients undergoing continent cutaneous diversions must physically be able to catheterize themselves on a routine basis. Those patients who are less concerned with body image, those who are socially isolated or prone to poor follow-up, and those with advanced age or significant comorbidities may be better served with a noncontinent urinary diversion.[22]

Absolute contraindications to continent urinary diversion are impaired renal function and severe hepatic dysfunction due to the metabolic complications associated with reabsorption of urine and electrolytes during periods of storage. There must be adequate renal function to address this reabsorption.

Patients with creatinine levels higher than 2.0 mg/dL or glomerular filtration rates lower than 35 mL/minute are not optimal candidates for continent diversion. Reabsorption of urinary components by the ileum and colon may lead to severe systemic electrolyte abnormalities in patients with limited renal function. In addition, free water loss occurs within continent reservoirs, which may lead to dehydration in those patients with impaired renal concentrating ability. Patients with severe hepatic dysfunction are at risk for hyperammonemia due to an impaired ability to process the ammonia absorbed by the reservoir.

Relative contraindications to continent cutaneous diversion are inflammatory bowel disease, an inability or unwillingness to self-catheterize, mental impairment, and prior colon cancer history if the colon is to be used for reconstruction. All patients who undergo continent urinary diversion need to receive detailed preoperative counseling and teaching regarding the planned reconstructive procedure. Patients must be aware that although the goal of reconstruction is to provide an acceptable substitute for the native bladder, there are inherent differences with continent diversions that the patient must be willing to accept long term.

ANATOMIC CONSIDERATIONS

Although any segment of bowel can be utilized to construct a urinary reservoir, factors such as the patient's renal function, history of prior abdominal surgery or radiation therapy, and the type of reconstruction planned will greatly impact the surgeon's choice of bowel segment. Each bowel segment has its own relative advantages and disadvantages including metabolic sequelae when used for urinary diversion.

The stomach is the least permeable and is associated with the lowest rates of bacteriuria of all intestinal segments due to the secretion of hydrochloric acid.[23] However, it is associated with a hypochloremic metabolic alkalosis secondary to the loss of protons and chloride in the urine. Those patients with impaired renal function may not be able to excrete sufficient bicarbonate to buffer this metabolic derangement. The secretion of excess acid in the urine may cause hematuria-dysuria syndrome in some patients. Typically, there is not an adequate volume of stomach than can be removed to form a complete urinary diversion; most commonly, the stomach is used in composite diversions or in children where it is utilized as an augment to the bladder. In addition, there are often limitations to the blood supply that limits the usefulness of stomach in pelvic urinary reconstruction.

The jejunum is not typically used for urinary diversion due to the high rates of symptomatic metabolic derangements observed with this bowel segment. Patients experience jejunal-conduit syndrome as a result of increased sodium and chloride excretion combined with potassium and hydrogen reabsorption. Patients develop a hyponatremic, hypochloremic, hyperkalemic metabolic acidosis that is associated with water loss and dehydration. The risk of metabolic derangements increases the more proximal the segment of jejunum used for the diversion. While the jejunum has the theoretical advantage of being less likely to have been within radiation fields administered to the pelvis, the relative disadvantages outweigh this theoretical benefit limiting its utility for diversions.

The ileum and colon are associated with the fewest electrolyte disturbances, have the greatest amount of redundancy, are easily mobilized to any portion of the abdomen or pelvis, and typically possess excellent blood supplies. Both segments are associated with the same metabolic abnormalities due to the absorption of ammonium chloride resulting in a hyperchloremic metabolic acidosis. Patients with impaired renal function are more susceptible to developing severe metabolic abnormalities and can develop lethargy, anorexia, weight loss, and long term are at risk for bone demineralization leading to osteopenia. Symptomatic metabolic acidosis can be treated with alkalinizing agents, maintaining good hydration, and minimizing dwell time of urine stored within the continent diversion. The terminal ileum is responsible for absorption of bile salts, fat-soluble vitamins (K, A, D, and E), and the absorption of vitamin B12. If excessive lengths of ileum are used for diversion, patients can develop steatorrhea, vitamin B12 deficiency, and dehydration. When the ileocecal valve is removed from bowel continuity, there is an increased risk of diarrhea due to the increased fluid load delivered to the colon.

Drugs excreted unchanged in the urine and absorbed by the urinary reservoir can be problematic, especially in those patients receiving adjuvant chemotherapy. Methotrexate toxicity has been described in patients with urinary diversions due to absorption.[24,25] To minimize the reabsorption of excreted drugs and/or metabolites, patients undergoing chemotherapy should have their reservoir or neobladder drained with a Foley catheter during treatment. Those patients taking phenytoin, theophylline, lithium, and certain antibiotics excreted in an active form into the urine should be closely monitored.[26-28]

PREOPERATIVE PREPARATION

Box 12-1 KEY SURGICAL INSTRUMENTATION

- 80-mm linear stapler with 3.5-mm staples
- 90-mm transverse stapler with 3.5-mm staples
- 7 or 8 French single-J ureteral stents
- 3-0 polyglycolic sutures

A thorough understanding of the patient's medical and surgical history is necessary when deciding upon the type of diversion planned after complete urinary bladder resection. As discussed, those patients with renal or severe hepatic insufficiency are not candidates for continent diversions. Adjuvant or a remote history of radiation therapy may influence the segment of bowel selected and the type of diversion planned. Patients should be assessed with respect to manual dexterity and be both willing and able to self-catheterize. Preoperative counseling and education by a wound-ostomy nurse is standard practice in our clinic.

All patients are marked prior to surgery for the possible stoma site in the case of intraoperative conversion to an incontinent diversion. Preoperative cardiovascular risk assessments are completed and patients undergo outpatient bowel preparation with an oral polyethylene glycol solution particularly if a colon-based reservoir is planned. Preparation for a small bowel-based reservoir does not require formal bowel preparation.

SURGICAL PROCEDURES

Box 12-2 MASTER SURGEON'S PRINCIPLES

- Gentle dissection of ureters with maximal preservation of blood supply
- In previously radiated patients, resect back to healthy ureter
- Consider using an extended limb of ileum to reach healthy, vascularized ureter rather than placing the ureter on stretch to reach its anastomosis
- Stented and tension-free ureterointestinal anastomoses
- Internal drainage of the diversion with a large caliber catheter

Continent Cutaneous Reservoir (Indiana Pouch)

The ascending colon and terminal ileum are isolated from the enteric tract. A 25- to 30-cm length of right colon is needed for the reservoir, and in some patients this may require taking a portion of the proximal transverse colon. A 7- to 10-cm segment of terminal ileum beyond the ileocecal valve is taken with the right colon and used as the catheterizable limb of the pouch (Figure 12-1). A deep division within the mesentery between the terminal superior mesenteric artery and ileocolic arterial branches facilitates mobility to the reservoir segment. Bowel continuity is restored in the standard fashion and the cecum and ascending colon are opened anteriorly along the antimesenteric border between the colonic tenia. Removal of the appendix is not required but advocated by many surgeons.[3] The appendix could be removed routinely by the authors if it is not to be used as a catheterizable limb. The terminal ileum is tapered over a 14 French red rubber catheter placed through the ileum into the open pouch. Babcock clamps are placed serially along the antimesenteric border of the ileum to hold the excess ileum to be removed away from the catheter. A straight gastrointestinal anastomosis (GIA) stapler is placed in the groove between the red rubber catheter and the Babcock clamps and the excess ileum is removed with the stapling device. Stapling is stopped just prior to reaching the ileocecal valve to avoid damage to the continence mechanism (Figure 12-2). Interrupted Lembert sutures are used to plicate the funnel-shaped terminal ileum at the ileocecal valve to bolster and support the continence mechanism. Classically, 3

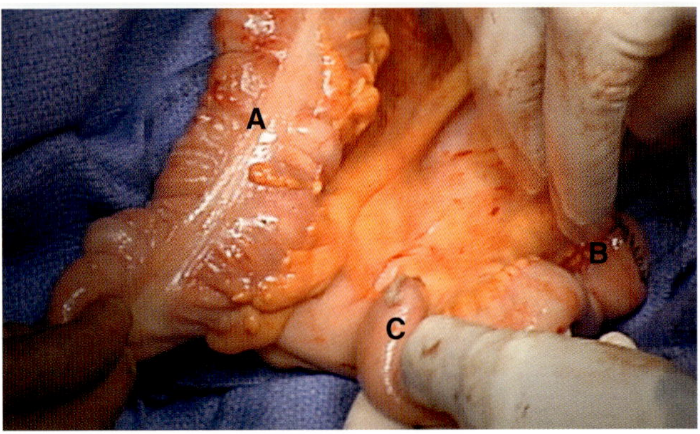

Fig. 12-1. The classic Indiana pouch utilizes the cecum and ascending colon (A) to form the continent reservoir and the terminal ileum (B) as the catheterizable limb. One modification of the classic Indiana reservoir that can be used to replace lost ureteral length or serve to substitute discarded distal-radiated ureteral segments uses a tubularized ileal segment as a ureteral substitution. A 10- to 14-cm segment of more proximal distal ileum is used to replace the desired ureteral length (C). The segment of ileum immediately proximal to the catheterizable limb is used.

to 4 Lembert sutures are required and placed along the cecum to tighten the ileocecal junction; however, additional sutures may be used to buttress the mechanism. The sutures are placed closest to the ileocecal valve initially and subsequent sutures moving away from the ileocecal valve should be placed wider than the previous to narrow the ileocecal junction (Figure 12-3). This portion of the reconstruction is done with the pouch open to allow for visualization of the internal aspect of the

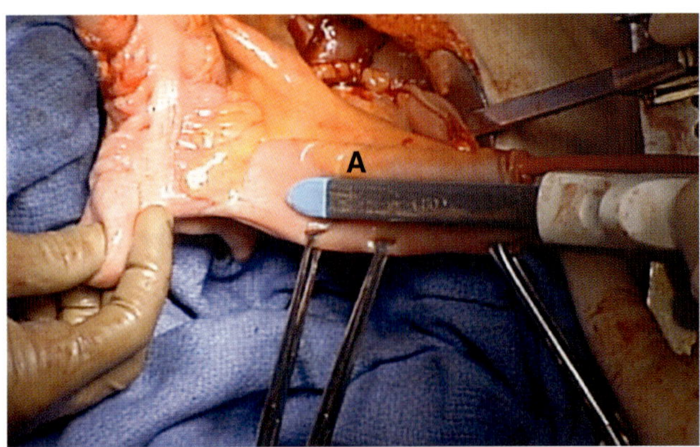

Fig. 12-2. The terminal ileum (A) is tapered over a 14 French red rubber catheter placed through the ileum into the open pouch. Babcock clamps are placed serially along the antimesenteric border of the ileum to hold the excess ileum to be removed away from the catheter. A straight gastrointestinal anastomosis (GIA) stapler is placed in the groove between the red rubber catheter and the Babcock clamps and the excess ileum is removed with the stapling device. Stapling is stopped just prior to reaching the ileocecal valve to avoid damage to the continence mechanism.

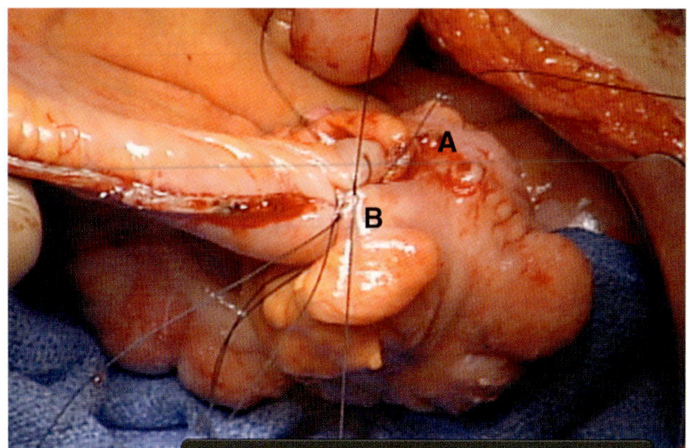

Fig. 12-3. Interrupted Lembert sutures are used to plicate the funnel-shaped terminal ileum (A) at the ileocecal valve to bolster and support the continence mechanism. Classically, 3 to 4 Lembert sutures are required and placed along the cecum to tighten the ileocecal junction; however, additional sutures may be used to buttress the mechanism (B). The sutures are placed closest to the ileocecal valve initially and subsequent sutures moving away from the ileocecal valve should be placed wider than the previous to narrow the ileocecal junction.

ileocecal junction and to allow for direct inspection of the catheter moving in and out of the pouch.

After the tapering of the terminal ileum is completed, the limb is catheterized with a 14 or 16 French catheter under direct visualization. The catheter should pass smoothly and only meet minimal resistance at the ileocecal junction. If the catheter does not pass smoothly, then it may be necessary to remove plicating sutures that may be too tight. If the channel is not straight or there is an outpouching along its course, then additional plication sutures may be required to correct any angulation.

Once catheterization is felt to be optimal, the detubularized colon is folded upon itself to create a spherical reservoir and the edges are closed with running 3-0 polyglycolic sutures. The reservoir may be closed completely at this time or following implantation of the ureters. Once the reservoir closure is completed, it is filled with saline through a catheter placed via the ileum to assess for watertight integrity. Any identified areas of leakage are closed with interrupted figure-of-eight absorbable sutures. A 24 French Malecot catheter is placed through the cecal portion of the reservoir and brought out through an abdominal incision later in the procedure.

The ureters can be anastomosed in a refluxing or nonrefluxing technique. Ureteroenteric stricture rates, however, may be higher by creating tunnels in the tinea of the cecum that are closed over the ureters than in an end-to-side refluxing manner. The authors prefer a direct anastomosis to the bowel without tunneling to minimize the risk of stricture. This would be performed prior to closure of the reservoir. The left ureter is passed through an avascular portion of the mesentery to reach the posteromedial aspect of the reservoir. The right ureter will easily reach the reservoir and should be reimplanted where a tension-free anastomosis can be completed. The ureteral anastomoses are performed over single-J ureteral stents that are passed out of the pouch adjacent to the cecostomy drainage catheter.

The stoma site can be placed within the umbilicus or on the side of the abdomen that will be most accessible to the patient for self-catheterization. The limb should be oriented as straight as possible between the skin and ileocecal valve; most commonly this will be on the right side of the abdominal wall. A 1.5-cm trephine is created though all layers of the abdominal wall, and the tapered ileum is brought to the skin surface. The limb is secured at the level of the fascia and any excess ileum beyond the level of the skin is removed to create a flush stoma. The ileal stoma is matured at the skin level with interrupted 3-0 polyglycolic sutures. A 16 French Foley catheter is passed to ensure ease of catheterization and the reservoir is filled to assess for leakage from the stoma. The catheter is replaced and closed suction drains are positioned dependent to the reservoir and adjacent to the uretero-intestinal anastomoses. The cecostomy drainage catheter and ureteral stents are brought out separately through the skin.

One modification of the classic Indiana reservoir that could be used to replace lost ureteral length or serve to substitute discarded distal-radiated ureteral segments would involve the use of a tubularized ileal segment as a ureteral substitution. A 10- to 14-cm segment of more proximal distal ileum would be used to replace the desired ureteral length. The segment of ileum immediately proximal to the catheterizable limb is used (Figure 12-4). The ureters are connected to the proximal portion of this tubularized limb in a similar fashion used for an ileal conduit (Figure 12-5). The distal end of the tubularized segment is then connected to the pouch in the region of the base of the cecum (Figure 12-6). By using bowel to replace radiated segments of distal ureter, the stricture/complication rate related to the ureteroenteric connection may be minimized.[5]

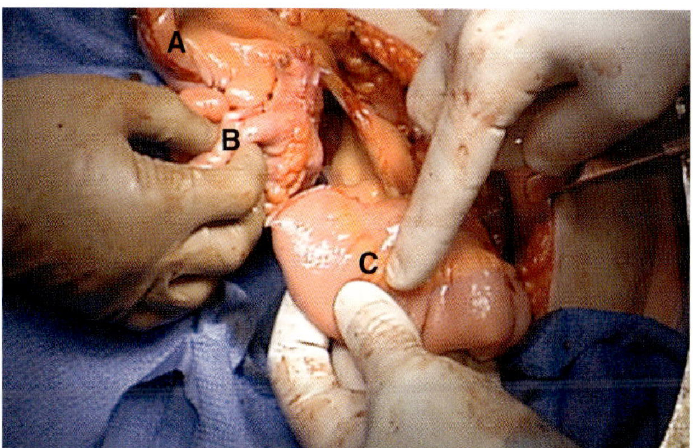

Fig. 12-4. The 10- to 14-cm segment of distal ileum to be used for ureteral substitution (A) is aligned for anastomosis to the cecum (B) in a position away from the ileocecal valve after the catheterizable limb (C) has been constructed.

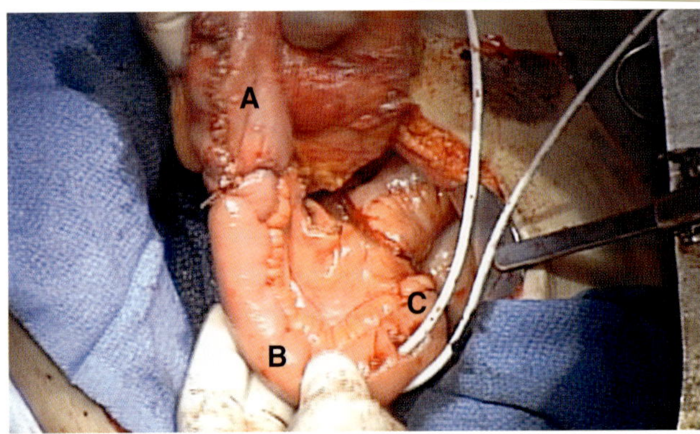

Fig. 12-5. The ureters are connected to the proximal portion of this tubularized limb in a similar fashion used for an ileal conduit. (A) Pouch. (B) Ureteral substitution limb. (C) Ureteral stents marking site of ureterointestinal anastomosis.

Ureteroileocecal Appendicostomy Urinary Reservoir

Use of the appendix as the continent catheterizable limb has been successfully used in large series of patients undergoing continent cutaneous urinary diversion. The appendix mechanism has proven to be reliably continent and may lead to fewer major reservoir-related complications that require revisionary surgery. The appendix is inspected for adequate length, luminal diameter, and structural integrity. An appendiceal length of 4 cm is necessary for tunneling and formation of a cutaneous catheterizable stoma. After the tip of the appendix is incised, the lumen of the appendix is sequentially dilated to 14 French.

The anterior tinea of the cecum is injected with an epinephrine solution diluted to 1:100,000 and an incision approximately 3 to 4 cm in length is made. The lateral flaps of the incision are developed to form a trough wide and deep enough to accommodate the proximal appendix.

A total of 3 to 4 windows are made in the appendiceal mesoappendix (Windows of Deaver) with care taken to prevent injury to the appendiceal artery. Serial seromuscular sutures are placed through the openings in the mesoappendix and the appendix is folded in a jack-knife fashion cephalad into the trough created in the cecal tinea. The sutures are tied, thus securing the appendix in a submucosal tunnel that will act as the continence mechanism for the reservoir.

The ascending colon is transected at the junction with the transverse colon with care taken to preserve the marginal artery blood supply. Similarly, the terminal ileum is divided at the junction between the superior mesenteric artery and ileocolic arteries. In general, a 15-cm segment of terminal ileum should be sufficient; however, in those patients requiring replacement of additional ureteral length due to radiation changes a longer segment of ileum can be used. Bowel continuity is restored (ileum to transverse colon) and the ascending colon and cecum are detubularized along the anterior antimesenteric border between the colonic tinea. The colon is fashioned into a spherical reservoir either by folding the distal detubularized segment onto its proximal cut edge or by folding the segment into a U shape and folding once again into a sphere.

End to side, refluxing anastomoses are formed between the ureters and tubularized ileal segment. Distal ureteral segments that show any signs of radiation damage are resected and mobilization of the remaining normal proximal portions of the ureters is minimized to limit any devascularization. The tubularized terminal ileum is brought to the ureters rather than mobilizing the ureters to reach the ileum for anastomosis. The ureters are spatulated in the standard fashion and anastomosed to the terminal ileum with multiple absorbable sutures. Bilateral single-J ureteral stents are placed prior to completion of the anastomosis and are exteriorized separately through the pouch and skin at the completion of the surgery.

The appendiceal stoma is preferentially positioned at the umbilicus, but can be placed in the right lower quadrant if necessary. The umbilicus is separated from the anterior rectus fascia and a Y-shaped incision is created at its base. The appendiceal stomal is matured to the edges of the Y incision and multiple absorbable sutures are placed to secure the reservoir to the posterior rectus fascia and peritoneum. A 24 French cecostomy drainage catheter is placed into the pouch through a separate incision for irrigation and a 14 French catheter is routed through the appendiceal stoma to support the stoma during healing. This catheter can be opened to drainage or capped to simply serve as a stent of the appendiceal stoma during healing. Closed suction drains are placed adjacent to the reservoir and the ureterointestinal anastomoses.[5]

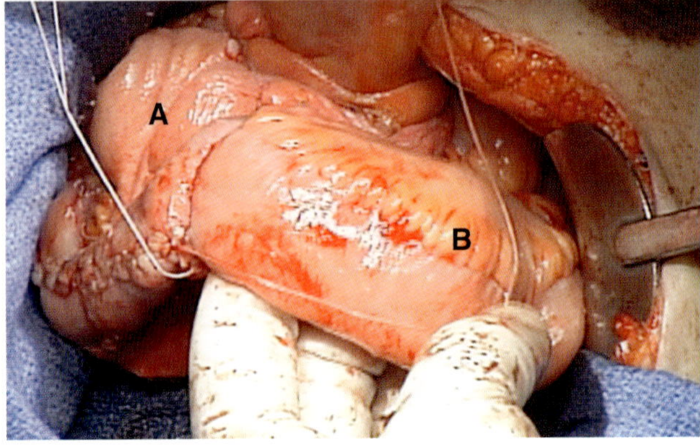

Fig. 12-6. The distal end of the tubularized segment is then connected to the pouch in the region of the base of the cecum. (A) Pouch. (B) Ureteral substitution limb.

Heavily pretreated patients are at risk for stomal complications and obstruction or leakage at the ureterointestinal anastomosis. The risk of developing these complications is associated with preoperative radiation therapy and is felt to be secondary to damage to the vascular endothelium and poor tissue viability that accompanies excessive mobilization of the irradiated ureters. Bochner et al[5] described the construction of a modified right colon reservoir employing a submucosally tunneled appendiceal valve and the terminal ileum as a ureteral substitute. They found the appendiceal-based continence mechanism to be very reliable even in their radiated patient population. The rate of stomal stenosis using the appendix is higher compared with ileal-based limbs; however, the risk of stomal leakage and difficulty catheterizing due to limb angulation is less. In addition, the use of the ureteral substitution segment has lowered the rates of ureteroenteric complications.

POSTOPERATIVE CARE

Box 12-3 PERIOPERATIVE MORBIDITY

- Ileus vs small bowel obstruction
- Deep venous thrombosis
- Pulmonary embolism
- Anastomotic leak
- Pelvic abscess

The use of standardized clinical pathways has been shown to reduce postoperative complications, decrease length of hospital stay, and provide cost-effective care for patients undergoing radical cystectomy. In our institution, a standardized clinical pathway is used for all patients undergoing complete bladder resection and urinary diversion. The pathways delineate milestones anticipated on each postoperative day and order sets are available to standardize the care such that all members of the team caring for the patient know what to expect on subsequent days of admission. The order sets are used a guidelines for the physician and nursing staff and clinical judgment may dictate removing a patient from the prescribed pathway. The nasogastric tube is routinely removed either prior to extubation in the operating room or upon arrival to the recovery room. Pain control is managed with either an epidural or intravenous patient-controlled analgesic pump according to surgeon preference. All patients receive prophylaxis against deep venous thrombosis with pneumatic compression devices and low-molecular weight heparin; in rare cases, prophylactic placement of inferior vena cava filters has been performed. Proton pump inhibitors are prescribed to reduce the risk of gastric ulcers and promotility agents such as metoclopramide are prescribed once bowel sounds have returned. Incentive spirometry, aggressive pulmonary therapy regimens, and early, frequent ambulation are prescribed for all patients.

At the time of surgery, at least 1 drainage catheter is placed within the continent reservoir to assist with decompression and irrigation of the urinary diversion during its period of healing. The reservoir is irrigated every 4 hours daily beginning on the day of surgery to clear any accumulated mucous. The percutaneous drainage catheter is typically removed after 3 weeks after reservoir formation. Routine fluoroscopy to assess for integrity of the reservoir or neobladder is not necessary if there is no evidence of urinary leakage perioperatively. In heavily radiated patients, a pouchogram to confirm complete reservoir healing is reasonable.[29]

Once the catheters are removed, patients are instructed to empty their reservoirs every 2 to 3 hours even at night. Patients can expect to gradually increase the interval as the capacity of the reservoir increases.[30] With continent cutaneous reservoirs, there is a lack of the sensation of fullness that was present with the native bladder, and patients must be instructed to catheterize on a time schedule or more frequently depending on the volumes of urine emptied. Patients may experience a sense of fullness with filling; however, despite the attempt to recapitulate the native bladder the new urinary diversion will not function entirely in the same manner.

LONG-TERM OUTCOMES

Box 12-4 DELAYED COMPLICATIONS

- Urinary incontinence
- Urinary retention
- Ureterointestinal strictures
- Urinary tract infections
- Vitamin deficiency
- Metabolic complications
- Reservoir rupture
- Urinary tract stones

Urinary Continence

Incontinence with a continent cutaneous reservoir typically occurs as a result of pressure within the reservoir overwhelming the resistance to outflow at the level of the continence mechanism. This may result from high reservoir pressures or low outlet resistance. Urodynamics should be performed prior to any surgical repair to assess the capacity and compliance of the reservoir. Surgical approaches to address leakage can include reinforcing Lembert sutures to bolster the ileocecal valve, augmentation of the reservoir in the case of a high-pressure system, or reconstruction of the catheterizable limb/continence mechanism. Incontinence with an appendix-based ileocecal reservoir is less common and typically occurs when there is loss of the reinforced tunnel supporting the appendix. Surgical repair is the most likely means of addressing leakage in a continent cutaneous reservoir, although attempts at endoscopic bulking can be made prior to open surgery. Alternatively, some patients may elect to use an external collection device, such as an ostomy appliance, rather than undergo surgical repair.

Ureterointestinal Strictures

As reviewed earlier in this chapter, ureterointestinal strictures occur in 3% to 29% of patients depending on the anastomotic technique used and the length of follow-up reported. Most strictures are felt to be due to ureteral ischemia and will occur within the first 1 to 2 years after surgery irrespective of the type of anastomosis performed. These strictures are typically asymptomatic and only identified by changes in creatinine levels over time or on surveillance imaging studies.[30-33] Minimizing mobilization and devascularization of ureters is of paramount importance in reducing the risk of postoperative strictures. Care must be taken in routing the left ureter under the descending colon that an adequate mesentery window must be created to eliminate excessive angulation or place the anastomosis on tension.

Antegrade and retrograde endoscopic as well as open surgical approaches have been described to address ureterointestinal strictures. Open surgical approaches have success rates approaching 90% but are the most invasive. Both dilation and incision of strictures have been described with success rates of 20.0% to 50.0% versus 44.4% to 63.0%, respectively. Dilation alone has been associated with higher rates of recurrence.[33-38] Length of the stricture and whether prior radiation damage has been incurred to the ureter are major predictors of success to endoscopic management of ureteroenteric strictures.

Urinary Tract Infections

Urinary diversions lack the immunologic defenses of the bladder mucosa and prostatic secretions; however, it is important to distinguish between bacterial colonization and symptomatic urinary tract infections in this patient population. Rates of chronic bacteriuria in urinary diversions range from 12% to 79%.[39] In the absence of symptoms, such as fever, flank pain, abdominal pain, purulent urine, leukocytosis, or high clinical suspicion, bacteriuria in a urinary diversion patient should not be treated to minimize the development of antibiotic resistance and potential medication adverse events. Clinical evaluation to determine if a symptomatic infection is present should be completed prior to initiation of antibiotic therapy. Routine cultures or urinalysis in asymptomatic patients will identify evidence of bacteriuria in most patients; however, in general, this should not lead to treatment in the absence of symptoms.

Vitamin Deficiency

The use of the terminal ileum for construction of either a continent cutaneous reservoir or orthotopic neobladder can place the patient at risk for vitamin B12 deficiency. Vitamin B12 absorption occurs primarily in the terminal ileum and deficiency can result in irreversible neurologic and hematologic derangements. From baseline levels vitamin B12 depletion is a slowly occurring event after loss of the terminal ileum, often taking 3 to 5 years to drop to a level sufficiently low enough to produce symptoms.[23,39-41] It is our practice to monitor B12 levels on an annual basis and to replace on a yearly basis beginning at year 3 after urinary diversion.

METABOLIC COMPLICATIONS

Chronic acidosis after urinary diversion occurs in 5.5% to 13.3% of patients at a mean follow-up of 51 months and can result long term in bone demineralization and osteomalacia.[42] Decreased intestinal absorption of calcium can occur with resection of longer segments of ileum. Bone minerals, such as calcium and carbonate, act as buffers against hydrogen ions, leading to decreased skeletal calcium content. Chronic acidosis will induce vitamin D deficiency, resulting in bone mineralization defects, and finally the acidic environment activates resorption of bone by osteoclasts.[43-46] Laboratory values may show elevated alkaline phosphatase and reduced serum calcium and phosphate levels.[44,47] Patients can present with a range of presentations related to bone demineralization ranging from being asymptomatic to pain in weight-bearing joints to having fractures. Women and those patients undergoing urinary diversion at a young age when bone growth is not yet complete appear to be at highest risk for the complications associated with bone demineralization. Patients with impaired renal function are at risk for acidosis, which may be worsened after urinary diversion. Radiographic evidence of bone demineralization may take years to develop. Serial measurements of bone mineral density by DEXA scan may demonstrate subtle alterations over time but this needs to be further studied in prospective manner in this cohort of patients. Symptomatic patients should have their acid-base status corrected as a first step, which may also result in remineralization of the bone. However, those patients failing to respond should be managed with calcium supplements and vitamin D.[48-50] Oral sodium bicarbonate should be considered for patients with a base deficit of −2.5 mmol/L to reduce the likelihood of developing bone sequelae from chronic acidosis.

Reservoir Rupture

Rupture of a continent reservoir is most commonly due to acute or chronic overdistension of the diversion. Catheter trauma and mucous plugging may rarely place the patient at risk for pouch rupture. This must be considered high on the differential diagnosis of any patient with a continent diversion who presents with acute abdominal pain. The diagnosis is established with either fluoroscopic or computed tomography (CT) cystography. CT offers the advantage of delayed imaging which may demonstrate extravasation of contrast-enhanced urine within the peritoneum. Patients who are hemodynamically stable without evidence of sepsis may be managed conservatively with catheter drainage and close observation. Open repair is mandatory in septic patients and those with an acute abdomen.

Urinary Tract Stones

Pouch stones are common in continent cutaneous diversions due to high volumes of retained urine after catheterization and bacterial colonization. Most pouch stones are radio-opaque and patients should undergo yearly imaging to rule out the presence of stones. Those patients who form stones are at increased risk for developing future stones and should be encouraged to increase fluid intake, reduce the interval between catheterizations, and may benefit from potassium citrate.[30,51] The natural history of pouch stones is continual growth, thus surgical intervention is warranted when they are identified. Standard endoscopic techniques or extracorporeal shock-wave lithotripsy may be employed to address small- to medium-sized stones. Open or percutaneous approaches may be necessary for larger stones or when endoscopic access is limited by anatomy, such as in a continent cutaneous reservoir or an appendix-based ileocecal reservoir where the continence mechanism can be damaged by excessive manipulation.

Quality of Life

Measuring quality of life (QoL) after total urinary bladder removal and urinary diversion can be problematic. Until the recent use of accepted standardized questionnaires, many reports were based upon ad hoc surveys generated by researchers and lacked validated instruments from which to draw conclusions. Regional and cultural influences may further introduce differences that may not allow results obtained in one country to be fully applicable in another. Lastly, there may be a change in a patient's perception of QoL longitudinally over time that makes comparisons challenging. The introduction of validated surveys measuring mental and psychological stress, cancer-specific surveys, and even bladder-cancer-specific instruments have helped to move this standardize reporting of QoL outcomes. Kulaksizoglu[52] found that the period of adaptation is about 1 year in most patients after urinary diversion, suggesting that QoL measures should not be assessed sooner. In a prospective study comparing patients undergoing incontinent versus continent diversions, Hardt et al[53] reported perceived global satisfaction was high for both conduit and continent cutaneous reservoirs and most patients would elect to have the same procedure performed again. Henningsohn et al[54] identified sexual dysfunction as the most distressing QoL issue for patients after radical cystectomy regardless of the type of diversion performed (whether continent or incontinent). McGuire et al[55] noted on self-survey that patients with continent diversions did not differ from a control group of normal patients in degree of mental stress, although those with conduit diversions ranked higher than the general population. It is our feeling that although the available literature does not demonstrate clear superiority of one type of diversion over the others, it is likely that there is significant selection bias associated with preoperative matching of patients to the type of diversion they ultimately received. In the absence of prospective studies randomizing equal groups of patients to different diversion types there are limitations to applicability in the available literature. For the motivated and well-counseled patient desiring a continent diversion, there are no identifiable domains in QoL that appear to preferentially suffer after this type of reconstruction.

MINIMALLY INVASIVE SURGICAL APPLICATIONS

Minimally invasive approaches to radical cystectomy are being increasingly utilized; however, only small series have described the intracorporeal construction of continent urinary diversions.[56,57] Most series report on the outcomes of robot-assisted radical cystectomy followed by extracorporeal construction of the diversion through the celiotomy created with removal of the bladder specimen. At this time, there are insufficient data on the safety and efficacy of minimally invasive intracorporeal continent urinary diversions, and the role of this procedure is limited.

SUMMARY

Urinary diversion after complete urinary bladder resection presents challenges to both the surgeon and patient. A complete understanding of the principles of urinary diversion construction, the metabolic consequences associated with the choice of bowel segment, and the options for construction in a previously radiated patient is necessary during preoperative planning. The patient's underlying medical conditions, manual dexterity, mental acuity, and motivation are additional factors to consider. Continent diversions have an excellent track record of safety and should be considered for patients well suited to this type of reconstruction. Patients need adequate preoperative and postoperative education in how to catheterize or void with their newly formed reservoirs. Long-term follow-up is required not only for oncologic purposes, but also to monitor for the late complications such as ureterointestinal strictures, renal deterioration, pouch stones, infections, and voiding dysfunction.

REFERENCES

1. Gilchrist RK, Merricks JW, Hamlin HH, Rieger IT. Construction of a substitute bladder and urethra. *Surg Gynecol Obstet*. 1950;90(6):752-760.
2. Mitrofanoff P. [trans-appendicular continent cystostomy in the management of the neurogenic bladder]. *Chir Pediatr*. 1980;21(4):297-305.
3. Bihrle R. The indiana pouch continent urinary reservoir. *Urol Clin North Am*. 1997;24(4):773-779.
4. Gburek BM, Lieber MM, Blute ML. Comparison of studer ileal neobladder and ileal conduit urinary diversion with respect to perioperative outcome and late complications. *J Urol*. 1998;160(3 Pt 1):721-723.
5. Bochner BH, McCreath WA, Aubey JJ, et al. Use of an ureteroileocecal appendicostomy urinary reservoir in patients with recurrent pelvic malignancies treated with radiation. *Gynecol Oncol*. 2004;94(1):140-146.
6. Studer UE, Zingg EJ. Ileal orthotopic bladder substitutes. What we have learned from 12 years' experience with 200 patients. *Urol Clin North Am*. 1997;24(4):781-793.
7. Paquin AJ, Jr. Ureterovesical anastomosis: The description and evaluation of a technique. *J Urol*. 1959;82:573-583.

8. Hutch JA. Vesico-ureteral reflux in the paraplegic: Cause and correction. *J Urol.* 1952;68(2):457-469.
9. Hodson CJ, Maling TM, McManamon PJ, Lewis MG. The pathogenesis of reflux nephropathy (chronic atrophic pyelonephritis). *Br J Radiol.* 1975;Suppl 13:1-26.
10. Berglund B, Kock NG. Volume capacity and pressure characteristics of various types of intestinal reservoirs. *World J Surg.* 1987;11(6):798-803.
11. Peters CA, Skoog SJ, Arant BS, Jr., et al. Summary of the aua guideline on management of primary vesicoureteral reflux in children. *J Urol.* 2010;184(3):1134-1144.
12. Stein JP, Stenzl A, Grossfeld GD, et al. The use of orthotopic neobladders in women undergoing cystectomy for pelvic malignancy. *World J Urol.* 1996;14(1):9-14.
13. Hobisch A, Tosun K, Kinzl J, et al. Quality of life after cystectomy and orthotopic neobladder versus ileal conduit urinary diversion. *World J Urol.* 2000;18(5):338-344.
14. Hautmann RE, de Petriconi R, Gottfried HW, Kleinschmidt K, Mattes R, Paiss T. The ileal neobladder: Complications and functional results in 363 patients after 11 years of followup. *J Urol.* 1999;161(2):422-427; discussion 427-428.
15. Henningsohn L, Steven K, Kallestrup EB, Steineck G. Distressful symptoms and well-being after radical cystectomy and orthotopic bladder substitution compared with a matched control population. *J Urol.* 2002;168(1):168-174; discussion 174-165.
16. Hart S, Skinner EC, Meyerowitz BE, Boyd S, Lieskovsky G, Skinner DG. Quality of life after radical cystectomy for bladder cancer in patients with an ileal conduit, cutaneous or urethral kock pouch. *J Urol.* 1999;162(1):77-81.
17. Mansson A, Caruso A, Capovilla E, et al. Quality of life after radical cystectomy and orthotopic bladder substitution: A comparison between italian and swedish men. *BJU Int.* 2000;85(1):26-31.
18. Kock NG. Ileostomy without external appliances: A survey of 25 patients provided with intra-abdominal intestinal reservoir. *Ann Surg.* 1971;173(4):545-550.
19. Henriet MP, Neyra P, Elman B. Kock pouch procedures: Continuing experience and evolution in 135 cases. *J Urol.* 1991;146(1):16-20.
20. Abol-Enein H, Ghoneim MA. A novel uretero-ileal reimplantation technique: The serous lined extramural tunnel. A preliminary report. *J Urol.* 1994;151(5):1193-1197.
21. Stein JP, Lieskovsky G, Ginsberg DA, Bochner BH, Skinner DG. The t pouch: An orthotopic ileal neobladder incorporating a serosal lined ileal antireflux technique. *J Urol.* 1998;159(6):1836-1842.
22. Montie JE. Ileal conduit diversion after radical cystectomy: Pro. *Urology.* 1997;49(5):659-662.
23. McDougal WS. Metabolic complications of urinary intestinal diversion. *J Urol.* 1992;147(5):1199-1208.
24. Bowyer GW, Davies TW. Methotrexate toxicity associated with an ileal conduit. *Br J Urol.* 1987;60(6):592.
25. Fossa SD, Heilo A, Bormer O. Unexpectedly high serum methotrexate levels in cystectomized bladder cancer patients with an ileal conduit treated with intermediate doses of the drug. *J Urol.* 1990;143(3):498-501.
26. Davidsson T, Akerlund S, White T, Olaisson G, Mansson W. Mucosal permeability of ileal and colonic reservoirs for urine. *Br J Urol.* 1996;78(1):64-68.
27. Ekman I, Mansson W, Nyberg L. Absorption of drugs from continent caecal reservoir for urine. *Br J Urol.* 1989;64(4):412-416.
28. Alhasso A, Bryden AA, Neilson D. Lithium toxicity after urinary diversion with ileal conduit. *BMJ.* 2000;320(7241):1037.
29. Ankem MK, Han KR, Hartanto V, et al. Routine pouchograms are not necessary after continent urinary diversion. *Urology.* 2004;63(3):435-437.
30. Hautmann RE. Urinary diversion: Ileal conduit to neobladder. *J Urol.* 2003;169(3):834-842.
31. Pantuck AJ, Han KR, Perrotti M, Weiss RE, Cummings KB. Ureteroenteric anastomosis in continent urinary diversion: Long-term results and complications of direct versus nonrefluxing techniques. *J Urol.* 2000;163(2):450-455.
32. Schwaibold H, Friedrich MG, Fernandez S, Conrad S, Huland H. Improvement of ureteroileal anastomosis in continent urinary diversion with modified le duc procedure. *J Urol.* 1998;160(3 Pt 1):718-720.
33. Roth S, van Ahlen H, Semjonow A, Oberpenning F, Hertle L. Does the success of ureterointestinal implantation in orthotopic bladder substitution depend more on surgeon level of experience or choice of technique? *J Urol.* 1997;157(1):56-60.
34. Abol-Enein H, Ghoneim MA. Functional results of orthotopic ileal neobladder with serous-lined extramural ureteral reimplantation: Experience with 450 patients. *J Urol.* 2001;165(5):1427-1432.
35. De Carli P, Micali S, O'Sullivan D, et al. Ureteral anastomosis in the orthotopic ileal neobladder: Comparison of 2 techniques. *J Urol.* 1997;157(2):469-471.
36. Kristjansson A, Bajc M, Wallin L, Willner J, Mansson W. Renal function up to 16 years after conduit (refluxing or anti-reflux anastomosis) or continent urinary diversion. 2. Renal scarring and location of bacteriuria. *Br J Urol.* 1995;76(5):546-550.
37. Osman Y, Abol-Enein H, Nabeeh A, Gaballah M, Bazeed M. Long-term results of a prospective randomized study comparing two different antireflux techniques in orthotopic bladder substitution. *Eur Urol.* 2004;45(1):82-86.
38. Studer UE, Danuser H, Thalmann GN, Springer JP, Turner WH. Antireflux nipples or afferent tubular segments in 70 patients with ileal low pressure bladder substitutes: Long-term results of a prospective randomized trial. *J Urol.* 1996;156(6):1913-1917.
39. Wood DP, Jr., Bianco FJ, Jr., Pontes JE, Heath MA, DaJusta D. Incidence and significance of positive urine cultures in patients with an orthotopic neobladder. *J Urol.* 2003;169(6):2196-2199.
40. Yakout H, Bissada NK. Intermediate effects of the ileocaecal urinary reservoir (charleston pouch 1) on serum vitamin b12 concentrations: Can vitamin b12 deficiency be prevented? *BJU Int.* 2003;91(7):653-655; discussion 655-656.
41. Pfitzenmaier J, Lotz J, Faldum A, Beringer M, Stein R, Thuroff JW. Metabolic evaluation of 94 patients 5 to 16 years after ileocecal pouch (mainz pouch 1) continent urinary diversion. *J Urol.* 2003;170(5):1884-1887.
42. Alcini E, D'Addessi A, Racioppi M, et al. Results of 4 years of experience with bladder replacement using an ileocecal segment with multiple transverse teniamyotomies. *J Urol.* 1993;149(4):735-738.
43. Bettice JA, Gamble JL, Jr. Skeletal buffering of acute metabolic acidosis. *Am J Physiol.* 1975;229(6):1618-1624.
44. McDougal WS, Koch MO, Shands C, 3rd, Price RR. Bony demineralization following urinary intestinal diversion. *J Urol.* 1988;140(4):853-855.
45. Lee SW, Russell J, Avioli LV. 25-hydroxycholecalciferol to 1,25-dihydroxycholecalciferol: Conversion impaired by systemic metabolic acidosis. *Science.* 1977;195(4282):994-996.
46. Arnett TR, Dempster DW. Effect of ph on bone resorption by rat osteoclasts in vitro. *Endocrinology.* 1986;119(1):119-124.
47. Mundy AR, Nurse DE. Calcium balance, growth and skeletal mineralisation in patients with cystoplasties. *Br J Urol.* 1992;69(3):257-259.
48. Hossain M. The osteomalacia syndrome after colocystoplasty; a cure with sodium bicarbonate alone. *Br J Urol.* 1970;42(2):243-245.
49. Siklos P, Davie M, Jung RT, Chalmers TM. Osteomalacia in ureterosigmoidostomy: Healing by correction of the acidosis. *Br J Urol.* 1980;52(1):61-62.
50. Perry W, Allen LN, Stamp TC, Walker PG. Vitamin d resistance in osteomalacia after ureterosigmoidostomy. *N Engl J Med.* 1977;297(20):1110-1112.
51. Terai A, Arai Y, Kawakita M, Okada Y, Yoshida O. Effect of urinary intestinal diversion on urinary risk factors for urolithiasis. *J Urol.* 1995;153(1):37-41.
52. Kulaksizoglu H, Toktas G, Kulaksizoglu IB, Aglamis E, Unluer E. When should quality of life be measured after radical cystectomy? *Eur Urol.* 2002;42(4):350-355.
53. Hardt J, Filipas D, Hohenfellner R, Egle UT. Quality of life in patients with bladder carcinoma after cystectomy: First results of a prospective study. *Qual Life Res.* 2000;9(1):1-12.

54. Henningsohn L, Wijkstrom H, Steven K, et al. Relative importance of sources of symptom-induced distress in urinary bladder cancer survivors. *Eur Urol.* 2003;43(6):651-662.
55. McGuire MS, Grimaldi G, Grotas J, Russo P. The type of urinary diversion after radical cystectomy significantly impacts on the patient's quality of life. *Ann Surg Oncol.* 2000;7(1):4-8.
56. Gill IS, Kaouk JH, Meraney AM, et al. Laparoscopic radical cystectomy and continent orthotopic ileal neobladder performed completely intracorporeally: The initial experience. *J Urol.* 2002;168(1):13-18.
57. Abreu SC, Fonseca GN, Cerqueira JB, Nobrega MS, Costa MR, Machado PC. Laparoscopic radical cystectomy with intracorporeally constructed y-shaped orthotopic ileal neobladder using nonabsorbable titanium staples exclusively. *Urology.* 2005;66(3):657.

Chapter 13. Bladder and Ureteral Substitution and Augmentation

Luis M. Chiva, MD, PhD,
Fernando Lapuente, MD,
Sonsoles Alonso, MD, and
Matias Jurado, MD, PhD

Iatrogenic harm to the urinary tract can be caused by any surgeon operating in or around the pelvis and the retroperitoneal abdominal space, with an overall incidence of 0.3% to 1.5%.[1] This applies to gynecologists, general surgeons, urologists, vascular surgeons, neurosurgeons, and orthopedic surgeons.

The anatomy of the lower urinary tract and its close connection with gynecologic organs makes it vulnerable to be affected by gynecologic tumors, adjuvant local treatment such as pelvic radiation, and surgical injuries at the time of dissection. More specifically, gynecologic oncologists have to often deal with a surgical scenario that includes urinary tract involvement by tumor, inflammation and, or fibrosis. It is not rare that, during the resection of a gynecologic tumor, a decision has to be made regarding whether or not to remove a portion of the ureter, bladder, or both. Furthermore, most pelvic exenterative procedures are performed in patients who have received high doses of pelvic radiation. Typically, in such situations, total cystectomy must be performed to accomplish complete tumor removal.

The goal of this chapter is to explain the general principles and different surgical tools that a trained gynecologic oncologist has to master in order to reconstruct the urinary tract when needed. Continent and incontinent reservoirs are discussed in Chapters 11 and 12 of this book. In this chapter we will discuss the surgical procedures utilized to reconstruct the ureter as well as to enlarge or substitute for the urinary bladder after any surgical injury or after a radical resection.

URETERAL SUBSTITUTION AND REPAIR

Background

The urinary tract is particularly susceptible to intraoperative injury for a variety of reasons. Operating in difficult situations, such as that encountered with surgery for recurrent malignancy, extensive inflammation and bulky tumors, places the urinary tract at even greater risk. Injuries to the ureter are the most common urinary tract injuries, because the ureter is similar in appearance to vascular structures, is difficult to identify as a result of its close adherence to the posterior peritoneum, and can be encountered at virtually any level in the retroperitoneum and upper pelvis. When these facts are studied, along with the intrinsic difficulties with the occasional unforeseen congenital anomalies, such as ureteral duplication or retrocaval ureter, it is easy to understand how easily ureteral injury can occur. Consequently, it is essential that each surgeon operating in this region be familiar with the specific anatomy of this structure.

Ureteral injury is most commonly iatrogenic in origin. Urological surgeons are the group most frequently causing ureteric injuries particularly with the use of rigid and flexible ureteroscopy. The ureter is at greatest risk for injury from ureteroscopy at the ureterovesical junction, pelviureteric junction, and the pelvic brim. Most injuries are limited to the mucosa and easily managed by the insertion of a ureteral stent.[2]

The majority of significant operative ureteric injuries occur during hysterectomy procedures by gynecologists.[3] Risk factors include:

a. Gynecologic malignancy
b. Endometriosis
c. Pelvic inflammatory disease
d. Pelvic organ prolapse
e. Previous pelvic surgery

The injury usually occurs where the ureter crosses inferior to the uterine artery and may be due to transection, suture ligation, or thermal damage. Unrecognized injury occurs in up to 80% of cases. Low anterior resection and abdominoperineal resection of the colon are the most common general surgical procedures associated with ureteric injuries. The left ureter is more commonly damaged than the right due to the relation with the sigmoid mesentery. Vascular bypass surgery, mainly aortoiliac and aortofemoral, can result in injury to the mid and distal third of the ureter. Devascularization during surgery is a cause of late stricture. Finally, it is fair to conclude that gynecologic oncologic procedures notably increase the risk of ureteral damage.[1-3]

Ureteral reconstruction aims to preserve renal function and ensure urinary continuity. This is achieved using similar principles of reconstruction as applied to other organs. These include ensuring good vascular supply, complete excision of pathologic lesions, good drainage, and a wide spatulated and tension-free anastomosis of mucosa to mucosa. The availability of another ureter and the similar transitional epithelial lining of the ureters and bladder allows for various functional options for reconstruction.

Indications and Clinical Applications

1. Iatrogenic ureteric injuries

Iatrogenic injuries occur typically during pelvic surgery and therefore the injury is predominantly to the distal ureter. The best outcomes are obtained when the injury is recognized and dealt with at the time of surgery. Unfortunately, unrecognized injury is common resulting in delayed presentation and diagnosis. Excessive fluid drainage from operatively placed drains, fever, nausea, vomiting, and flank pain due to infection, urinoma, fistula formation, or ureteric obstruction are all worrisome signs of late presentation. A high index of suspicion is necessary to avoid missing the injury. The measurement of creatinine on fluid from drains is a rapid and accurate way of confirming the absence or presence of postoperative urinary leakage.[4]

From a surgical perspective, the ureter is divided into the abdominal and pelvic portions. The renal pelvis is the upper border of the abdominal ureter and the iliac vessels are the inferior border. The pelvic ureter extends from the iliac vessels to the bladder. A total of 80% of all gynecologic-related ureteral injuries occur below the pelvic brim.

Many ureteral injuries can be repaired endoscopically with a combination of internaureteral stenting and percutaneous nephrostomy tube drainage.[5] For the rest, a variety of open and laparoscopic surgical techniques have been utilized, depending on the level of injury.

Evaluation depends mainly on the surgical approach and time of presentation. If the abdomen is open, then mobilization and direct inspection of both ureters in the area of suspected injury is recommended. If direct inspection is not possible, then retrograde pyelography is very sensitive for identifying the injury and will allow stenting if possible. If the presentation is delayed, then an intravenous pyelogram or a computed tomography (CT) urography is recommended to identify the location and number of injuries. Any drain fluid should be sent for analysis for creatinine to confirm the presence of urine.

Operative repair of ureteral injuries requires meticulous techniques and should be performed at the time of the injury when is recognized. Minimizing ureteral trauma and preservation of adequate blood supply are essential steps for a successful outcome. The ureter should be handled gently to avoid ischemia.

The ureter should be mobilized with a generous amount of periureteral tissue to preserve its collateral circulation. The level of ureteral injury dictates the type of surgical repair feasible for a successful outcome. Although a midureteral injury can be repaired with ureteroureterostomy, a distal ureteral injury should not be reconstructed in this fashion, as the distal ureteral stump will be at risk for being devascularized.[6]

2. Planned oncologic ureteral resections

The same principles of repair apply when an indicated oncological resection of the ureter has to be carried out. In these circumstances a preoperative plan for the repair should be considered in advance. In these cases, patients must be informed preoperatively of the nature of the reconstructive procedure and the potential negative outcomes.

Anatomic Considerations

The ureters, approximately 25 cm long, descend from the renal pelvis to the bladder along the anterior surface of the psoas muscle in the retroperitoneum. In the posterior aspect of the peritoneal cavity, the colonic mesentery rests anteriorly and gonadal vessels lie medial to the ureters. At the pelvic brim, the gonadal vessels cross the ureter at the level of the division of the common iliac vessels. The ureters course over the division of the common iliac vessels from lateral to medial running medial to the internal iliac vessels and turning further medially to enter the posterior wall of the bladder. In the pelvis the ureter passes under the vas deferens in the male, and under the uterine artery in the female (Figures 13-1 and 13-2).

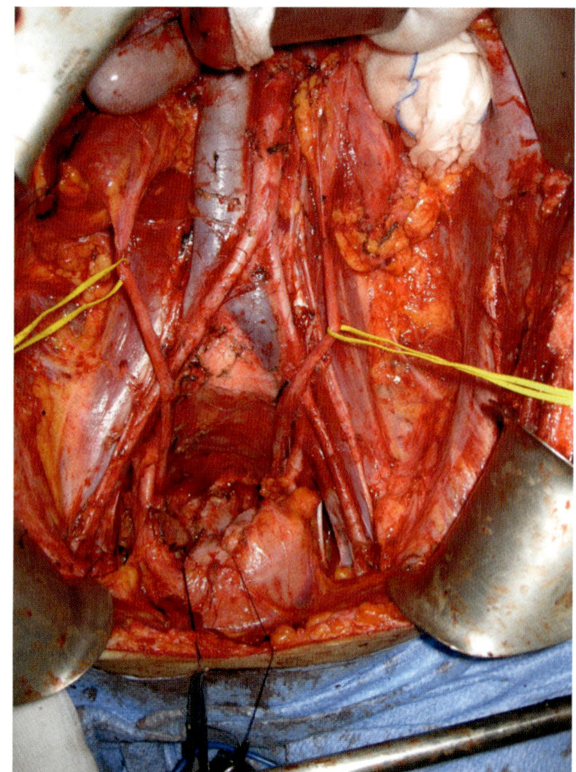

Fig. 13-1. Retroperitoneal course of the upper ureter. (Reproduced with permission from Luis Chiva.)

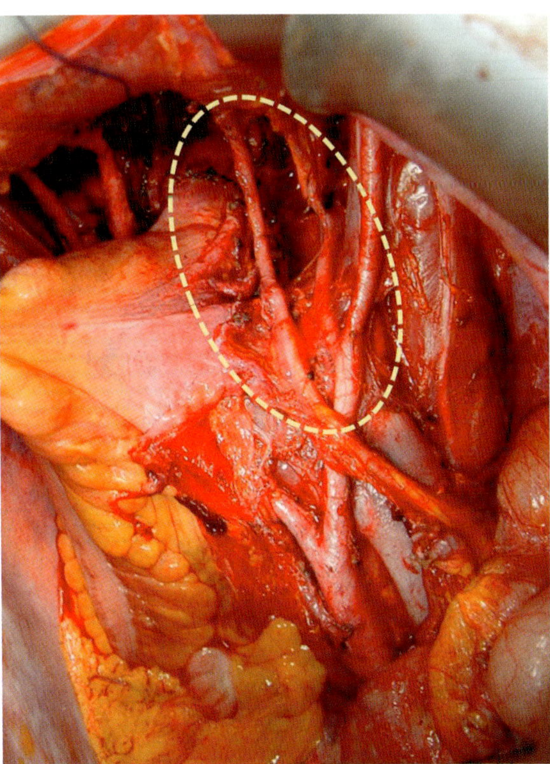

Fig. 13-2. Retroperitoneal course of the lower ureter. (Reproduced with permission from Luis Chiva.)

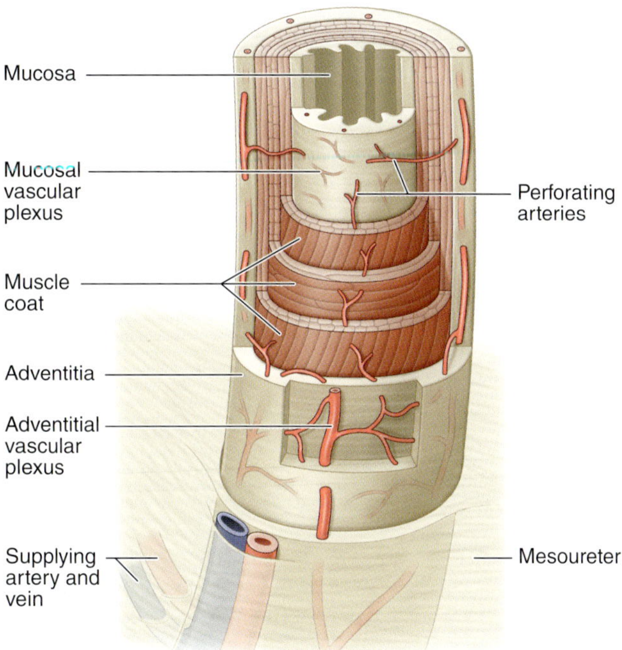

Fig. 13-3. Vascular network of the ureteric wall distributed from the adventitia. 1. Mucosa. 2. Muscle coat. 3. Adventitia. 4. Mesoureter. 5. Supplying artery and vein. 6. Adventitial vascular plexus. 7. Perforating arteries. 8. Mucosal vascular plexus. (Adapted with permission from Stephan Spitzer, Medical Illustrator.)

The blood supply to the ureter comes from the renal artery, gonadal artery, lumbar arteries, and aorta proximally and the internal iliac artery and its branches distally. A delicate network of sub-adventitial vessels supplies the whole course of the ureter (Figure 13-3).

The lumen of the ureter is coated with urothelium, an epithelium lying on the lamina propria. This mucous membrane contains a finely entwined mucosal vascular plexus. The muscle layer, responsible for the bilateral alternating peristaltic movements of the ureter, consists primarily of twisted arranged smooth muscle bundles. In cross section, the bundles form 2 muscle layers joined by connective tissue. The inner layer is longitudinal in arrangement, and in the outer layer the muscle bundles are ordered circularly (Figure 13-4). Near the bladder the intrinsic musculature is separated from a third layer, the muscular layer of Waldeyer; it consists of longitudinally arranged muscle bundles, which emerge from the bladder wall into the ureter. The connective tissue of the adventitia, the ureteric cover, contains the adventitial vascular plexus responsible for supplying the ureteral wall. It is divided into an outer and an inner vascular network. The inner network is characterized by a dense complex of vessels, with small perforating arteries running superficially and obliquely through the intrinsic musculature and continuing to the mucosal vascular plexus. The outer network, which is reticulated, contains longitudinal vessels with multiple anastomoses. It is a crucial point that the adventitial vascular network allows the ureter to be extensively mobilized without ischemia if the vascular supply is preserved.[7] To illustrate this concept, one can consider how the ureter is completely isolated from its vascular vessels at the time of a conventional renal transplant.

Preoperative Preparation

Box 13-1 KEY SURGICAL INSTRUMENTATION

- Basic table-fixed retractor
- Basic laparotomy set
- Magnification system if needed
- DeBakey atraumatic vascular tissue forceps
- Pott scissors
- Thin vascular needle holders
- 6-8 F double-J stents
- Sensor tip guidewire
- 3-lumen Foley catheter will comfortably fit the urethra after calibration
- 5/0, 3/0, and 2/0 absorbable polidaxone or monofilament sutures
- Soft suction drain

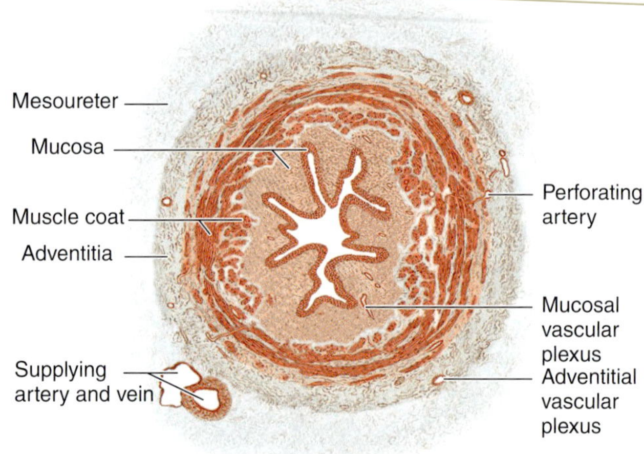

Fig. 13-4. Anatomic section of the ureter. 1. Mucosa. 2. Muscle coat. 3. Adventitia. 4. Mesoureter. 5. Supplying artery and vein. 6. Adventitial vascular plexus. 7. Perforating arteries. 8. Mucosal vascular plexus. (Adapted with permission from Stephan Spitzer, Medical Illustrator.)

Any patient being prepared for a surgical resection with suspected involvement of the ureter on CT or magnetic resonance imaging should have a cystoscopy performed. The patient should be informed in detail about the findings and the possible outcomes during and after surgery, including the various options for ureteric stenting, reconstruction, or both. Written informed consent should be obtained that includes the different surgical options available and the specific procedure preferred by the patient, their drawbacks and limitations, and typical complications before and after surgery. We consider bowel preparation a necessity for all patients possibly undergoing ileal or colon surgery in order to reduce the incidence of complications like fistula formation or infection. After 1 day on a low-residue diet, the patient drinks a bowel-cleansing solution until clear stools are obtained. We do not use oral antibiotics, but strongly advocate intravenous antibiotics during and after surgery (gentamicin plus metronidazole) for 3 days.

Surgical Procedures

After assessing the injury or the length of resection, repair should be based on the extent and location of the injury, the patient's overall status and associated injuries. In the unstable patient, a more conservative approach, such as ureteric ligation and nephrostomy drainage may be most appropriate. Concomitant bowel injuries are not a contraindication to ureteral reconstruction. Endourological techniques, either antegrade or retrograde, may be able to bridge partial or minor defects with a stent.

Most ureteric injuries are short transections and can be repaired with debridement and ureteroureterostomy in the proximal and midureter or with ureteroneocystostomy in the distal ureter. The psoas hitch is a very useful adjunct to creating a tension-free repair in distal ureteric reconstructions.

The principles of ureteral repair are:

1. Mobilization of the ureter preserving the adventitia.
2. Debridement of nonviable tissue.
3. Spatulation and a tension-free anastomosis with absorbable sutures.
4. An internal stent and separate retroperitoneal drain.
5. Omental interposition to separate the repair from associated intra-abdominal injuries or suture lines is recommended.

The different surgical options to achieve these basic principles are outlined in Tables 13-1 and 13-2. More than 1 technique may be used if necessary.

Table 13-1. Surgical procedures to manage upper ureter injuries.

Location	Technique
Proximal ureter	Ureteroureterostomy
	Transureteroureterostomy
	Ileal interposition
	Renal autotransplantations

Reconstructive Procedures on the Upper Ureter

1. Ureteroureterostomy

Primary anastomosis of ureteral injuries is feasible when the defect is short. Injuries to the upper and middle ureter are ideal for primary ureteroureterostomy. In cases of necrosis or thermal damage, the ureter should be débrided to viable tissue. As much periureteral tissue as possible should be left attached to the ureter during dissection to preserve ureteral blood supply. Both ends of the divided ureter are spatulated on opposite sides for 1 cm. Spatulation may not be essential in cases where the ureters are dilated. Sutures of 5:0 polydioxanone (PDS) or polyglactin on an avascular atraumatic needle are inserted from the apex of one ureter to the corner of spatulation of the other ureter. A watertight anastomosis of the ureteral wall is then accomplished using either interrupted or running sutures of 5:0. A total of 6 to 8 sutures are usually

Table 13-2. Surgical procedures to manage lower ureter injuries.

Location	Technique
Distal ureter	Ureteroureterostomy (refluxing or tunnelled)
	Psoas hitch
	Boari flap

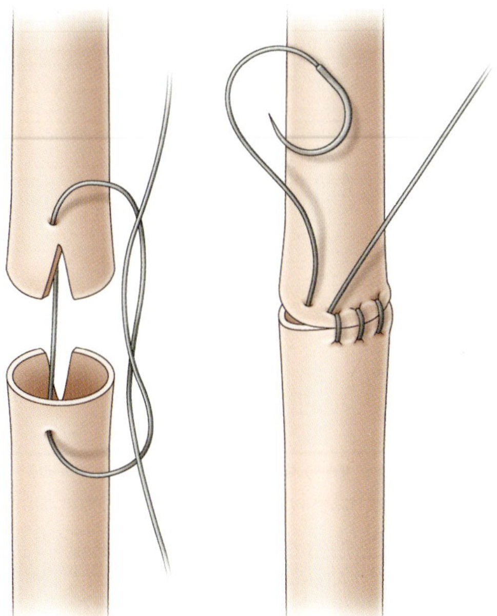

Fig. 13-5. Spatulation and repair of the defect by ureteroureterostomy.

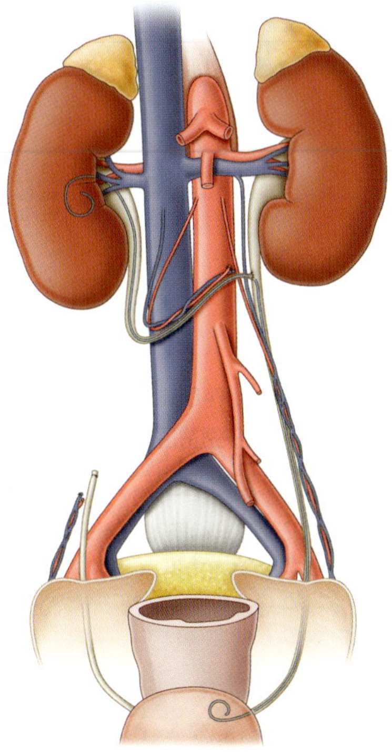

Fig. 13-6. Final surgical view after transureteroureterostomy. (Adapted with permission from Stephan Spitzer, Medical Illustrator.)

sufficient. A double-J stent is inserted after completion of one side of the ureteral anastomosis. In cases of concomitant abdominal surgery, the greater omentum can be mobilized and wrapped around the ureteral anastomosis. A surgical drain is elective and is removed postoperatively when drainage disappears. The double-J stent is removed in 4 to 8 weeks (Figure 13-5).

2. Transureteroureterostomy

There are certain conditions that might exclude the accomplishment of a traditional ureteric reconstruction. For example, extensive resection of a tumor-infiltrated ureter may be necessary in order to maintain curative intent.[8] In such cases, techniques such as the psoas hitch or the Boari flap might be impossible due to thickening of the bladder wall, for example, after previous radiation treatment. One can argue that this would be an ideal case for an ileal ureteral replacement; however, prior radiation or concomitant inflammatory bowel disease may make this reconstructive strategy unattractive as well. In these cases, transureteroureterostomy may be contemplated.[9] The use of this technique was popularized in the 1960s; however, significant adverse effects have been reported. In subsequent years, there has been a clear reluctance among reconstructive surgeons to perform this technique, which could endanger both renal units (Figure 13-6).

3. Ileal interposition

Since its first description in 1906 by Shoemaker and later popularization by Goodwin et al in the late 1950s, the use of ileal segments for ureteral replacement have become a valued procedure when reconstructing the ureter. Although it was initially described for tuberculosis ureteral obstruction, more recently the indications for its use have broadened. The main advantage of reconstructing the ureter with ileum is the long-term avoidance of nephrostomy tubes, ureteral stents, and nephrectomy.[10] Furthermore, the ileal ureter requires no external devices, preserves renal function, and has the advantage of using an uncompromised blood supply in irradiated cases. In cases of total ureteral avulsion or when a long segment is unhealthy or damaged, a segment of ileum can be used to reconstruct the urinary system. Candidates for this operation should have relatively normal kidney function.[11] An ileal segment 20 to 25 cm in length is mobilized 15 to 20 cm in length proximal to the ileocecal valve. Bowel continuity is re-established. The isolated ileal segment is then positioned posteriorly in an isoperistaltic fashion. An end-to-end anastomosis between the renal pelvis and the proximal ileal segment is done using running or interrupted 3:0 PDS or polyglactin sutures. If the proximal ureteral segment is healthy, then anastomosis can be performed between the ureter and the ileal segment in an end-side fashion using interrupted 4:0 PDS or polyglactin suture. A double-J stent is inserted in the ureter prior to completion of the anastomosis. Distally the ileal segment is anastomosed to the posterior wall of the bladder. The bladder is mobilized and an anterior cystotomy is done. An end-side ileovesical anastomosis is done on the posterior bladder wall. A circular opening on the posterior bladder wall is removed and the ileum tunneled through the defect. The anastomosis is then done in 2 layers. The inner layer of interrupted or continuous 3:0 reabsorbable sutures inserted through the full thickness of bladder and ileum from within the bladder (through the anterior cystotomy). An outer strengthening layer of interrupted seromuscular sutures is then placed from outside the bladder. The anterior cystotomy is then closed in 1 or 2 layers. Alternatively, the anastomosis between the distal ileal segment and the bladder can be done in the anterior bladder wall. A direct one layer, nontunneled anastomosis with interrupted or continuous 3:0 reabsorbable sutures is placed circumferentially. A large Foley or suprapubic catheter is inserted. Drains are inserted close to all anastomotic sites. The Foley catheter, nephrostomy tube, or both are maintained on dependent drainage for at least 1 week. The bladder catheter may need frequent irrigation. A cystogram is obtained 7 to 10 days postoperatively to ensure there is no extravasation (Figures 13-7 and 13-8).

4. The Yang–Monti procedure

The feasibility of constructing a long tube from short segments of ileum was first introduced in 1993 by Yang[12] and later verified and reproduced by Monti[13] in 1997. The basic principle entails isolation of a vascularized segment of ileum 2 to 3 cm in length. An incision on the antimesenteric border will form a rectangular strip. If this strip is folded over its longitudinal axis, then a 6-cm length tube will be created. If more than one ileal ring are joined together, we obtain a tube whose length is 18 cm long (Figure 13-9). A number of authors have reported their experience with remarkable functional outcomes.[14] Furthermore, video radiographic studies have demonstrated that the reconfigured tube is capable of active antegrade propulsion of urine from the renal pelvis down to the bladder. This tailoring of the bowel segment has been suggested to improve the functional outcome of this operation by increasing the propulsion of the urine, limiting the absorptive surface area, and decreasing the formation of mucus. More studies are needed to recommend this surgical operation as a standard reconstructive approach in these cases.

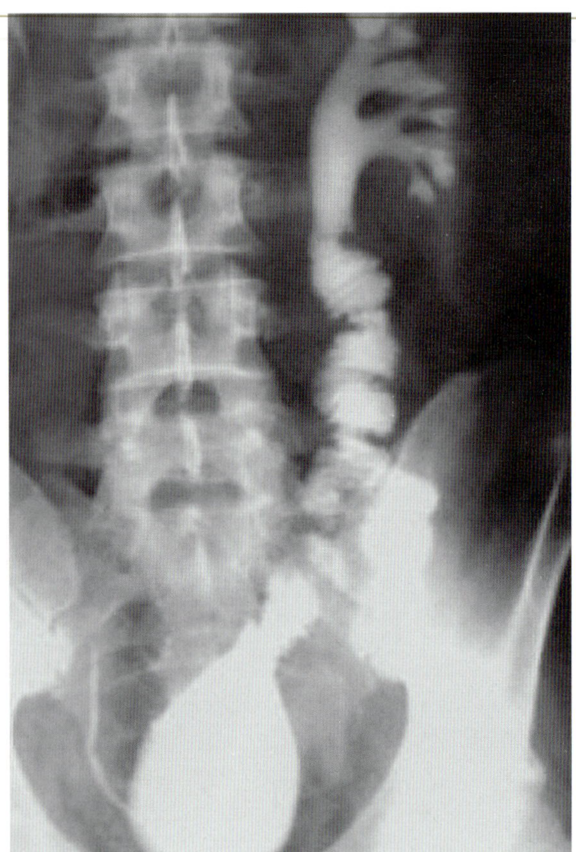

Fig. 13-8. Urography showing a left ileal interposition.

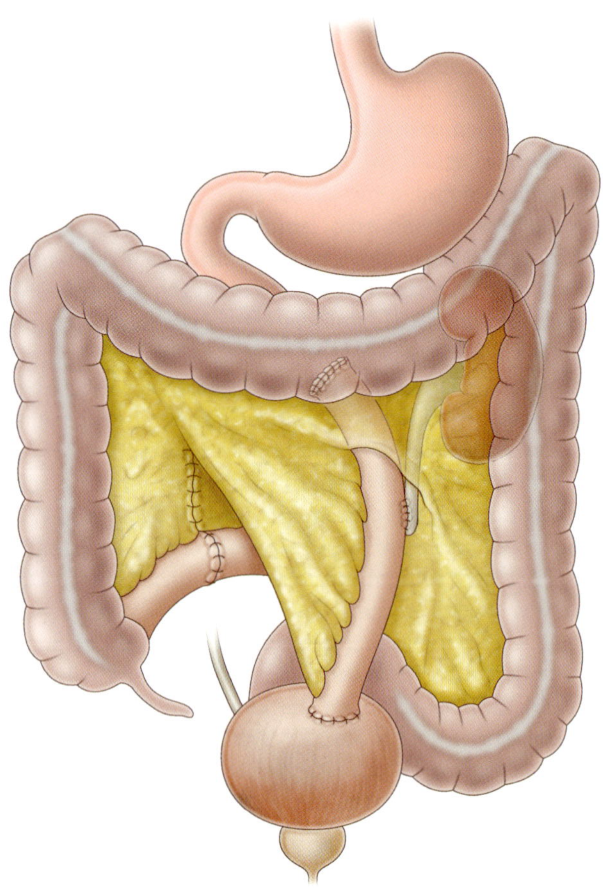

Fig. 13-7. Schema showing the ileal interposition. (Adapted with permission from Robert J. Stein, Glickman Urological and Kidney Institute, Cleveland Clinic.)

5. Renal mobilization

In specific circumstances, surgical mobilization of the kidney from its neighboring tissue allows the surgeon to gain up to 3 cm which may allow for a tension-free anastomosis. In these cases, special attention must be paid to avoid torsion of the renal pedicle.

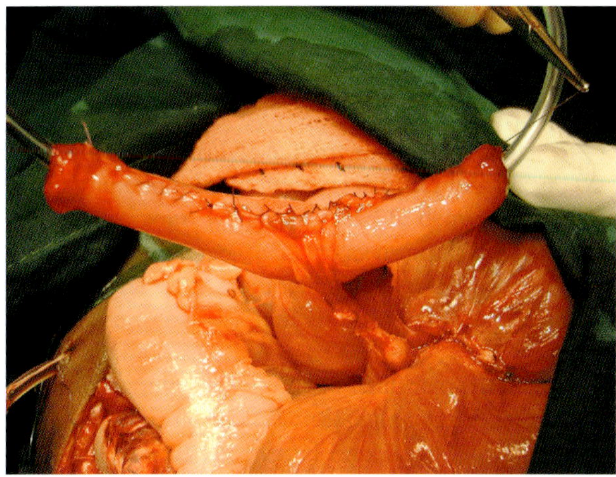

Fig. 13-9. Development of a ileal ureter following the Yang-Monti procedure. (Reproduced with permission from Abu Obaidah, MS.)

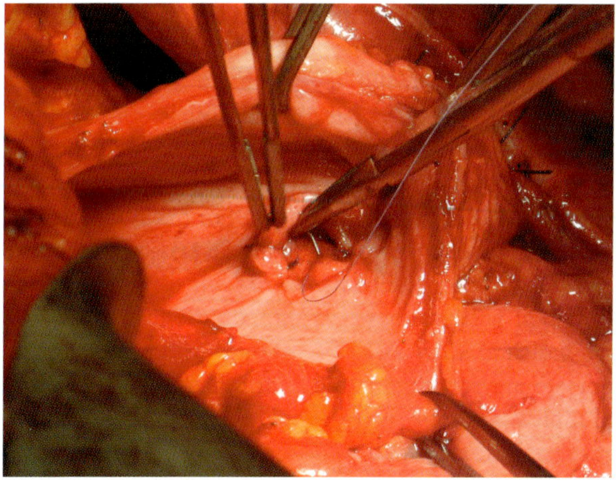

Fig. 13-10. Suturing the ureter to the bladder at the time of ureteroneocystostomy.

6. Renal autotransplantation

Renal autotransplantation is an alternative to ureteral interposition in cases of complete ureteral avulsion or a long diseased ureteral segment. Renal autotransplantation is best reserved for patients with solitary kidney or compromised renal function.[15]

Reconstructive Procedures on the Lower Ureter

1. Ureteroneocystostomy

Ureteroneocystostomy is best utilized for injuries involving the distal 3 to 4 cm of the ureter.[16] The ureter is mobilized with generous periureteral tissue. The ureter is spatulated and anastomosed to the bladder in an anterior extravesical or intravesical technique. Following the extravesical technique, the bladder musculature is cut, exposing the bladder mucosa over the entire length of the incision. A 1-cm circle of bladder mucosa is removed. The ureter is anastomosed to the bladder using continuous or interrupted 5:0 PDS sutures approximating full thickness of the ureteral wall to the bladder mucosa. A double-J stent is inserted prior to the conclusion of the anastomosis. The bladder muscle is then closed on top of the ureter using interrupted 3:0 absorbable sutures to accomplish an antireflux mechanism. Care should be taken to avoid stricture of the ureter. Otherwise, an intravesical technique can be used. The bladder is opened through an anterior cystotomy. An incision is made on the mucosa in the posterolateral aspect of the bladder. A submucosal tunnel of 2 cm in length is developed. At the end of the tunnel, the bladder wall is perforated and the ureter is taken across the incision under the submucosal tunnel.[17]

The ureter that was spatulated is now anastomosed to the bladder with 6 to 8 interrupted 4:0 or 5:0 absorbable sutures. The distal sutures are inserted deeply into the muscularis, and the remaining sutures are placed only through the bladder mucosa. The cystotomy incision is closed in 2 separate layers (Figures 13-10 to 13-12).

2. Psoas hitch

When the distal ureteral injury is more proximal but still below the pelvic entrance, a psoas bladder hitch can be used to mobilize the bladder more proximal to allow the completion of an ureteroneocystostomy.[11] A psoas hitch can provide an additional 5 cm of length as compared with ureteroneocystostomy alone. A preoperative cystogram is helpful but not mandatory in assessing bladder anatomy. The space of

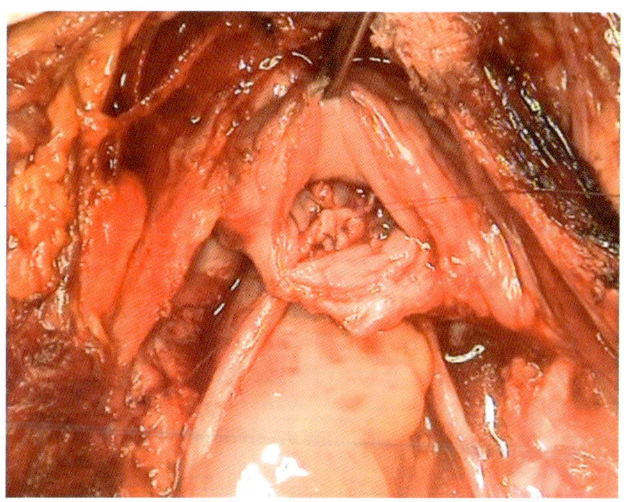

Fig. 13-11. Bilateral ureteroneocystostomy after an ovarian cancer debulking.

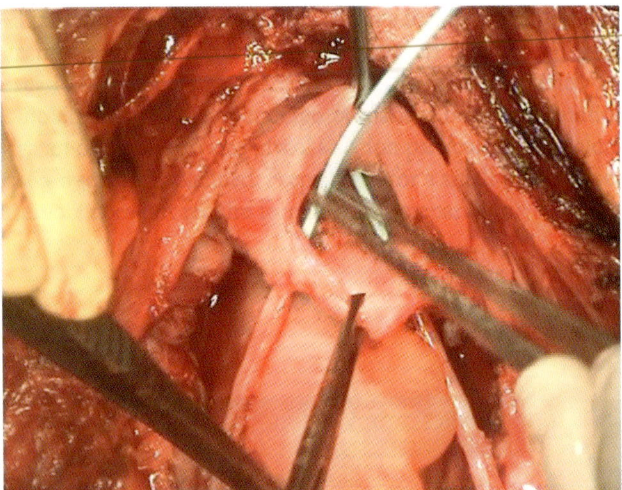

Fig. 13-12. Ureteroneocystostomy. The left stent is placed after finishing both ureteral anastomoses to the bladder.

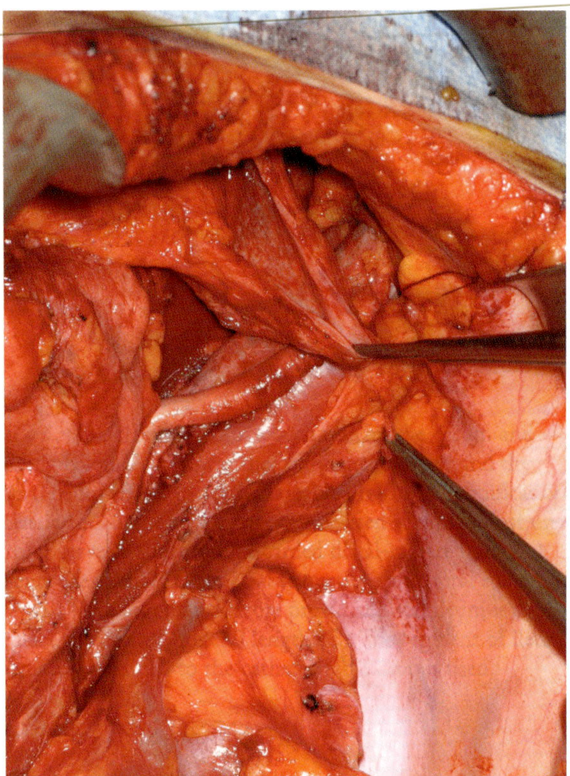

Fig. 13-13. Psoas hitch. The bladder has been mobilized and it is approximated ton right psoas muscle.

Retzius and both paravesical spaces are developed and the bladder is extensively mobilized. The dome of the ipsilateral bladder should be able to reach superior to the iliac vessels. The contralateral superior vesicle artery can be divided to gain more mobility. The ureter is dissected, cut back to healthy tissue and spatulated. The bladder is opened with a parallel incision to the psoas muscle on the side toward the mobilization is planned. The ipsilateral roof is sutured to the lateral psoas muscle using several interrupted sutures of 2:0 polydioxanone. Sutures are placed through the full thickness of the posterolateral bladder wall to the psoas muscle. Care should be taken to avoid injury to either the genitofemoral or the femoral nerve that rest beneath the psoas muscle. The ureter is anastomosed to the superolateral aspect of the bladder dome with or without a submucosal tunnel using interrupted of 5:0 or 4:0 absorbable sutures. A double-J stent is inserted. The bladder is then closed in 2 layers (Figures 13-13 to 13-18).

3. Boari flap

Injuries to the mid to low ureter with large defects not amenable for primary ureteroureterostomy can be repaired with an anterior bladder wall flap as described by Boari.[18,19] A ureteral defect 10 to 15 cm in length can be joined with this technique (Figure 13-19). Using this technique and the development of curved flaps, it is possible to reach the renal pelvis. Generally, Boari flaps are most successful when the injury is below the level of the common iliac artery. A small, irradiated bladder is a contraindication for a Boari flap. Bladder capacity and anatomy need to be assessed with a preoperative cystogram. The bladder, again, is mobilized from its peritoneal attachment as in the psoas hitch procedure. Special care must be taken to avoid unnoticed damage to the ipsilateral superior vesical artery. A U-shaped full-thickness bladder wall flap is usually developed. The length of the flap depends upon the distance between the posterior lateral bladder wall and the distal ureter. If a longer segment is needed, the flap can be shaped into an L shape by extending the tip laterally at the anterior bladder wall. The base of the flap should be at least 2 cm wider than the top to ensure good blood supply.

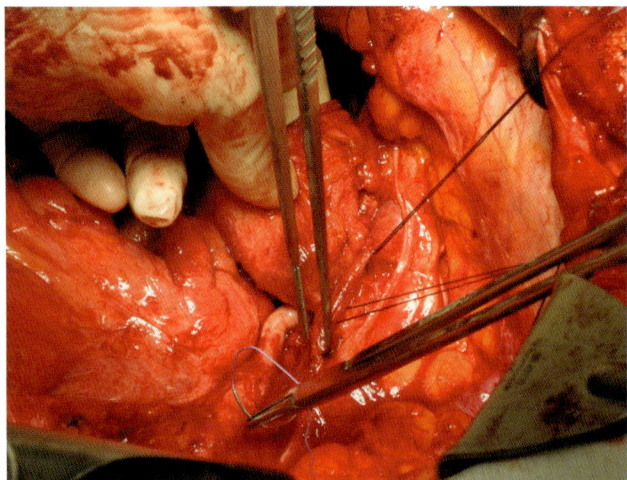

Fig. 13-14. Psoas hitch. The bladder is sutured to the muscle by 3 interrupted stitches but avoiding the bladder mucosa yet noting that the femoral nerve runs just beneath the psoas muscle.

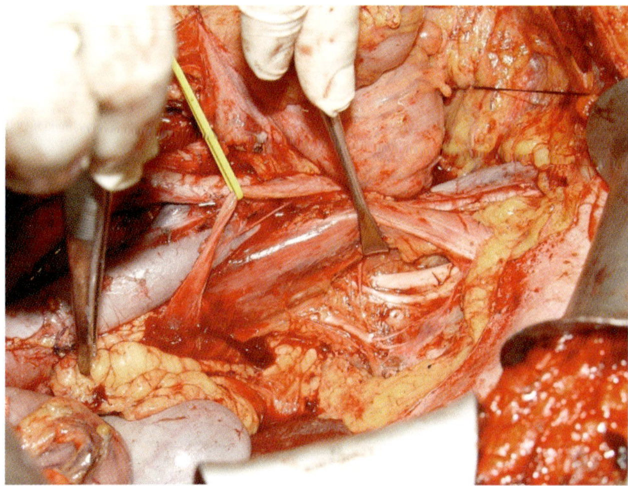

Fig. 13-15. Psoas hitch. The picture shows the anatomic relationship between the psoas muscle and the femoral nerve. A retractor is elevating the external aspect of the right psoas muscle.

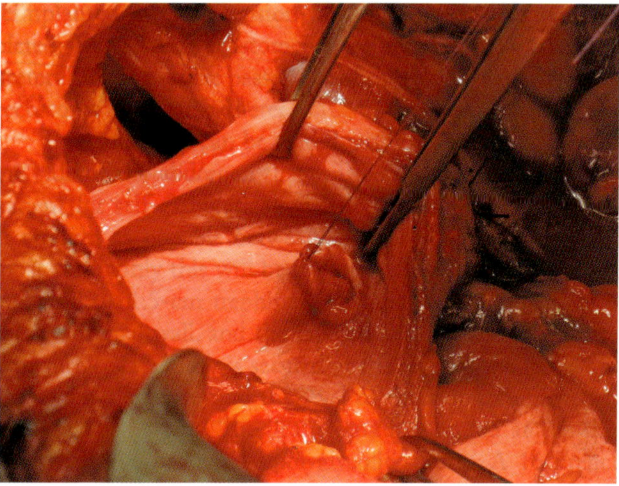

Fig. 13-17. Psoas hitch. When anastomosing the ureter, we usually use 5-0 absorbable interrupted sutures and 6 stitches between the full thickness of the ureteral wall and the mucosa of the bladder.

The width of the flap should be 3 to 4 times the diameter of the ureter. The vertex of the flap is secured to the psoas muscle with interrupted absorbable sutures. The spatulated ureter is subsequently anastomosed to the bladder flap in direct fashion or via a submucosal tunnel. Anastomosis avoiding any tension is performed with interrupted absorbable sutures of 4:0 chromic or 5:0 absorbable sutures. The flap is sutured and rolled into a tube using two layers of absorbable sutures. A double-J stent is inserted prior to bladder closure. A drain is placed. The Foley catheter remains for 7 to 10 days. A cystogram is performed prior to removal of the Foley catheter. The stent is removed in 4 to 8 weeks (see Figure 13-18).

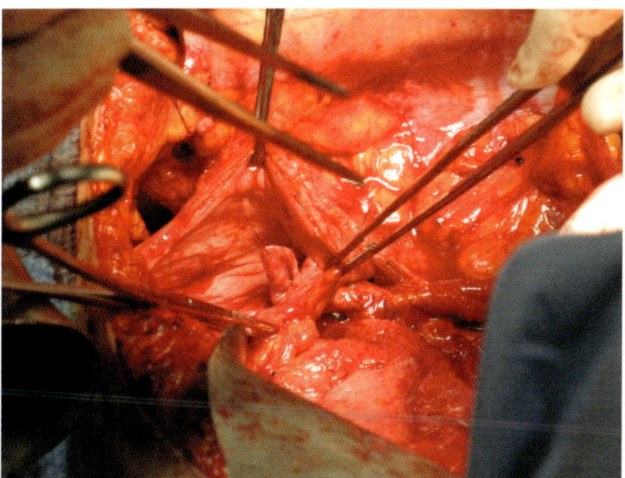

Fig. 13-16. Psoas hitch. After spatulating the ureter, it is passed through the bladder wall directly or using a submucosal antireflux tunnel.

Postoperative Care

Box 13-2 MASTER SURGEON'S PRINCIPLES

1. Mobilize the ureter preserving the adventitia
2. Remove all nonviable tissue
3. Perform ureteral spatulation and a tension-free anastomosis with absorbable sutures
4. **Never underestimate the need of stenting a ureter. Wide is better than narrow**
5. Leave a soft suction drain close to the repaired area
6. Consider an omental interposition to separate the repair from associated intra-abdominal injuries or suture lines

After the procedure the care must be taken to avoid the obstruction of the Foley catheter. In nonirradiated patients, remove the Foley catheter after 10 to 14 days. A cystogram is performed prior to removal of the Foley catheter to confirm the bladder has healed and there is no leak. Special attention must be taken to the drains close to the bladder. If there is any suspicious leakage, then a creatinine level can be measured in the drainage fluid to confirm assess for a urinary leak and a cystogram must be ordered. The ureteral stents usually are removed 2 months after the procedure.

Long-term Outcomes

Box 13-3 PERIOPERATIVE MORBIDITY

1. Bladder fistula
2. Wound infection

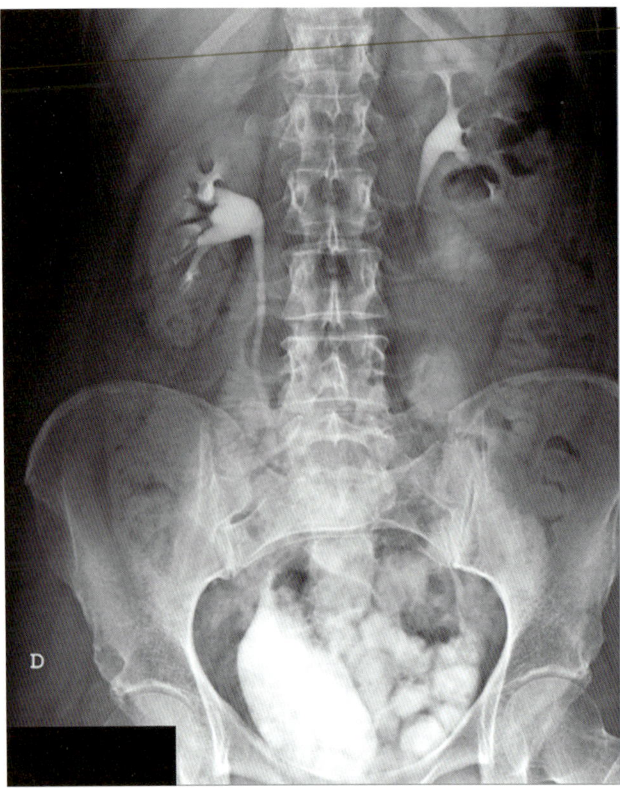

Fig. 13-18. Psoas hitch. Image showing the urocytogram after the surgical procedure.

3. Small bowel obstruction
4. Bleeding requiring reoperation

Reconstruction of ureteral injuries is generally successful in experienced hands; however, the evidence base is limited. The incidence of complications after the repair of the iatrogenically injured ureter has not been reported.

Minimally Invasive Surgical Applications

During the last few years there has been a growing interest in the literature regarding the feasibility and success of laparoscopic approaches to ureteral reconstruction at the time of early and delayed diagnosis of ureteral injuries.[20] Furthermore, there are many articles reporting successful ureteral reconstructive procedures with robotics.[21] Although the instrumentation may differ with these minimally invasive approaches, the surgical principles, such as removing nonviable tissue, preserving the adventitia, spatulating the ureters, and performing a tension-free anastomosis, all remain the same.

Summary

The principles and techniques for ureteral reconstruction have remained unaltered throughout the years. Of particular importance are adequate exposure, identification of anatomic landmarks, meticulous dissection, and a tension-free anastomosis. Preventative strategies and a high degree of suspicion are paramount to preventing morbidity. There are certain interesting innovations emerging in this field of reconstructive surgery. Several authors have recently carefully evaluated ureteral replacement with bowel, and the results are relatively impressive. However, complication rates in these recent reports are still appreciably high, perhaps making such reconstructive techniques salvage procedures only to be chosen when more conservative surgical measures, not requiring segments of bowel, have been ruled out.

BLADDER AUGMENTATION

Background

Augmentation cystoplasty is a reconstructive technique for creating a large capacity urinary storage unit to protect the upper urinary tract and to provide urinary continence when more conservative management does not work. The standard enterocystoplasty comprises anastomosing an adequate-sized and well-vascularized patch of bowel with the urinary bladder. Different segments of the digestive tract can be selected from stomach, ileum, cecum, and ascending and sigmoid colon. Nevertheless, no intestinal segment is a perfect physiologic substitute for a natural bladder. All of them have the hypothetical risk of potential complications, including urinary tract

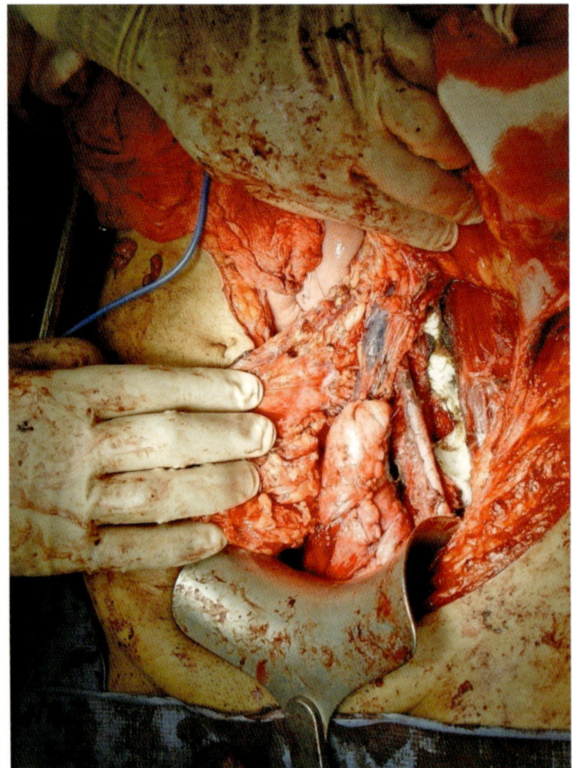

Fig. 13-19. Ureteric reconstruction with a Boari flap.

infection, stone formation, small bowel obstruction, metabolic complications, fistula formation, and more infrequently, tumor cancer tumor growth. The choice of the bowel segment is based on the primary clinical necessities of the patient and the secondary predilection of the surgeons. Recently, among urologists, the laparoscopic approach to bladder augmentation has become the primary approach for bladder augmentation procedures.

In the late 1800s, Tizzoni and Foggi[22] first described augmentation cystoplasty by augmenting the bladder of a dog by anastomosing an ileal loop to the bladder neck. Enterocystoplasty was first performed in humans by von Mikulicz in 1899,[23] and then was popularized by Couvelaire[24] in the 1950s for the treatment of small contracted bladders infected by the Koch bacillus. Bladder augmentation cystoplasty procedures were later introduced as surgical alternatives for cases of refractory detrusor hyperactivity and related urgency incontinence as well as for patients with neurogenic bladder dysfunction resulting from myelomeningocele, bladder exstrophy, spinal cord injury, multiple sclerosis, and myelodysplasia.[25] The introduction of clean intermittent self-catheterization was very helpful in increasing the indications for bladder augmentation techniques for patients incapable of spontaneous voiding. The rationale in augmentation cystoplasty is that by opening a poorly compliant, small capacity bladder and placing an intestinal segment, it is possible to create a bladder with an increased functional capacity and a lower filling pressure. Because bladder augmentation is an invasive procedure that involves discontinuation of the intestinal tract and incorporation of a segment of bowel or ureter into the bladder, it is accompanied by significant associated risks and complications.

Indications and Clinical Applications

In gynecologic oncology, the most common indications for this procedure are radiation cystitis, interstitial cystitis, and in surgical situations that require a partial cystectomy and when it is anticipated that the remaining bladder will be unable to store adequate amounts of urine.

Typical contraindications include intrinsic bowel disease (Crohn disease, congenital anomalies such as cloacal exstrophy, and bowel enteritis), or conditions resulting in short or abnormal bowel, whereby removal of a segment will produce further deleterious effects. Significant renal impairment is a relative contraindication.

Preoperative Preparation. (Same preparation as in ureteral reconstruction)

Box 13-4 KEY SURGICAL INSTRUMENTATION

- Basic table-fixed retractor
- Basic laparotomy set
- Magnification system if needed
- DeBakey 'Atraugrip' vascular tissue forceps
- Allis clamps
- Pott scissors
- Thin vascular needle holders
- 6-8 F double-J stents
- Sensor tip guidewire
- Three-lumen Foley catheter will comfortably fit the urethra after calibration
- 5/0, 3/0, and 2/0 absorbable polidaxone or monofilament sutures
- Soft suction drain

Surgical Procedure

Box 13-5 MASTER SURGEON'S PRINCIPLES

1. Check that the isolated bowel is perfectly viable and easily reaches the bladder
2. Avoid any tension
3. Test the water-tightness of the sutures
4. **Do not underestimate the need for a cystostomy catheter to wash out the mucus**
5. Always leave soft suction drains close to the sutured area
6. Avoid obstruction of the Foley
7. Keep in mind the use of an omental interposition if possible

The most widely used bowel segment for bladder augmentation is a detubularized patch of ileum. Ideally, it is taken 25 to 40 cm from the ileocecal value to reduce the risk of metabolic disorders. Other bowel segments are less commonly used. The sigmoid is generally detubularized as a flat patch or a cup patch, and is the most common alternative to the ileum for an uncomplicated augmentation. The sigmoid has several advantages. Its thick muscular wall, large lumen, and abundant mesentery guarantee adequate bladder capacity. The potential disadvantages are the higher risk of urinary infections and larger amounts of mucus production and a theoretically higher long-term risk of malignancy.

The cecum can be used in its original tubular shape or, more commonly, as a detubularized patch to prevent spontaneous colonic contractions and avoid associated rises in bladder pressure. The cecum is most commonly used in conjunction with the terminal ileum as ileocecocystoplasty. The cecum can be used as detubularized patch with the distal part utilized to anastomose the ureters; if the ileocecal valve is competent, then this might provide an antireflux mechanism. Its mobility permits tension-free ureteral anastomoses; however, the diarrhea and malabsorption associated with resection of the ileo-cecal valve is often significant and most authorities avoid this segment for bladder augmentation if possible.

When bowel is unavailable or inadequate and in those patients with chronic metabolic acidosis, stomach can be used as an alternative to bowel. The advantages include reduced secretion of mucus, reduced infection risk, and reduced malabsorption of electrolytes.

In addition, the stomach secretes hydrochloric acid that has bactericidal properties. Disadvantages include the hematuria-dysuria syndrome in particular; with reports of up to 70% of patients requiring histamine 2 receptor blockers and or hydrogen pump inhibitors to control symptoms. Other problems include peptic ulceration of the bladder, perforation of the gastric segment, hypochloremic hyponatremic alkalosis, and hypergastrinemia. There are also complications associated with partial gastrectomy including early satiety and poor feeding, dumping syndrome, and exacerbation of preexisting peptic ulcer disease or gastroesophageal reflux. With the publication of long-term outcomes of gastrocystoplasty, there is a concerning increase in the incidence of malignancies. The combination of these problems, but particularly the hematuria dysuria syndrome, has reduced the use of the stomach for bladder augmentation.

To carry out the procedure, the bladder is opened with an inverted Y or "Mercedes logo" incision being extended close to the trigone to obtain a large circumference for bowel anastomosis and to avoid a strangulation phenomenon (Figure 13-20).

For ileocystoplasty, approximately 25 to 30 cm of ileum are divided from its bowel continuity where the mesentery can easily reach down to the bladder. An adequately vascularized segment of the ileum should be ensured. The ileal segment is opened adequately at the opposite side of the mesentery after being cleaned with saline. Folding in a U shape and suturing the ileal segment with 3/0 running absorbable sutures forms the ileal plate (Figure 13-21). For cases with a very tiny bladder, a longer ileal segment (45 cm) is divided and may be sutured in an S shape. The ileal patch then is sutured to the open bladder with full thickness 3/0 running absorbable sutures (Figure 13-22).

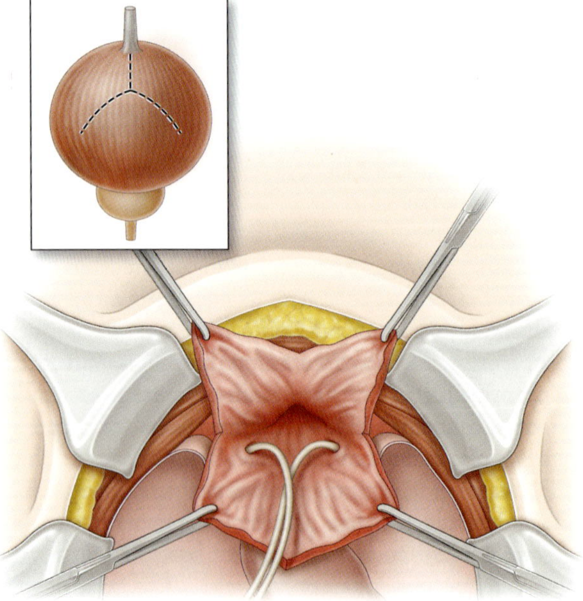

Fig. 13-20. Augmentation enterocystoplasty. Inverted "Y" shape incision is used to open the bladder. (Adapted with permission from Stephan Spitzer, Medical Illustrator.)

Interrupted sutures are placed to reinforce the anastomosis. Suturing starts on each side posterolaterally. Stenting of the ureters is not necessary in enterocystoplasty without ureteric reimplantation. In addition to the transurethral Foley catheter, a suprapubic cystostomy catheter is placed through the anterior bladder wall and fixed to it with a 4/0 rapidly absorbable suture. The cystostomy catheter is placed to irrigate the bladder and wash out the mucus secreted by the intestinal patch. A drain is positioned at the anastomosis site.

Postoperative Care

Box 13-6 PERIOPERATIVE MORBIDITY

1. Bladder fistula
2. Wound infection
3. Small bowel obstruction and leak
4. Bleeding requiring reoperation

The oral-gastric decompression tube is removed before extubation. The pelvic drain is removed when the drainage is less than 25 mL or fluid chemistries suggest peritoneal fluid. Discharge criteria are met when the patient is afebrile and able to eat without abdominal distention or symptoms of nausea and vomiting; the first meal is usually started on the first postoperative day. Patients are discharged with the indwelling urethral catheter used for bladder drainage and daily bladder irrigation with 100 mL of sterile saline. At that time the urinary catheter is removed and intermittent catheterization is initiated.

Long-Term Outcomes

Box 13-7 DELAYED COMPLICATIONS[27] (TABLE 13-3)

1. Voiding dysfunction
2. Malignant transformation
3. Bowel activity/urinary leakage
4. Bowel dysfunction
5. Calculi formation
6. Metabolic disturbance
7. Mucus formation
8. Urinary tract infection

Table 13-3. Most common complications related to the gastrointestinal segments used for bladder augmentation.

Intestinal segment	Risk of malignancy	Bowel dysfunction	Peristaltic activity/ urinary leakage	Metabolic disturbance	Mucus production	Calculi formation	Urinary tract infections	Other
Ileum	+	++	+	Metabolic acidosis +	++	++	+	Perforation ++
Sigmoid colon	++	+	++	Metabolic acidosis ++	+++	++	++	Perforation ++
Stomach	+		+	Metabolic alkalosis ++	+	+	+	Hematuria/ dysuria syndrome, peptic ulceration, perforation +

Reproduced with permission from Sountoulides P, Laguna MP, de la Rosette JJ: *Cent European J Urol* 2009;62:216.

In addition to the delayed complications listed in Box 13-7, outcomes from a 10-year follow-up study after augmentation cystoplasty showed that 20% of patients demonstrated deterioration in renal function.[26] The most common reason for this decline in renal function was chronic retention or infection caused by inadequate catheterization in poorly compliant patients.[26]

Summary

Bladder augmentation is the surgical treatment of choice for the few selected patients with a high pressure and low compliance bladder. However, augmentation cystoplasty is a major abdominal intervention with hypothetically severe complications. It requires careful patient selection, lifetime patient follow-up, and physician alert for the prevention and identification of complications.

It is probably true that the variety and incidence of complications following augmentation cystoplasty is more a matter of the segment of bowel chosen rather than a special surgical technique.

BLADDER SUBSTITUTION

Background

In gynecologic oncology there are a number of circumstances where the entire bladder has to be removed at the time of a radical surgical procedure. Most of the indications of radical cystectomy in gynecologic oncology occur within the scenario of recurrent cancer and a radiated pelvis. In complicated procedures such as pelvic exenteration, especially, when the patient has received radiation, it is usually necessary to remove the urinary bladder along with the tumor.

In these cases, it is often impossible to preserve healthy bladder tissue with adequate bladder function while trying to obtain safe oncological margins. Therefore, in exenterative surgery for years the classic reconstruction procedure after cystectomy has been a continent or incontinent urinary diversion. Very often, to eliminate the tumor, the entire urethra needs to be removed. Nevertheless, in a select number of patients the urethra may be preserved. These cases include patients who undergo a supralevator exenteration where the urethra could be free of any tumor involvement. In these patients, we may consider the option of an orthotopic bladder reconstruction, which spares the patient from the need for a urostomy or external appliance, and the consequent improvement in quality of life.

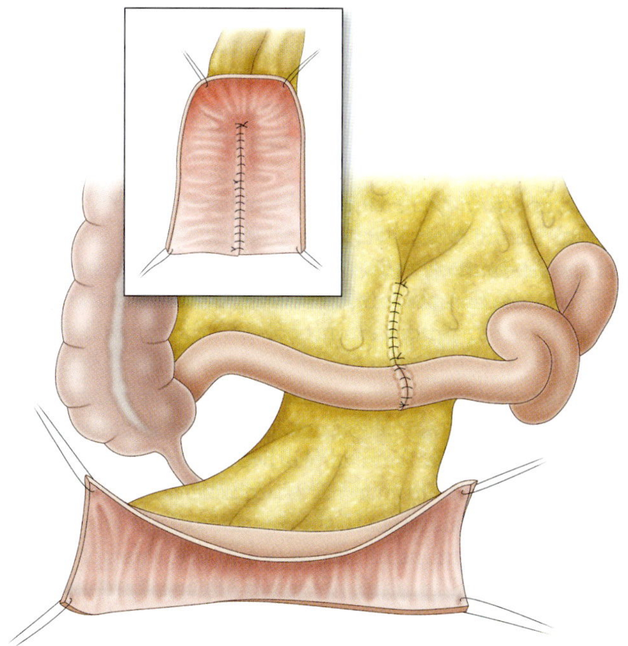

Fig. 13-21. Augmentation enterocystoplasty. Isolation of the selected loop of ileum and detubulation.

The rationale for recommending orthotopic neobladder reconstruction includes the fact that sparing the urethra does not compromise the oncologic outcome, as evidenced by the literature dealing with bladder cancer.[28]

Since Bricker first described his procedure in 1950,[29] the ileal conduit has been for many years the gold standard for urinary diversions after cystectomy for bladder cancer or after exenteration for gynecologic malignancies. The Bricker ileal conduit is still performed by many oncology surgeons around the world. There is a global perception that the ileal conduit is a safer procedure because of its technical simplicity. According to a consensus conference on bladder cancer that reviewed the literature on urinary diversion, the orthotopic bladder replacement and continent urinary diversion constituted up to 70% of all procedures.[30] But this review did not show any superiority of orthotopic neobladder over the other options of transposed intestinal segment surgery in regard of quality of life, and the committee's decision relied heavily on expert opinion and single-institution retrospective series.[30]

The orthotopic bladder reconstruction is associated with an approximately 80% rate of urinary continence.[31] Diurnal and nocturnal continence rates are acceptable in irradiated patients, although we must expect worse functional results compared to nonirradiated patients.[32]

With orthotopic urinary reconstruction, it is possible to attain a functional lower urinary tract. But this advantage can be counteracting by an increased rate of complications because of the major technical complexity of the procedure. For some authors, complications after neobladder creation are actually similar to or lower than the complication rates after conduit formation, which is in contrast to the popular view that conduits are simple and safe.[33]

In bladder cancer, orthotopic reconstruction of the lower urinary tract in males has almost been a standard operation for over the last decade with an acceptably low local recurrence rate. Up to the early 1990s, orthotopic lower-tract reconstruction was contraindicated in females. It was thought that to maintain continence, it was necessary to preserve bladder neck and the entire urethra; and this approach could be oncologic risky with a high rate of recurrence. Now that we know that the relapse rates are similar to men it is felt by many that the orthotopic neobladder is an oncologically safe option for women with pelvic tumors with negative intraoperative margins.[34] By contrast, historically it was reported that the remaining rhabdomyosphincter in the female was insufficient to provide adequate urinary continence. There is growing evidence demonstrating the oncologic safety and technical feasibility of neobladder reconstruction in females[35-37] and there are anatomic studies on the female rhabdosphincter that support its ability to provide urinary continence. The preservation of the somatic innervation of the urethra enables good continence rates and spontaneous micturition. To use the urethra for the neobladder, only about 80% should be preserved.[39] These studies formed the basis for recommending orthotopic neobladder as the diversion type of choice both in male and female patients with bladder cancer.

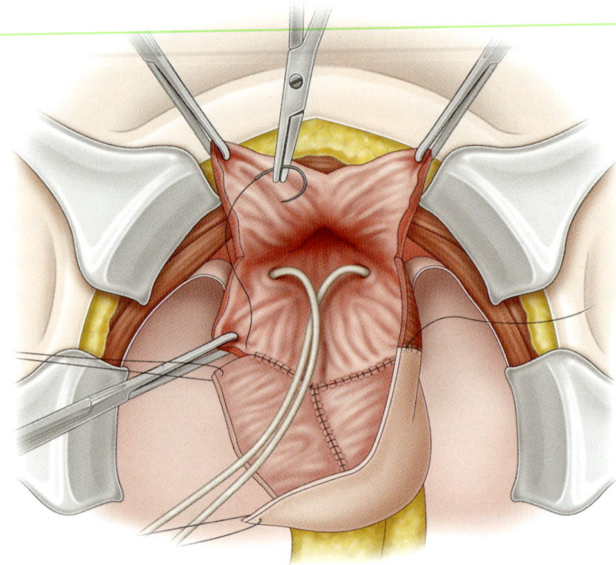

Fig. 13-22. Augmentation enterocystoplasty. The detubulized ileum is sutured to the bladder.

In gynecologic oncology, there is a very limited experience with orthotopic reconstruction of the bladder. Ungar and Palfalvi[40] reported the first large series of gynecological cancer patients who underwent anterior or total pelvic exenteration and then had urinary reconstruction without external urinary diversion. These authors described their experience with a colonic orthotopic neobladder in 13 women who underwent an exenteration after irradiation for cervical cancer. In this series, 30% of patients experienced fistula formation, while 70% achieved adequate daytime continence.

We recently published our experience with a Y-shaped ileal neobladder performed at the time of pelvic exenteration for patients with recurrent pelvic tumors who have previously undergone pelvic irradiation.[41]

Preoperative Preparation

Box 13-8 KEY SURGICAL INSTRUMENTATION

- Basic table-fixed retractor
- Basic laparotomy set
- Magnification system if needed
- DeBakey 'Atraugrip' vascular tissue forceps
- Allis clamps
- Pott scissors
- Thin vascular needle holders
- 6-8 F double-J stents
- Sensor tip guidewire
- 3-lumen Foley catheter will comfortably fit the urethra after calibration

- Reloadable linear stapler device
- 5/0, polidaxone or monofilament sutures for anastomosing the ureters
- 4/0 polidaxone or monofilament sutures for attaching the stents to the neobladder
- 3/0 polidaxone or monofilament sutures for the bowel anastomosis
- 2/0 polidaxone or monofilament sutures for anastomosing the urethra
- Soft suction drain

The preoperative orders are the same as that for a standard pelvic exenteration, ie, mechanical preoperative bowel preparation and subcutaneous prophylaxis for deep venous thrombosis. Patients wear compression stockings and are mobilized on the day after surgery. Antibiotic prophylaxis with aminoglycoside and metronidazole is started during surgery; combination aminoglycoside/metronidazole is continued for 48 hours. Patients are shaved just before surgery. Typically, four units of cross-matching blood are ordered in advance.

Surgical Procedure

Box 13-9 MASTER SURGEON'S PRINCIPLES

- All the surgical principles applied to ultra radical procedures such as careful coagulation, debridement of any necrotic tissue, and tension-free anastomoses should be followed.
- A pelvic drain must be placed in every case.
- The most threatening part of the operation is the anastomosis between the neobladder and the radiated urethra. Fistula formation at this level must be prevented by ensuring the diversion of the urethral flow and by keeping patent at all times both ureteral catheters coming out through the abdominal wall.
- Assure patency of the transurethral Foley catheter and avoid any mucous plugs or accidental traction that might avulse the anastomosis.

Even though there are a variety of different techniques described to create a neobladder, the 3 most performed are the Camey,[42] the Studer,[43] and the Hautman[44] neobladder. Our technique is a variation of the technique described by Lilien and Camey[42] and later modified by Fontana et al.[43] Briefly, the objective is to create a Y-shaped neobladder with detubularized ileum.

Once the exenterative part of the surgical procedure is completed, the loop of ileum that most easily reaches the urethra is chosen to create the neobladder (Figure 13-23). An approximately 50-cm segment of ileum, sparing the distal 20 cm of terminal ileum, is isolated with a linear stapler device.

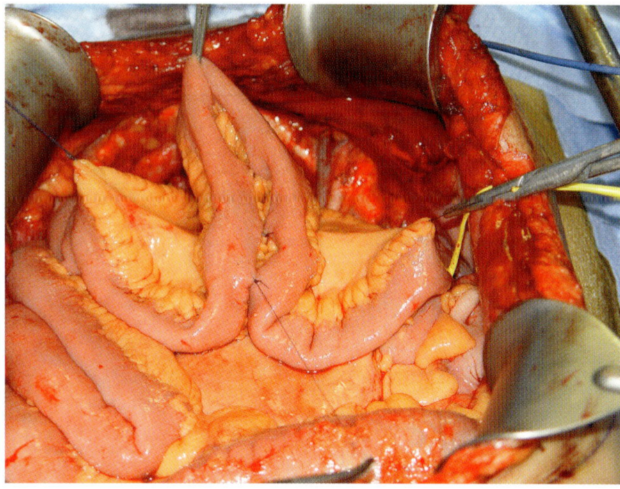

Fig. 13-23. Bladder substitution. A total of 40 to 50 cm of terminal ileum has been isolated to create the neobladder. The loop of bowel is folded, simulating a letter Y. The horizontal arm will be sutured to the urethra and both lateral arms will be anastomosed to both ureters.

A small incision is made in the distal loop of the ileal segment on the antimesenteric part of the bowel. The same linear stapler device is inserted through this incision and used to detubularize the ileum and create the vertical arm of the neobladder that will be connected to the proximal urethra. Two passes of 7.5 cm each are needed to obtain a sufficiently long ileal neobladder (Figure 13-24).

The ileal–urethral anastomosis is initiated on the posterior aspect of the anastomosis with three 2-0 reabsorbable

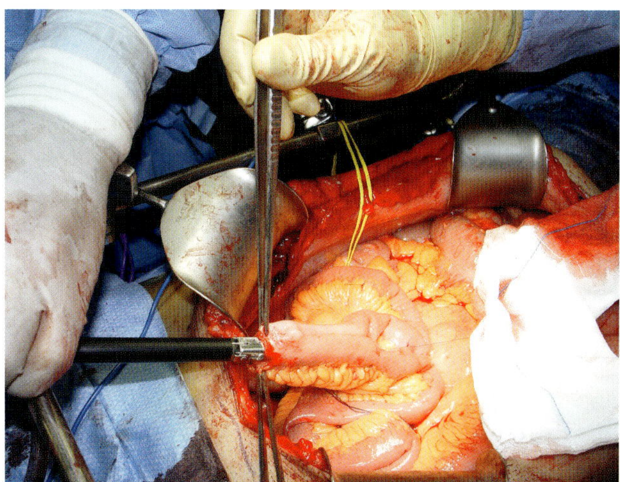

Fig. 13-24. Bladder substitution. Using in this case an endo gastrointestinal anastomosis (GIA) (blue loading units, 35 mm in height, 45 mm in length) with nonabsorbable staples, the horizontal arm is detubularized by firing several times the stapler device up to obtain a central arm of 12- to 14-cm length.

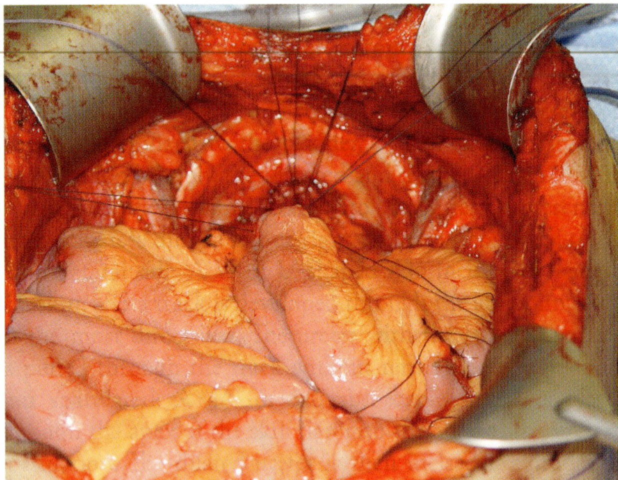

Fig. 13-25. Bladder substitution. The ileal-urethral anastomosis is the critical step of the procedure, particularly in radiated patients. A meticulous care must be taken when suturing the urethra to the ileum. Urologists carry out this suture in different ways, we typically prefer to use 6 to 8 2-0 Vicryl interrupted sutures.

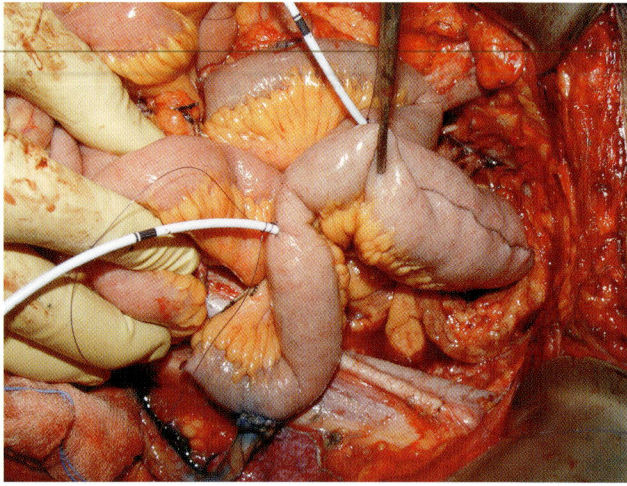

Fig. 13-26. Bladder substitution. This picture shows a full view of the Y-shaped neobladder. Observe the omental collar wrapping the urethral anastomosis. It can be note how both ureteral catheters are coming out from the neobladder ready to be exteriorized to the skin. They have been secured to the ileal serosa by tiny purse string suture.

interrupted sutures. After that, a Foley catheter is introduced into the neobladder, and the anterior aspect is completed with three new interrupted sutures of the same type (Figure 13-25). Once the anastomosis is completed, an omental J-flap is developed. The omental flap is then used to cover the anastomosis circumferentially. Subsequently, both ureters will be anastomosed to the ipsilateral arm of the Y-shaped neobladder. Each ureter is spatulated with Potts scissors, and then is catheterized with a 25-cm, 8-French, simple-pigtail catheter that is taken out through the abdominal wall trying to divert the urinary flow from the urethral anastomosis (Figure 13-26). The anastomosis between both ureters and the lateral arms of the neobladder is performed following the same technique as previously discussed. The integrity of the neobladder anastomoses is evaluated by injecting methylene blue through the Foley catheter into the neobladder.

Finally, a latero-lateral mechanical anastomosis is accomplished on both ends of the loop of ileum that was used for the neobladder creation. It is highly recommend patients who have a neobladder and a colorectal anastomosis must also have a protective temporary ileostomy.

Postoperative Care

Box 13-10 PERIOPERATIVE MORBIDITY

- Intermittent ileus or small bowel obstruction
- Urinary tract infections
- Postoperative fistulas
- Urinary leakage (ureteric, neobladder, urethral anastomosis)
- Pelvis abscess, seromas, or hematomas
- Metabolic acidosis

The suprapubic and transurethral catheters need to be irrigated and aspirated with saline 0.9% every 8 hours to prevent any catheter blockage, which may lead to a rupture of the neobladder. In our institution, we commend total parenteral nutrition on the first postoperative day and stop as soon as oral intake is established. The exteriorized ureteral catheters can also be manually irrigated if there is suspected blockage and ureteral obstruction. Four weeks after surgery, we routinely obtain a cystogram to confirm the absence of any urinary leak (Figure 13-27). After confirmation, both ureteral catheters are removed and 1 week later the Foley catheter is taken out. After catheter removal, the patient is at increased risk for metabolic acidosis. Patients will complain of lethargy, fatigue, nausea, vomiting, and anorexia associated with epigastric burning. The acidosis is monitored using the base excess estimated by venous blood gas analysis. The base excess needs to be corrected if it is negative. Virtually all patients will require sodium bicarbonate treatment (2–6 g/day), which can be stopped 2 to 6 weeks later. A salt-losing syndrome of the bladder substitute can cause hypovolemia, dehydration, and a loss of body weight. Patients should therefore consume 2 to 3 L of fluids per day, which is supplemented with increased salt intake in their diet; body weight should also be monitored each day.

After the Foley catheter is removed, the following voiding schedule is suggested to patients: week 1, void every 2 hours during the day and every 3 hours at night; week 2, void every 3 hours during the day and every 4 hours at night; week 3, void every 4 hours during the day and every 5 hours at night;

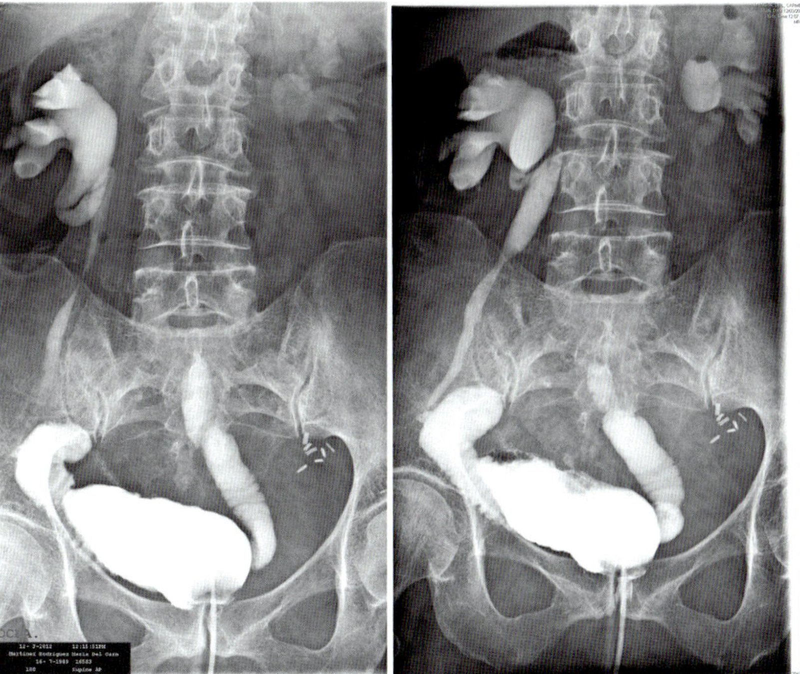

Fig. 13-27. Bladder substitution.

week 4, void every 5 hours during the day and every 6 hours at night; week 5, void every 6 hours day and night. Patients are trained to do self-catheterization of the neobladder, to measure the postvoid residual urine volume, and to clean any mucus plug that forms in the neobladder. For patients who complain of mucous plug formation, we recommend oral *N*-acetyl-*L*-cysteine (200 mg every 8 hours) to decrease the viscosity of ileal neobladder mucus. Renal sonography is performed 1 to 2 months after the pigtail catheters are removed to exclude hydronephrosis due to ureteral stricture, and excretory urography and cystography are performed at 6 and 12 months after surgery to test the ureteral patency and bladder capacity.

Long-Term Outcomes

Box 13-11 DELAYED COMPLICATIONS

- Ureteroenteric stricture
- Vesicourethral stricture
- Neobladder calculi
- Metabolic acidosis
- Incisional hernia
- Neobladder rupture

Long-term results in a growing number of female patients with orthotopic bladder substitution have verified that removing the bladder neck and a small portion of adjacent urethra but leaving a large portion of the urethra will not compromise oncological outcome.[46] Diurnal and nocturnal continence rates ranging from 82% to 95% and 72% to 86%, respectively,[47] were comparable with male patients. There is an observed increased rate of urinary retention seen in female compared to male neobladder patients. In an early series of women undergoing cystectomy without removing the entire bladder neck and subsequent orthotopic bladder substitution a majority of patients went into urinary retention.[48]

There are very few reported cases of neobladder procedures performed in gynecologic patients after irradiation to definitively conclude if is a feasible procedure in this setting.

Summary

In conclusion, bladder substitution after cystectomy has been a challenge for the urological oncologist, with several attempts in the last 2 decades to develop a method that preserves continence, self-image, and a better quality of life, without compromising the oncologic outcomes of radical surgery. For the gynecologic oncologist, it is even a greater enterprise because most of the indications for cystectomy occur in patients with recurrent disease within a radiated pelvis. The technical objectives are to create low-pressure reservoirs, which preserve the upper tracts, avoiding metabolic dysfunction, and warranting near-complete emptying on voiding. Orthotopic neobladder substitution has emerged as a gold standard after radical cystectomy for bladder cancer and has acceptable complication rates in properly selected patients. However, in the radiated patient, it must be considered as an experimental procedure with a greater-than-expected rate of complications.

REFERENCES

1. De Cicco C, Ret Davalos ML, Van Cleynenbreugel B, Verguts J, Koninckx PR. Iatrogenic ureteral lesions and repair: a review for gynecologists. *J Minim Invasive Gynecol.* 2007;14:428-435.
2. Abboudi H, Ahmed K, Royle J, Khan MS, Dasgupta P, N'dow J. Ureteric injury: a challenging condition to diagnose and manage. *Nat Rev Urol.* 2012;10(2):108-115.
3. Cirstoiu M, Munteanu O. Strategies of preventing ureteral iatrogenic injuries in obstetrics-gynecology. *J Med Life.* 2012;5(3):277-279.
4. Klap J, Phé V, Chartier-Kastler E, Mozer P, Bitker MO, Rouprêt M. Aetiology and management of iatrogenic injury of the ureter: a review. *Prog Urol.* 2012;22(15):913-919.
5. Aungst MJ, Sears CL, Fischer JR. Ureteral stents and retrograde studies: a primer for the gynecologist. *Curr Opin Obstet Gynecol.* 2009;21(5): 434-441.
6. Park JH, Park JW, Song K, Jo MK. Ureteral injury in gynecologic surgery: a 5-year review in a community hospital. *Korean J Urol.* 2012;53(2):120-125.
7. Fröber R, Surgical Atlas: Surgical anatomy of the ureter. *BJU Int.* 2007;100:949-965.
8. Iwaszko MR, Krambeck AE, Chow GK, Gettman MT. Transureteroureterostomy revisited: long-term surgical outcomes. *J Urol.* 2010;183(3):1055-1059.
9. Richter S, Kollmar O, Lindemann W, Schilling MK. Transureteroureterostomy allows renal sparing radical resection of advanced malignancies with rectosigmoid invasion. *Int J Colorectal Dis.* 2007;22(8):949-953.
10. Elkas JC, Berek JS, Leuchter R, Lagasse LD, Karlan BY. Lower urinary tract reconstruction with ileum in the treatment of gynecologic malignancies. *Gynecol Oncol.* 2005;97(2):685-692.
11. Stief CG, Jonas U, Petry KU, et al. Ureteric reconstruction. *BJU Int.* 2003;91(2):138-142.
12. Yang, W-H. Yang needle tunneling technique in creating antireflux and continent mechanisms. *J Urol.* 1993;150:830.
13. Monti PR, Lara RC, Dutra MA, de Carvalho JR. New techniques for construction of efferent conduits based on the Mitrofanoff principle. *Urology.* 1997;49:112.
14. Ali-el-Dein B, Ghoneim MA. Bridging long ureteral defects using the Yang-Monti principle. *J Urol.* 2003;169(3):1074-1077.
15. Milonas D, Stirbys S, Jievaltas M. Successful treatment of upper ureteral injury using renal autotransplantation. *Medicina (Kaunas).* 2009;45(12):988-991.
16. Png JC, Chapple CR. Principles of ureteric reconstruction. *Curr Opin Urol.* 2000;10(3):207-212.
17. Slagt IK, Klop KW, Ijzermans JN, Terkivatan T. Intravesical versus extravesical ureteroneocystostomy in kidney transplantation: a systematic review and meta-analysis. *Transplantation.* 2012;94(12):1179-1184.
18. Peeker R. Ureteric reconstruction and replacement. *Curr Opin Urol.* 2009;19:563-570.
19. Shaba A, Sharma D. Ureteric injury and reconstruction. *Urol News.* 2008;(6):27-29.
20. Rassweiler JJ, Gözen AS, Erdogru T, Sugiono M, Teber D. Ureteral reimplantation for management of ureteral strictures: a retrospective comparison of laparoscopic and open techniques. *Eur Urol.* 2007;51(2):512-522.
21. Musch M, Hohenhorst L, Pailliart A, Loewen H, Davoudi Y, Kroepfl D. Robot-assisted reconstructive surgery of the distal ureter: single institution experience in 16 patients. *BJU Int.* 2013.
22. Tizzoni G, Foggi A. Die wiederhestellung der harnblase. *Centralbl F Chir.* 1888;15:921-923.
23. Mikulicz J. Zur Operation der angeborenen Blasenspalte. *Z bl f Chir.* 1899;22:641.
24. Couvelaire R. The "little bladder" of genito-urinary tuberculosis; classification, site and variants of bladder-intestine transplants. *J Urol Medicale Chir.* 1950;56:381-434.
25. Stein R, Schröder A, Thuroff JW. Bladder augmentation and urinary diversion in patients with neurogenic bladder: Surgical considerations. *J Pediatr Urol.* 2012;8:153-161.
26. Fontaine E, Leaver R, Woodhouse CR: The effect of intestinal urinary reservoirs on renal function: a 10-year follow-up. *BJU Int.* 2000;86(3):195-198.
27. Sountoulides P, Laguna M, Rosette JJ. Complications following augmentation cystoplasty; prevention and management. *Central Eur J Urol.* 2009;62(4):216-221.
28. Stenzl A, Bartsch G, Rogatsch H. The remnant urothelium after reconstructive bladder surgery. *Eur Urol.* 2002;41(2):124-131.
29. Bricker EM. Bladder Substitution after pelvic evisceration. *Surg Clin North Am.* 1950;30:1511-1521.
30. Hautmann RE, Abol-Enein H, Hafez K, et al. World Health Organization (WHO) consensus conference on bladder cancer. Urinary diversion. *Urology.* 2007;69(1 suppl):17-49.
31. Hautmann RE, Volkmer BG, Schumacher MC. Long-term results of standard procedures in urology: the ileal neobladder. *World J Urol.* 2006;24(3):305-314.
32. Hautmann RE. 15 years experience with the ileal neobladder: what have we learned? *Urologe A.* 2001;40:360-367.
33. Hautmann RE. Urinary diversion: ileal conduit to neobladder. *J Urol.* 2003;169:834-842.
34. Stenzl A, Jarolim L, Coloby P, et al. Urethra-sparing cystectomy and orthotopic urinary diversion in women with malignant pelvic tumors. *Cancer.* 2001;02(7):1864-1871.
35. Gerber WL. Is urethral sparing at cystectomy a safe procedure? *Urology.* 1990;36:303-304.
36. Stenzl A, Draxl H, Posch B, Colleselli K, Falk M, Bartsch G. The risk of urethral tumors in female bladder cancer: can the urethra be used for orthotopic reconstruction of the lower urinary tract? *J Urol.* 1995;153:950-955.
37. Stein JP, Penson DF, Lee C, Cai J, Miranda G, Skinner DG. Long-term oncological outcomes in women undergoing radical cystectomy and orthotopic diversion for bladder cancer. *J Urol.* 2009;181:2052-2058.
38. Colleselli K, Stenzl A, Eder R, Strasser H, Poisel S, Bartsch G. The female urethral sphincter: a morphological and topographicalstudy. *J Urol.* 1998;160:49-54.
39. Stenzl A, Colleselli K, Bartsch G. Update of urethra sparing approaches in cystectomy in women. *World J Urol.* 1997;15:134-138.
40. Ungar L, Palfalvi L. Pelvic exenteration without external urinary or fecal diversion in gynecological cancer patients. *Int J Gynecol Cancer.* 2006;16:364-368.
41. Chiva LM, Lapuente F, Núñez C, Ramirez PT. Ileal orthotopic neobladder after pelvic exenteration for cervical cancer. *Gynecol Oncol.* 2009;113:47-51.
42. Lilien OM, Camey M. 25-year experience with replacement of the human bladder (Camey procedure). *J Urol.* 1984;132:886-891.
43. Studer UE, Spiegel T, Casanova GA, et al. Ileal bladder substitute: antireflux nipple or afferent tubular segment? *Eur Urol.* 1991;20: 315-326.
44. Hautmann RE, Paiss T, de Petriconi R. The ileal neobladder in women: 9 years of experience with 18 patients. *J Urol.* 1996;155(1):76-81.
45. Fontana D, Bellina M, Fasolis G, et al. Y-neobladder: an easy, fast, and reliable procedure. *Urology.* 2004;63(4):699-703.
46. Wu SD, Simma-Chang V, Stein JP. Pathologic guidelines for orthotopic urinary diversion in women with bladder cancer: a review of the literature. *Rev Urol.* 2006;8:54-60.
47. Bhatta Dhar N, Kessler TM, Mills RD, Burkhard F, Studer UE. Nerve-sparing radical cystectomy and orthotopic bladder replacement in female patients. *Eur Urol.* 2007;52:1006-1014.
48. Hautmann RE. The ileal neobladder to the female urethra. *Urol Clin North Am.* 1997;24:827-835.

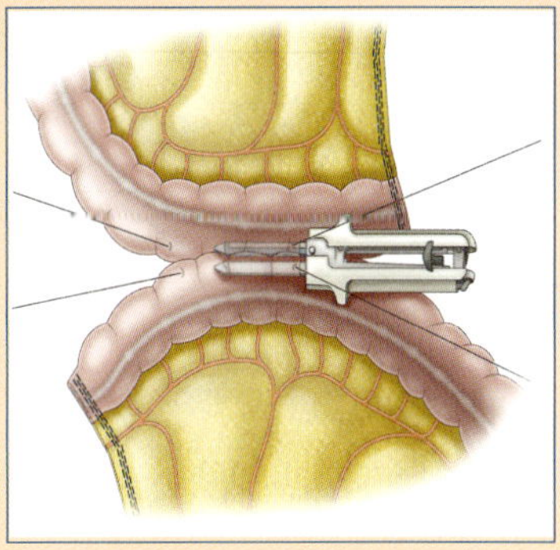

Section B Gastrointestinal Tract

Chapter 14. Colorectal Anastomosis, Colostomy, and Small Bowel Anastomosis

John P. Geisler, MD,
Katherine L. Wood, MD, and
Kelly J. Manahan, MD

BACKGROUND

The first step in understanding any surgery is achieving a clear overall picture of the patient. If the patient is healthy enough medically, nutritionally, and mentally to undergo debulking surgery, then the surgeon must have a concrete understanding of the anatomy involved.[1] Without a thorough understanding of the anatomy, many pitfalls and complications may occur. The anatomy of the entire abdomen needs to be under the purview of the gynecologic oncologist. Because gynecologic cancers do not remain confined to the pelvis, our anatomic knowledge cannot remain confined to the pelvis.

Morrow and Curtin[2] have previously elegantly illustrated that certain conditions must be met prior to creating any bowel anastomosis. First, healthy tissue with good blood supply needs to be used in both the afferent and efferent bowel limbs. If blood supply is questionable, then fluorescein dye with a wood's lamp can be used to visualize the blood supply.[3] Second, an adequate, nonstrictured, water-tight, hemostatic lumen must be created. Third, the anastomosis should be free of tension. Fourth, an anastomosis should not be created in the presence of *established* peritonitis. Applying these guidelines to any bowel anastomosis is crucial.

INDICATIONS AND APPLICATIONS

The stomach at the proximal end of the small bowel is a site frequently involved with disease extending over from the lesser or greater omentum. Infrequently, disease is large enough to require wedge resection for complete cytoreduction or gastrojejunostomy for palliation secondary to a large node or mass obstructing the pylorus or proximal duodenum.[4,5] Hoffman et al[6] described cases in which en bloc resection of the left upper quadrant intra-abdominal contents (including 2 cases of partial gastrectomy), was able to leave the patient with minimal residual disease. In a larger series, Walter et al[4] have shown that partial gastrectomy (or wedge resection) can be safely performed in radical debulking of ovarian cancer.

The most common surgery performed on the small bowel (jejunum and ileum) in gynecologic oncology is small bowel resection with primary reanastomosis. This can be performed for a variety of reasons by gynecologic oncologists. The resection may be for obstruction by cancer, debulking of cancer, radiation damage causing fistula or stricture, or for dead or damaged bowel as a complication of therapy.

Bristow et al[7] demonstrated the safety and utility of colorectal resection and reanastomosis in women with ovarian cancer. Three years later, Hoffman[8] built upon their study and echoed the safety of similar procedures. Both of these papers showed that large resections of the colon could be safely performed to aid in cytoreduction. Silver and Walter separately have shown that subtotal colectomies can be safely performed in achieving complete cytoreduction.[9,10] These extensive resections with pouches (Figure 14-1) are associated with complications but are tolerated well by patients.[11] Once the protective ostomy is reversed, patients will have continence but increased fecal frequency.[9] This topic will be covered more extensively in Chapter 15.

ANATOMIC CONSIDERATIONS

Pertinent anatomic figures are provided in Chapter 2. The stomach is the most proximal abdominal organ of the digestive tract. It lies asymmetrically in the abdomen to the left of midline and is comprised of 4 parts: cardia, fundus, body, and pyloric antrum. The cardia surrounds the cardiac orifice where the stomach attaches to the esophagus just inferior to the lower esophageal sphincter. The cardiac notch or angle of His lies between the esophagus and fundus, and approximates the location of the gastroesophageal (GE) junction. The horizontal

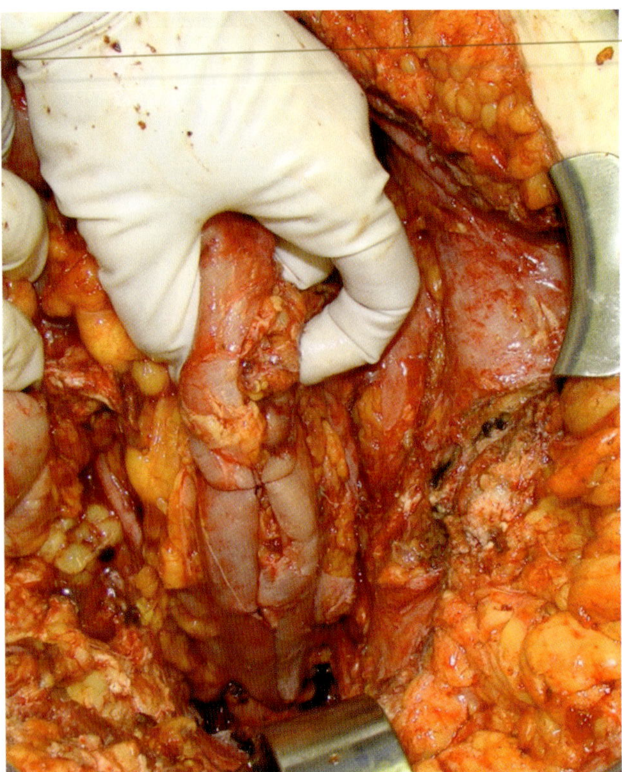

Fig. 14-1. Example of a ascending colonic J-pouch with low colorectal anastomosis.

plane of the GE junction marks the inferior border of the distensible fundus, which is bounded superiorly by the left dome of the diaphragm and laterally by the spleen. The fundus is the most superior aspect of the stomach. The largest portion of the stomach is the body, which is located between the fundus and the pyloric antrum. It is bound on the right by the lesser curvature and on the left by the greater curvature. The sharp angle of the lesser curvature, the angular incisure, identifies the junction of the body and the pyloric antrum. Distally, the pylorus connects the antrum to the proximal duodenum.

The stomach is anteriorly related to diaphragm, left lobe of the liver, and anterior abdominal wall. The posterior surface of the stomach forms the anterior wall of the omental bursa. The gastrosplenic ligament attaches the proximal greater curvature to the spleen. Inferiorly, the stomach is attached to the transverse colon by the gastrocolic omentum as it courses along the greater curvature to the left colic flexure (splenic flexure). The lesser curvature is attached to the liver by the hepatogastric ligament (part of the lesser omentum).

The duodenum is the most proximal segment of the small intestine, lying partially in the retroperitoneum. It is also the shortest segment of small intestine, only 25 cm in length. It has a C-shaped course around the head of the pancreas, beginning just distal to the pylorus and ending at the ligament of Treitz (duodenojejunal junction). It is divided into 4 parts: superior, descending, inferior, and ascending. Proximally, the superior part is attached to the hepatoduodenal ligament (lesser omentum) containing the portal triad. The descending portion curves around the head of the pancreas and is entirely retroperitoneal. The inferior part courses horizontally and is crossed by the superior mesenteric artery and the root of the mesentery of the jejunum and ileum. Posteriorly, the inferior part is related to the inferior vena cava, aorta, and right ovarian vessels. The ascending part of the duodenum curves anteriorly to join the jejunum at the duodenojejunal flexure.

The main blood supply to the stomach comes from the celiac axis and its branches. The lesser curvature is supplied by anastomoses formed between the right and left gastric arteries, arising from the hepatic artery and celiac trunk, respectively. An anomalous hepatic artery can arise from the left gastric artery 15% to 20% of the time, which occasionally is the only arterial flow to the left hepatic lobe. The gastroduodenal artery arises from the hepatic artery and supplies the right portion of the greater curvature along with part of the omentum (through the right gastroepiploic). The splenic comes either off a named branch or directly off the celiac trunk giving blood supply to the proximal greater curvature and fundus via short gastrics, and blood to the omentum and greater curvature through the left gastroepiploic before supplying the named organ. The duodenum is supplied by the superior and inferior pancreaticoduodenal arteries, via the celiac trunk (branch of gastroduodenal artery) and superior mesenteric artery, respectively. The veins of the stomach and duodenum parallel the arteries and drain into the hepatic portal vein either directly or indirectly via the superior mesenteric vein and splenic vein.

Because of its length (15–30 feet, with the female average of 21 feet), the small bowel is a frequently involved area with tumor or complications from therapy. The jejunum and ileum comprise the intraperitoneal portion of the small intestine, beginning at the duodenojejunal junction and extending to the ileocecal junction. It can be difficult to grossly distinguish between the ileum and jejunum as there is no distinct anatomic marking identifying them. Most of the jejunum lies in the left upper quadrant of the infracolic compartment of the abdomen, comprising about two-fifths of the small bowel. The ileum primarily resides in the right lower quadrant and makes up the remaining three-fifths of the small bowel. The jejunal mucosa is thicker with more prominent plicae circulares. The mesenteric vessels form one or two arcades with long, straight vasa recta. The ileum has a thinner wall with slightly smaller caliber, more prevalent mesenteric arcades and short vasa recta. There is also increased mesenteric fat in the ileum.

The superior mesenteric artery with its numerous branches is the main blood supply to the small bowel (embryologic midgut). It can be found arising from the aorta just posterior to the pancreas. The pancreaticoduodenal is the first branch followed by a variable number of jejunal and ileal branches (12–15). Next come the ileocolic, right colic, and middle colic vessels. The ileocolic and right colic may branch of together from the aorta before dividing, and so this is an anatomic variation.

The colon has 4 parts: ascending, transverse, descending, and sigmoid. The ascending colon is approximately 15 cm in length and is a secondarily retroperitoneal continuation of the cecum, extending between the level of the ileocecal valve and the right colic flexure. The transverse colon, the longest (45 cm) and most mobile part of the large intestine, is suspended between the hepatic and splenic flexures and attached to the greater omentum along its superior aspect. Like the ascending colon, the descending colon is also secondarily retroperitoneal, beginning at the splenic flexure and extending approximately 25 cm to the left iliac fossa. It is fixed against the retroperitoneum posteriorly with the lateral and anterior surfaces as true intraperitoneal structures. The white line of Toldt is the lateral peritoneal reflection that can be used as a guide to mobilize the colon. It should be noted that this lies in close proximity to the left ureter and ovarian vessels. At the level of the pelvic brim, the descending colon transitions to the S-shaped sigmoid colon with a mesentery (pelvic mesocolon) that is fixed to the posterior pelvic wall. It is highly variable in length (15–50 cm) and smaller in caliber than the descending colon. The sigmoid colon terminates at the rectosigmoid junction at the level of the sacral promontory, as do the characteristic markings of the colon—teniae, haustra, and omental appendices.

The rectum extends approximately 12 to 15 cm into the true pelvis and is mostly extraperitoneal. The posterior rectal wall is covered in a thin fascia propria (visceral layer) opposed by a thicker, presacral fascia (parietal layer) that covers presacral veins. A fine areolar fascia is present between the anterior surface of the parietal layer and the posterior surface of the visceral layer of the rectum. The Waldeyer's fascia is formed by fusion of these 2 layers just superior to the coccyx. Anteriorly, Denonvilliers fascia, a bilaminar fascial layer, separates the anterior rectum from the vagina. It is also known as the rectovaginal septum and is continuous with the uterosacral folds.

The ascending and transverse colon is supplied by branches of the superior mesenteric artery, including ileocolic, right colic, and middle colic arteries. Beginning at the splenic flexure, the remainder of the colon and rectum is supplied by branches of the inferior mesenteric artery, including the superior and inferior left colic arteries, multiple sigmoid arteries, and the middle rectal artery. The posterior wall of the rectum is also supplied by branches of the median sacral artery. One area of confusion that continues until today regarding the blood supply of the colon is caused by the different names used for vessels. The central anastomotic artery of the mesocolon is sometimes referred to as the arc of Riolan and sometimes as the marginal artery of Drummond. The key point to understand is that this vessel extends from the ileocolic artery to the lowest sigmoid vessel (Figure 14-2).

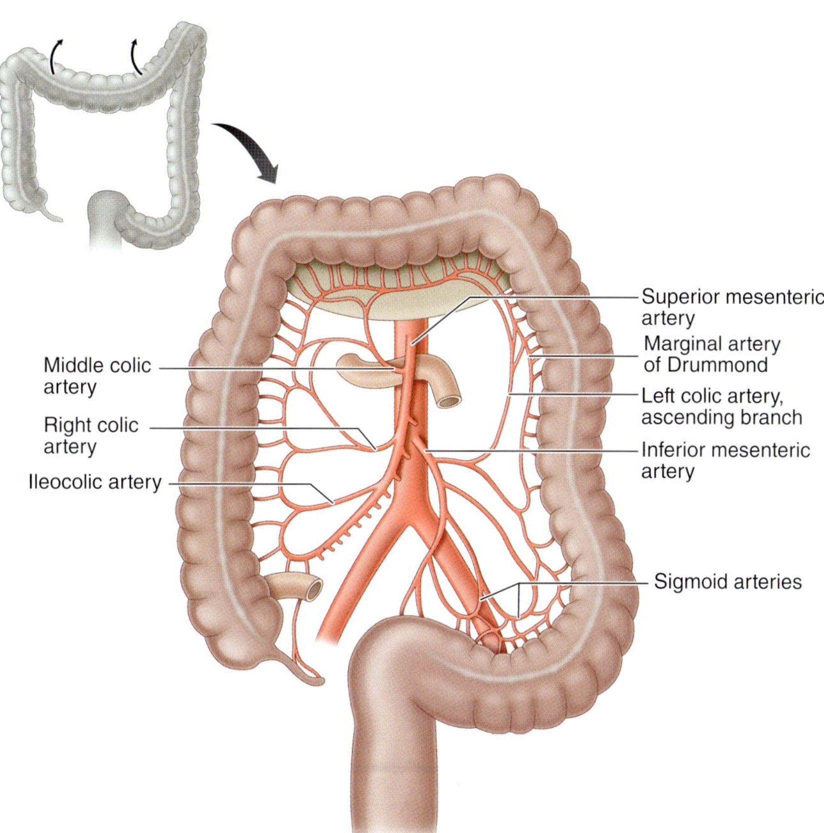

Fig. 14-2. Diagram of colorectal blood supply with special attention to arc of Riolan (marginal artery of Drummond).

PREOPERATIVE PREPARATIONS

Box 14-1 KEY SURGICAL INSTRUMENTATION

- 60- to 80-mm linear stapler/cutter with 3.5- to 4.8-mm staple
- 45- to 60-mm endoscopic linear stapler/cutter
  - 2.0-mm staple for vascular pedicles
  - 3.0- to 3.5-mm staple for bowel
- 21- to 33-mm circular stapler/cutter with 3.5–4.8 mm staple-size
- 30- to 60-mm linear stapler with 3.5–4.8 mm load
- 3-0 monofilament, delayed-absorbable suture on taper needle
- Argon beam coagulation device

At our institution, before performing any surgical procedure on a woman with a pelvic mass albumin and prealbumin are checked.[12] If the prealbumin level is below 10 mg/dL, then patients are started on parenteral nutrition even if tolerating supplemental enteral feeds. If the prealbumin does not increase to at least 10 mg/dL after 7 to 10 days, the patient will undergo paracentesis or percutaneous biopsy to attempt to get a cancer diagnosis. Once the diagnosis is made, they will be offered neoadjuvant chemotherapy because of the increased risk of morbidity and mortality when operating on women with a low prealbumin level.[1] All patients with a starting prealbumin from at least 10 to 18 mg/dL are placed on postoperative supplementation with oral supplements being preferred.

Although the redundant blood supply of the stomach makes the stomach a forgiving organ on which to operate, several points exist about which to be aware when operating on the stomach. Surgical adventures to the patient's right of the angular notch can turn into misadventures if the biliary tree is damaged. If performing gastrostomy, then it is best to sew the stomach to the anterior wall to decrease the chances of spilling gastric contents into the abdomen.

Preservation of the blood supply of the small bowel is paramount. Careful surgical manipulation of the mesentery and bowel wall is of utmost importance. Although the small bowel can be stripped of its mesentery in creating an ileostomy for up to 6 cm, this is often not necessary and potentially harmful if done incorrectly.[13,14]

While operating on the colon, several key points must be considered. First, while the small intestine's arcades allow up to 6 cm of bowel to be devascularized, the colon's vascular redundancy is more proximal; therefore, only 2 cm can be devascularized without necrosis. Next, operating on the left colon near the splenic flexure and sigmoid near Sudeck point, can be precarious if the surgeon is not aware of the vascular watershed areas. It is best to create anastomoses proximal or very distal to these points.

A further point of caution has recently been illustrated.[15] It is critical for good outcomes when performing ovarian cancer cytoreduction, especially bowel resections and anastomoses, to not allow hypothermia to occur. Patients in whom core temperatures dropped below 96.8°F (36°C) had increased complications compared to those in whom hypothermia did not occur.[15]

Bowel resections are performed in gynecologic oncology most commonly for either debulking or obstruction. Each of these is fraught with potential pitfalls for the unwary. Also, each is more quickly performed if the surgeon is knowledgeable of the surgical anatomy, surgical techniques, and surgical tools. Over the past few decades, the paradigm has shifted away from preoperative oral antibiotic bowel preparation and mechanical bowel preparation to using just parenteral antibiotics one hour before incision. The paradigm may be shifting again. Recent data demonstrate that the best combination to achieve the lowest surgical site infection rate in patients undergoing elective colon surgery is the combination of preoperative oral antibiotic bowel preparation, mechanical bowel preparation, and parenteral antibiotics within 1 hour of incision.[16]

If an ostomy is being considered preoperatively, then enterostomal therapy is consulted to talk with the patient and mark optimal sites. In any patient that receives an ostomy, enterostomal therapy is consulted immediately postoperatively to begin patient education.

Currently, most intestinal anastomoses are performed using mechanical surgical devices and endomechanical surgical devices.[17] These are supplied by a variety of companies. The specific devices associated with each procedure are discussed in the related section along with device sizes and staple diameters.

SURGICAL PROCEDURES

Box 14-2 MASTER SURGEON'S PRINCIPLES

- Healthy tissue with good blood supply needs to be used in both the afferent and efferent bowel limbs (test with fluorescein dye if unsure)
- An adequate, nonstrictured, water-tight, hemostatic lumen must be created
- Anastomosis should be free of tension
- Anastomosis should not be created in the presence of *established* peritonitis without a proximal diversion

Stomach

1. Wedge resection

Even after an infragastric omentectomy, the redundancy of the gastric blood supply allows wedge resection to be safely performed. To avoid a key area of complication when working with the lesser omentum or lesser curvature, the surgeon must stay to the patient's left of the hepatoduodenal ligament in the hepatogastric area of the lesser omentum. The key anatomic point to recognize is the stomach's angular notch. Damage to the biliary tree can be safely avoided if the surgeon stays to the patient's left of this anatomic point on the lesser curvature. Using a laparoscopic gastrointestinal linear stapler/cutter (Figure 14-3), a full thickness resection can be safely and easily accomplished using a 45- to 60-mm long stapler with a 3- to 3.5-mm thick staple. A second load is used to create a wedge around the tumor and crossing the original line to seal the stomach (Figure 14-4). This type of resection can be undertaken on either the greater or lesser curvature. The staple line from an endoscopic linear stapler/cutter has 3 rows of staples so oversewing is not usually necessary (see Figure 14-3).

Alternatively, a smaller lesion can be resected with a football or elliptical-shaped resection of the gastric serosa (with or without muscularis and mucosa as indicated). This may result in the stomach mucosa (and the gastric contents momentarily being open. The site should be closed with a delayed absorbable 3-0 monofilament suture (polyglyconate or polydioxanone) on a taper needle. A running or Connell stitch can be used. Recent studies have even demonstrated that a running stitch using a barbed suture is equivalent to a running stitch using a delayed absorbable suture.[18] Whether or not a second imbricating layer is used depends on the patient's history and status, as well as surgeon preference. A small resection can also be accomplished by pulling the tumor up to be resected, then placing an endoscopic 45- to 60-mm long stapler with a 3- to 3.5-mm staple, and firing it. This results in a closed resection without any exposure of the abdomen to gastric contents.

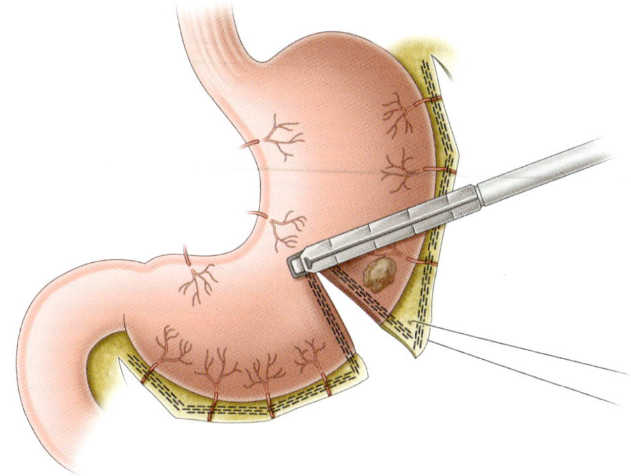

Fig. 14-4. Diagram of wedge resection with overlapping staple lines from a Laparoscopic gastrointestinal linear stapler/cutter.

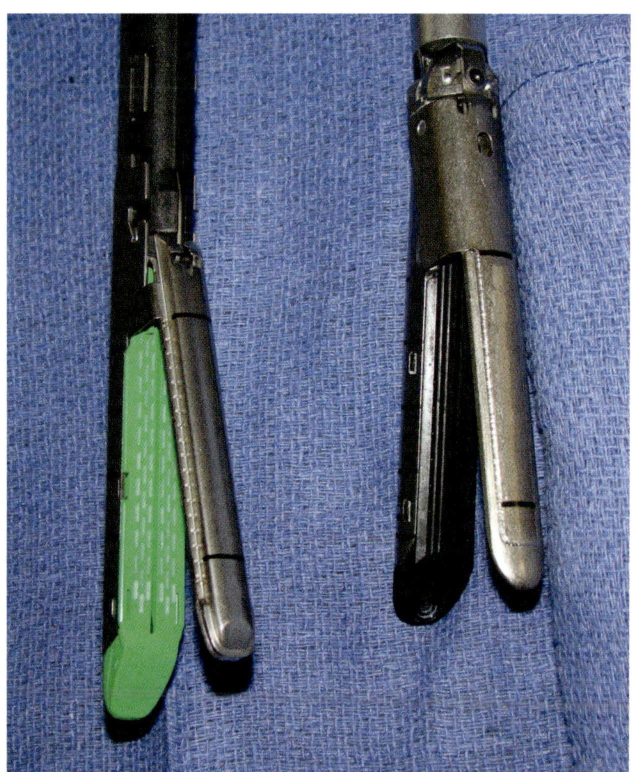

Fig. 14-3. Laparoscopic gastrointestinal linear stapler/cutter with a 45-mm long stapler and 3.5-mm thick staple.

Small Bowel

1. Gastrojejunostomy

In women with ovarian cancer, the infragastric omentum should already have been surgically resected at the initial debulking, so one difficulty with the gastrojejunostomy in other patients is absent. When performing the procedure, a decision has to be made whether the jejunum is going to be anastomosed to the anterior stomach, the greater curvature, or posterior stomach. If the plan is to perform an anastomosis to the anterior stomach or greater curvature, the jejunum is brought over the transverse colon. If a posterior attachment is planned, then the jejunum is passed through the transverse colon mesentery through a window of Dever.

Either way, the anastomosis is most easily performed using a 60- to 80-mm long linear stapler/cutter (Figure 14-5) with a 2.5- to 3.8-mm staple. For example, the jejunum is placed with its antimesenteric border against the greater curvature. Stabilizing sutures can be placed before small incisions are made in the stomach and the jejunum. Alternatively, the two bowel segments can just be carefully aligned or even held with Allis clamps. A small hole is made in the stomach and the jejunum on the antimesenteric side. The linear stapler/cutter is placed with one piece in each lumen and fired (Figure 14-6). The remaining opening can be then closed with a linear stapler (3.5- to 4.8-mm staple) or sewn closed with a 3-0 delayed absorbable suture.

Another surgery performed in women with ovarian cancer is a Stamm gastrostomy procedure.[19] This procedure used to be performed more commonly than it is today because

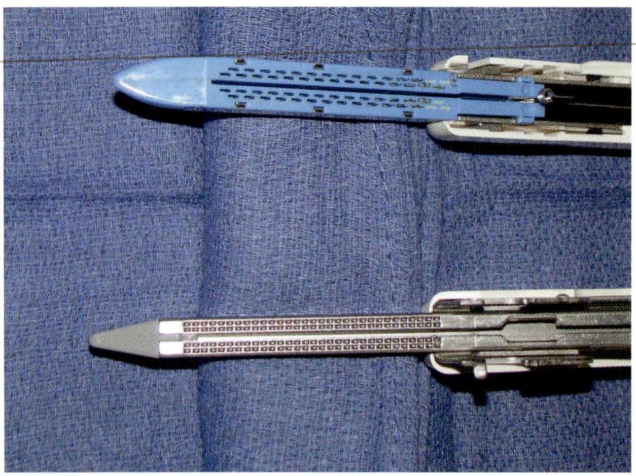

Fig. 14-5. linear stapler/cutter with 60-mm load with a 2.5-3 mm staple.

percutaneous endoscopic gastrostomy tubes (PEG) can be placed safely in many patients without the need for a laparotomy or laparoscopy.[20,21] In ovarian cancer patients, gastrostomies are used palliatively because of obstruction or tumor ileus rather than for feeding. Because of the specific need, occasionally tumor or ascites prevent percutaneous placement. When still performed, a Stamm gastrostomy can be performed through a 7- to 8-cm upper midline or left subcostal incision. The tube itself can be a standard PEG tube, a Foley catheter or a Mallinckrodt catheter of large gauge. The stomach is grasped on the anterior mid surface near the greater curvature with a Babcock clamp. Two purse string sutures of 3-0 delayed absorbable monofilament are placed around the Babcock clamp with needles left attached. The tube is brought through the anterior wall away from the incision. It is placed through a small puncture wound in the stomach. The purse sutures are closed inner first and then outer, and then the sutures are sewn to the anterior abdominal wall. The tube can be connected to suction or can be left capped only to be opened when needed. Alternatively, a permanent tube can be made from the anterior gastric wall and brought as a gastrostomy through the anterior abdominal wall. The defects are closed with a 3-0 delayed absorbable suture. Complications from this approach include the possibility of gastric contents getting on the skin.

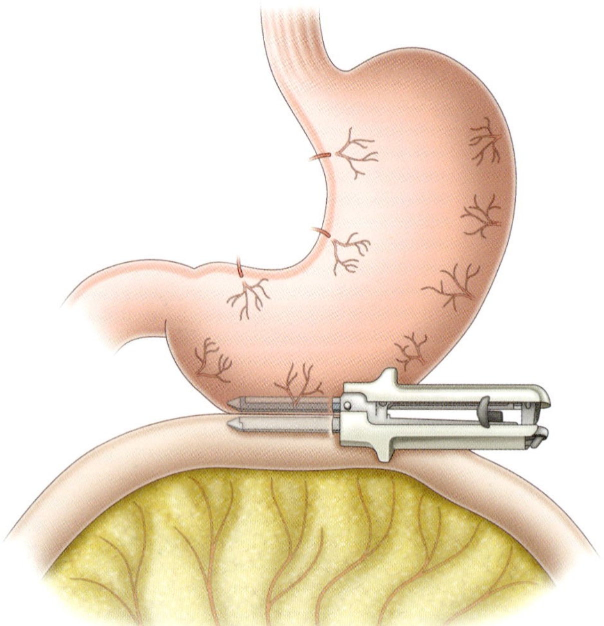

Fig. 14-6. Diagram of gastrojejunostomy with linear stapler/cutter placed with one side in each lumen and fired.

2. Small bowel resection

The actual resection of the bowel can be accomplished using bowel clamps or using a 60- to 80-mm open linear stapler/cutter. The mesentery can be resected by hand with clamps, scissors, and ties; by endoscopic linear stapler/cutter with a 2- to 2.5-mm staple load; or by a vessel-sealing device. A smaller diameter staple is used on mesenteric vascular tissue than on the adjacent bowel to seal the vessels. If this same diameter staple was used on bowel, then the staples could cause local necrosis and failure of the staple line.[22] The linear staple/cutter is passed through the avascular window just below the bowel edge (Figure 14-7) in a healthy area of bowel proximal to the area to be resected. The linear staple/cutter is closed (Figure 14-8), and the bowel is divided giving 2 fresh staple lines (Figure 14-9) closing the bowel lumen on both sides. If a linear stapler alone was used, then one side of the bowel would be open. A similar procedure is performed in a healthy area of bowel distal to the site being resected. The mesentery can then be resected quickly with either an endoscopic linear staple/cutter with vascular loads (staple 2–2.5 mm) or a vessel-sealing device. After completion of the anastomosis, the mesentery should be closed with 3-0 delayed absorbable suture.

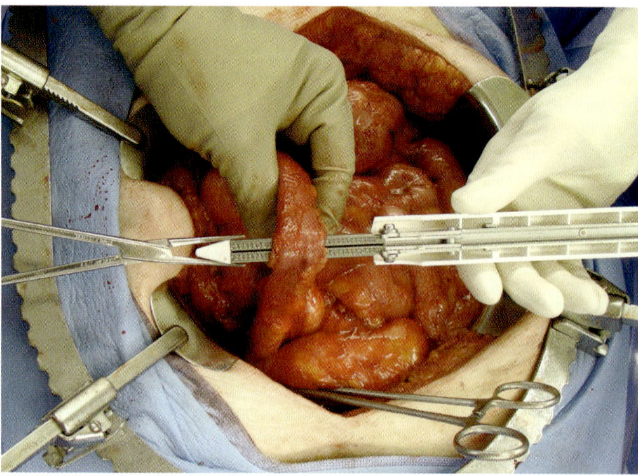

Fig. 14-7. linear staple/cutter through the avascular window just below the bowel edge in a healthy area proximal (and distal) to area to be resected.

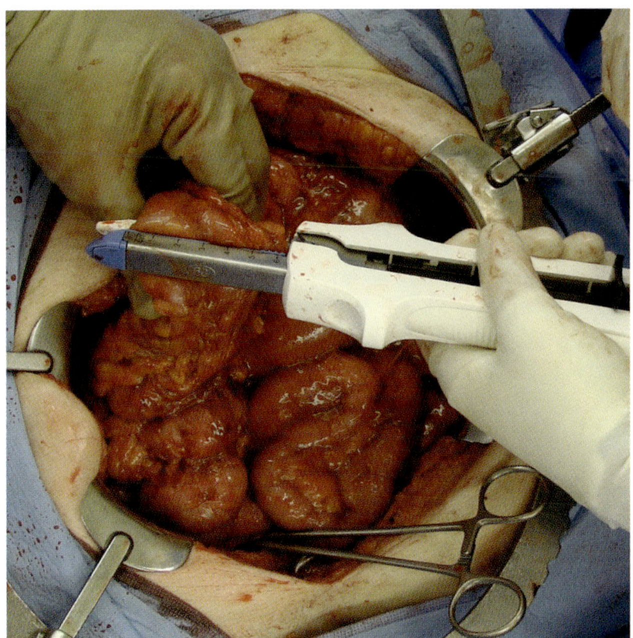

Fig. 14-8. A 60-mm linear stapler/cutter has been passed through an avascular window on the mesenteric side of the ileum and has been closed with the other part of the linear stapler/cutter. When looking closely at the bowel coming through the device, notice that the device had to be repositioned prior to firing. Although in this picture the entire bowel would have been appropriately stapled, the bowel extended past the "cut" line and so would be sealed but not cut.

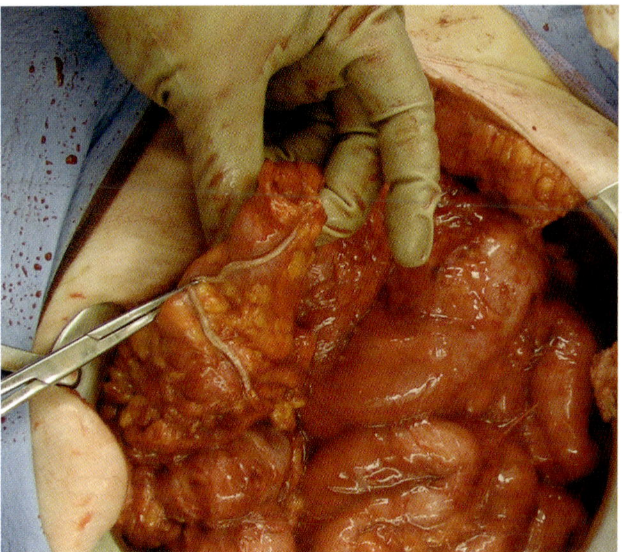

Fig. 14-9. The previously shown piece of ileum has been stapled and divided as intended. A hemostat is shown hold the apex.

The next decisions that need to be made are what type of anastomoses and whether to use staplers or sew by hand. Two main types of anastomoses performed in the small bowel currently are the more common side-to-side functional end-to-end anastomoses and the less common end-to-end anastomosis.

If a side-to-side anastomosis is being performed, then the 60- to 80-mm linear stapler/cutter is then used to recreate the lumen. The 2 bowl limbs that are to be joined are placed antimesenteric to antimesenteric side. The antimesenteric corners of the staple lines on both limbs are cut open with heavy-curved scissors. One side of the linear stapler/cutter is placed in each lumen (Figure 14-10A). If needed, stay sutures can be place to stabilize the bowel. The bowels are now connected in a side-to-side functional end-to-end anastomosis. The right side of the figure demonstrates the residual opening after creating the anastomosis (Figure 14-10B). The edges of the opening are grasped carefully with Allis or Babcock clamps and are brought above the future staple line of the linear stapler. The residual opening is closed with a linear stapler 30 to 60 mm in length with a 3.5 or 4.8 mm load (Figure 14-11A). Any tissue above the staple line is removed with a pair of heavy scissors. Figure 14-11B shows an already fired 45-mm linear stapler with 3.5-mm staples. As can be seen, there are two rows of alternating staplers and no knife or knife ridge to cut the tissue. This type of instrument only seals one side of bowel. Therefore, it should not be used in a procedure where you are dividing bowel and want both proximal and distal lumens closed unless another load is used immediately adjacent to the first.

An end-to-end anastomosis can be performed by hand-sewn closure or be an end-to-end anastomotic circular cutter/stapler (Figure 14-12). As can be seen in Figure 14-12, the end-to-end anastomotic circular stapler/cutter has 2 concentric rings of staples with an inner circular knife. An end-to-end anastomosis can be performed of varying inner diameter based on the size of the smallest piece of bowel being connected. An analogous procedure will be described in the section on colorectal procedures. An even less common procedure is an end-to-side anastomosis. This type is usually performed in the situation where a bowel bypass, rather than a bowel resection, is being performed. This is also quickly performed with an end-to-end anastomotic circular stapler/cutter.

3. Ileostomy formation

Ileostomies may be placed in patients to protect more distal anastomoses or as an end ostomy. The more distal the ostomy is in the small bowel, the less the chance of electrolyte and fluid problems. Often, vitamin K must be supplemented if the ostomy is prior to the terminal ileum. Diverting ostomies can either be an end or a loop ileostomy. Loop ostomies add the benefit that a closure of the ostomy to reintroduce bowel continuity can be performed through just the ostomy site, minimizing the incision size for the patient.

A loop ostomy is made by first creating a quarter-size opening in the skin with the cut mode of the electrosurgical unit. The subcutaneous tissue is not removed and it is just pushed to the sides. The assistant or the nondominant hand pushes up from inside the abdomen and a cruciate incision is

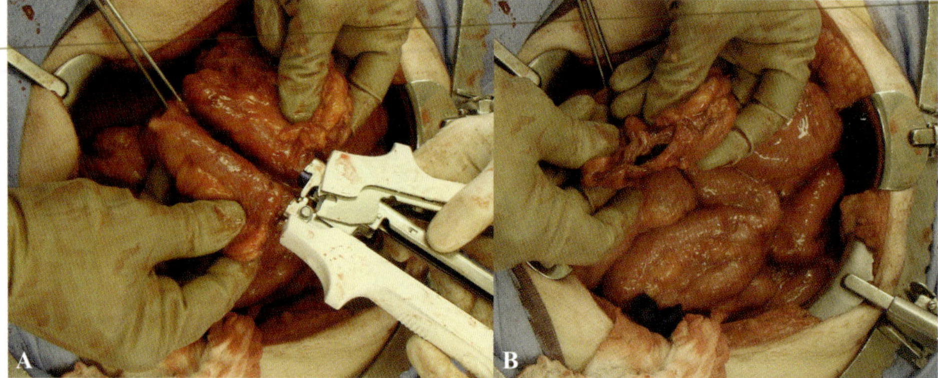

Fig. 14-10. (A) The 2 antimesenteric sides of the bowel to be anastomosed are lined up with a linear stapler/cutter in position to join the bowels in a side-to-side functional end-to-end anastomosis. (B) The residual opening is shown after the bowel has been anastomosed.

made in the fascia. A cruciate incision is used to decrease the chances of the fascia constricting the bowel. The fibers of the rectus are pushed apart (and not cut) to decrease parastomal hernia. The site for the opening in the bowel is marked by bluntly passing a vessel loop or small diameter Penrose drain through the mesentery just below the bowel wall. The previously identified site in the ileum is gently brought through the ostomy site using a combination of pushing from below and gentle traction with either a Babcock clamp or the vessel loop from above. Once the bowel is brought up through the ostomy above the skin level (5–6 cm), an ostomy bar is used to replace the vessel loop. The shortest possible ostomy bar should be used to facilitate appliance placement. The bar is sewn to the skin edge with an absorbable monofilament. Previously, authors have thought that sewing the small bowel to the skin created more problems, but this has been demonstrated not to be true. It is safe to create a rosebud ostomy with small intestine. The rosebud is created at the cardinal points with either a 3-0 absorbable monofilament (poliglecaprone 25 or glycolide/dioxanone/trimethylene carbonate) or 3-0 absorbable braided (polyglycolic acid or polyglactin) suture. The afferent loop will produce the effluent and the efferent limb acts as a mucous fistula.

4. Ileostomy closure

Closure of a diverting ileostomy can be performed in a variety of ways. Classically, surgeon preference dictates which of the following 3 techniques is chosen: hand-sewn anastomosis without bowel resection, hand-sewn anastomosis with bowel resection, and stapled anastomosis. Gustavsson et al[23] showed in a large series of patients that stapled anastomoses had a shorter hospital stay and less chance of small bowel obstruction than either of the hand-sewn methods.

The skin around the ostomy is incised with the electrical surgical unit on cut. The subcutaneous tissues are carefully dissected off of the bowel sparing the ileal mesentery. Once the fascia is reached, the bowel is carefully separated from the rectus fascia. This dissection allows mobilization of enough bowel to allow creation of a new lumen and restitution of bowel continuity in most cases. After mobilization, the ileum is pulled up and the antimesenteric edges are placed next to

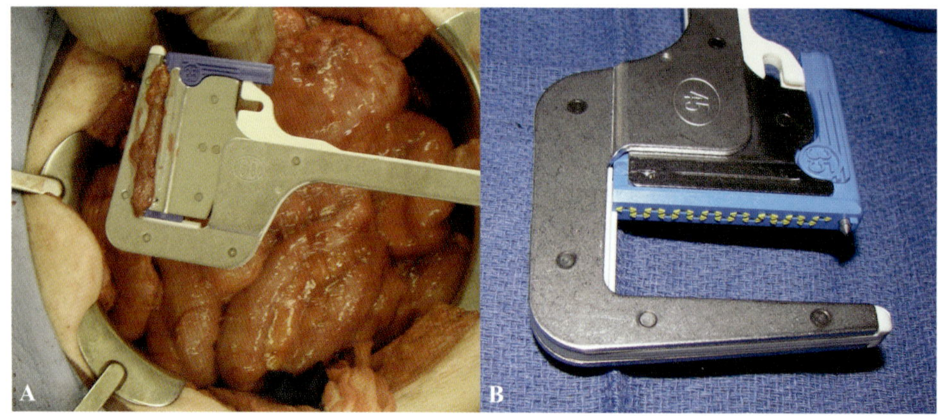

Fig. 14-11. (A) Linear stapler is used to close opening from Figure 14-8B. Tissue protruding above device is trimmed away prior to loosening the device. (B) A close-up of an already used linear stapler. Note that there are only 2 rows of stable and no blade to cut.

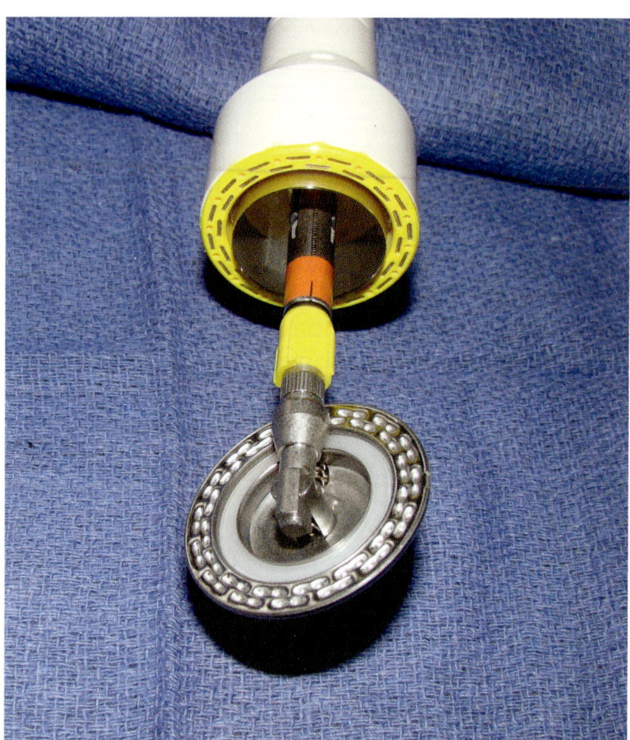

Fig. 14-12. A circular stapler/cutter for end-to-end anastomosis is demonstrated in this picture. In gynecologic oncology, these devices are most frequently used to anastomose colon to rectum or anus during a debulking with low anterior resection. Two rows of staples are seen with a circular blade closer to the center.

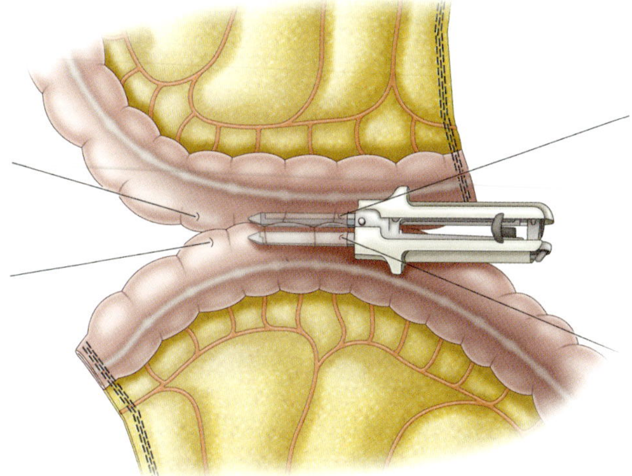

Fig. 14-13. Afferent and efferent limbs of the bowel are placed parallel to each other with their antimesenteric borders. Stay sutures of a 3-0 delayed monofilament suture are placed to ease the procedure. Side-to-side anastomosis is performed with linear stapler cutter (shown). The residual opening of the bowel is closed either a linear stapler (3.5–4.8 mm staple) or sewn closed with a 3-0 delayed absorbable suture in a careful running fashion.

each other. Analogous to Figure 14-10, the 60- to 80-mm linear stapler/cutter (with a 2.5–3.8 mm staple load) is placed (one part in each lumen). Once the alignment is correct, the instrument is fired and a new anastomosis is created. The residual opening is again closed with a 30- to 60-mm linear stapler with a 3.5- to 4.8-mm staple load. Residual tissue is resected above the staple line.

If an end ileostomy is being reversed, a midline incision is first made. The ostomy is mobilized as above with the reversal of the loop ostomy. The ostomy itself is either closed with a linear stapler (Figure 14-11), or closed with a delayed absorbable 3-0 monofilament suture. This closure decreases chances of spilling succus entericus into the abdomen. Some surgeons prefer to leave the ostomy open. After mobilization (and closure) of the ostomy, the ileum is brought into the open abdomen. The distal bowel to which the segment will be reanastomosed is identified. Any adhesions are takedown with cautery or sharp dissection to allow there to be no tension on the anastomosis. The continuity of the bowel is restored as a side-to-side functional end-to-end anastomosis as previously described. Occasionally, the patient's anatomy is more conducive to placing the proximal and distal bowel parallel to each other with their antimesenteric borders touching although this is more common in the colon (Figure 14-13). Stay sutures of a 3-0 delayed monofilament suture are placed to ease the procedure. This side-to-side anastomosis is performed similarly to the previously described gastrojejunostomy. Again the residual opening of the bowel is closed either a linear stapler (3.5–4.8 mm staple) or sewn closed with a 3-0 delayed absorbable suture in a careful running fashion.

5. Ileocolic resection

In Hoskins' 1987 description of right ileocolic resection for radiation injury,[24] a hand sewn end-to-end anastomosis was the most common type performed. As staplers have improved, this trend has changed and more stapled anastomoses are being performed.[25] Most of these stapled anastomoses are side-to-side functional end-to-end anastamoses.[25] Key steps in the resection are mobilization of the right colon by finding the white line of Toldt on the right. This overlap of the visceral and parietal peritoneum allows the colon to be medialized and pulled off of Gerota fascia of the kidney, off the duodenum, and off the right ureter. If resecting the entire right colon, then the right lateral omentum must be mobilized off the transverse colon if not previously removed. In addition, the hepatocolic ligament will be incised to free the colon. The ileocolic and right colic arteries should be identified and transected. All of this is done with constant awareness of the location of the right ureter.

A side-to-side functional end-to-end anastomosis is performed by aligning the distal and proximal bowels' 2 antimesenteric sides that are to be connected. These can be held in place with stay sutures or just carefully approximated. A small opening is made through the previous staple lines on the side closest to the other piece of bowel with heavy scissors. A 60- to 80-mm linear stapler/cutter is used to recreate the lumen (Figure 14-10A, B). The right side of the figure demonstrates the residual opening. The bowels are now connected in a side-to-side functional end-to-end anastomosis. The edges of the opening are grasped carefully with Allis or Babcock clamps, and all the edges are brought above the future staple line of the linear stapler. The residual opening is closed with a linear stapler 30- to 60-mm in length with a 3.5- or 4.8-mm load (see Figure 14-10B). Again any tissue above the staple line is removed with a pair of heavy scissors.

Alternatively, the whole procedure can be done by hand. A Cochrane Database review of hand-sewn versus stapled anastomoses in cancer patients has shown that stapled techniques lead to fewer anastomotic leaks.[26,27] This difference was more important in small bowel and small bowel to colon surgery than in colorectal surgery.

Another option is an end-to-end anastomosis with a combination of hand sewing and stapled triangular closure. The area to be resected is identified. Good, healthy areas of bowel are identified proximal and distal to the site to be resected. A window is made just below the bowel wall and bowel clamps (Figures 14-14 and 14-15) are carefully passed just below the bowel edge. A total of four bowel clamps are used so that there is minimal spillage of succus entericus. The bowel is divided with heavy scissors or an electrosurgical unit on cut. The bowel is clamped, cut, and tied with 2-0 or 3-0 braided silk suture on a passing instrument. The resected piece is now handed off and attention is paid to the area to be hand-sewn. A 3-0 delayed absorbable suture is used on the posterior aspect (mesenteric side) of the area to be anastomosed. The bowel wall is inverted. A running suture technique is used for the posterior aspect (one-third to one-half of anastomosis). These stitches are full thickness. The knots can be extraluminally or intraluminally tied. The remaining portion of the anastomosis is sewn with full thickness bites, inverting the mucosa. If the anastomosis appears to be too small, a slit can be made full thickness in the antimesenteric portion of both limbs (spatulating the bowel; Figure 14-16). A triangular closure is then used. The linear stapler linear 30 to 60 mm in length with a 3.5- or 4.8-mm load is used to close 3 times starting on the mesenteric side with the mucosa raised (Figure 14-17). This side has the only staple line on the inside of the lumen. The other parts of the triangle are closed with overlapping staple lines on the external surface (Figures 14-18 and 14-19). This allows the anastomosis to be larger diameter than the actual bowel, which is being joined. Imbricating delayed absorbable sutures can be placed to protect the anastomotic integrity if desired by the surgeon.

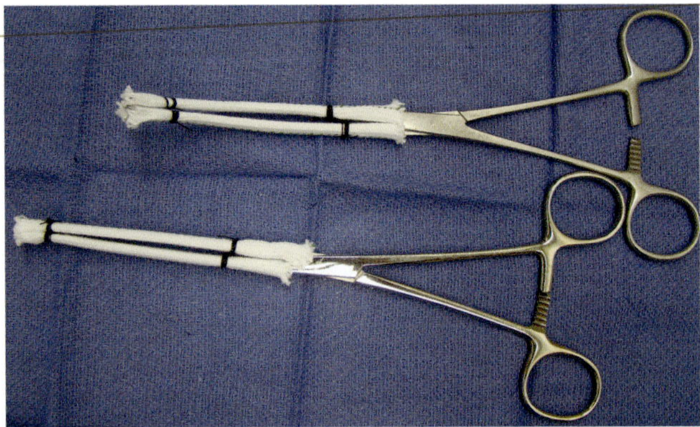

Fig. 14-14. Curved (upper) and straight (lower) linen shod bowel clamps. The linen helps protect the bowel from crush injury.

Large Bowel

1. Right hemicolectomy/ileocolic resection

A right hemicolectomy (ascending colectomy) with ileotransverse anastomosis is described in the section on ileocolic resection above. The resection and anastomosis can be performed either with staplers or by hand.

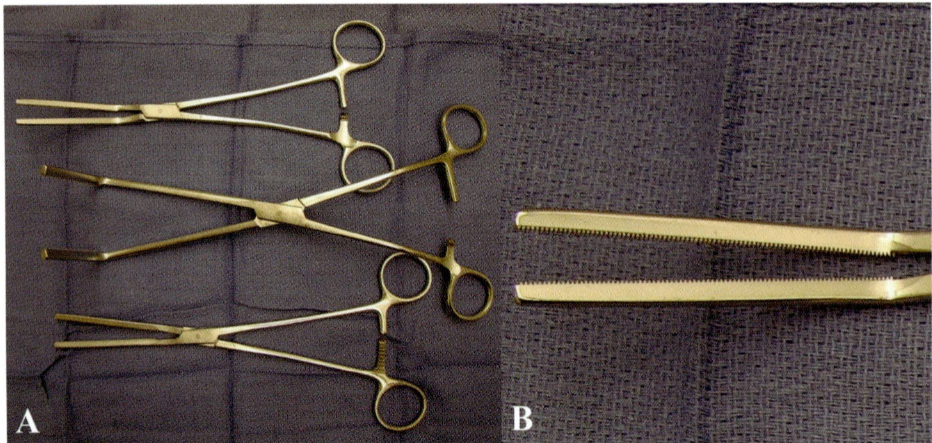

Fig. 14-15. (**A**) Three different Glassman-type bowel clamps are shown. The upper is angled at < 45 degrees. The center clamp is at a right angle. The lower clamp is straight. (**B**) A close up of the small nonpenetrating teeth on the Glassman-type bowel clamps.

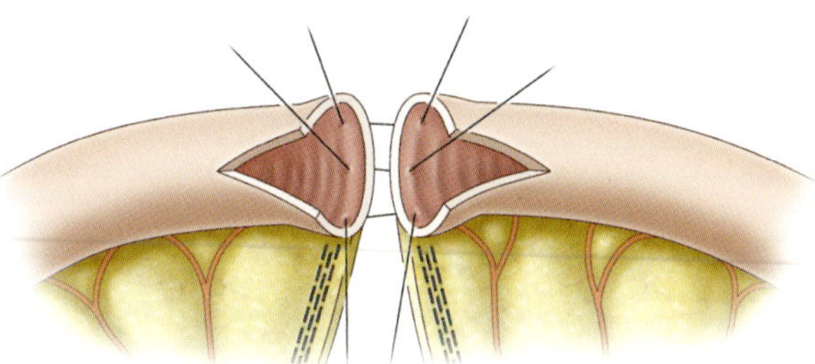

Fig. 14-16. The steps involved in a triangulation technique used to anastomose pieces of bowel that are at risk for stricture is shown in this figure and Figures 14-17 to 14-19. This illustration shows the spatulation of the bowel by cutting an antimesenteric slit to expand the surface being connected.

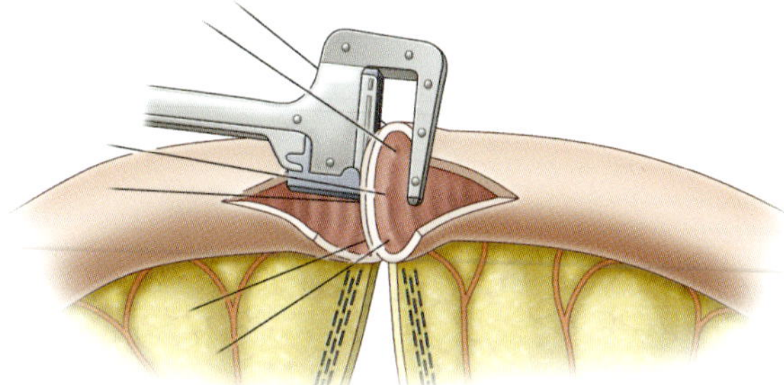

Fig. 14-17. The 2 lengths of bowel are brought together with stay sutures prior to the closure of the base of the triangle (mesenteric side of bowel). Both limbs of bowel have an inverted portion that will be stapled together. Note that this is the only staple line that will be intraluminal.

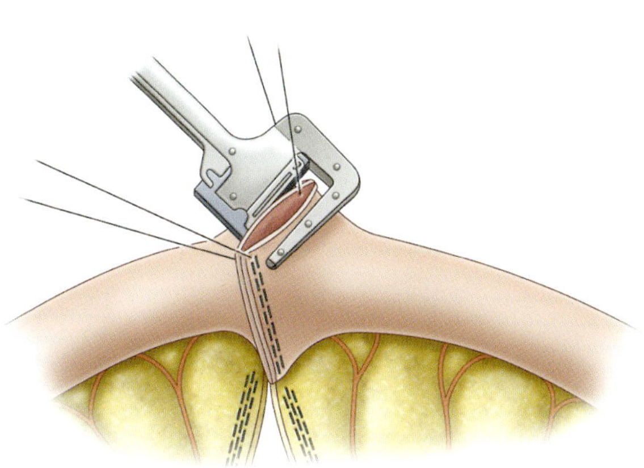

Fig. 14-18. Two sides of the triangular closure are completed. The unseen posterior aspect is intraluminal. A linear stapler has been used to close side 2, and the linear stapler is in place with another load ready to close the final portion of the new anastomosis.

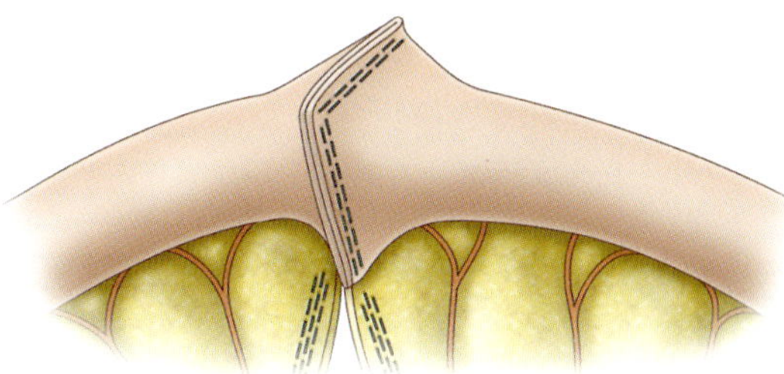

Fig. 14-19. The new anastomosis created in this manner (antimesenteric slits with triangular closure) is larger than either bowels diameter.

2. Transverse colectomy

A transverse colectomy with right-left colonic anastomosis can be performed for debulking or creation of transverse colon incontinent urinary diversion (discussed in Chapter 11). In either situation, if the omentum is present, it must be taken off the colon by going through the avascular plane connecting the omentum to the transverse colon. The hepatocolic and the splenocolic ligaments are transected mobilizing the hepatic and splenic flexures, respectively. The transverse colon is pulled up by gently grasping the bowel with a gloved hand or a gloved hand wrapped with a surgical laparotomy sponge. The middle colic vessels are identified and the area to be resected is identified. Care is made to make sure that the resection margins have a good blood supply. For debulking of a gynecologic malignancy, the middle colic vessels are resected as distally as possible so as not to compromise blood flow to the remaining bowel.

3. Left hemicolectomy

A left hemicolectomy is very similar to a right hemicolectomy but mobilization is even more important so that there is no tension on the anastomosis. Key steps in the resection are mobilization of the left colon by finding the white line of Toldt on the left. If this resection is being performed with a primary debulking of ovarian cancer, then the white line is most easily found by cephalically extending the opening of the posterior broad ligament. This overlap of the visceral and parietal peritoneum allows the colon to be medialized and pulled off of Gerota fascia of the kidney and off the left ureter. If resecting the entire left colon, then the left lateral omentum must be mobilized off the transverse colon if not previously removed. In addition, the splenocolic ligament will be transected to free the colon. Performing the above-described efforts of mobilization will help dramatically when it comes time to anastomose the colon. The inferior mesenteric artery (IMA) and its tributaries are identified. The vessels are ligated as distal as possible since this surgery is for debulking and not for resection of a primary colon cancer. This preservation helps maintain the vascular integrity of the colon. All of this is done with constant awareness of the location of the left ureter. With the descending (left) colon placed medially, the procedure can be performed predominantly from the lateral/ retroperitoneal perspective.

4. Sigmoid colectomy

While general surgeons often take an intraperitoneal approach, we find a retroperitoneal approach is very quick and allows us to identify the ureters most easily. The retroperitoneum is entered by ligating the round ligaments or by tenting up the peritoneum of the pelvis and entering it. The paravesical and pararectal spaces are opened bilaterally. This action identifies the ureters, isolates the sigmoid, and ascertains the position of the sigmoidal vessels. The 60- to 80-mm linear stapler/cutter with a 2.5- to 3.8-mm stapler is fired at the distal resection margin after placing it carefully through a window just below the serosal edge of the bowel. This allows the bowel to remain closed and decreases chance of spillage. If the pelvis is too small to allow a linear stapler/cutter to be used, then a linear stapler 45 to 60 mm in length with 3.5- to 4.8-mm staples can be used. This would have to be used twice and the bowel cut in between the placement of the 2 loads because this device does not have a knife. Alternatively, the surgeon could choose to leave the resected area open and just cut proximal to the distal staple line. Attention is then paid to the proximal point of resection. Ideally, this proximal resection should take place upstream to the critical area of Sudeck. This point where the last branch of the IMA is joined by the superior hemorrhoidal artery from the internal iliac artery is a watershed area and an area of possible ischemia. A 60- to 80-mm linear stapler/cutter with a 2.5- to 3.8-mm stapler is placed and fired at the proximal margin of resection. The mesentery of the sigmoid is resected and the specimen is sent to pathology (Figure 14-20).

5. Low colorectal resection (Low anterior resection)

In gynecologic oncology, a low colorectal resection/low anterior resection may be performed for a variety of reasons, including debulking, bowel obstruction, fistula repair, and pelvic exenteration.[28,29] To most easily perform this operation, the patient should be in low lithotomy position with Allen-type stirrups. The vertical abdominal incision is extended from the pubic symphysis into the upper abdomen. Small bowel is packed away. As described in the section of sigmoid colectomy, the retroperitoneum is entered and the paravesical and pararectal spaces are created. The procedure can either be performed en bloc with the uterus or independently. The rectum needs to be isolated posteriorly, laterally, and anteriorly. Only the anterior dissection is changed by the presence of the uterus. With the opening of the retroperitoneum, the dissection is made much easier. Posteriorly, the rectum is separated from Waldeyer's fascia. This is most easily accomplished by dividing the rectococcygeal ligament (anterior-posterior orientation) with an endoscopic linear stapler/cutter 45-60 mm long with a 2.5-mm staple load. Bilaterally, the rectal pillars comprise the rectal (hemorrhoidal) vessels and the corresponding ligaments. These are isolated with gentle blunt dissection anterior and posteriorly on each side and an endoscopic linear stapler/cutter 45 to 60 mm long with a 2.5-mm staple is placed and fired on both sides. This action is repeated until the caudal extent of the dissection is reached. Anteriorly, if the uterus is being spared, the posterior peritoneum just below the cervix is entered. Denonvilliers fascia is identified and pushed anteriorly separating the vagina from the rectum. Once the caudal margin of resection is identified a linear stapler 45 mm in length with a 3.5- or 4.8-mm load is placed and fired. If the surgeon wants the bowel closed, then the 45-mm linear stapler with a 3.5- or 4.8-mm load is placed and fired, and the bowel is cut with scissors in between the staple lines. The specimen is then sent to pathology for examination.

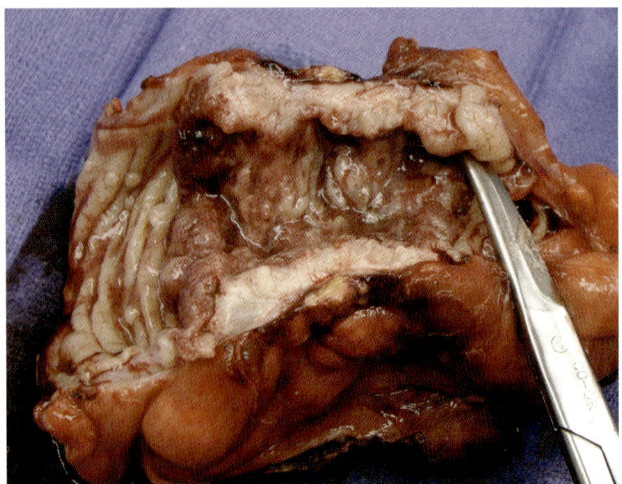

Fig. 14-20. Small section of sigmoid colon is shown. Near the left side (away from scissors) is a circumferential ovarian cancer metastasis to the bowel mucosa.

6. Colorectal anastomosis

End-to-end anastomosis can be performed for low anterior resection with colorectal re-anastomosis. Although a large meta-analysis demonstrated no difference in anastomotic leak rated comparing staplers to hand-sewn, the same analysis did show that stapled anastomoses are performed more quickly.[27] A sizing device from 25 to 31 mm is used to determine the correct size that should be used. The circular stapler/cutters used for end-to-end anastomoses range from an external diameter of 21 to 33 mm with staples from 3.5 to 4.8 mm. Too large a diameter device will thin the bowel and lead to breakdown. Too small a diameter device will lead to stricture. Figure 14-12 shows the anvil, which is placed in the proximal bowel lumen. The opening is then closed with a 3-0 monofilament suture in a purse string technique. Because this suture will be removed by the anastomosis, it does not matter whether the monofilament suture is absorbable or not. The end of the hand piece with the spike retracted is gently advanced through anus and into the rectum. It is guided until the ring of the hand piece can be seen near the previous distal limb staple line. The spike in the hand piece is advanced until it passes either through or near the previous staple line. Once it is fully advanced, the sharp spike can be carefully removed and the anvil (in the proximal loop of bowel) and receiving piece attached to the hand piece are engaged with an audible click. The device is then closed by twisting until a green line appears in the window of the hand piece. At this point the stapler/cutter is fired, and the device is carefully opened approximately one and one half turns. The device is removed along with the anvil from the proximal limb of bowel by gently rotating the hand piece 90 to 180 degrees back and forth until the entire device is removed from the rectum and anus. Now the two tissue rings or "doughnuts" are examined to make sure they are complete. The "flat tire test" is performed to check the integrity of the anastomosis by filling the pelvis above the level of the anastomosis with warm water. The bowel proximal to the ring anastomosis is occluded with a hand gently. A red rubber catheter with a large 60 to 120 mL wide mouth syringe is advanced to just distal to the anastomosis. Air in the syringe is pushed quickly into the bowel lumen, and the presence of an anastomotic leak will be detected by bubbles appearing in the water. This can be performed 1 to 3 times to be certain. If a leak is detected, an imbricating layer of 3-0 delayed absorbable sutures can be placed and the flat tire test repeated. Alternatively, the anastomosis can be taken down and redone if the leak is more than 25% of the anastomotic diameter.[30]

If a large portion of the rectum or the entire rectum is resected, then a j-pouch can be made using colon or ileum (see Figure 14-1).[9] To do this type of anastomosis, the remaining colon is mobilized until the residual proximal large intestine can be brought without tension into the pelvis. The apex to which the distal bowel is going to be anastomosed to is identified. This technique will be described in further detail in Chapter 15.

7. Colostomy formation

Colostomies, like ileostomies, may be placed in patients to protect more distal anastomoses or as an end ostomy. Similar to the small intestine, diverting ostomies can either be an end or a loop ileostomy. Loop ostomies add the benefit that a closure of the ostomy to reintroduce bowel continuity can be performed in a minimally invasive manner through just the ostomy site.

A loop ostomy is made by first creating a quarter-size opening in the skin with the cut mode of the electrosurgical unit. The subcutaneous tissue is not removed and it is just pushed to the sides. The assistant or the nondominant hand pushes up from inside the abdomen and a cruciate incision is made in the fascia. A cruciate incision is used to decrease the chances of the fascia constricting the bowel. The fibers of the rectus are pushed apart (and not cut) to decrease parastomal hernia. The site for the opening in the bowel is marked by bluntly passing a vessel loop or small diameter Penrose drain through the mesentery just below the bowel wall. The previously identified is gently brought through the ostomy site using a combination of pushing from below and gentle traction with either a Babcock clamp or the vessel loop from above. Once the bowel is brought up through the ostomy above the skin level (5–6 cm), an ostomy bar is used to replace the vessel loop. As small a length bar as possible is used to ease ostomy appliance placement. The bar is sewn to the skin edge with an absorbable monofilament. Often, the ostomy is not matured until the vertical skin incision is closed. The rosebud is created at the cardinal points with either a 3-0 absorbable monofilament or a 3-0 absorbable-braided suture.

8. Colostomy closure

The closure of a diverting or end colostomy is very similar to the closure of the analogous ileostomy and is covered in that section. A few minor differences exist. First, the larger length linear stapler/cutter with thick staples is often needed.

POSTOPERATIVE CARE

Box 14-3 PERIOPERATIVE MORBIDITY

- Ileus/gastroparesis/Ogilvie syndrome
- Small bowel obstruction
- Pelvic abscess/anastomotic leak

Bowel Obstruction or Ileus

Either a mechanical bowel obstruction or a paralytic ileus can occur after any surgery in the abdominal cavity. Although ileus is a loss of functional activity anywhere from the stomach to the colon, bowel obstruction is a mechanical blockage. These mechanical obstructions are often caused by adhesive scar tissue. The use of hyaluronic acid/carboxymethyl cellulose membrane reduces the incidence, extent, and severity of adhesions in the abdomen. However, it does not decrease the rate of intestinal obstruction or need for operative intervention. Hyaluronic acid/carboxymethyl cellulose membrane should not be wrapped around an anastomosis because there may be an increased risk of leak.[31]

Ileus in the stomach is often referred to as gastroparesis. It is especially common in women with glucose intolerance, hyperglycemia, or overt diabetes. Some level of postoperative gastroparesis exists in most patients after exploratory laparotomy for 24 to 48 hours after surgery. For mild-to-moderate cases, dietary management (small amounts at a time) is the mainstay of treatment.[32]

After elective major gynecologic abdominal surgery, it has been shown that oral intake may be safely started on postoperative day 1.[33] Starting feeding results in quicker release from the hospital, but may also result in increased postoperative nausea. Because bowel obstruction and adynamic ileus are both significant causes of prolonged hospital stay and increased cost, many trials have been performed utilizing the routine use of prokinetic agents. In general, the routine use of erythromycin, cholecystokinin, cisapride, dopamine-antagonists, propranolol, or vasopressin has not been shown to be effective or the side effects are too great (cisapride).[34] More data are needed regarding the routine use of neostigmine or intravenous lidocaine. Evidence does support the use of neostigmine 2 mg intravenously for the specific treatment of Ogilvie syndrome.[35]

Identification of ileus versus small bowel obstruction can be undertaken by the use of computed tomography (CT) or flat plate roentgenograms. CT not only gives better resolution in diagnosis, but it may offer a therapeutic benefit when water soluble contrast is used.[36,37] Once ileus is diagnosed, the current mainstay of treatment is use of nasogastric tube, intravenous fluids, or parenteral nutrition if without food for at least 7 days, and patience. Some data have shown benefit to the therapeutic ingestion of water-soluble contrast.[36]

When a bowel obstruction is diagnosed, the acuity of the patient needs to be determined. If the patient is stable and does not require emergent surgical intervention, then patience is the operative word along with a nasogastric tube and either intravenous fluids or parenteral nutrition if without food for at least 7 days. CT with water-soluble contrast can be performed 3 to 5 after diagnosis of the obstruction.[37] Conflicting data exist as to how long one can wait for spontaneous resolution to occur, in general, patience and time can be used for resolution if the patient's acuity does not change.

Abscesses and Anastomotic Leaks

The actual reported rate of intestinal anastomotic leaks varies greatly by the reports and whether the paper is describing testing all anastomoses with water soluble contrast (≤ 50% leaks found) or leaks that present themselves clinically (1%–30%).[2] So, although a small leak may be present in up to half and not clinically significant, a clinically significant leakage should be treated with broad spectrum and percutaneous drainage. If this fails after 24 to 48 hours, then repeat water-soluble contrast-based CT imaging should be repeated. If further CT guided drain placement is not of value, or peritonitis develops, then laparotomy and drainage is required for a patient who would survive the repeat surgery.

Abscesses can develop postoperatively because of anastomotic leaks, anastomotic hemorrhage, fecal spill at surgery, or hematoma formation. The most common time of formation is 1 to 2 weeks but they have been reported up to 6 weeks after anastomosis. Typical signs and symptoms at presentation are abdominal pain; malaise; intermittent fever; diarrhea, constipation, or ileus; elevated or severely decreased white blood count; a poor defined pelvic mass. Again, CT with water-soluble oral and rectal contrast allows both identification and possible placement of a drain if feasible. Broad-spectrum antibiotics are used until cultures identify a more specific choice. Surgery can now usually be avoided due to radiologic placement of drains. Strictures can develop on their own or after a complication such as these and so one should watch for them after a complication.

LONG-TERM OUTCOMES

Box 14-4 DELAYED COMPLICATIONS

- Malabsorption
- Fistulas
  - Enterocutaneous
  - Enterovaginal
  - Enterovesical

Delayed Complications

Absorption problems can arise if too much distal ileum has to be removed for obstruction or debulking. Because the terminal portion of the ileum is responsible for absorption of fat-soluble vitamins (A, D, E, K) plus vitamin B12, patients may need parental supplementation of these vitamins if resected. If the patient further develops a difficulty in absorbing high-molecular-weight fats (especially after pelvic radiation), intractable diarrhea can ensue. Diarrhea can also occur for a different reason if a large amount of colon is removed. Walter and Silver have both discussed the role of bulking agents and antidiarrheals in this patient to decrease stool frequency and increase control.[9,10]

Enterocutaneous, enterovaginal, and/or enterovesical fistulas are uncommon complications that are dreaded by most surgeons. Once a fistula is considered, a patient is started on intravenous broad-spectrum antibiotics to decrease infection. The patient is not allowed to eat (NPO) pending results of the work-up. The first step in working up a fistula from the gastrointestinal tract is determining the site of origin. Because fistulas can be either simple (bowel directly to skin or vagina) or complex (bowel to cavity to skin or vagina), one cannot always tell the origin of the fistula by the appearance of the effluent. We recommend starting with a Gastrografin enema or CT of the abdomen and pelvis with intravenous, water-soluble oral, and water-soluble rectal contrast. If you do not start with rectal contrast, then it may be days before you are able to tell if it is a colonic fistula.

If a small intestine fistula is found, then the next step is determining the amount of output. Low output fistulas (< 100 mL/day) may heal rapidly with complete bowel rest, either intravenous fluids or parenteral nutrition if without food for at least 7 days, and careful isolation of the effluent in an ostomy appliance if possible. It is much easier to control the effluent in an enterocutaneous than an enterovaginal fistula. High output fistulas can be changed into low output fistulas by the use of subcutaneous or intravenous somatostatin or somatostatin analogues.[38] Using low doses of the somatostatin analogues do not appear to be effective in helping close a fistula, but high doses (up to 1500 mcg subcutaneous every 8 hours) can be tolerated and effective knowing that hyperglycemia may occur.[38] Rahbour et al[39] have shown in a large meta-analysis that intravenous continuous

Table 14-1. Reasons for failure of a fistula to close without surgery.

F	Foreign bodies
R	Radiation injury
I	Infection or inflammation
E	Epithelialization of the tract
N	Neoplasia
D	Distal obstruction

somatostatin may be better than separate subcutaneous, intravenous, or intramuscular somatostatin analogue (ie, octreotide) injections but this needs to be confirmed by randomized trial.

If a fistula does not close either spontaneously or with bowel rest and somatostatin, then the reason for failure need to be considered (Table 14-1). This simple mnemonic "FRIEND" explains the common reasons for failure of a fistula to close. Often in bowel surgery, a staple in an anastomotic line may be the foreign body causing the fistula to remain open. If the reason can be reversed, then the fistula can be closed. There are currently multiple options available for attempted closure from open surgical to laparoscopic to endoscopic or percutaneous closure. Little data other than case reports and case studies exist, so the gynecologic oncologist at this point should rely on experience to determine the best method for their patient.

SUMMARY

The optimal treatment for women initially presenting with epithelial ovarian, fallopian tube, or peritoneal cancer is radical debulking followed by adjuvant chemotherapy.[40] Although some recommendations regarding CT features suggestive of unresectability exist, there are no readily agreed upon objective criteria that enable gynecologic oncologists to determine whom would be best directed to undergo neoadjuvant chemotherapy because of a high risk of major morbidity or mortality from primary debulking.[41] To maximally debulk, bowel resections are often needed. With proper patient selection, preoperative, intraoperative, and postoperative care, multiple bowel resections can be tolerated by the patient.

REFERENCES

1. Geisler JP, Linnemeier GC, Thomas AJ, Manahan KJ. Nutritional assessment using prealbumin as an objective criterion to determine whom should not undergo primary radical cytoreductive surgery for ovarian cancer. *Gynecol Oncol.* 2007;106:128-131.
2. Morrow CP, Curtin JP. *Gynecologic Cancer Surgery.* New York: Churchill Livingstone, New York.; 1996.
3. Geisler JP, Stowell MJ, Melton ME, Maloney CD, Geisler HE. Extramammary Paget's disease of the vulva recurring in a skin graft. *Gynecol Oncol.* 1995;56:446-447.
4. Walter AC, Manahan KJ, Geisler JP. Morbidity of partial gastrectomy in primary ovarian cytoreduction. *J Gyn Surg.* 2010;46:243-245.
5. Chi DS, Diaz JP, Jamagin WR. Distal partial gastrectomy and gastrojejunal anastomosis for recurrent ovarian cancer. *Gynecol Oncol.* 2007;104:S33-S36.
6. Hoffman MS, Tebes SJ, Sayer RA, et al. Extended cytoreduction of intraabdominal metastatic ovarian cancer in the left upper quadrant utilizing en bloc resection. *Am J Obstet Gynecol.* 2007;197:209.e1-209.e5.
7. Bristow RE, del Carmen MG, Kaufman HS, Montz FJ. Radical oophorectomy with primary stapled colorectal anastomosis for resection of locally advanced epithelial ovarian cancer. *J Am Coll Surg.* 2003;197: 565-574.
8. Tebes SJ, Cardosi R, Hoffman MS. Colorectal resection in patients with ovarian and primary peritoneal carcinoma. *Am J Obstet Gynecol.* 2006;195:585-589.
9. Walter AC, Manahan KM, Geisler JP. Total colectomy in primary ovarian cytoreduction. *Eur J Gynecol Oncol.* 2011;23:487-490.
10. Silver DF, Zgheib NB. Extended left colon resections as part of complete cytoreduction for ovarian cancer: tips and considerations. *Gynecol Oncol.* 2009;114:427-430.
11. Sagar PM, Pemberton JH. Intraoperative, postoperative and reoperative problems with ileoanal pouches. *Brit J Surg.* 2012;99:454-468.
12. Ronco DA, Manahan KJ, Geisler JP. Ovarian cancer risk assessment: a tool for preoperative assessment. *Eur J Obstet Gynecol Reprod Biol.* 2011;158:325-329.
13. Turnbull RB, Weakley FL. *Atlas of Intestinal Stomas.* St. Louis, MO: CV Mosby; 1967.
14. Fazio VW, Church JM, Chu JW. *Atlas of Intestinal Stomas.* New York: Springer; 2012.
15. Moslemi-Kebria M, El-Nashar SA, Aletti GD, Cliby WA. Intraoperative hypothermia during cytoreductive surgery for ovarian cancer and perioperative morbidity. *Obstet Gynecol.* 2012;119:590-596.
16. Cannon JA, Altom LK, Deierhoi RJ, et al. Preoperative oral antibiotics reduce surgical site infection following elective colorectal resections. *Dis Colon Rectum.* 2012;55:1160-1166.
17. Choy PYG, Bissett IP, Docherty JG, Parry BR, Merrie A, Fitzgerald A. Stapled versus handsewn methods for ileocolic anastomoses. *Cochrane Database Syst Rev.* 2011;(9):CD004320.
18. Demyttenaere SV, Nau P, Henn M, et al. Barbed suture for gastrointestinal closure: a randomized control trial. *Surg Innov.* 2009;16:237-242.
19. Ruge J, Vazquez RM. An analysis of the advantages of Stamm and percutaneous endoscopic gastrostomy. *Surg Gynecol Obstet.* 1986;162: 13-16.
20. Winter WE, McBroom JW, Carlson JW, Rose GS, Elkas JC. The utility of gastrojejunostomy in secondary cytoreduction and palliation of proximal intestinal obstruction in recurrent ovarian cancer. *Gynecol Oncol.* 2003;91:261-264.
21. Pothuri B, Montemarano M, Gerardi M, et al. Percutaneous endoscopic gastrostomy tube placement in patients with malignant bowel obstruction due to ovarian carcinoma. *Gynecol Oncol.* 2005;96:330-334.
22. Myers SR, Rothermel WS Jr, Shaffer L. The effect of tissue compression on circular stapler line failure. *Surg Endoscop.* 2011;25:3043-3049.
23. Gustavsson K, Gunnarsson U, Jestin P. Postoperative complications after closure of a diverting ileostoma—differences according to closure technique. *Int J Colorect Dis.* 2012;27:55-58.
24. Hoskins WJ, Burke TW, Weiser EB, Heller PB, Grayson J, Park RC. Right hemicolectomy and ileal resection with primary reanastomosis for irradiation injury of the terminal ileum. *Gynecol Oncol.* 1987;26:215-224.
25. Leung TT, MacLean AR, Buie WD, Dixon E. Comparison of stapled versus handsewn loop ileostomy closure: a meta-analysis. *J Gastro Surg.* 2008;12:939-944.
26. Choy PYG, Bissett IP, Docherty JG, Parry BR, Merrie A, Fitzgerald A. Stapled versus handsewn methods for ileocolic anastomoses. *Cochrane Database Syst Rev.* 2011;(9):CD004320.
27. Neutzling CB, Lustosa SAS, Proenca IM, da Silva EMK, Matos D. Stapled versus handsewn methods for colorectal anastomosis surgery. *Cochrane Database Syst Rev.* 2012;(2):CD003144.

28. Geisler JP, Wiemann MC, Geisler HE. Optimal cytoreductive surgery in the elderly woman with stage IIIc serous cystadenocarcinoma of the ovary. *J Pelvic Surg.* 1995;1:2-5.
29. Geisler JP, Wiemann MC, Geisler HE. Pelvic exenteration in the elderly female. *J Pelvic Surg.* 1995;1:204-209.
30. Fouda E, El Nakeeb A, Magdy A, Hammad EA, Othman G, Farid M. Early detection of anastomotic leakage after elective low anterior resection. *J Gastro Surg.* 2011;15:137-144.
31. Kumar S, Wong PF, Leaper DJ. Intra-peritoneal prophylactic agents for preventing adhesions and adhesive intestinal obstruction after non-gynaecological abdominal surgery. *Cochrane Database Syst Rev.* 2009.
32. Keld R, Kinsey L, Athwal V, Lal S. Pathogenesis, investigation and dietary and medical management of gastroparesis. *J Hum Nutr Diet.* 2011;24:421-430.
33. Charoenkwan K, Phillipson G, Vutyavanich T. Early versus delayed oral fluids and food for reducing complications after major abdominal gynaecologic surgery. *Cochrane Database Syst Rev.* 2007.
34. Traut U, Brügger L, Kunz R, et al. Systemic prokinetic pharmacologic treatment for postoperative adynamic ileus following abdominal surgery in adults. *Cochrane Database Syst Rev.* 2008.
35. Ponec RJ, Saunders MD, Kimmey MD. Neostigmine for the treatment of acute colonic pseudo-obstruction. *N Engl J Med.* 1999;341:137-141.
36. Abbas S, Bissett IP, Parry BR. Oral water soluble contrast for the management of adhesive small bowel obstruction. *Cochrane Database Syst Rev.* 2007.
37. Maung AA, Johnson DC, Piper GL, et al. Evaluation and management of small-bowel obstruction: an Eastern Association for the Surgery of Trauma practice management guideline. *J Trauma Acute Care Surg.* 2012;73:s362-s369.
38. Geisler JP, Manahan KJ. Increasing somatostatin analogues until effective. *Gynecol Oncol.* 2005;96:906.
39. Rahbour G, Siddiqui MR, Ullah MR, Gabe SM, Warusavitarne J, Vaizey CJ. A meta-analysis of outcomes following use of somatostatin and its analogues for the management of enterocutaneous fistulas. *Ann Surg.* 2012;56:946-954.
40. Chi DS, Eisenhauer EL, Lang J, et al. What is the goal of primary cytoreductive surgery for bulky stage IIIC epithelial ovarian carcinoma (EOC)? *Gynecol Oncol.* 2006;103:559-564.
41. Lee SJ, Kim BG, Lee JW, Park CS, Lee JH, Bae DS. Preliminary results of neoadjuvant chemotherapy with paclitaxel and cisplatin in patients with advanced epithelial ovarian cancer who are inadequate for optimum primary surgery. *J Obstet Gynaecol Res.* 2006;32:99-106.

Chapter 15. Ileal Pouch Anal Anastomosis

David F. Silver, MD and
Beman Khulpateea, MD

BACKGROUND

The ileal pouch anal anastomosis (IPAA) procedure, also known as ileoanal anastomosis or restorative proctocolectomy, was developed in the 1970s by Sir Alan Parks in London. It was offered as an alternative to performing a Brooke end ileostomy for patients who underwent total colectomies for a variety of diagnoses, most commonly inflammatory bowel disease.[1,2] The Parks' procedure offered important advantages over the previously used ileoanal end-to-end anastomosis (without a pouch reservoir), which resulted in poor functional outcomes, including higher fecal frequency, urgency, and incontinence rates.[3-5] With the addition of a pouch that serves as a lower pressure reservoir, patients are offered the quality-of-life advantage of restoring the continuity of their intestinal tracts, which obviates the need for permanent abdominal wall stomas (and ostomy appliances). When performed on properly selected patients, high rates of fecal continence and patient satisfaction can be expected.[6,7]

Over the past several decades minor modifications in the IPAA procedure have been suggested; however, the basic principles of the surgery have been maintained. Parks' original reservoir was created as an S-shaped (or 3-limbed) ileal pouch.[2] Alternatives to the 3-limbed S-pouch are the 4-limbed W-pouch and the 2-limbed J-pouch (Figure 15-1). Because fecal continence rates are equal in all the pouch designs, and the 2-limbed approach offers the greatest amount of surgical ease and a lower complication rate, the J-pouch ileoanal anastomosis is most commonly used and is our preferred technique. Other modifications have included the addition of an anorectal mucosectomy (important for primary colonic disorders such as colon cancer, polyposis, or inflammatory bowel disease) and the use of hand-sewn versus stapled techniques.[8-10] We believe that the most appropriate technique for patients who undergo an IPAA following radical pelvic resections for gynecologic cancers is a stapled ileal J-pouch anal anastomosis. It is a complex procedure that should be performed by experienced surgeons.

INDICATIONS AND CLININCAL APPLICATIONS

The IPAA is most commonly performed after total colectomy for patients with ulcerative colitis or familial adenomatous polyposis.[6,11,12] Although Crohn disease is a relative contraindication to performing this procedure due to concerns for the development of Crohn enteritis and higher risks for pouch complications, patients with Crohn disease can be cautiously offered this option if total colectomy is required.[13-15] Toxic megacolon is another indication for colectomy and IPAA.[16] Patients with colon cancer may also be offered this restorative procedure following colectomy if appropriate counseling with regard to the potential risk of recurrent cancer to the remaining bowel is provided.[17-19]

There is very little published data with respect to the use of the IPAA in patients who undergo radical surgical procedures for gynecologic cancers.[20] Although total (or subtotal) colectomy is rarely indicated for gynecologic cancer resections, selected patients with advanced ovarian, fallopian tube, peritoneal, or endometrial carcinomas may benefit from radical cytoreductive surgeries that include extended colectomies.[20-23] Such surgical procedures are performed with curative intent in well-selected patients. In most cases, resection of the entire rectum below the pelvic peritoneal reflection is not necessary to achieve the goal of completely debulking visible metastatic disease. Therefore, subtotal—rather than total—colectomy is usually employed in such instances when visible cancer involves the serosal surfaces of all segments of the colon. If complete surgical cytoreduction is achieved, which is associated with a relatively high rate of survival, it is reasonable to perform IPAA to provide these women with restored bowel continuity and maintenance of quality of life.

ANATOMIC CONSIDERATIONS

Superior Mesenteric Artery

The superior mesenteric artery (SMA) arises from the aorta behind the inferior edge of the pancreas and crosses over the duodenum anteriorly (where the duodenum transitions from its third to its fourth segment) to enter the root of the small bowel mesentery. The superior mesenteric artery trunk extends toward the terminal ileum at a location approximately 15 to 20 cm proximal to the cecum. At this location it forms an anastomosis with a branch of one of its own arterial branches—the ileal branch of the superior mesenteric artery. Prior to (and more proximal to) joining the ileal branch of the ileocolic artery, the superior mesenteric artery gives rise to a dozen or so jejunal and ileal branches, which subsequently anastomose

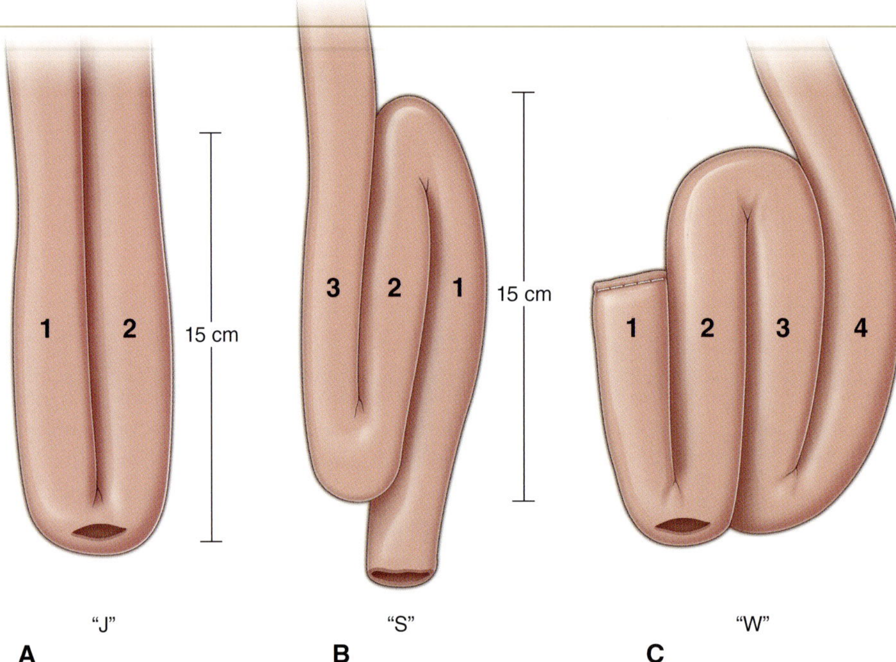

Fig. 15-1. Pouch design options. The 2-limbed J-pouch, 3-limbed S-pouch, and 4-limbed W-pouch are depicted.

to form arcades, which then give rise to the vasa recta, that provide the capillary blood supply to the small intestine.

Ileocolic Artery

The ileocolic artery typically branches from the superior mesenteric artery approximately 3 to 5 cm from its origin and travels within the small bowel mesentery toward the junction of the ileum and cecum. As described above, one of its terminal branches is the ileal branch which doubles back to travel proximally through the ileal mesentery to anastomose with the superior mesenteric artery. The ileal branch of the ileocolic artery travels parallel to and approximately 3 to 4 cm from the serosal surface of the ileum. It provides the terminal ileum with its blood supply via the vasa recta. Knowing this blood supply is imperative to accomplishing an adequate mobilization of the small bowel to ensure a tension-free pouch-anal anastomosis (Figure 15-2).

Duodenum, Pancreas, and Surrounding Structures

On occasion, when additional mobilization of the small bowel is required, a Kocher maneuver may be performed. When utilizing this maneuver, an understanding of the anatomy surrounding the first 3 segments of the duodenum and its neighboring retroperitoneal structures is needed. The first part of the duodenum arises from the gastric pylorus to travel toward the right and posteriorly. The second and third segments travel inferiorly and then toward the left and are overlapped by the head of the pancreas. At the distal end of the third segment of the duodenum (where it becomes the fourth and final segment), the superior mesenteric vessels can be found crossing anteriorly. It should be recognized that the bile duct passes posterior to the first part of the duodenum to join the pancreatic duct where they empty into the duodenal (or hepatopancreatic) ampulla in the medial aspect of the second part of the duodenum. The vena cava and aorta are located posterior to the first 3 parts of the duodenum and the head of the pancreas. At this level the celiac trunk arises from the aorta posterior to the superior edge of the pancreas and the superior mesenteric artery arise between the posterior edge of the pancreas and the third and fourth segments of the duodenum.

PREOPERATIVE PREPARATION

Box 15-1 KEY SURGICAL INSTRUMENTATION

- 80-mm linear stapler with 3.5-mm staple size
- 60-mm thoracoabdominal stapler with 3.5-mm staple size
- 28- to 29-mm circular stapler with 3.5-mm staple size
- LigaSure (Valleylab, Boulder, Colorado) device or 45-mm linear stapler with 2.0-mm staple size
- 3-0 monofilament, delayed-absorbable suture

Extent of Disease

Although it is well established that there is no preoperative imaging test that accurately details the extent of disease for

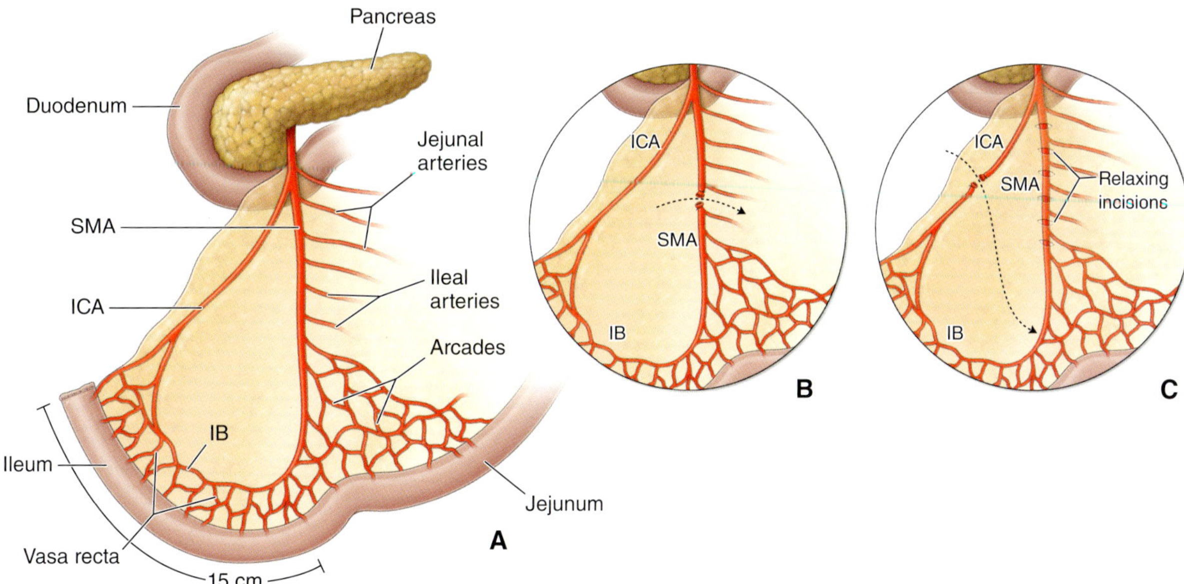

Fig. 15-2. Anatomy of the small bowel mesentery and mobilization options. (**A**) Normal structures relevant to surgical anatomy. (**B**) The SMA is divided and ligated distal to the last jejunal branch. A window is created in the mesentery by dividing it perpendicular to the SMA. The dotted line depicts the line of surgical division. (**C**) The ICA is divided and ligated proximal to its IB. The mesentery is then divided parallel to the ileum toward the SMA. The dotted line depicts the line of surgical division. If further mobilization is required then relaxing incisions are made on the peritoneum along the mesenteric path of the SMA. IB = ileal branch of the ICA, ICA = ileocolic artery, SMA = superior mesenteric artery.

patients with metastatic gynecologic carcinomas, it is advisable to establish whether the disease is confined to the peritoneal cavity prior to attempting a complete and radical cytoreductive surgery in most situations. On our service, preoperative computed tomography (CT) of the chest, abdomen, and pelvis is obtained. If thoracic metastases are identified, then we would advocate a maximal thoracic and intraperitoneal cytoreductive effort on selected patients, however, would not recommend an IPAA because there are not enough published data to establish that survival rates are as good as with complete cytoreduction of intraperitoneal disease alone. If preoperative imaging does not identify metastatic disease beyond the peritoneal cavity and intraoperative assessments determine that an extended colectomy is necessary for complete cytoreduction, then the option of performing IPAA is entertained.

Performance Status

For patients undergoing radical resections with or without reconstructive surgical procedures such as the ileal pouch anal anastomosis, outcomes are directly related to preoperative performance status.[22,24] In addition to evaluating the immediate preoperative performance status, we also inquire about the performance status 1 month prior to presentation. IPAA procedures are considered for women who have an immediate preoperative Gynecologic Oncology Group performance status of 0 to 1. Although there is no validation to the predictive value of a remote performance status, in our experience patients with immediate preoperative performance statuses equal to 1 who had a 1-month preoperative performance status equal to 0 have outcomes similar to those with immediate preoperative performance statuses equal to 0.

Medical and Nutritional Status

Blood work, including a comprehensive metabolic panel and complete blood count, are obtained. Electrolyte derangements and anemia are corrected as needed. Medical and cardiac clearance is obtained on selected patients, depending on their medical history and current well being. If the patient is malnourished with albumen levels less than 2.0 mg/dL, then perioperative nutritional counseling is recommended and the possibility of nutritional supplementation and total parenteral nutrition in the postoperative period is discussed (although it is not necessary for the pouch anal anastomosis procedure specifically). Due to the catabolic nature of advanced malignant disease, it is usually not effective or advisable to delay surgery to attempt to restore nutritional status preoperatively in these patients.

Anal Sphincter Competence

Although anodynamic testing can be utilized to document appropriate anal sphincter pressures and continence, it is not possible to accurately select those patients who will require subtotal colectomies as part of their radical gynecologic cancer procedure. Therefore, a simple history of bowel function and fecal continence along with an interactive rectal examination is performed on all gynecologic cancer patients in the preoperative setting. This will determine with reasonably good accuracy which patients have adequate sphincter competence when considering an IPAA as part of their reconstruction after radical surgery.

Bowel Preparation and Enterostomal Therapy Consultation

A complete mechanical bowel preparation is recommended prior to surgery that may include colon resection with or without IPAA. Appropriate prophylactic antibiotics should be administered preoperatively and may be continued up to 23 hours postoperatively at the discretion of the surgeon. The combination of subcutaneously administered heparin and pneumatic compression stockings are used for deep venous thrombosis (DVT) prophylaxis perioperatively. Because the decision to create an IPAA is ultimately made at the time of surgery and since the procedure is frequently performed in 2 stages, it is beneficial to consult the enterostomal therapist to appropriately counsel the patient about life with a stoma and to mark the abdomen for temporary or permanent stomas dependent on intraoperative determinations.

SURGICAL PROCEDURE

Box 15-2 MASTER SURGEON'S PRINCIPLES

- Mobilization of the small intestine for the creation of a tension-free pouch-anal anastomosis
  - Divide all small bowel mesenteric attachments along the right side of the mesentery, up to and including the attachments to the third part of the duodenum
  - Consider dividing the ileocolic artery
  - Alternatively, consider dividing the superior mesenteric artery
  - Relaxing incisions on the peritoneal surface of the mesentery along the path of the superior mesenteric artery (if the SMA is left intact)
  - Kocher maneuver

Mobilization of the Small Intestine

The peritoneal pattern of metastatic spread of adnexal, peritoneal, and endometrial adenocarcinomas rarely involves the anus or rectum below the pelvic peritoneal reflection. Therefore, if the serosal surfaces of the cecum, ascending, transverse, and descending colon are involved with substantial metastases, a subtotal colectomy should adequately remove all visible disease without resecting the anus or significant length of the extraperitoneal rectum. If a subtotal colectomy is required for maximal cytoreduction, then other radical procedures are likely to be needed as part of the same surgical effort. Upon completion of the tumor-resection-phase of surgery, if the colon was removed and the patient is deemed a reasonable candidate for reconstructive procedures, then the ileal J-pouch anal anastomosis is considered.

The ileal pouch will be constructed from the distal 30 cm of the terminal ileum, creating a 15-cm long reservoir with double the circumference of the ileum. The distal (or efferent) end of the pouch will be anastomosed to the rectum (or anus). By grasping the ileum 15 cm from its distal end with an atraumatic clamp (such as a Babcock) the segment can be pulled deep into the pelvis to the rectal stump to evaluate the feasibility of establishing a tension-free anastomosis. In some instances, the distal loop of terminal ileum falls easily into the pelvic hollow, requiring no further mobilization. However, if this is not the case, there are several maneuvers that can facilitate the mobilization needed to perform an anastomosis without tension.

The small bowel mesentery should be mobilized by dividing its right-sided peritoneal attachments all the way to and including the junction of the mesenteric root to the third part of the duodenum. The 2 most obvious lines of tension are (1) the mesentery along the path of the ileocolic artery and (2), more proximally, along the path of the superior mesenteric artery. When the mesentery is transilluminated, these 2 vascular bundles can be visualized. As discussed previously, the distal ileum is supplied by the vasa recta arising from the ileal branch of the ileocolic artery, which connects the ileo colic artery to the distal end of the superior mesenteric artery in the mesentery approximately 3 to 4 cm below the ileum. Due to this arterial connection, either the ileocolic or the superior mesenteric vessels (but not both) can be sacrificed without compromising the terminal ileum (see Figure 15-2A).

With gentle traction on the ileum 15 cm from its distal end, the primary point of tension may be a short mesentery restricted by the superior mesenteric vascular supply. In this case, the superior mesenteric artery is identified using transillumination. It is divided and ligated distal to its last jejunal branch and a window is made in the mesentery by dividing it perpendicular to the axis of the superior mesenteric artery (see Figure 15-2B). By doing this the vascular connections between the jejunal and proximal ileal arcades, the distal superior mesenteric vessels, and the ileal branch of the ileocolic vessels remains intact to preserve the vascular integrity of the terminal ileum. Prior to dividing the superior mesenteric vessels, the integrity of the ileocolic artery and the vascular connections is tested by placing a bulldog clamp on the superior mesenteric artery for at least 5 minutes. By dividing the superior mesenteric vessels, an additional 5 cm of length may be provided to the ileal mesentery facilitating adequate mobilization for a tension-free anastomosis.

More commonly, the most obvious point of tension in the ileal mesentery is along the path of the ileocolic vasculature. In this case, the ileocolic vessels are divided proximal to the ileal branch. Once the ileocolic vessels are divided and ligated, the mesentery below and parallel to the ileal branch of the ileocolic artery is divided toward the superior mesenteric vessels (see Figure 15-2C). The mesentery is divided with either the LigaSure or a linear stapling device with 2.0-mm staple size. Either of these tools provides excellent hemostasis and prevents the bunching of suture-ligated mesenteric pedicles, which can shorten the small bowel length and prohibit maximum mobilization. This maneuver allows for mobilization of the distal terminal ileum providing approximately 3 cm of extension toward the pelvis.

If tension still remains in the small bowel mesentery and the superior mesenteric artery has not been ligated and divided, then the next step is to make relaxing incisions in the peritoneum perpendicular to and superficial to the superior mesenteric vascular bundle. The incisions can be made 1 to 3 cm in length using DeBakey forceps (or a right angle clamp) to lift the peritoneum off the underlying vessels prior to incising it with electrocautery. Incisions can be made 1 cm apart along the entire path of the superior mesenteric vessels from the root of the mesentery until approximately 4 cm from the ileal serosa on both the anterior and posterior aspects of the mesentery (see Figure 15-2C). In our experience, 4 to 6 relaxing incisions can provide an additional 2 to 3 cm of mesenteric extension. Transillumination is very helpful in avoiding vascular injury.

Occasionally, transecting the ileocolic vessels, mobilizing the distal terminal ileum, and making serial relaxing incisions in the peritoneum along the superior mesenteric vessels does not adequately mobilize the ileum to allow for a tension-free ileal pouch anal anastomosis. In this scenario, an additional 2 cm of extension of the ileal mesentery can be obtained by performing a Kocher maneuver. A Kocher maneuver is more commonly performed to expose the retroperitoneal structures behind the duodenum and the head of the pancreas to safely control upper abdominal bleeding. However, a consequence of performing this maneuver is that when the duodenum is mobilized, it provides a degree of laxity to the superior mesenteric vessels that allows the root of the small bowel mesentery to relax inferiorly toward the pelvis. To accomplish this maneuver, the peritoneum lateral to the second part of the duodenum is incised with electrocautery to enter the retroperitoneal space. The incision is then carried inferiorly and to the left to elevate the second and third segments of the duodenum exposing the vena cava and aorta. Next, while extending the peritoneal incision superiorly around the first portion of the duodenum toward the pylorus, take care to avoid the bile duct as it passes posteriorly to the duodenum. Once the peritoneum is divided around the first 3 segments of the duodenum, it is gently lifted off the vena cava and aorta along with the head of the pancreas, providing the extra mobility needed to bring the ileum a couple of centimeters deeper into the pelvis.

Creation of the J-Pouch Reservoir

The distal 15 cm of ileum is folded back onto itself, creating a 30-cm segment. Synthetic absorbable suture is used to plicate the antimesenteric surfaces of the 2 limbs together (Figure 15-3). A linear enterotomy incision is made along the antimesenteric side of the ileum at the fold. The location of the enterotomy will become the distal (efferent) end of the J-pouch. The enterotomy incision is large enough to allow the passage of a linear stapling device, which is used to staple the 2 limbs together and open the bowel wall between them, creating a lumen with twice the circumference of the ileum (see Figure 15-3). We choose to utilize 80-mm long linear staplers with 3.5-mm staple size (100-mm long linear staplers can also be used). Because the J-pouch is 15 cm in length, a second stapler is used to complete the proximal (afferent) portion of the pouch. Although some surgeons apply the second staple line via the previously made enterotomy incision at the efferent end of the pouch, we prefer to make separate small enterotomies on the antimesenteric surfaces of the 2 limbs of ileum at the afferent end of the pouch to place the second stapler (see Figure 15-3). By doing this, the surgeon's finger can be placed into the pouch through the efferent incision to guide the precise placement of the proximal staple line along the antimesenteric side to meet the distal staple line and complete the pouch. The enterotomy at the afferent end of the pouch (see Figure 15-3) is then repaired with monofilament, delayed-absorbable suture, or a 30-mm thoracoabdominal stapler.

J-Pouch Anal Anastomosis

At this point, the ileum has been fully mobilized and the J-pouch has been created. Although hand-sewn anastomoses between the pouch and the anus or rectum can be performed, we prefer the ease and security of a stapled anastomosis using a transanal circular stapling device. A purse-string suture is placed around the edges of the enterotomy at the efferent end of the J-pouch. The anvil from a 28- to 29-mm circular stapler is placed into the pouch through the enterotomy and the purse string suture is cinched down snuggly around the stem of the anvil and tied (Figure 15-4). The stapling device is placed transanally and the spike is advanced through the anus into the peritoneal cavity just posterior to the anal staple line. The stem of the anvil is snapped onto the spike, the device is closed and the end-to-end stapled anastomosis is completed (see Figure 15-4). We prefer to reinforce the staple line with interrupted monofilament, delayed-absorbable suture. All staple lines are checked for air leaks by submerging the pouch in saline and filling it with air transanally via proctoscopy.

Diverting Loop Ileostomy

Although a single-staged IPAA is offered to selected patients who undergo total colectomies for other indications, patients who undergo extended colectomies as part of radical surgery for advanced gynecologic malignancies generally have multiple comorbidities secondary to their age, the extent of their disease, and the extent of the surgical procedure they endured. In addition, patients with advanced gynecologic cancers will likely require postoperative adjuvant chemotherapy to maximize their survival, and many will be candidates for intraperitoneal chemotherapy. Although data do not suggest that there are fewer anastomotic leaks detected radiologically

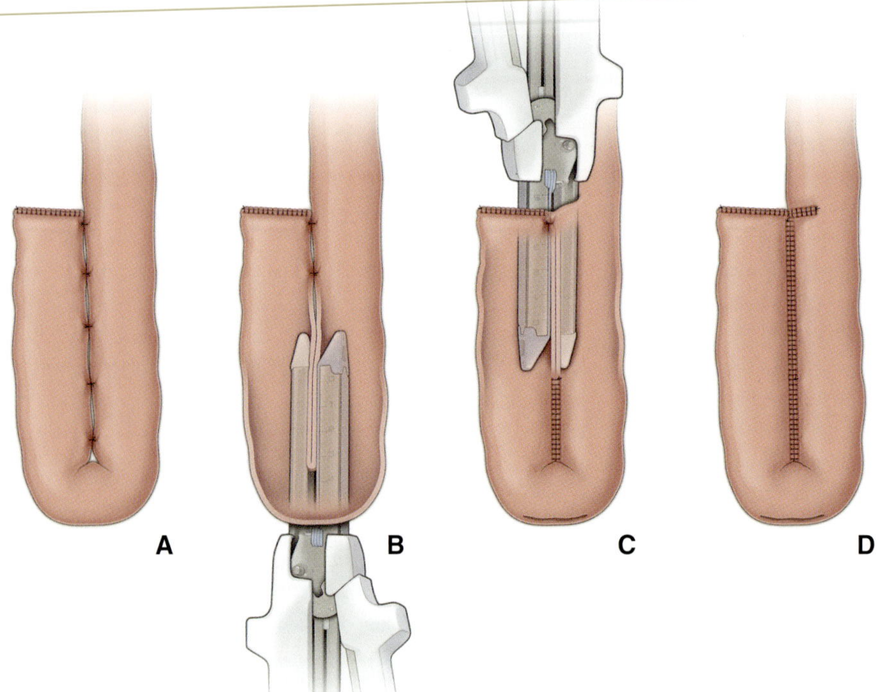

Fig. 15-3. Creating the pouch reservoir. **(A)** The distal 15 cm of ileum is folded back onto itself. Its antimesenteric surfaces are plicated together with 3-0 synthetic absorbable suture. **(B)** The 80-mm linear stapler with 3.5-mm staple size is placed through an enterotomy made at the efferent end of the pouch (where the small bowel is folded back onto itself). The efferent portion of the pouch is stapled creating a lumen with twice the circumference as the ileum. **(C)** A second 80-mm linear stapler is placed through small enterotomies made on the antimesenteric surfaces of the 2 limbs of ileum to create the afferent portion of the pouch. An index finger (not seen) is placed into the pouch via the efferent enterotomy to guide the stapling device to meet the previously made efferent staple line. **(D)** This completes the pouch reservoir. Both the efferent and afferent staple lines have been placed and the pouch reservoir now has a lumen circumference equal to twice that of the ileum. The enterotomy seen at the afferent end of the pouch is then closed with 3-0, monofilament, delayed-absorbable suture, or a thoracoabdominal stapler with a 3.5-mm staple size.

when diverting stomas are used, diverting stomas have been shown to decrease the rate of clinically relevant, symptomatic leaks.[25,26]

At our center, a 2-staged procedure is preferred. Creating a diverting ileostomy to allow the ileal J-pouch anal anastomosis to heal without the continuous passage of enteric contents prevents postoperative complications related to symptomatic anastomotic leaks. This avoids undesirable chemotherapy delays. Although, the second-staged surgery to reverse the loop ileostomy can be performed 6 weeks after the initial operation, we prefer to wait until the completion of chemotherapy to take down the ileostomy to avoid setbacks during the treatment period.

A loop of ileum proximal to the pouch reservoir is used. We select a loop that easily extends to an appropriate location on the abdominal wall where a temporary ileostomy stoma can be matured. A circular skin incision is made at the marked stoma site. This is carried down to the fascia. A cruciate incision is made through the musculofascial layers of the abdominal wall and through the peritoneum. The opening is made large enough to tightly fit 2 examining fingers. Using a Babcock clamp, the loop of ileum is pulled through the abdominal incision. We do not plicate the bowel serosa to either the peritoneum or the fascia because this stoma is meant to be temporary.

Some surgeons choose to mature the diverting stoma 24 to 72 hours postoperatively at the bedside. In this situation the loop of ileum is supported above the skin by placing a rod through a small mesenteric window made just beneath the ileal loop. The rod is slipped out approximately 1 week postoperatively at the bedside. We prefer to mature the stoma immediately. Before the abdominal incision is closed, 2 closed suction drains are placed in the pelvis—1 anterior and 1 posterior to the pouch reservoir—to guard the staple lines. After the surgical procedure is completed and the laparotomy incision is closed and covered to avoid wound contamination, a linear enterotomy incision measuring approximately 4 to 5 cm is made on the antimesenteric surface of the small bowel loop. Using synthetic absorbable suture, the edges of the enterotomy are plicated back onto

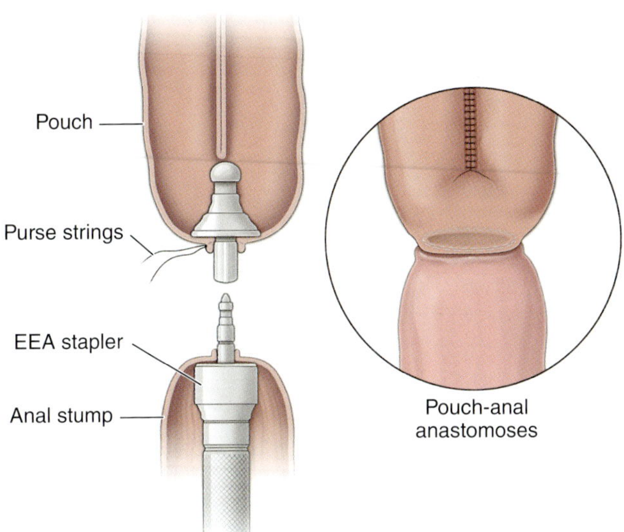

Fig. 15-4. Creating the pouch-rectal anastomosis. After a purse-string is placed around the edges of the efferent enterotomy, the anvil from a 29-mm circular stapling device is placed into the efferent end of the pouch leaving the stem of the anvil exposed. The purse string is tied snuggly around the stem of the anvil. The circular stapler is placed transanally and the spike is advanced to perforate through the rectal stump just posterior to the rectal staple line. The stem of the anvil is snapped onto the spike. The stapling device is closed to staple the efferent end of the pouch to the rectum completing the ileal pouch anal anastomosis.

the bowel serosa and then to the skin edge in a rosette fashion. Approximately 8 to 10 sutures are required to mature the entire circumference of the loop ileostomy stoma (Figure 15-5). An ostomy appliance is placed prior to leaving the operating room.

Reversal of the Loop Ileostomy

At least 6 weeks following the IPAA, a barium enema is performed to evaluate the integrity of the reservoir staple lines. If no leak is identified, then the patient is scheduled for takedown of her ileostomy. This is usually accomplished through a circular (or elliptical) incision around the stoma. In rare cases a midline laparotomy is performed due to extensive adhesions. Hand-sewn closures can be performed; however, we prefer a stapled technique. Using a 60-mm linear stapler with 3.5-mm staple size, the antimesenteric sides of the 2 limbs of the loop ileostomy are stapled together and divided. Closure is completed with a 60-mm thoracoabdominal stapler with 3.5-mm staple size. The loop of bowel is replaced into the peritoneal cavity and the abdominal wall fascia is closed transversely using monofilament, delayed absorbable suture. The subcutaneous tissue is irrigated and the skin is reapproximated with skin clips or subcuticularly with absorbable, monofilament suture.

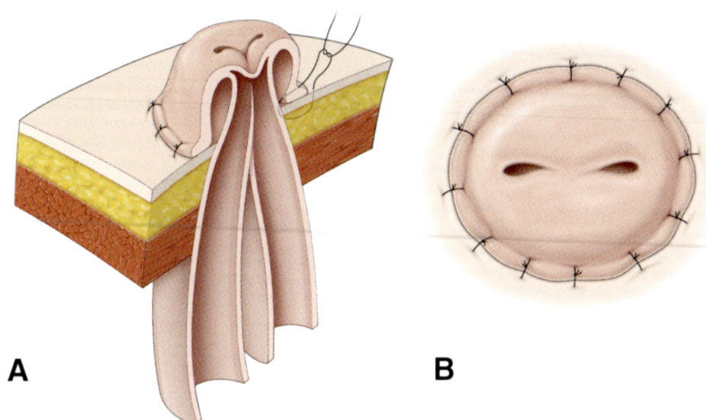

Fig. 15-5. Loop ileostomy. (A) Loop of ileum brought through a separate incision on the abdominal wall. A rosette stitch plicating the edge of the ileum back onto the seromuscular surface of the bowel wall and then to the skin edge to ensure that the stoma is elevated over the surface of the skin for ease of ostomy bag application. (B) Finished loop ileostomy stoma.

POSTOPERATIVE CARE

Box 15-3 PERIOPERATIVE MORBIDITY

- Staple line hemorrhage
- Staple line disruption (leak or fistula)
- Pelvic abscess/sepsis
- Small bowel obstruction

Immediate

Women who undergo extended colectomies and IPAA as part of radical gynecologic cancer surgery have inevitably endured an extensive surgical experience. The decision to admit the patient to the intensive care unit postoperatively is dependent on the length and extent of surgery and the intraoperative stability of the individual patient. To avoid postoperative emesis and aspiration pneumonitis, a nasogastric tube is placed intraoperatively and maintained for 1 to 2 days. Immediately upon removal of the nasogastric tube, a clear liquid diet may be instituted and advanced as tolerated the following day. Although closed suction drains are probably not necessary if a loop ileostomy is created, we prefer to leave the drains in place to guard the pouch staple lines until a significant amount of ileostomy output is observed. Consultation and frequent visits with an enterostomal therapist is an important postoperative consideration. Patients should not be discharged from the hospital prior to developing reasonable comfort with stomal care.

First 6 Weeks

In the first 6 weeks of the postoperative period, high output through the ileostomy should be expected. With high enteric output and the lack of colonic absorption, the patient must be monitored closely for signs and symptoms of dehydration and electrolyte derangements. These include thirst, lassitude, fatigue, nausea, and headache. This is particularly important for those who are preparing for chemotherapy treatments. Diets high in fat or nutritional fiber should be avoided as well as carbonated, alcoholic, or caffeinated beverages. Patients should be encouraged to imbibe large volumes of fluids and may require electrolyte supplementation during this phase of recovery. Loperamide can be started at a dose of 4 mg (2 tablets) 2 to 4 times a day and is effective at creating a more formed ileostomy output.

After 6 Weeks

After the first 6 weeks, and certainly after the ileostomy is reversed, if the patient is still experiencing high, watery output, adding psyllium-based bulking agents can be effective not only to help in reducing risks of dehydration, but also to prevent watery fecal urgency and incontinence. With time, the small intestine functionally accommodates the loss of the colon and in most cases patients may explore a more normal dietary intake.

LONG-TERM OUTCOMES

Box 15-4 DELAYED COMPLICATIONS

- Anal anastomotic stricture
- Pouchitis
- Cuffitis
- Irritable pouch syndrome
- Pouch failure

Long-term outcomes are ultimately quite good with high patient satisfaction. However, the surgeon must be cognizant of a number of potential risks and complications. Since data describing complications related to IPAA are predominantly on patients with inflammatory bowel disease or polyposis, it is difficult to extrapolate meaningful information relevant to the same procedure performed for reconstruction after radical gynecologic cancer surgery.

Hemorrhage

During the postoperative period minor self-limited bleeding from pouch staple lines may occur, but the incidence of hemorrhage is only 1.5% to 3.5%.[27,28] Fortunately, the use of adrenaline (1:200,000) irrigations is effective at controlling the pouch bleeding in 80% of cases. If hemorrhage persists or the patient is unstable, reexploration is warranted—either anoscopically or via laparotomy. If specific sites of bleeding can be identified endoscopically, then they can be cauterized, clipped, or injected with epinephrine successfully. It is rare that the pouch must be disconnected from the anal anastomosis in order to control hemorrhage.

Staple Line Disruptions

The risks of staple line leak and fistula formation (to the vagina or perineum) is 5% and 7%, respectively.[29] Multiple retrospective studies have demonstrated high-dose steroids to be an independent risk factor and likely cause for most of these staple line disruptions as well as a postoperative diagnosis of Crohn disease.[30-33] In our experience with IPAA and diverting loop ileostomy after radical gynecologic cancer surgery over the last 12 years, we have yet to see a symptomatic staple line leak or fistula. Because gynecologic cancer patients rarely use high-dose steroids, staple line disruptions are unlikely to occur in this population of patients if meticulous technique results in a tension-free anastomosis. If staple line disruptions do occur and pelvic sepsis or abscesses develop, then CT scans or MRIs may be used to identify and guide the percutaneous drainage of collections. If disruptions occur with major leaks in the absence of a diverting ileostomy, then considerations for creating a proximal diverting ileostomy or simply exteriorizing the pouch should be made. If the pouch is grossly ischemic, then resection and end ileostomy is required.

Bowel Obstruction and Anastomotic Stricture

Small bowel obstructions requiring surgical interventions have been reported in 4% to 5% of patients undergoing IPAA for inflammatory bowel disease.[34,35] The vast majority of these small bowel obstructions are due to adhesion formation. Some develop at the afferent end of the pouch as a result of formation of a flap valve due to angulation of the pouch from pelvic adhesions. Most obstructions can be released without resection of the pouch. If extensive adhesiolysis is required, then cautious dissection should be performed around the pouch to avoid subsequent pouch complications.

Outlet strictures of the anal anastomosis are reported in the literature with an incidence of 10% to 40%. Risk factors include pelvic sepsis, anastomotic tension or ischemia, Crohn disease, hand-sewn technique, and stapler size, among others.[34,36-40] The diagnosis may be made 6 to 9 months after surgery. Patients will have symptoms of crampy abdominal pain, watery stools, straining, and the feeling of incomplete emptying. In most instances they can be remedied with simple dilation. In a gynecologic cancer population this complication has not been observed.

Pouch-Related Inflammatory Conditions

1. Pouchitis

Pouchitis, a long-term inflammatory complication of uncertain pathogenesis, occurs in 16% to 48% of ileal pouch anal anastomoses.[6,28,41,42] However, its predominance in patients with inflammatory bowel disease makes it highly unlikely in our patient population.[6,42] Symptoms include crampy abdominal pain, increased frequency, urgency and liquid consistency of stool, and anal bleeding. Although most diagnoses are made empirically, an objective diagnostic scale has been established and verified. It incorporates endoscopic, histologic, and symptomatic factors and is known as the Pouchitis Disease Activity Index.[43] Pouchitis responds well to a 14-day course of either ciprofloxacin or metronidazole.

2. Cuffitis

Because many extended colectomies performed as part of a radical gynecologic cancer surgery are subtotal colectomies that retain a portion of the rectal cuff above the dentate line of the anus, an inflammatory complication of the rectal cuff, clinically similar to pouchitis can arise, known as cuffitis. Rectal cuffitis is best treated with topical steroids or suppositories.

3. Irritable pouch syndrome

A third overlapping inflammatory complication of IPAA is irritable pouch syndrome. It is symptomatically similar to the other 2 conditions excluding rectal bleeding and has no histologic or endoscopic evidence of inflammation.[44,45] It is a diagnosis of exclusion and seems to respond to therapeutic approaches recommended for irritable bowel syndrome. These include antispasmodics, antidiarrheal agents, and antidepressants.

Pouch Function and Patient Satisfaction

Pouch failure, defined as the need for indefinite defunctioning or excision of a pouch due to unmanageable complications, is reported to have an incidence that varies from 3% to 30%.[6,28,46,47] Because most complications related to ileal pouch anal anastomoses have higher incidences in patients with inflammatory bowel disease, symptomatic staple line disruptions, or pelvic sepsis, it is reasonable to expect that failures occur relatively infrequently in patients with a gynecologic cancer diagnoses.

Ultimately, long-term functionality and patient satisfaction are excellent. The frequency of bowel movements is 6 to 7 times a day.[48,49,51] From a very practical perspective, most postmenopausal women are in the bathroom more often than that to empty their bladders. When surveys were included, reports demonstrate satisfaction in 91% to 98% of patients.[38,49-51] These consistent quality of life end points, demonstrate the value of considering this reconstructive procedure for selected patients who undergo extended colectomies as part of a radical surgery for advanced gynecologic malignancies.

MINIMALLY INVASIVE SURGICAL APPLICATIONS

Women with gynecologic malignancies requiring radical resection, including an extended colectomy are rarely considered as candidates for minimally invasive surgical techniques. However, with advancements in instrumentation and skill sets, it should be acknowledged that selected women are and will be appropriately offered radical resections of this extent using laparoscopic or robotic techniques. Hand-assisted laparoscopic total colectomy and IPAA is being used by many institutions in the treatment of inflammatory bowel disease and adenomatous polyposis.[52] The stapled J-pouch procedure is performed with similar techniques and outcomes as described using the standard laparotomy approach.[53] Although long-term data are emerging, short-term results on minimally invasive IPAA are comparable with standard techniques and seem to provide for shorter postoperative hospitalizations and decreased pain.[54,55] With greater experience in the use of minimally invasive options for radical surgical procedures, the evolution toward their use for reconstructive procedures should be expected.

SUMMARY

Radical gynecologic cancer resections rarely include the performance of a subtotal colectomy. However, in selected patients who require this extent of surgery to accomplish a surgical outcome consistent with curative intent, consideration for an IPAA is important in restoring quality of life along with survivorship. Although the list of complications is lengthy, they are largely attributable to factors unrelated to the gynecologic cancer population such as high-dose steroid use and inflammatory bowel disease. Performing a 2-staged procedure with a temporary loop ileostomy can minimize the risk of clinically relevant untoward events. It is of utmost importance to obtain a tension-free anastomosis between the pouch reservoir and the rectal stump. If this is not possible, then we have a low threshold for creating an end ileostomy. A broad perspective of the overall patient situation is imperative, recognizing that postoperative complications will result in treatment delays that are potentially detrimental to overall survival, nullifying any quality-of-life benefits the procedure was intended to provide. In our experience, with meticulous attention to surgical detail, thoughtful small bowel mobilization, and tensionless anastomoses, serious complications directly related to this procedure are rare, and high rates of satisfaction are expected.

REFERENCES

1. Parks AG, Nicholls RJ, Belliveau P. Proctocolectomy with ileal reservoir and anal anastomosis. *Br J Surg*. 1980;67(8):533-538.
2. Parks AG, Nicholls RJ: Proctocolectomy without ileostomy for ulcerative colitis. *Br Med J*. 1978;2:85-88.
3. Pemberton JH, Phillips SF, Ready RR, Zinsmeister AR, Beahrs OH. Quality of life after brooke ileostomy and ileal pouch – anal anastomis. *Ann Surg*. 1989;209(5):620-626.
4. Taylor BM, Beart RW, Dozois RR, Kelly KA, Phillips SF. Straight ileoanal anastomosis v ileal pouch - anal anastomosis after colectomy and mucosal proctectomy. *Arch Surg*. 1983;118(6):696-701.
5. Taylor BM, Cranley B, Kelly KA, Phillips SF, Beart RW, Dozois RR. A clinico- physiological comparison of ileal pouch- anal and straight ileoanal anastomosis. *Ann Surg*. 1983;198(4):462-468.
6. Fazio VW, Kiran R, Remzi F, et al. Ileal pouch anal anastomosis – analysis of outcome and quality of life in 3707 patients. *Ann Surg*. 2013;257(4):679-685.
7. Berndtsson I, Lindholm E, Oresland T, Borjesson L: Long term outcome after ileal pouch- anal anastomosis: function and health-related quality of life. *Dis Colon Rectum*. 2007;50(10):1545-1552.

8. Ziv Y, Fazio VW, Church JM, Lavery IC, King TM, Ambrosetti P. Stapled ileal pouch anal anastomoses are safer than handsewn anastomoses in patients with ulcerative colitis. *Am J Surg*. 1996;171(3):320-323.
9. Lovegrove RE, Constantinides VAHeriot AG, et al. A comparison of hand-sewn versus stapled ileal pouch anal anastomosis (IPAA) following proctocolectomy: a meta-analysis of 4183 patients. *Ann Surg*. 2006;244(1):18-26.
10. Becker JM. What is the better surgical technique in ileal pouch-anal anastomosis? Mucosectomy. *Inflamm Bowel Dis*. 1996;2(2):151-154.
11. Kornbluth A, Sachar DB. Ulcerative colitis practice guidelines in adults: American college of gastroenterology, practice parameters committee. *Am J Gastroenterol*. 2010;105(3):501-523.
12. Vasen HFA, Moslein G, Alonso A, et al. Guidelines for the clinical management of familial adenomatous polyposis (FAP). *Gut*. 2008;57(5):704-713.
13. Le Q, Melmed G, Dubinsky M, et al. Surgical outcome of ileal pouch-anal anastomosis when used intentionally for well-defined crohn's disease. *Inflamm Bowel Dis*. 2013;19(1):30-36.
14. Melton GB, Fazio VW, Kiran RP, et al. Long-term outcomes with ileal pouch-anal anastomosis and crohn's disease – pouch retention and implications of delayed diagnosis. *Ann Surg*. 2008;248(4):608-616.
15. Hartley JE, Fazio VW, Remzi FH, et al. Analysis of the outcome of ileal pouch-anal anastamosis in patients with chron's disease. *Dis Colon Rectum*. 2003;47(11):1808-1815.
16. Ausch C, Madoff RD, Gnant M, et al. Aetiology and surgical management of toxic megacolon. *Colorectal Dis*. 2005;8(3):195-201.
17. Radice E, Nelson H, Devine RM, et al. Ileal pouch-anal anastomosis in patients with colorectal cancer: long-term functional and oncologic outcomes. *Dis Colon Rectum*. 1998;41(1):11-17.
18. Ziv Y, Fazio VW, Strong SA, Oakley JR, Milsom JW, Lavery IC. Ulcerative colitis and coexisting colorectal cancer: recurrence rate after restorative proctocolectomy. *Ann Surg Oncol*. 1994;1(6):512-515.
19. Holder-Murray J, Fichera A. Anal transition zone in the surgical management of ulcerative colitis. *World J Gastroenterol*. 2009;15(7):769-773.
20. Silver DF, Zgheib NB. Extended left colon resections as part of complete cytoreduction for ovarian cancer: tips and consideration. *Gynecol Oncol*. 2009;114(3):427-430.
21. DF Silver. Left-sided subtotal colectomy for advanced serous carcinoma of the ovary or uterus. *J Pelvic Med Surg*. 2005;10(6):323-327.
22. Bristow RE, Zerbe MJ, Rosenshein NB, Grumbine FC, Montz FJ. Stage IV endometrial carcinoma: the role of cytoreductive surgery and determinants of survival. *Gynecol Oncol*. 2000;78(2):85-91.
23. Hoffman MS, Zervose E. Colon resection for ovarian cancer: intraoperative decisions. *Gynecol Oncol*. 2008;111(2Suppl):S56-S65.
24. Bristow RE, Montz FJ, Lagasse LD, Leuchter RS, Karlan BY. Survival impact of surgical cytoreduction in stage IV epithelial ovarian cancer. *Gynecol Oncol*. 1999;72(3):278-287.
25. Marusch F, Koch A, Schmidt U, et al. Value of a protective stoma in low anterior resections for rectal cancer. *Dis Colon Rectum*. 2002;45(9):1164-1171.
26. Pakkastie TE, Ovaska JT, Pekkala ES, Luukkonen PE, Jarvinen HJ. A randomized study of colostomies in low colorectal anastomoses. *Eur J Surg* 1997;163(12):929-933.
27. Lian L, Serclova Z, Fazio VW, Kiran RP, Remzi F, Shen B. Clinical features and management of postoperative pouch bleeding after ileal pouch-anal anastomosis (IPAA). *J Gastrointest Surg*. 2008;12(11):1991-1994.
28. Fazio VW, Ziv Y, Church JM, et al. Ileal pouch-anal anastomoses complications and function in 1005 patients. *Ann Surg*. 1995;222(2):120-127.
29. Fazio VW, Tekkis PP, Remzi F, et al. Quantification of risk for pouch failure after ileal pouch anal anastomosis surgery. *Ann Surg*. 2003;238(4):605-614.
30. Ferrante M, D'Hoore A, Vermeire S, et al. Corticosteroids but not infliximab increase short term postoperative infectious complications in patients with ulcerative colitis. *Inflamm Bowel Dis*. 2009;15(7):1062-1070.
31. Reese GE, Lovegrove RE, Tilney HS, et al. The effect of crohn's disease on outcomes after restorative proctocolectomy. *Dis Colon Rectum*. 2006;50(2):239-250.
32. Brown CJ, MacLean AR, Cohen Z, MacRae HM, O'Connor BI, McLeod RS. Crohn's disease and indeterminate colitis and the ileal pouch-anal anastomosis: outcomes and pattern of failure. *Dis Colon Rectum*. 2002;48(8):1542-1549.
33. Heuschen UA, Hinz U, Allemeyer EH, et al. Risk factors for ileoanal J pouch-related septic complications in ulcerative colitis and familial adenomatous polyposis. *Ann Surg*. 2002;235(2):207-216.
34. MacLean AR, Cohen Z, MacRae HM, et al. Risk of small bowel obstruction after the ileal pouch-anal anastomosis. *Ann Surg*. 2002;235(2):200-206.
35. Marcello PW, Roberts PL, Schoetz DJ, Coller JA, Murray JJ, Veidenheimer MC. Obstruction after the ileal pouch– anal anatomosis: a preventable complication? *Dis Colon Rectum*. 1993;36(12):1105-1111.
36. Lewis WG, Kuzu A, Sagar PM, Holdsworth PM, Johnston D. Stricture at the pouch-anal anastomosis after restorative proctocolectomy. *Dis Colon Rectum*. 1994;37(2):120-125.
37. Kirat HT, Kiran RP, Lian L, Remzi FH, Fazio VW. Influence of stapler size used at ileal pouch-anal anastomosis on anastomotic leak, stricture, long-term functional outcomes, and quality of life. *Am J Surg*. 2010;200(1):68-72.
38. Michaelassi F, Lee J, Rubin M, et al. Long-term functional results after ileal pouch anal restorative proctocolectomy for ulcerative colitis – a prospective observational study. *Ann Surg*. 2003;238(3):433-441.
39. Fleshman JW, Cohen Z, McLeod RS, Stern H, Blair J. The ileal reservoir and ileoanal anastomosis procedure; factors affecting technical and functional outcome. *Dis Colon Rectum*. 1988;31(1):10-16.
40. Hahnloser D, Pemberton JH, Wolff BG, Larson DR, Crownhart BS, Dozois RR. Results at up to 20 years after ileal pouch-anal anastomosis for chronic ulcerative colitis. *Br J Surg*. 2007;94(3):333-340.
41. Hoda KM, Collins JF, Knigge KL Deveney KE. Predictors of pouchitis after ileal pouch- anal anastomosis: a retrospective review. *Dis Colon Rectum*. 2008;51(5):554-560.
42. Seidel SA, Peach SE, Newman M, Sharp KW. Ileoanal pouch procedures: clinical outcomes and quality-of-life assessment. *Am Surgeon*. 1999;65(1):40-46.
43. Sandborn WJ, Tremaine WJ, Batts KP, Pembertom JH, Phillips SF. Pouchitis after ileal pouch- anal anastomosis: a pouchitis disease activity index. *Mayo Clin Proc*. 1994;69(5):409-415.
44. Shen B, Achkar JP, Lashner BA, et al. Irritable pouch syndrome: a new category of diagnosis for symptomatic patients with ileal pouch- anal anastomosis. *Am J Gastroenterol*. 2002;97(4):972-977.
45. Shen B, Sanmiguel C, Bennett AE, et al. Irritable pouch syndrome is characterized by visceral hypersensitivity. *Inflamm Bowel Dis*. 2011;17(4):994-1002.
46. Meagher AP, Farouk R, Dozois RR, Kelly KA, Pemberton JH. J ileal pouch- anal anastomosis for chronic ulcerative colitis: complications and long term outcome in 1310 patients. *Br J Surg*. 1998;85(6):800-803.
47. Delaney CP, Remzi FH, Gramlich T, Dadvand B, Fazio VW. Equivalent function, quality of life and pouch survival rates after ileal pouch-anal anastomosis for indeterminate and ulcerative colitis. *Ann Surg*. 2002;236(1):43-48.
48. Farouk R, Pemberton JH, Wolff BG, Dozois RR, Browning S, Larson D. Functional outcomes after ileal pouch-anal anastomosis for chronic ulcerative colitis. *Ann Surg*. 2002;231(6):919-926.
49. Fazio VW, O'Riordain MG, Lavery IC, et al. Long term functional outcome and quality of life after stapled restorative proctocolectomy. *Ann Surg*. 1999;230(4):575-584.
50. Pemberton JH, Kelly KA, Beart RW, Dozois RR, Wolff BG, Ilstrup DM. Ileal pouch-anal anastomosis for chronic ulcerative colitis – long term results. *Ann Surg*. 1987;206(4):504-513.
51. Bullard KM, Madoff RD, Gemlo BT. Is ileoanal pouch function stable with time? Results of a prospective audit: *Dis Colon Rectum*. 2002;45(3):299-304.

52. Maartense S, Dunker MS, Slors JF, et al. Hand assisted laparoscopic versus open restorative proctocolectomy with ileal pouch anal anastomosis—A randomized trial. *Ann Surg*. 2004;240(6):984-991.
53. Hasegawa H, Watanbe M, Baba H, Nishibori H, Kitajima M. Laparoscopic restorative proctocolectomy for patients with ulcerative colitis: *J Laparoendosc Adv Surg Tech*. 2002;12(6):403-406.
54. Fichera A, Silvestri MT, Hurst RD, Rubin MA, Michelassi F. Laparoscopic restorative proctocolectomy with ileal pouch anal anastomosis: a comparative observational study on long-term functional results. *J Gastrointest Surg*. 2009;13(3):526-532.
55. Sylla P, Chessin D, Gorfine SR, Roth E, bub DS, Bauer JJ. Evaluation of one-stage laparoscopic-assisted restorative proctocolectomy at a specialty center: comparison with the open approach. *Dis Colon Rectum*. 2009;52(3):394-399.

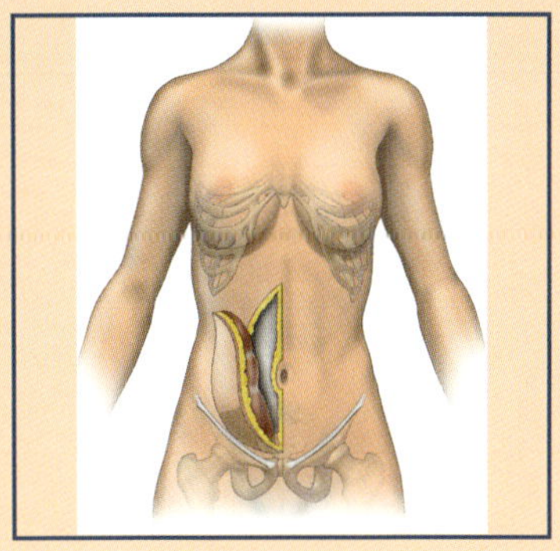

Section C Vulvovaginal and Pelvic Floor Reconstruction

Chapter 16. Skin Grafts, Omental Flaps, Advancement and Rotational Flaps

Jonathan M. Winograd, MD,
John O. Schorge, MD, and
Edward M. Kobraei, MD

BACKGROUND

The condition and appearance of a woman's genitalia strike at the core of her identity. Many patients experience severe sexual dysfunction, disturbed body image, and deranged pelvic anatomy after pelvic cancer surgery that compromise quality of life. Despite these important concerns, vulvovaginal reconstruction after pelvic cancer resection is not currently considered standard therapy.

Competent, safe, and functional vulvovaginal reconstructions are essential components of the care of patients with pelvic malignancies. The reconstruction cannot be achieved by doing a few standard procedures; it requires specialists familiar with general principles of reconstructive surgery to select the most appropriate among many possible techniques for each individual patient. To this end, the plastic and reconstructive surgeon should play an integral role in the care of the patient with pelvic cancer.

The surgeon and patient's therapeutic partnership is central to the outcome of the reconstruction. Operations in this anatomic region have a significant bearing on quality of life, and patients and families should be involved in decision making when appropriate. Patients must be educated about their disease, prognosis, treatment options, and the likely deficits in structure and function that can result from their cancer operation. Reconstructive options must be thoroughly described along with reasonable expectations about future sensibility, function, and aesthetic outcome. It cannot be overemphasized that joint oncologic-reconstructive endeavors are first and foremost for cancer treatment; barring unique circumstances, oncologic resection should never be compromised to facilitate reconstructive efforts.

The overarching goal of vulvovaginal reconstruction is the anatomic and functional restoration of these structures in an oncologically safe fashion that minimizes the risk of morbidity while optimizing the cosmetic outcome. Improved integration of reconstruction with primary treatment will improve aesthetic and functional results, and, thus, the quality of life of patients with pelvic neoplastic diseases. In this chapter, we explore the role of 3 essential tools in the armamentarium of plastic and reconstructive surgeons; skin grafts, omental flaps, and advancement and rotational flaps in vulvar and vaginal reconstructive surgery.

INDICATIONS AND CLINICAL APPLICATIONS

Squamous cell carcinoma is the most common histologic type of vulvar malignancy and the most frequent setting in which vulvar reconstruction occurs. It is diagnosed in 2 women per 100,000 every year in developed countries, and the age at diagnosis is most commonly in the sixth and seventh decades of life. Vulvar intraepithelial neoplasia (VIN) grade III represents a precursor lesion characterized by cellular atypia and abnormal maturation of the vulvar epithelium; it is typically found in a much younger patient population (around the fourth decade). VIN grade III is a surgical diagnosis, given that a 9% incidence of invasive carcinoma has been observed in untreated patients.

Primary carcinoma of the vagina is rare, accounting for about 1% of reproductive cancers in women, with squamous cell carcinoma being the most common histologic type. Vaginal resection occurs much more commonly due to advanced and recurrent malignancies in the adjacent organs, including cervix, endometrium, vulva, urethra, and most frequently bladder and rectum. Because the vaginal anatomy may be variably affected by resection, versatile methods are paramount to achieving successful reconstruction.

The most widely used, oncologically safe, and cosmetically acceptable methods in vulvovaginal reconstruction are included in the discussion that follows. Skin grafting alone for neovaginal reconstruction has largely been supplanted by more modern techniques; however, skin grafting remains a viable option for coverage of thin resection beds in vulvar reconstruction. Neovaginal reconstruction with omental flaps may proceed in conjunction with skin grafting to create a neovaginal canal. The omental flap has also proven to be an excellent solution to the problem of pelvic dead space following pelvic exenteration and resection for anorectal malignancy. An exciting and rapidly evolving area in vulvovaginal reconstruction relates to applications of advancement and rotational flaps. An impressive assortment of V-Y advancement flaps has been developed to reconstruct vulvar defects, combining a favorable aesthetic and functional outcome with reduced donor site morbidity. Emerging methods such as abdominoplasty advancement flaps will be discussed briefly. The Singapore flap for neovaginal reconstruction provides an excellent illustration of a rotational flap that continues to find use today.

SKIN GRAFTS AND OMENTAL FLAPS IN VULVOVAGINAL RECONSTRUCTION

Anatomic Considerations

Successful reconstruction of vulvovaginal defects is predicated on a careful appreciation of the specific surgical defect. This includes an assessment of exactly which structures were removed and which remain, along with their postresection configuration. Numerous classification systems have been developed to help characterize residual defects and propose optimal reconstructive options. The system devised by Cordeiro et al[1] is still widely used today and divides vaginal defects into either type I or II (Figure 16-1). Höckel and Dornhöfer[2] outline an algorithm of vulvovaginal reconstruction

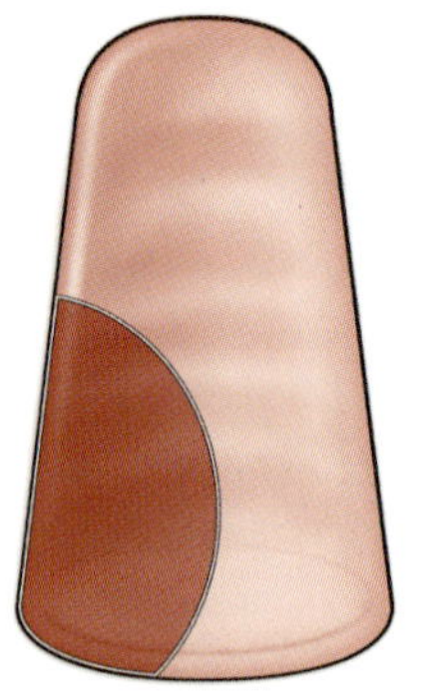

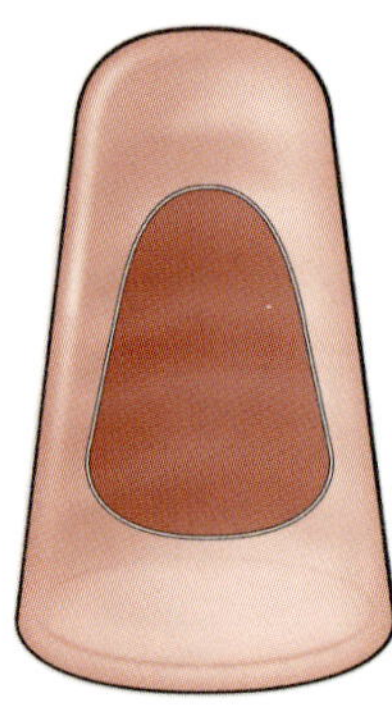

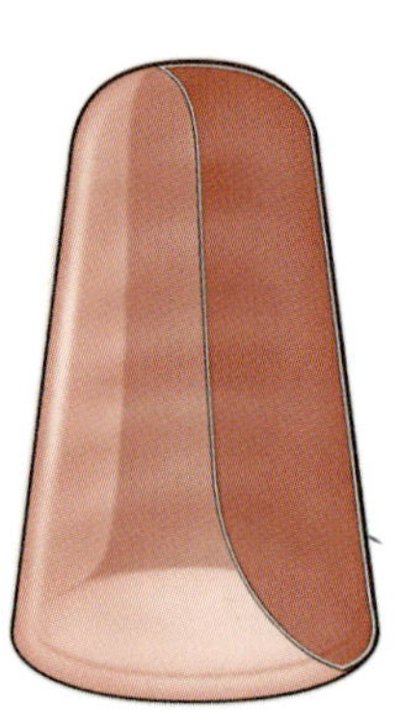

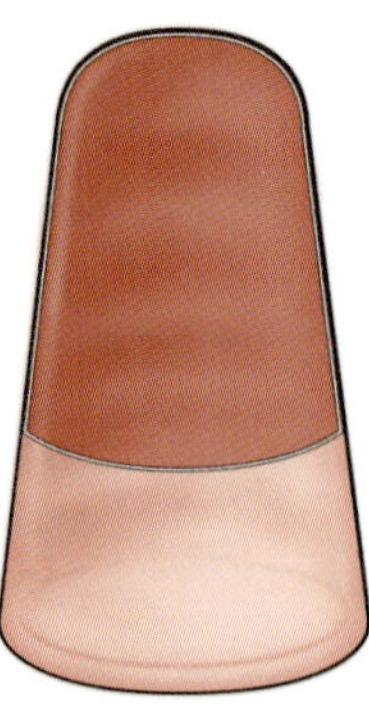

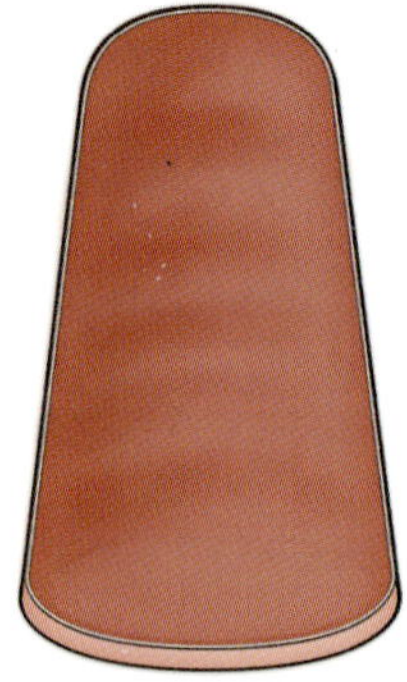

Fig. 16-1. Type IA defects are partial defects of the anterior and/or lateral vaginal wall, frequently resulting from resection of urinary tract malignancies or primary malignancies of the vaginal wall. Type IB defects involve the posterior vaginal wall and result from resections of locally advanced colorectal carcinoma. Type IIA defects are circumferential and include the upper two-thirds of the vagina, most commonly resulting from resection for uterine and cervical disease. Type IIB defects represent circumferential, total vaginal resection frequently seen in the setting of pelvic exenteration. (Reproduced with permission from Cordeiro PG, Pusic AL, Disa JJ. A classification system and reconstructive algorithm for acquired vaginal defects. *Plast Reconstr Surg*. 2002;110(4):1058-1065.)

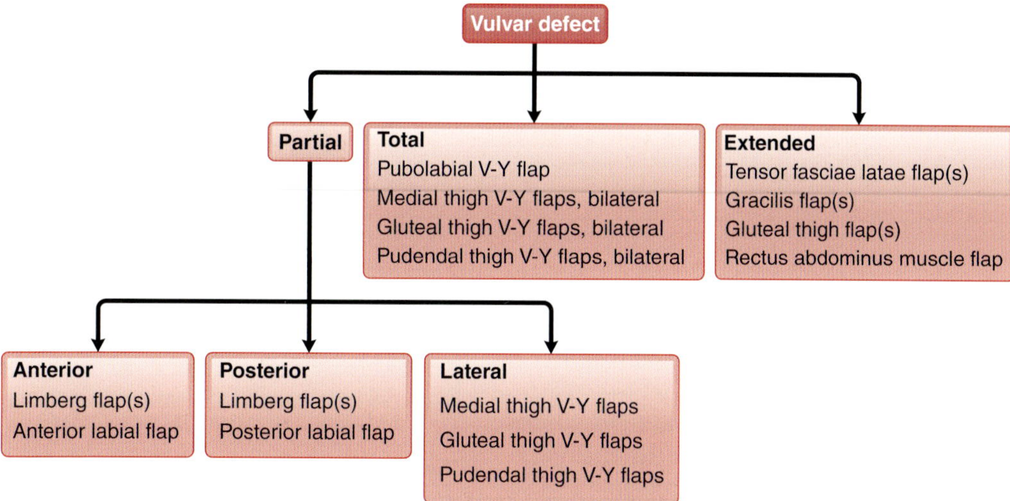

Fig. 16-2. Classification scheme of vulvar defects and proposed reconstructive options. (Reproduced with permission from Höckel M, Dornhöfer N. Vulvovaginal reconstruction for neoplastic disease. *Lancet Oncol*. 2008;9(6):559-568.)

in which vulvar and vaginal defects are divided into partial, total, and extended defects. Each defect is accompanied by a number of suggested reconstruction options (Figures 16-2 and 16-3).

Among the first methods of vaginal reconstruction was the application of full and partial-thickness skin grafts for creation of a neovagina. First described by Abbe[3] in 1898 for treatment of congenital absence of the vagina, these methods marked a new era in vaginal reconstruction that would find applications for acquired defects. In 1938, McIndoe et al[4] would use prosthetic vaginal stents lined with skin grafts to avert the problems with stenosis and shaping in earlier methods, which became known as the McIndoe technique. Local and regional flap techniques have since been developed to address more complex pelvic surgical procedures, and skin grafting for vaginal reconstruction remains mostly of historic interest today, except used in conjunction with omental flaps (discussed below).

Two types of skin graft are widely used in vulvar reconstruction. These include full-thickness skin grafts (FTSGs) and partial or split-thickness skin grafts (STSGs). Full-thickness skin grafts contain the epidermis and entire dermis and, therefore, leave a residual defect at the donor site exposing subcutaneous tissue. This defect must be

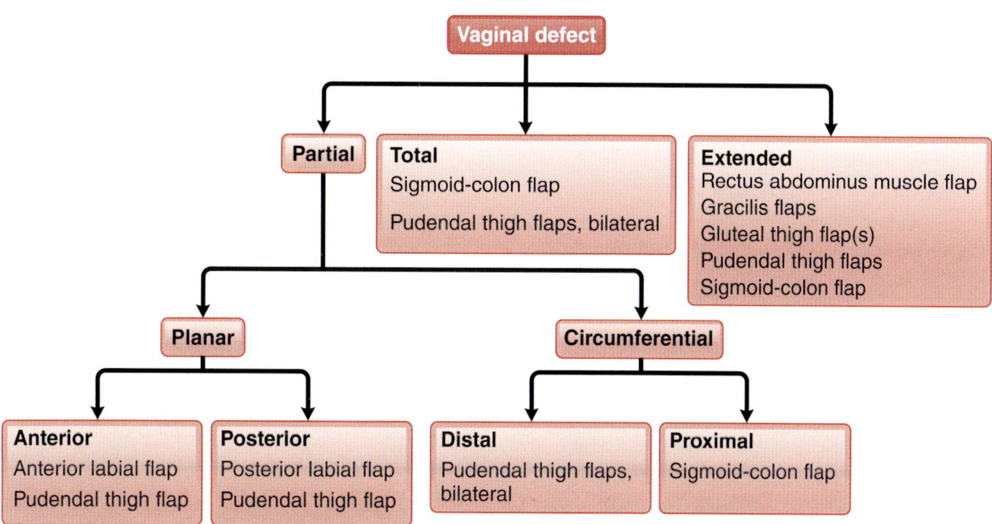

Fig. 16-3. Classification scheme of vaginal defects and proposed reconstructive options. (Reproduced with permission from Höckel M, Dornhöfer N. Vulvovaginal reconstruction for neoplastic disease. *Lancet Oncol*. 2008;9(6):559-568.)

Table 16-1. Characteristics of split and full-thickness skin grafts.

Characteristic	STSG	FTSG
Graft thickness	Usually uniform	May be variable
Secondary contraction[a]	Considerable, particularly in thin grafts	None
Pigmentation considerations	Prone to hyperpigmentation	Color/texture match more similar to normal skin
Donor site morbidity	Minimal, can be reused proportional to dermal thickness	Complete skin excision, donor site must be closed/covered and cannot be reused
Durability	More prone to shear injury, trauma	More durable
Donor site selection	Great flexibility, most commonly upper thigh, buttock	Often harvested in areas where skin is thin and lax to permit primary closure
Graft survival	More likely than FTSG	Less likely than STSG

[a]Secondary contraction: graft contraction over period of 6 to 18 months due to myofibroblast activity. FTSG = full-thickness skin graft, STSG = split-thickness skin graft.

closed primarily or covered at the time of graft harvest. By contrast, STSGs contain a variable amount of dermis, and remaining hair follicles and epithelial appendages ultimately regenerate the overlying epidermis. The differences between these 2 types of skin grafts have important implications for operative planning and outcomes and are highlighted in Table 16-1.

Skin grafts rely entirely on the vascularity of the recipient bed, and grafting onto contaminated or infected wounds, bare tendons without paratenon, or bone without periosteum is generally unsuccessful. It is also important to consider that skin grafts do not provide a significant protective barrier for vital underlying structures and should not be applied over great vessels, nerves, or bone.

Early animal studies by Senn[5] in 1888 were among the first to document the use of the greater omentum in surgery, where it was applied for protection and support of healing intestinal anastomoses. Later, in 1937 Graham[6] would uncover its utility in closing perforated duodenal ulcers. However, the value of omental flaps in extraperitoneal surgery was not appreciated until the mid-20th century. Since that time the omentum has been used in the reconstruction of defects all over the body, including chest wall and head and neck wounds, breast reconstruction, and for the treatment of rectovaginal and vesicovaginal fistulae.

The omentum is a thin apron of fat-containing peritoneum, attaching to the greater curvature of the stomach and transverse colon. It drapes the anterior surface of the small intestine, extending inferiorly almost to the level of the pelvis. An omental flap can be based on either the right or left gastroepiploic artery and the omental vascular arcade, and may be designed in a pedicled or free fashion. Most commonly, it is harvested as a pedicle flap, and the right gastroepiploic artery is usually dominant with regard to caliber and length. A right gastroepiploic artery pedicle generally permits a greater arc of rotation than the left.

Preoperative Preparation

Box 16-1 KEY SURGICAL INSTRUMENTATION

Skin grafts

- Dermatome
- Skin graft mesher
- Light bolster dressing or negative pressure therapy device
- 3-0 or 4-0 chromic sutures

Omental flaps

- Laparoscopic equipment setup (trocars, graspers, video monitors; if laparoscopic harvest)
- Vascular clamps, vessel clips, or silk ties
- Bowel retractors
- Vaginal stent
- Dermatome

Skin grafts may be used to cover large perineal resection beds for anatomic reconstruction following superficial "skinning" vulvectomy, commonly performed for VIN grade III and carcinoma in situ. These defects are amenable to skin grafts because they are superficial and often have healthy, vascular wound beds. For these reasons, skin grafting of vulvar defects can be used in the setting of pre- or postoperative radiation with excellent outcomes. Vulvar skin grafts are useful when tissue bulk is not required for optimal reconstruction, or when patient preferences dictate that more anatomic or functional methods be avoided. In such cases primary closure of the vulvectomy defect may be reasonable if a tension-free closure can be accomplished (Figure 16-4).

The omental flap is unique among the reconstructive methods described here in that it necessitates violation

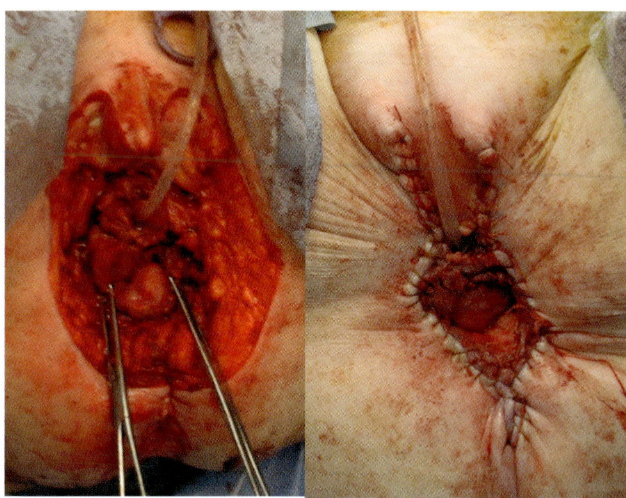

Fig. 16-4. (*Left*) Intraoperative photograph of perineum after vulvectomy. (*Right*) Intraoperative photograph after primary closure of vulvectomy defect.

of the peritoneal cavity. Flap harvest usually requires no additional incisions given that a laparotomy or other large exposure incision is necessitated by the pelvic cancer operation. In cases in which reconstruction is performed in a delayed or staged fashion, the omentum can be harvested through transdiaphragmatic or laparoscopic and minimally invasive techniques in addition to the standard open abdominal approach. Contraindications to the use of omental flaps include adhesions, concomitant abdominal disease, or evidence of any peritoneal or omental metastasis. Both reconstructive and oncologic teams should be keenly aware of oncologically safe technique during joint operations. This can be facilitated by having 2 or more separate scrub tables in the operating room, each with several extra pairs of gloves and ample sterile equipment to avoid any possible contamination of healthy tissues with malignant cells.

Surgical Procedure

1. Skin grafting

Box 16-2 MASTER SURGEON'S PRINCIPLES

Skin grafts

- Débride ischemic or threatened tissue at the recipient site prior to grafting
- Choose donor sites that can be closed primarily or well concealed by normal clothing
- A preset graft thickness of 0.014–0.018 in. is preferred
- Consider meshing or pie-crusting sheet graft to increase surface area or allow fluid egress
- A bolster or negative pressure wound dressing should cover the skin graft
- The donor site should be covered with nonadherent petrolatum gauze or similar dressing

Omental Flaps

- The right gastroepiploic artery is often preferred due to greater size and rotation
- Omental fixation at the pelvic rim allows for optimal neovaginal positioning
- A vaginal stent with draining capacity should be used and continued postoperatively
- The J portion of the omental flap must completely envelop the dermal side of the skin graft
- Stent migration is prevented by suturing stent to the labia and placing mattress sutures at the skin graft apex

Recipient Site Preparation. Prior to skin graft harvest, the recipient wound must be thoroughly assessed. The exact dimensions of the wound should be recorded, and the wound inspected for its degree of perfusion (capillary refill, skin blanching, or discoloration) or any evidence of infection. Ischemic or necrotic tissue at the wound edges should be sharply excised with the use of a tenotomy scissor, 15-blade, or other fine tissue-cutting instrument. The wound base may also be sharply debrided to establish a uniform thickness, and the wound is copiously irrigated with saline solution and gently dabbed dry with sterile gauze. Lightly moistened gauze is then gently placed over the wound bed and attention is directed to the donor site.

Donor Site Preparation. Options for the skin graft donor site should be discussed with the patient preoperatively; however, patient positioning, skin quality and availability, and preexisting skin lesions all factor into the final donor site selection. Common STSG donor sites include the lower abdomen, suprapubic region, lateral hairless inguinal region, upper medial and lateral thigh, and buttocks. For FTSGs, the groin is often the donor site of choice.

After the donor site is selected, a marking pen is used to outline a rectangle of skin, with dimensions slightly exceeding the recipient site in both length and width. Harvesting of the STSG is most easily accomplished with the use of a dermatome. One should bear in mind that using a dermatome restricts the maximum width of STSG that can be harvested at any given time, although there is no such restriction on the length of graft harvested. Scarring will ultimately occur at the donor site, and grafts should be arranged so as to minimize scar exposure in regular clothing if possible.

Graft Harvest and Care. It is critical to assess the integrity and function of the dermatome prior to each use; failure to do so is frighteningly common and may have catastrophic results. Verify that the appropriate blade is securely attached and that there are no mobile parts on the dermatome. The blade is set to a predefined thickness; for most STSGs, a thickness of approximately 0.014 to 0.018 in. is preferred. The dermatome motor is tested by turning it on for a several seconds before harvesting the graft.

A layer of mineral oil is placed over the outlined donor site. To harvest the graft, the dominant hand should hold the dermatome, while the nondominant hand provides traction on the surrounding skin to create a flat surface conducive to harvesting a graft of uniform thickness. The dermatome is turned on and approaches the skin directly in line with the outlined donor skin at an angle of approximately 45 degrees. The skin is contacted firmly and gentle pressure is maintained as the dermatome is advanced along the skin, without changing the angle. Once the end of the donor site is encountered, the dermatome is gently lifted away from the skin, and a toothed forceps is used to very carefully remove the skin graft from the dermatome.

Sheet grafts may be meshed to significantly increase skin graft surface area and facilitate fluid egress; however, this may result in increased secondary contraction and a suboptimal aesthetic outcome. Pie-crusting the sheet graft (the placement of intermittent slit incisions in a skin graft) may be used to permit fluid egress and allow assessment of structures deep to the graft with less compromise of the final aesthetic result.

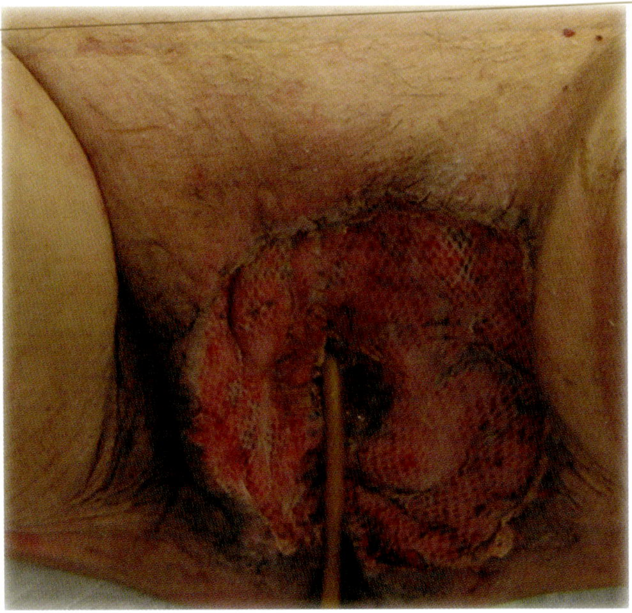

Fig. 16-5. Perineum of an elderly woman with multiple medical comorbidities and Bowen disease following radical vulvectomy and split-thickness skin graft reconstruction, with 95% skin graft incorporation. The radical vulvectomy wound was initially closed primarily with subsequent wound breakdown requiring debridement and wound vacuum-assisted closure (VAC) therapy for 1 week before skin graft coverage.

Handling and Securing the Graft. The skin graft is carefully inset into the recipient wound. Care should be taken to prevent any traction or tearing of the skin graft. It is important to maintain awareness of skin graft sidedness, such that the epidermal side is placed facing outward and the dermal side facing the recipient wound bed. Redundant edges are trimmed such that the skin graft is tailored to the wound. The skin graft is then sutured in place from skin graft to bordering native skin in a running fashion with a 3-0 or 4-0 chromic suture (Figure 16-5). Although practices vary widely, it is common to place a monolayer sheet of nonadherent petrolatum gauze dressing directly over the skin graft. The graft is then secured in place with a bolster or other light pressure dressing to closely approximate the graft to the recipient bed and prevent mechanical disruption, hematoma, or seroma. To do this, several 2-0 or 3-0 Nylon sutures are placed in a symmetrical fashion in the skin immediately adjacent to the graft. A separate stitch should be used for each interrupted suture and the suture tied but not cut, leaving 2 very long tails associated with each suture. The needle of each stitch is removed, and opposing paired suture tails are tied firmly over a mineral oil–soaked cotton ball (or multiple cotton balls) forming the bolster dressing on top of the graft. More recently, negative pressure wound dressings are being placed over skin grafts in the place of bolsters to facilitate egress and promote graft take.

Donor Site Dressing. FTSG sites must be either closed primarily, skin-grafted, or temporarily covered with a dressing. The approach to coverage of STSG donor sites varies widely among surgeons; it is our practice to cover the donor site with a monolayer of Xeroform that is gently sutured in place with interrupted 3-0 or 4-0 chromic sutures at the corners and middle of the dressing (sutured in place at ~ 6 points). As the suture absorbs and the donor site recovers, the Xeroform will ultimately slough off at which point a dressing is no longer required over the donor site. Some surgeons prefer to spray the donor site with thrombogenic agents to promote hemostasis or cover the donor site with alternative sterile nonadherent dressings and abdominal pads, with or without overlying circumferential 4-in. gauze and elastic bandage wrappings.

2. Omental flaps

Omental Flap Mobilization. Three methods have been described for the mobilization of a pedicled omental flap (Figure 16-6). The 2 safest and most widely used involve isolation of the right or left gastroepiploic artery as the pedicle; pedicled omentoplasty based on the epiploic arcade fails to provide adequate mobilization. The greater omentum is first elevated from the transverse colon, and the left and right gastroepiploic arteries are identified. Each pedicle results in a unique arc of rotation. On the right side, the flap rotates about the first portion of the duodenum; on the left side the flap pivots at the splenocolic ligament. The desired pedicle is selected and the other side tied off with nonabsorbable suture tie.

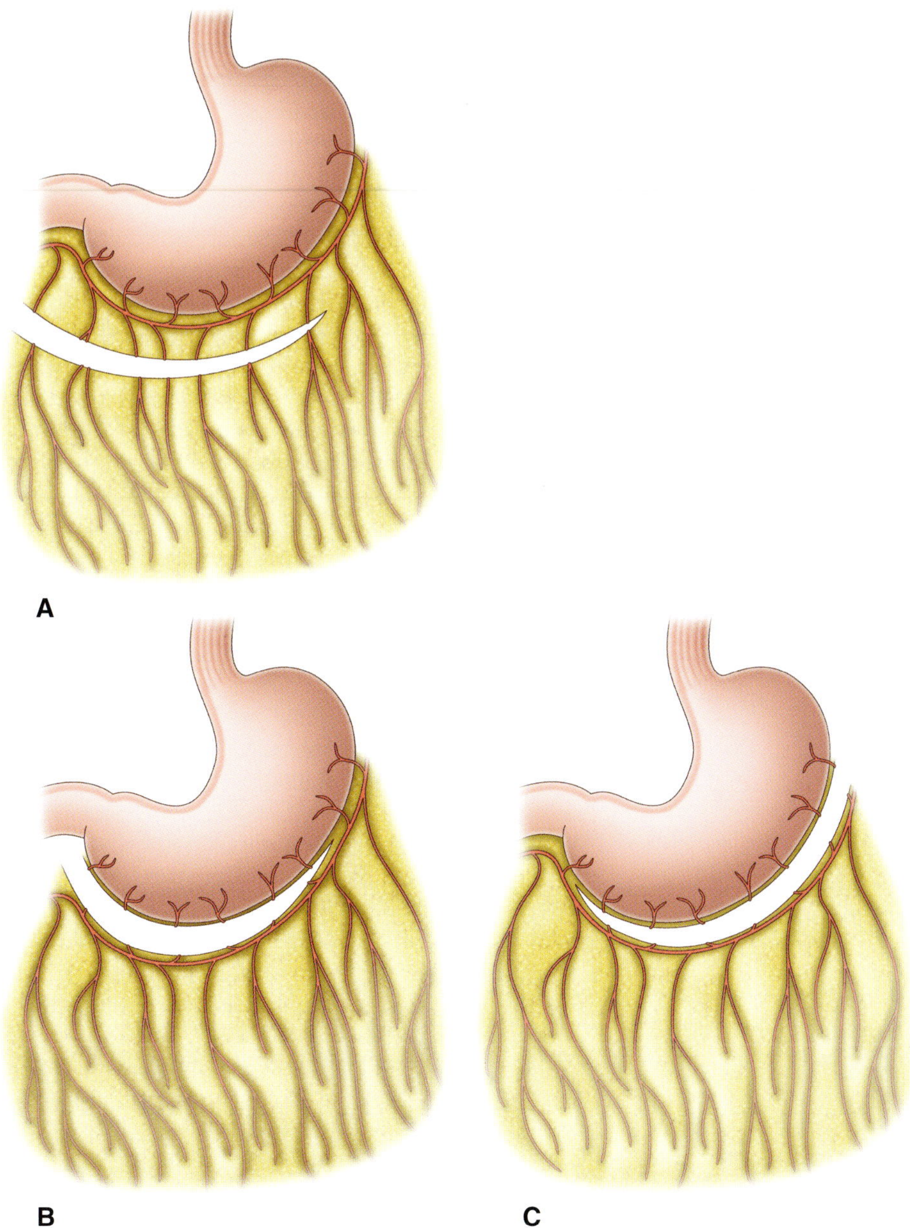

Fig. 16-6. Techniques for mobilizing an omental flap. (**A**) Mobilization based on the epiploic arcade, which is not commonly used in pelvic reconstruction. (**B**) Pedicled omentoplasty based on the left gastroepiploic vessels. (**C**) Pedicled omentoplasty based on the right gastroepiploic vessels. (Adapted and reproduced with permission from O'Leary DP. Use of the greater omentum in colorectal surgery. *Dis Colon Rectum.* 1999;42(4):533-539.)

The remaining attachments of the pedicle are carefully divided to completely mobilize the flap, protecting the pedicle at all times. The omentum is then tunneled into the pelvis along either the right or left paracolic gutters or in a retrocolic fashion, where it lines the pelvic sidewalls and fills the pelvic floor.

Omental J Flap Neovaginal Reconstruction. In a procedure similar to the McIndoe technique described earlier, Wheeless[7] and later Kusiak and Rosenblum[8] described a method of neovaginal reconstruction using a skin graft-lined vaginal stent; the critical distinction from the McIndoe technique is the use of an omental flap to completely envelop and nourish the skin graft. Use of an omental flap in this method emerged out of the necessity to ensure "take" of the skin graft; patients undergoing total pelvic exenteration may not have surrounding structures like urinary bladder or rectum, which are conducive for skin graft incorporation.

In this technique the omentum is fashioned as a J-shaped flap, oriented first downward along the paracolic gutter before

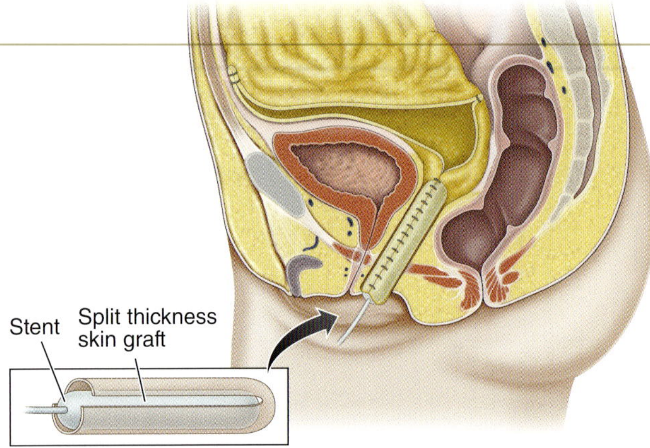

Fig. 16-7. Neovaginal reconstruction with a split-thickness skin graft and omental J flap. (*Left*) A split-thickness skin graft is wrapped around the vaginal stent, with dermal side facing outward. This is depicted diagrammatically (*top*) and intraoperatively (*bottom*). (*Right*) Sagittal view diagram demonstrating omental cylinder flap supporting and wrapping the stent and skin graft, with omental fixation at the pelvic inlet.

being sutured directly to the periosteum along the iliopectineal line at the level of the pelvic rim. The distal aspect of the flap is allowed to curve toward to the introitus. An STSG is harvested and sutured circumferentially to a vaginal-shaped prosthetic stent, with the dermal side facing outward and the epidermal side contacting the stent. The vaginal stent itself can collect fluid and be attached to drainage tubing to promote fluid egress. At this point an apical cruciate incision can be made in the skin graft, permitting drainage through the stent and decreasing the risk of seroma formation. The curved J portion of the omental flap is then used to cylindrically wrap the skin graft–lined vaginal stent, creating the neovagina (Figure 16-7). The omental cylinder is closed on itself with polyglycolic acid suture, and several horizontal mattress sutures are placed at the apex of the skin graft to prevent migration of the stent deep into the pelvis. Interrupted absorbable sutures are used to secure the stent/skin-graft complex to the introitus. The attachment point of the vaginal stent drain is brought through the introitus, the tubing later removed once fluid egress subsides. Two 2-0 Nylon sutures are placed through the labia and stent bilaterally as another measure to prevent stent migration.

Omentum in Pelvic Floor Reconstruction. The use of the omental flap for reconstruction of pelvic floor defects is well established. Pelvic cancer operations often result in significant dead space, and the structural laxity and generous surface area of the omental flap are well suited to this purpose. Packing the pelvis with omentum after radical gynecologic resections raises the level of the lowest loop of small intestine, and appears to protect against intestinal complications of subsequent radiotherapy exposure. Pedicle omentoplasty in pelvic floor reconstruction theoretically provides neovascularization, improved lymphatic drainage, and protection from perineal hernia.

Postoperative Care

Box 16-3 PERIOPERATIVE MORBIDITY

Skin grafts
- Shear
- Infection
- Seroma
- Hematoma

Omental flaps
- Abdominal wall infection
- Hernia
- Fascial dehiscence
- Stent migration

Perineal skin grafts for vulvar reconstruction are fragile in the immediate postoperative period and experience shear stress with minimal movement. Prolonged postoperative immobilization is necessary to ensure appropriate graft take, with particular attention to avoiding abduction. It is prudent to maintain urinary catheterization postoperatively for this reason. Negative pressure wound dressings should be left in place for a minimum of 5 days postoperatively, after which they are not replaced assuming appropriate skin graft take.

When neovaginal reconstruction is performed with an omental J flap and skin graft, patients must remain immobilized with vaginal stent in place to permit graft take and neovaginal molding in the immediate postoperative period. Although practice varies widely, stents are often left in place for 1 week, followed by a return to the operating room in which the stent is removed. After this, multiple daily stenting intervals (around 20 minutes) commence that may continue for 6 months postoperatively to prevent graft contraction and stenosis.

Long-Term Outcomes

Box 16-4 DELAYED COMPLICATIONS

Skin grafts
- Graft failure

Omental flaps
- Vesico-neovaginal fistula
- Recto-neovaginal fistula
- Neovaginal stenosis

Complications following skin grafting in vulvar reconstruction are relatively rare. Seroma, hematoma, infection, mechanical shear, and failure of graft take are among the most common reasons for skin graft failure, and typically occur in the early postoperative period. Grafting onto irradiated or poorly vascularized wound beds increases the likelihood of graft failure, which is a devastating complication.

The low harvest morbidity rate, reliable blood supply, and immunologic and angiogenic properties of the omental flap promote excellent wound healing and low perioperative morbidity in these patients. The most common complications following omental flap harvest include abdominal wall infection, fascial dehiscence, and symptomatic hernia. Hultman et al[9] uncovered a beneficial effect of omental flaps on postoperative complications following pelvic exenteration and abdominoperineal resection. Specifically, pelvic abscess, urinoma, deep venous thrombosis, flap dehiscence, hernia, bowel obstruction, and fistula were all significantly less common when omental flaps were used in the reconstruction.[9] Reoperation for complications related to omentoplasty has been reported in the 0% to 7% range.

Not unsurprisingly, patient compliance with vaginal-stenting continues to be the chief deterrent to a successful reconstruction using the J flap method of neovaginal reconstruction. Complications following this procedure include fistulae between neovagina and bladder or rectum, graft failure, and reoperation.

ADVANCEMENT AND ROTATIONAL FLAPS IN VULVOVAGINAL RECONSTRUCTION

Anatomic Considerations

As early as the late 1960s and 70s, flaps found broad clinical application in vulvovaginal reconstruction. Pioneering work by McCraw et al[10] in the 1970s resulted in the gracilis and other myocutaneous flaps for the provision of tissue bulk with robust vascularity for vulvovaginal defects. Huge strides were made in the late 1980s and early 1990s after seminal vascular anatomic studies by Cormack et al led to rationally designed local fasciocutaneous and advancement flaps.[11,12] Most notable among these include fasciocutaneous flaps based on the internal pudendal vessels such as the neurovascular pudendal thigh flap (also known as the Singapore flap) for vaginal reconstruction and various V-Y advancement flaps for vulvar reconstruction. More recently, several techniques have been developed that take advantage of redundant abdominal tissue to reconstruct the vulva in an advancement flap fashion. These methods may combine abdominoplasty with additional flaps to reconstruct the vulva while simultaneously improving abdominal contour.

Local vascularized flaps in vulvar reconstruction are most appropriate when the surgeon is confronted with poorly vascularized, scarred, or radiated wound beds. They are also indicated for defects that are larger in three dimensions than can be adequately addressed by primary wound closure or skin grafting. In addition to providing bulk for padding or restoration, these flaps are well suited for potentially hostile environments resulting from fistulous drainage, chronic infection, or spillage of intestinal fluid. In cases in which radiation to the surrounding tissues precludes the use of these tissues in flap coverage, more distant sources of vascularized tissue must be considered.

The vascular organization within local flaps is of central importance and can be divided broadly into 2 types. Random pattern flaps are not based on distinct vascular territories and should have a length to width ratio of at least 2:1 to ensure adequate perfusion. Alternatively, axial pattern flaps are single-pedicle flaps that contain an anatomically recognizable arteriovenous system. This chapter contains examples of flaps with both types of vascular organization.

Preoperative Preparation

Box 16-5 KEY SURGICAL INSTRUMENTATION

V-Y advancement flaps

- Doppler probe for vascular mapping

Singapore flap

- Doppler probe for vascular mapping

Abdominoplasty advancement flaps

- Surgical drains
- Abdominal binder

The technique of V-to-Y advancement as a simple means to provide soft tissue coverage of defects throughout the body is well established. Except in cases where the soft tissue volume of muscle flaps is required, V-Y advancement flaps have become the preferred choice in vulvar reconstruction, avoiding the bulk, donor site morbidity, ischemic complications, and unsightly abdominal or leg scars associated with several muscle flaps. This is particularly true as recent trends in vulvar cancer surgery favor more conservative resections. The diversity of V-Y advancement flaps is tremendous. Despite this heterogeneity, these flaps share several important principles. They are each random pattern flaps, relying on a rich subcutaneous vascular network and muscular perforating arteries for their perfusion. Each involves creating a V-shaped flap of perineal soft tissue that may include fascia or muscle, depending on the particular technique or demands of the resection bed. The flaps may be oriented in several different directions, yet each is advanced toward the midline to close the vulvar defect. The donor site is closed in a V-Y fashion.

The Singapore or neurovascular pudendal thigh flap has proven to be an excellent rotational flap for vaginal reconstruction. Originally described in Singapore by Wee and Joseph in 1989,[13] the technique utilizes fasciocutaneous flaps of the thigh crease overlying the adductor musculature for partial or total neovaginal reconstruction. This flap remains a viable option in vaginal reconstruction today for several different types of vaginal defects (see Figure 16-3).

Surgical Procedure

1. V-Y advancement flaps

Box 16-6 MASTER SURGEON'S PRINCIPLES

V-Y advancement flaps

- Incorporate muscle into the flap when additional bulk is needed at the resection bed
- Divide the attachment of the gracilis to the tibia for considerably greater advancement
- The gluteal V-Y flap may be superior in flap advancement and cosmetic outcome

Singapore flap

- Avoid including hair-bearing tissue into flap design if possible
- Maximum flap dimensions generally 15 × 6 cm
- Flap should be centered on groin crease to permit excellent scar concealment on closure
- The epimysium of the adductors is included in the flap to the protect neurovascular structures
- The flap should be undermined in the subcutaneous plane to permit adequate rotation
- Tunnel each flap under the labia by elevating the labia or dividing their posterior attachments

Abdominoplasty advancement flaps

- Harvest of FTSG/STSG from resected abdominal pannus avoids donor site morbidity
- Abdominoplasty can be coupled with pannicular advancement to assist in vulvar coverage

V-Y Flap Orientation. V-Y flaps can be organized by flap donor site location and include pubolabial, medial thigh, and gluteal V-Y advancement flaps (Figure 16-8). V-Y advancement flaps have been widely advocated for both partial and total vulvar defects (see Figure 16-2). Pubolabial flaps have now largely been replaced by alternative methods and are not discussed here.

Medial Thigh V-Y Advancement Flaps. Medial thigh V-Y advancement flaps are useful for both total and lateral vulvar defects. At least 2 types of medial thigh V-Y advancement flap have documented efficacy in vulvar reconstruction: a subcutaneous island flap and a musculocutaneous flap that incorporates the gracilis muscle (Figure 16-9). Both techniques involve approaching the defect from lateral to medial and use the same island of skin and subcutaneous tissue. The patient is placed in the lithotomy position and a V-shaped incision is made, with the broad base of the flap facing the defect that is to be covered. Care is taken to avoid injury to the musculocutaneous perforators from the gracilis and adductor musculature, which supply the flap. Depending on the needs of the resection bed, the flap can incorporate fascia as a fasciocutaneous flap or the gracilis muscle forming a musculocutaneous flap. When additional advancement or tissue bulk is required, the musculocutaneous V-Y flap is an excellent option. In this case the dissection is carried deeper to the level of the gracilis muscle, with great care taken to protect the medial circumflex femoral artery. A separate incision is made near the attachment point of the gracilis to the tibia, where the tendon is divided. This critical step results in a significant gain in advancement and can allow for some skin redundancy to recreate the appearance of labia majora. The soft-tissue island is advanced medially, and the medial margin of the flap is sutured to the vaginal mucosa; the donor site is closed in the standard V-Y fashion.

Gluteal V-Y Advancement Flaps. Medial thigh V-Y advancement flaps are rivaled only by gluteal V-Y advancement flaps in terms of their breadth of application. These flaps are based on the skin and subcutaneous tissue overlying the gluteus maximus, and rely on a blood supply from the inferior gluteal and circumflex femoral arteries. The most notable of the gluteal V-Y advancement flaps is the gluteal fold V-Y advancement flap (Figure 16-10). Medial thigh V-Y flap advancement flaps have been criticized for conspicuous scars that are left along the medial thighs. Gluteal V-Y flaps overcome this problem with concealed scar placement in the gluteal fold and allow a greater degree of advancement due to the tissue redundancy of the gluteal region. Surgical technique for these procedures is very similar to that for the medial thigh V-Y advancement flaps.

2. Singapore flap

Singapore Flap Design. The Singapore flap is an axial pattern rotational flap based on the posterior labial artery, which is a continuation of the perineal artery (Figure 16-11). Its innervation is provided by the posterior labial branches of the pudendal nerve and the perineal branches of the posterior cutaneous nerve of the thigh. Flap design should incorporate the tissue just lateral to the hair-bearing area of the labia majora and the flap centered on the crease of the groin, which is crucial for scar concealment. The base of the flap is marked in transverse orientation at the level of the posterior end of the introitus, and a 15 × 6 cm roughly rectangular-shaped flap is ideally suited for adults. These flap dimensions allow for primary closure of the donor site and are appropriately sized for creation of the neovaginal canal.

Flap Elevation and Tunneling. Two key points are worth mentioning in regard to elevation and tunneling of

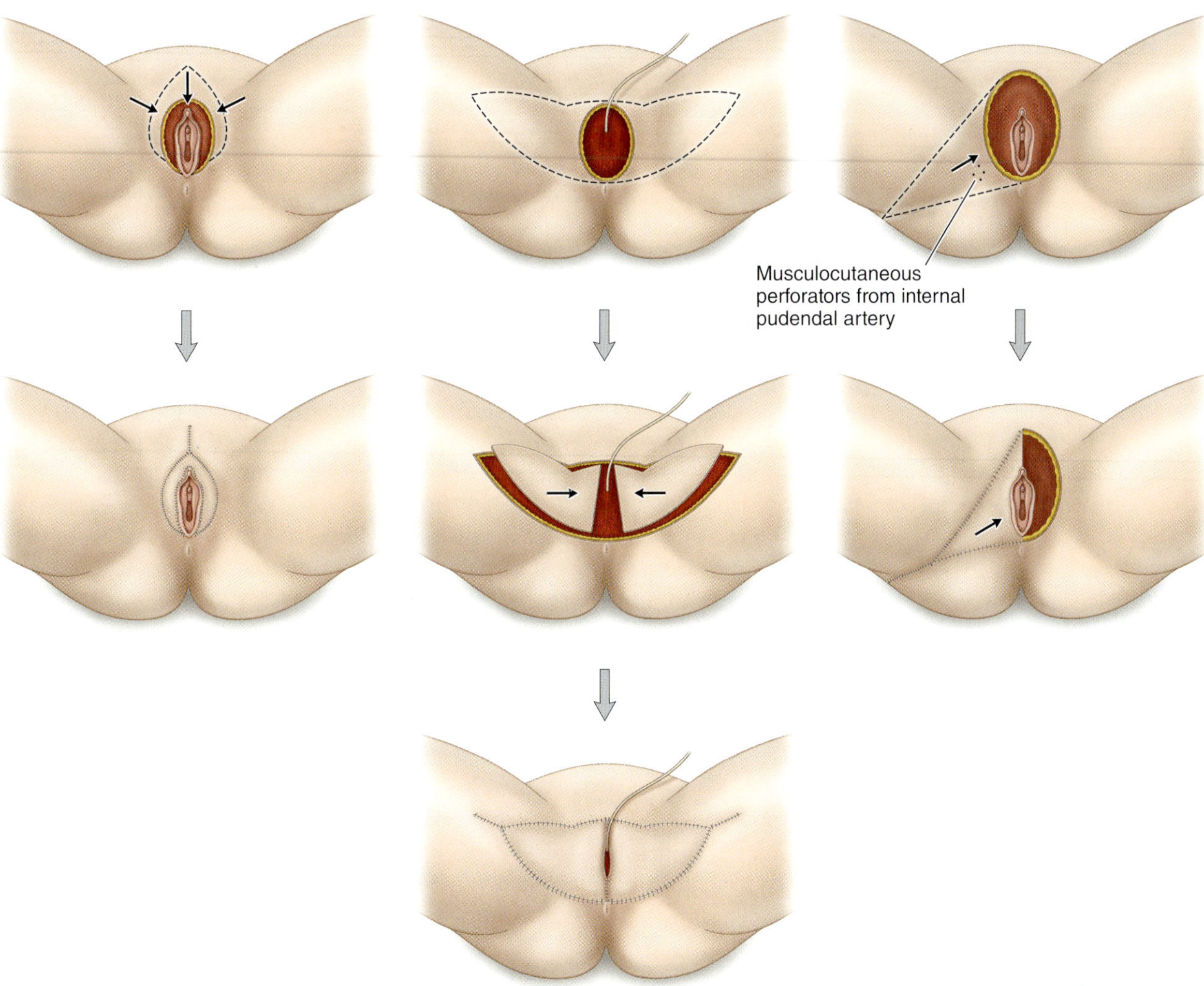

Fig. 16-8. Schematic representation of the differences among pubolabial, medial thigh, and gluteal V-Y advancement flaps. (*Left*) V-Y amplified sliding flap from the pubis, an example of a pubolabial V-Y advancement flap. Note that the 2 posterior flaps at the wound margin are rotated inferiorly and medially. (*Center*) Medial thigh V-Y advancement flap with base of triangular flap abutting the defect and apex extending along the medial thigh. (*Right*) Gluteal fold V-Y advancement flap, an example of gluteal V-Y advancement flap. Note that the base of the triangular flap also abuts the wound margin but the apex is oriented along the axis of the gluteal fold.

the Singapore flap. First, the flap is elevated with the deep fascia of the thigh and the epimysium of the adductor muscles, which adds an additional layer of protection of the neurovascular structures in the flap. After flap elevation, the base of the flap is undermined in the subcutaneous plane to facilitate 70 to 90 degrees of rotation, so that it may meet its contralateral counterpart in the midline. This is accomplished by making a 1- to 1.5-cm deep skin incision at the base down to the superficial subcutaneous tissue, and then undermining about 4 cm posteriorly in a plane parallel to the skin. These 2 critical maneuvers are demonstrated diagrammatically in Figure 16-12.

Each flap is then tunneled under the labia majora by first elevating the labia off the periosteum of the pubic rami and perineal membrane. The 2 flaps are sutured together in the midline to create a cul-de-sac, which is then invaginated and anchored to sacral periosteum, or rectum or bladder, if present. The vaginal opening is sutured to the mucocutaneous edge of the labia minora to complete the flap, and the donor site is closed primarily. The Modified Singapore flap differs only in that the labia majora are divided posteriorly, allowing easy anterior retraction of the labia majora. This maneuver facilitates tunneling and inset of the flaps with only minimal aesthetic loss (Figure 16-13).

3. Abdominoplasty advancement flaps

An alternative method of vulvar reconstruction incorporates concepts from “spare parts” surgery, in which redundant soft

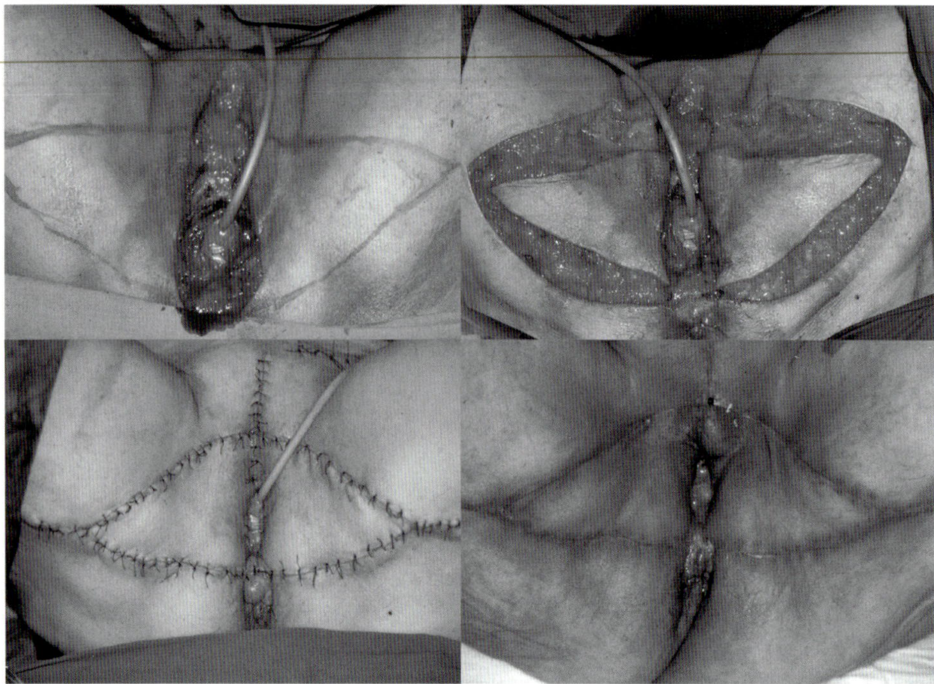

Fig. 16-9. Medial thigh V-Y advancement flap. (*Above, left*) Vulvar wound following radical vulvectomy and lymphadenectomy, with bilateral medial thigh V-Y advancement flaps outlined. (*Above, right*) Mobilization of bilateral triangular shaped island flaps. The gracilis muscle was not included in this flap. (*Below, left*) Immediate postoperative result. (*Below, right*) Result 2 months after operation. (Reproduced with permission from Tateo A, Tateo S, Bernasconi C, et al. Use of V-Y flap for vulvar reconstruction. *Gynecol Oncol.* 1996;62:203-207.)

tissue of the abdomen is used to reconstruct the vulva. While such methods have received little attention in the literature, they are particularly useful for coverage of mons pubis defects. One method is to combine abdominoplasty and pannicular advancement with other flap techniques to reconstruct the vulva (Figure 16-14). Another approach is to harvest full-thickness skin grafts from abdominal pannus for vulvar reconstruction followed by a panniculectomy style closure, which obviates concerns about closure or coverage of the skin graft donor site.

Postoperative Care

Box 16-7 PERIOPERATIVE MORBIDITY

V-Y advancement flaps
- Infection
- Poor wound healing
- Flap necrosis
- Wound dehiscence
- Scar contracture
- Temporary urinary stream deviation

Singapore flap
- Infection
- Poor wound healing
- Flap necrosis

Abdominoplasty advancement flaps
- Wound dehiscence
- Seroma
- Hematoma

Foley catheters are maintained postoperatively following V-Y advancement flap closure and the patient's mobility restricted for a variable interval. Practices vary widely, and drains are usually not needed in the vulvar region. Delays in local wound healing should be managed with a simple dressing regimen and daily cleansing. For all flaps involving the thigh and perineum, patients should avoid thigh abduction in the early postoperative period.

By contrast to the omental J flap method of neovaginal reconstruction, the Singapore flap method requires no vaginal stenting postoperatively. There is variation in postoperative mobility recommendations, but most patients are on bedrest with the thighs adducted in the early postoperative period. During this interval, operative drains and urinary catheterization are continued. The orientation of the flaps makes postoperative monitoring of its distal aspect difficult, but the pedicle and lower part of the flap can be monitored readily by physical examination and Doppler flow assessment.

Whenever panniculectomy or methods involving abdominoplasty are performed, patients should be maintained in a

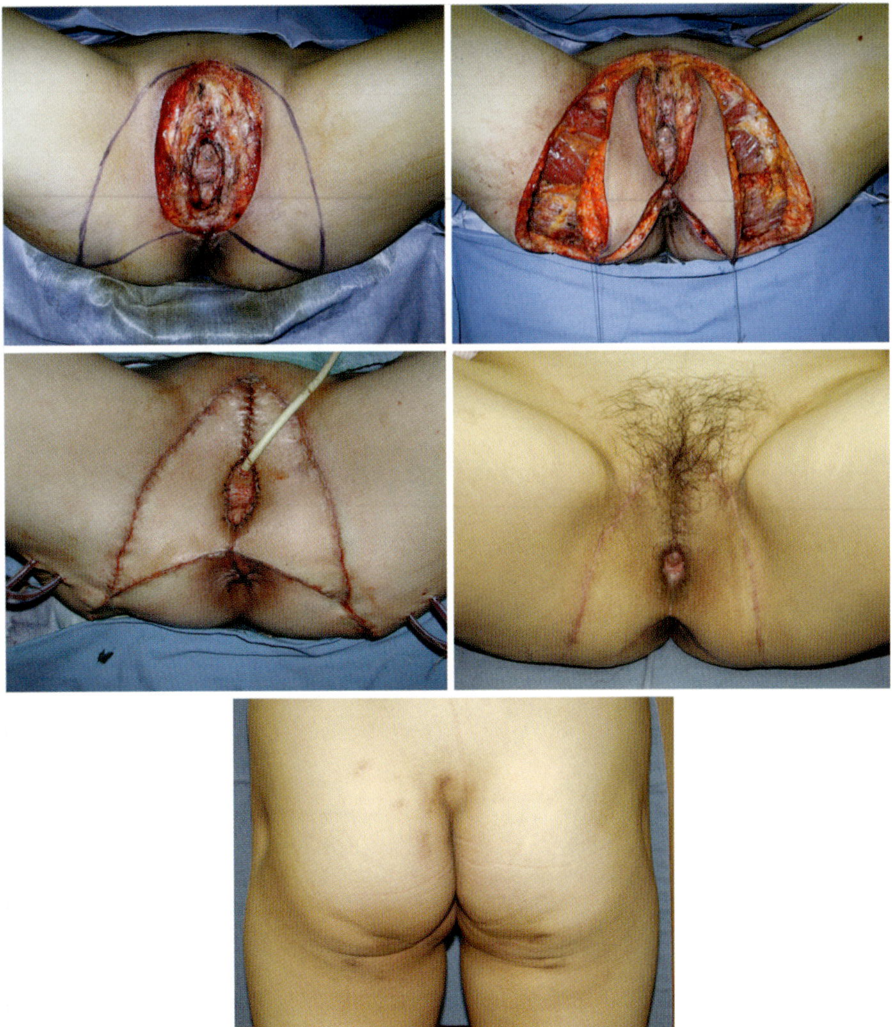

Fig. 16-10. Gluteal fold V-Y advancement flap. (*Above, left*) Simple vulvectomy defect in a 40-year-old woman with vulvar intraepithelial neoplasia. Gluteal fold V-Y flaps outlined bilaterally. Note base of triangular flaps at defect margin, with apex directed along the axis of the gluteal fold. (*Above, right*) Bilateral elevation fasciocutaneous flap islands. (*Center, left*) Flap advancement in a V-Y fashion with skin closure. (*Center, right*) Anterior view 6 months after surgery. (*Below*) Posterior view 6 months after surgery. (Reproduced with permission from Lee PK, Choi MS, Ahn ST, et al. Gluteal fold V-Y advancement flap for vulvar and vaginal reconstruction: a new flap. *Plast Reconstr Surg*. 2006;118:401-406.)

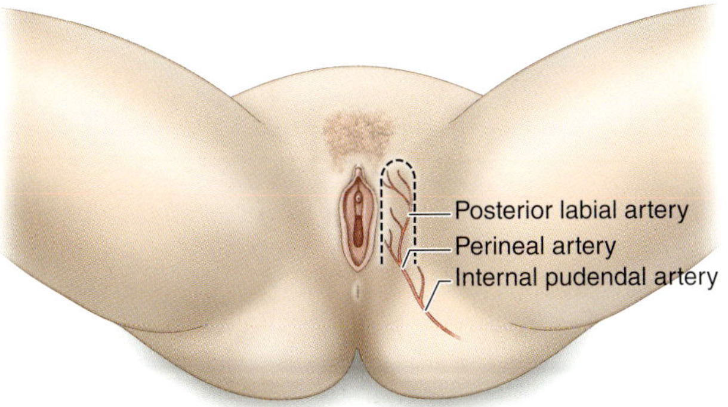

Fig. 16-11. Diagram of perineum illustrating the axial pattern blood supply of the Singapore flap. The flap is supplied by the posterior labial artery, a continuation of the perineal artery.

"beach-chair" position in the early postoperative period to avoid tension on the abdominal closure. At least 2 surgical drains are commonly used and patients may be placed in an abdominal binder to prevent seroma formation or excessive tension on surgical wounds.

Long-Term Outcomes

Box 16-8 DELAYED COMPLICATIONS

V-Y advancement flaps

- Suboptimal cosmesis
- Introduction of hairy skin to vaginal wall

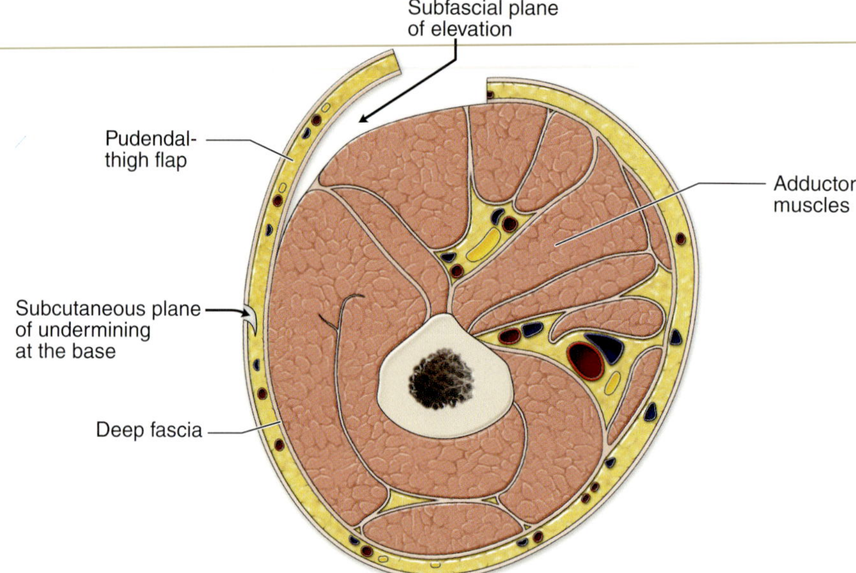

Fig. 16-12. Axial view diagram of the upper medial thigh demonstrating 2 key points for Singapore flap elevation. The plane of flap elevation is beneath the deep fascia and includes the epimysium of the adductor muscles. The base of the flap is incised superficially and undermined in the subcutaneous plane, in order to allow for medial rotation of the flap toward the midline.

Singapore flap

- Introduction of hairy skin to vaginal wall
- Vaginal vault shortening
- Vulvar pain during intercourse
- Apical necrosis

Abdominoplasty advancement flaps

- Poor wound healing
- Unfavorable scarring

No single V-Y advancement flap technique has been shown to be better than another. However, some techniques are more suited to particular vulvar defects, and each differs in their attendant donor site morbidity, ultimate scar position, flap orientation, and degree of advancement. The reconstructive surgeon must be fluent in many such methods to accommodate the preferences and reconstructive needs of each individual patient.

V-Y flaps have demonstrated remarkable resilience, very rare ischemic complications, retained sensation, and great potential for sexual function. Cosmetic outcomes are often excellent given that the skin used for reconstruction is well matched to the resected tissue, and scars can be placed in concealed locations. These are quickly performed procedures, involve little blood loss, and have a great record of success in patients receiving chemotherapy and radiation. Revisional procedures are rarely indicated.

Vulvar cancer may involve lymphatic spread, requiring radical resection with inguinal lymph node sampling for treatment. The oncologic safety of medial thigh V-Y advancement flaps was documented in a landmark study by Carramaschi et al,[14] where no increase in the recurrence rate of malignancy was noted following immediate flap reconstruction after resection for invasive vulvar carcinoma. Scar contracture, temporary urinary stream deviation, and introduction of hairy

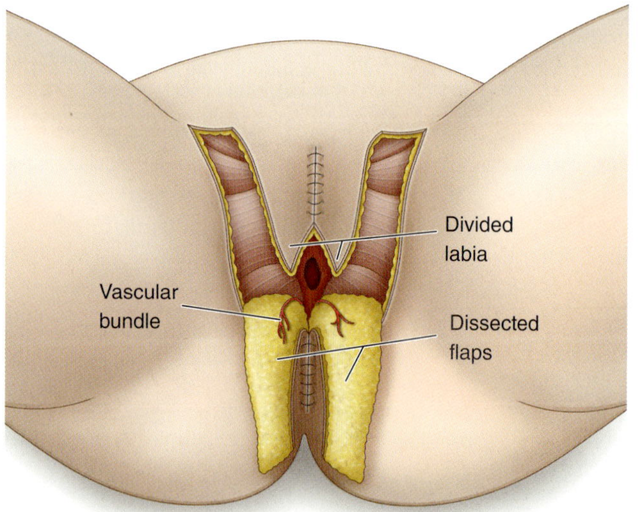

Fig. 16-13. Modified Singapore flap. (*Left*) Diagram depicting the posteriorly divided labia, which represents the major distinction from the Singapore flap. (*Right*) Intraoperative view demonstrating divided labia posteriorly, with flaps elevated in preparation for creating the neovaginal pouch.

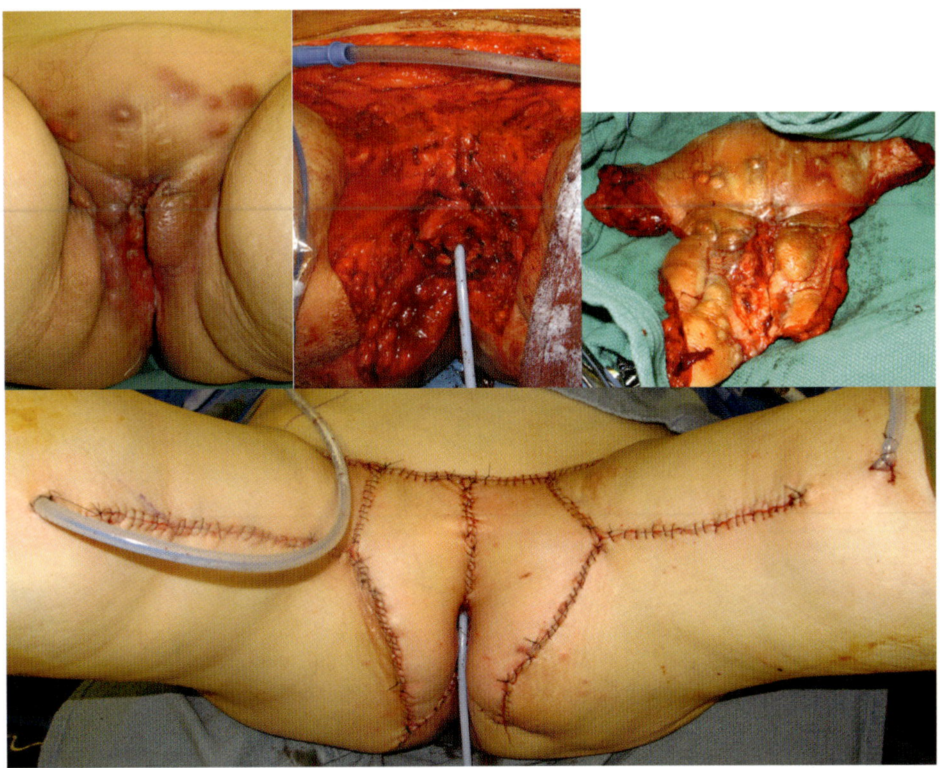

Fig. 16-14. (*Above, left*) Immediate preoperative photograph of a 57-year-old woman with a history of vulvar carcinoma status postresection in 2007 followed by chemoradiotherapy. She subsequently developed lesions consistent with carcinoma in situ and dysplasia. (*Above, center*) Perineum immediately after resection. (*Above, right*) Vulvectomy specimen, with significant suprapubic component. (*Below*) Elegant reconstructive solution incorporating bilateral gracilis myocutaneous flaps and abdominoplasty advancement flap.

skin of the remaining labia majora into the vaginal wall are infrequent but notable complications.

The Singapore flap introduced unprecedented ease, safety, and reliability to vaginal reconstruction and can yield excellent functional and cosmetic outcomes. It boasts numerous advantages, including a single-stage procedure with technical simplicity. It has a reliable blood supply and sufficient tissue thickness that allow for elimination of some dead space. The flap often retains its original pattern of innervation of the erogenous zones of the perineum and upper thigh, and is cosmetically acceptable to patients with scars strategically hidden in the groin and perineal creases. Success with postoperative sexual intercourse has been reported without prolapse or stenosis; however, vault shortening and vulvar pain may discourage this. As with many methods in vulvovaginal reconstruction, the data on outcomes following Singapore flap neovaginal reconstruction in the reported literature are limited. The rate of complete flap loss is less than 15%, but a higher risk for apical necrosis exists. The flap may transfer hair-bearing skin, which may become problematic postoperatively.

Even though data on outcomes following abdominoplasty advancement flaps in vulvovaginal reconstruction are lacking, complications in this setting can be extrapolated from the literature on abdominoplasty alone. The most common complications following abdominoplasty include seroma, infection, wound dehiscence, poor wound healing, and hematoma. Studies have documented the safety of combining abdominoplasty with other operations such as elective breast surgery, and complications in combined surgeries are not significantly different from those of abdominoplasty alone.[15] Those who smoke appear to be at increased risk for both wound-healing problems and infections.

SUMMARY

Reconstructive procedures using skin grafts, omental flaps, and advancement and rotational flaps have evolved to minimize morbidity, optimize function and appearance, and preserve quality of life for women undergoing radical surgery for gynecologic cancer. A multidisciplinary collaboration between gynecologic cancer surgeons and plastic surgeons forms the foundation for effective, contemporary treatment of vulvovaginal defects. Increasing emphasis is being placed on patient quality of life after radical surgery for gynecologic cancer, and additional research is needed to define optimal treatment paradigms.

REFERENCES

1. Cordeiro PG, Pusic AL, Disa JJ. A classification system and reconstructive algorithm for acquired vaginal defects. *Plast Reconstr Surg.* 2002;110(4):1058-1065.

2. Höckel M, Dornhöfer N. Vulvovaginal reconstruction for neoplastic disease. *Lancet Oncol*. 2008;9(6):559-568.
3. Abbe R. A new method of creating a vagina in a case of congenital absence. *Med Record NY*. 1898;54:836-838.
4. McIndoe AH, Bannister JB. An operation for the cure of congenital absence of the vagina. *J Obstet Gynaecol Br Emp*. 1938;45(3):490-494.
5. Senn N. An experimental contribution to intestinal surgery with special reference to the treatment of intestinal obstruction. *Ann Surg*. 1888;7:171-186.
6. Graham RR. Treatment of perforated duodenal ulcers. *Surg Gynecol Obstet*. 1937;64:235-238.
7. Wheeless CR. Neovagina constructed from an omental "J" flap and a split thickness skin graft. *Gynecol Oncol*. 1989;35(2):224-226.
8. Kusiak JF, Rosenblum NG. Neovaginal reconstruction after exenteration using an omental flaps and split-thickness skin graft. *Plast Reconstr Surg*. 1996;97(4):775-781.
9. Hultman CS, Sherrill MA, Halvorson EG, et al. Utility of the omentum in pelvic floor reconstruction following resection of anorectal malignancy: patient selection, technical caveats, and clinical outcomes. *Ann Plast Surg*. 2010;64(5):559-562.
10. McCraw JB, Dibbell DG, Carraway JH. Clinical definition of independent myocutaneous vascular territories. *Plast Reconstr Surg*. 1977;60(3):341-352.
11. Cormack GC, Lamberty BGH. A classification of fasciocutaneous flaps according to their patterns of vascularisation. *Br J Plast Surg*. 1984;37(1):80-87.
12. Wang TN, Whetzel T, Mathes SJ, Vasconez LO. A fasciocutaneous flap for vaginal and perineal reconstruction. *Plast Reconstr Surg*. 1987;80(1):95-103.
13. Wee JT, Joseph VT. A new technique of vaginal reconstruction using neurovascular pudendal-thigh flap: a preliminary report. *Plast Reconstr Surg*. 1989;83(4):701-709.
14. Carramaschi F, Ramos ML, Nisida AC, et al. V-Y flap for perineal reconstruction following modified approach to vulvectomy in vulvar cancer. *Int J Gynaecol Obstet*. 1999;65:157-163.
15. Buck DW II, Mustoe TA. An evidence-based approach to abdominoplasty. *Plast Reconstr Surg*. 2010;126(6):2189-2195.

Chapter 17. Rectus Abdominis Flaps and Pudendal Thigh and Related Flaps

Theresa Y. Wang, MD,
Michael Chu, MD, and
Colleen M. McCarthy, MD

BACKGROUND

Reconstruction of the vulvovaginal and pelvic region can be a complex and formidable undertaking. Defects from oncologic resection can be extensive and variable. The increasing use of adjuvant radiation therapy and chemotherapy further adds to the challenge of achieving uncomplicated wound healing. Trends indicate that patients are being diagnosed with gynecologic malignancies at younger ages, and with better treatments, long-term survival has increased.[1-4] Longer survival results in a higher risk of local recurrence, which can complicate reconstruction, because the operative field in such patients is often scarred and radiated. The goals of reconstructing vaginal defects are manifold: to restore normal anatomy, to facilitate primary wound healing, to fill in dead space in the pelvis with healthy tissue, to restore support of the pelvic floor, and to create a neovagina that allows for sexual activity.

Vaginal reconstruction comprises techniques designed to ameliorate defects not just from extirpative procedures but also from congenital vaginal agenesis. However, regardless of the cause of the defect, the ultimate goal is the same: to restore a vagina that maintains sexual function and body image. From the original nonoperative technique of stenting and dilatation by Frank[5] to skin graft inlay combined with stenting by McIndoe[6,7], to some of the more established flap techniques—including the gracilis myocutaneous flap,[8-12] the medial thigh flap, the rectus flap, the omentum, and various fasciocutaneous flaps—there is no one ideal method for reconstruction.[13-20] However, flaps must be able (1) to provide a reliable amount of skin and subcutaneous fat and/or muscle into the defect, to produce a functional outcome, (2) to provide a sensate flap, when needed, (3) to minimize donor site morbidity, and (4) to achieve an aesthetic outcome.

Vaginal defects can be reconstructed using a number of locoregional flaps. A detailed assessment of the wound must be performed before selection of the flap. To better visualize the range of vaginal defects, the vagina can be represented as a coned cylinder, as shown in Figure 17-1.[21,22] The opening of the cone is the introitus. The anterior wall of the vagina is adjacent to the bladder, the lateral walls are next to the pelvic musculature, and the posterior wall is in proximity to the rectum. Vaginal defects are classified, on the basis of these anatomic considerations, into 2 general categories: partial defects (type I) and circumferential defects (type II; see Figure 17-1). Type I defects are further classified as either anterior or lateral wall defects (type IA); these often result from bladder or urinary tract malignancies or from primary vaginal malignancies. Type IB defects are posterior wall defects and often are caused by colorectal cancers. Type II defects are circumferential defects and are further divided into type IIA, which are located in the upper two-thirds of the vagina and are usually caused by uterine and cervical malignancies, and type IIB, which result from total, circumferential vaginal resections related to pelvic exenterations.

INDICATIONS AND CLINICAL APPLICATIONS

A reconstructive algorithm can be used to simplify the choice of flap on the basis of the type of defect (Figure 17-2). Three regional flaps can be used to reconstruct the vast majority of vaginal defects. The Singapore or pudendal thigh fasciocutaneous flap is ideal for type IA defects, which involve the anterior or lateral wall.[13,23-28] This flap is well vascularized and reliable, and it is thin, which allows for easy insertion and insetting into the anterior/lateral defect. Type IB defects involve the posterior wall of the vagina, and the rectus abdominis flap provides well vascularized skin to cover the posterior vaginal wall and good muscle bulk to obliterate the dead space between the abdominal and pelvic cavities.[29,30] Type IIA defects can also be reconstructed using the rectus abdominis flap. For type IB defects, it provides a good skin paddle and good muscle bulk. However, for type IIA defects, this flap is best conformed into a rolled or tubed flap to form the neovagina. Type IIB defects, which result from circumferential

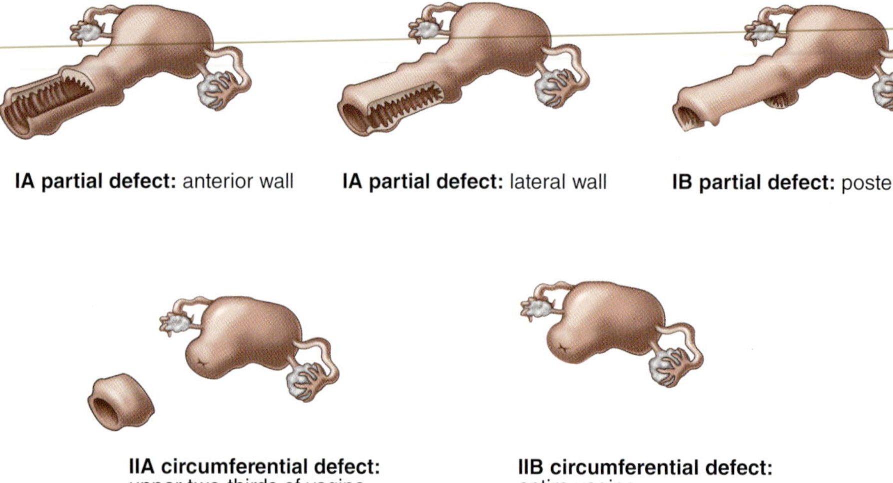

Fig. 17-1. To better visualize the range of vaginal defects, the vagina can be represented as a cylinder. Defects can be categorized as type I partial defects, which involve the anterior or lateral wall (type IA) or the posterior wall (type IB), or type II circumferential defects, which involve the upper two-thirds of the vagina (type IIA) or total vaginectomies (type IIB).

total vaginectomies, are best reconstructed using bilateral myocutaneous gracilis flaps. There is usually a large amount of vaginal surface area that needs to be replaced after a type IIB resection.

When selecting the flap for reconstruction, patient characteristics must also be taken into consideration. In patients who are obese, thin, pliable flaps such as the Singapore or pudendal thigh flap may be more optimal than the rectus flap, on account of the unreliable vascularity of the rectus flap's skin paddle in this population. For patients who smoke, careful consideration must be taken when selecting a regional flap to ensure reliability of the skin portion of the flap. In patients with prior vaginal reconstruction, the use of pedicled flaps may be limited. In radiated patients, because of scarring and the higher risk of problems with wound healing, the rectus flap may be used to fill pelvic dead space and to improve revascularization. For patients who do not plan to resume sexual activity, vaginal vault reconstruction can be excluded, and the rectus myocutaneous flap can be placed in the pelvis to obliterate dead space and to provide healthy, vascularized tissue to promote healing.

In patients with prior abdominal incisions, care must be taken when harvesting the flap to first ensure that the vascular pedicle is patent. For patients with a history of vascular surgery or inguinal hernia repairs (especially those in whom mesh was used), it may be prudent to obtain a preoperative angiogram to evaluate the inferior-based pedicle of the rectus flap.

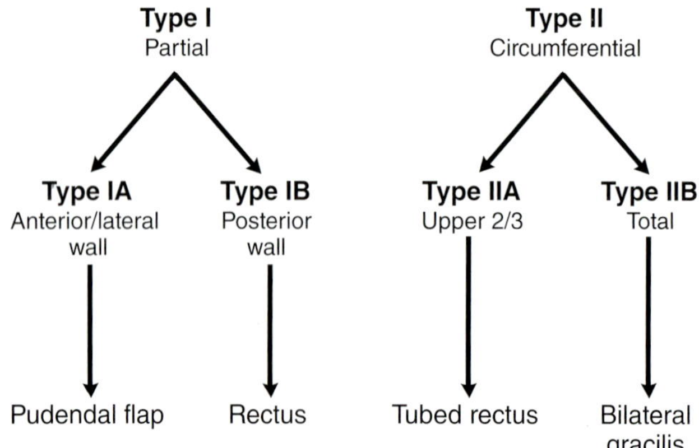

Fig. 17-2. An algorithm approach based on the type of vaginal resection.

RECTUS ABDOMINIS FLAP

Anatomic Considerations

The rectus abdominis is a long, flat muscle that extends vertically along the length of the anterior abdomen. Superiorly, the muscle inserts into the xiphoid process and attaches to the anterior surfaces of the fifth, sixth, and seventh costal cartilages. The paired rectus abdominis muscles are key postural muscles. Together they are responsible for flexing the lumbar spine when the muscles of the posterior trunk are relaxed. By contrast, when both the paired rectus and posterior trunk muscles contract, intra-abdominal cavity pressure is increased. Thus, the rectus muscles play an important role in coughing, defecation, and childbirth. Their dimensions measure approximately 26 cm in length and 6.6 cm in width. The muscle is enclosed by the anterior and posterior rectus sheaths, which are formed by the three fascial layers of the abdominal wall: the external oblique, the internal oblique, and the transversus abdominis. Of note, below the arcuate line, the anterior sheath is composed of aponeurotic contributions from all 3 fascial layers. However, there is no posterior sheath below the arcuate line; the posterior rectus muscle is separated from the peritoneal cavity by only the transversalis fascia. This is important to take into consideration when closing the fascia, once the muscle flap is harvested and inserted into the pelvis, in order to prevent herniation.

1. Blood supply and innervation

The rectus abdominis muscle is a class II muscle with a dual blood supply (Figure 17-3).[31-33] One dominant pedicle involves the superior epigastric artery and vein, which arise from the internal mammary vessels. This pedicle is approximately 2 cm in length and 1.8 mm in diameter. It lies beneath the muscle insertion at the costal margin and usually enters the muscle at the medial to midposterior third of the muscle. The other dominant pedicle involves the deep inferior epigastric artery and vein (DIEA/DIEV), which come from the external iliac artery and vein. This pedicle is approximately 5 to 6 cm in length and 2.5 mm in diameter. It enters the lateral edge of the muscle 4 cm superior to the groin origin. Minor pedicles that also contribute to the blood supply involve the subcostal and intercostal vessels. When using the pedicled rectus abdominis flap in pelvic and vaginal reconstruction, the muscle is usually detached superiorly at the costal margin, thereby making the deep inferior epigastric vessels the main blood supply to the flap.

The rectus muscles are innervated in a segmental fashion by intercostal nerves T7 through T12, which contain both motor and sensory fascicles. This segmental innervation prevents the use of this flap as an innervated muscle or sensory skin flap.

2. Skin territory

A musculocutaneous flap of varying dimensions can be designed along the entire length of the muscle and/or along any axis radiating from the umbilicus. The rectus muscle will perfuse a very wide vertical skin flap, with excellent reliability. The maximum width of the vertical island is typically dictated by the ability to obtain primary closure of the abdominal donor site (Figure 17-4); this is generally a width of 6 to 8 cm. Alternatively, a horizontal and/or oblique skin paddle can be placed anywhere along the length of the rectus abdominis muscle, but it is important to note that the concentration of perforators below the arcuate line is not as great. However, the flaps used for vaginal reconstruction are, in general, best

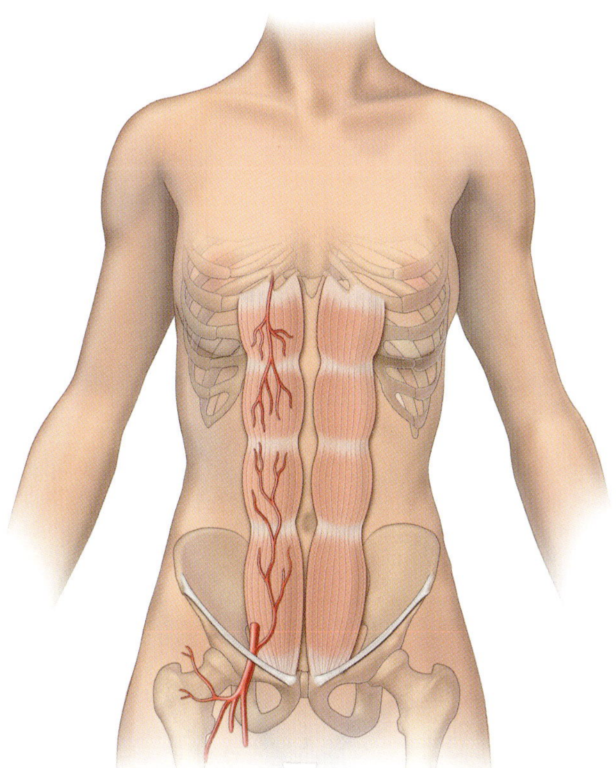

Fig. 17-3. The rectus abdominis muscle has a dual blood supply: superiorly from the internal mammary vessels and inferiorly from the deep inferior epigastric vessels.

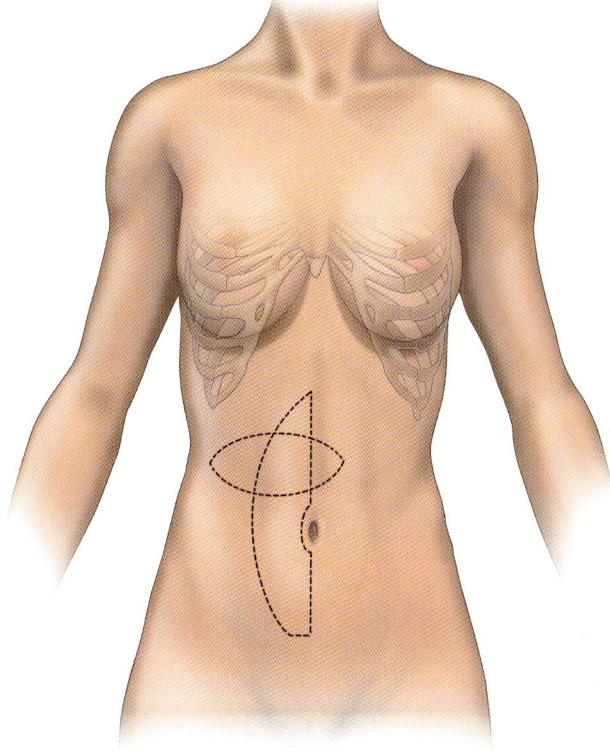

Fig. 17-4. A vertical or horizontal skin paddle can be designed over the rectus muscle.

designed either with muscle alone or with a vertical skin paddle and are, therefore, known as vertical rectus abdominis myocutaneous flaps. Perforating vessels arise along the course of both the superior epigastric and the deep inferior epigastric artery, piercing the anterior rectus abdominis fascia 2 to 3 cm from the lateral border of the muscle. A cluster of large (> 0.5 mm) periumbilical perforating vessels, representing terminal branches of the DIEA, is present within a rectangular area 2 cm cranial and 6 cm caudal to the umbilicus, and from 1 to 6 cm lateral to the umbilicus. A musculocutaneous flap should be designed to include at least one of these perforating vessels; thus, it is wise to make the skin island at least 6 cm in diameter and to include the direct periumbilical skin.

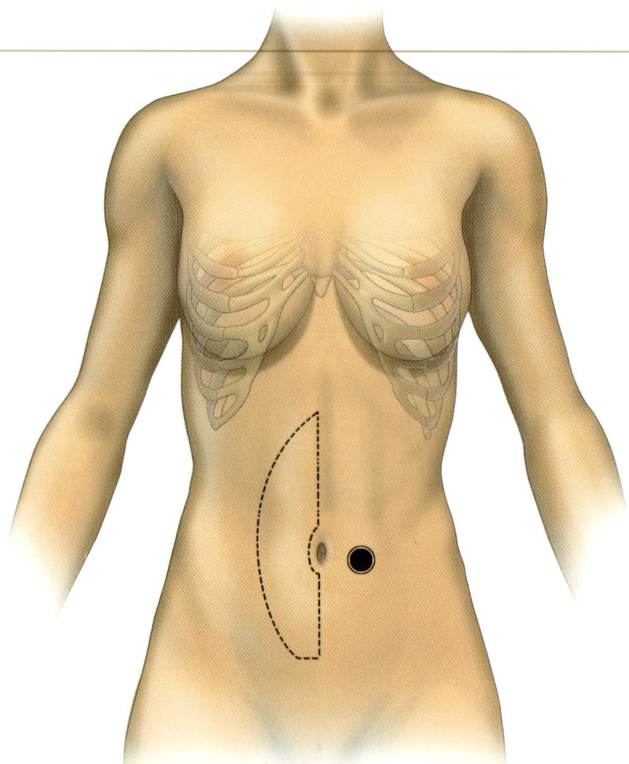

Fig. 17-5. The skin island should be on the side contralateral from the stoma site. The umbilicus should remain on the same side as the stoma.

Preoperative Preparation

Box 17-1 KEY SURGICAL INSTRUMENTATION FOR FLAP INSET

- A lighted retractor can be used in the pelvic region during flap inset for better visualization.
- The Lonestar retractor system can be used to help flap insetting in the vaginal wound and to allow for a simultaneous, 2-team approach for closing the abdomen while the flap is sutured in place and the perineal wound is closed.

The presence of long abdominal scars may interfere with flap design or preclude the use of the flap altogether. Furthermore, the placement of such scars may indicate that the vascular supply to the flap has previously been transected. For patients at risk for pulmonary complications and/or back pain or weakness, harvest of the flap should be carefully considered, because abdominal wall strength will be weakened following harvest of one or both rectus muscles. In cases in which ostomy sites are already present or are planned in the concurrent procedure, the contralateral muscle should ideally be harvested for the flap.

1. Muscle flap

The approximate location of the rectus abdominis muscle to be harvested is outlined. The lateral border of the muscle is indicated by a line drawn from the pubic tubercle, intersecting the midpoint of another line drawn from the anterior superior iliac spine, to the umbilicus. The medial border is typically represented by the midabdominal line, or linea alba; however, the border may lie more laterally, depending on the degree of diathesis between the paired rectus muscles. The arcuate line is located approximately midway between the umbilicus and the symphysis pubis or at the level of the anterosuperior iliac spine. Typically, a midline or paramedian vertical incision is planned.

2. Myocutaneous flap

A vertical cutaneous paddle can be designed over the rectus abdominis muscle. The flap is designed so that primary closure is permitted. The umbilicus should be maintained on the same side as the stoma. Therefore, the medial part of the vertical skin incision should be lateral to the umbilicus (Figure 17-5). The average flap width measures 5 to 6 cm, and the average length is 12 to 14 cm. The length of the skin paddle is determined according to the amount of vaginal wall surface area that is needed to be replaced after resection.

Surgical Procedure

Box 17-2 MASTER SURGEON'S PRINCIPLES

- Before flap elevation, the pedicle should be palpated at the iliac takeoff to ensure viable donor flap vessels. Retraction during the pelvic portion of the procedure should be performed without applying too much force and pressure, which can cause pedicle compression and thrombosis.
- To preserve the musculocutaneous perforators, elevation of the skin paddle of more than 1 cm on either side of the rectus muscle should be performed under direct vision.
- During flap elevation, the skin paddle can be sutured to the muscle to prevent shearing or separation of the skin island from the muscle underneath.

- To avoid pedicle tension and to prevent hernia formation, the fascia must be closed carefully—a breadth of 1 finger should be able to comfortably fit into the fascial defect at the flap base after primary closure.
- If the fascia is attenuated or if primary closure results in tearing of the fascia, mesh should be applied as reinforcement.

1. Muscle flap

Flap elevation is performed with the patient in the supine or lithotomy position. In general, for cases involving pelvic and vaginal reconstruction, the patient will already be in the lithotomy position from the oncologic resection portion of the case. The skin is incised, and subcutaneous tissue is dissected. Once the anterior rectus sheath is visualized along the length of the incision, the sheath is incised 1 cm lateral to the linea alba. This exposes the rectus abdominis muscle. The anterior rectus sheath is then sharply elevated from the anterior surface of the muscle. The muscle must also be freed from its close attachments to the anterior sheath at its inscriptions. The lateral border of the muscle is located. At a level just above the arcuate line, the rectus muscle is bluntly elevated from the posterior rectus sheath. Dissection is carefully continued distally to expose the vascular pedicle entering the posterior rectus sheath from a lateral direction. The DIEA and DIEV are readily seen coursing beneath the transparent transversalis fascia, approximately 3 to 4 cm below the level of the arcuate line.

Once the vascular pedicle has been visualized, attention can be turned to harvesting the muscle. Depending on the requirements of the recipient site, the rectus muscle is transected at or inferior to its sternocostal attachment. The muscle is then elevated from the posterior sheath, beginning superiorly and moving inferiorly. Segmental neurovascular structures are cut and ligated. At the level of the arcuate line, the vascular pedicle is traced from its point of entry into the muscle to the external iliac artery and vein. If a portion of the rectus muscle distal to the vascular pedicle is to be harvested, then the branch medial to this inferior muscle portion is preserved. Following transplantation, wound closure consists of careful approximation of both the anterior and the posterior sheaths of the anterior rectus sheath. Closed-suction drains are placed superficial to the fascial closure.

2. Myocutaneous flap

The lateral flap margin is incised, and the skin and subcutaneous tissues are elevated from the external oblique fascia, the linea semilunaris, and the lateral anterior rectus sheath, until the lateral row of musculocutaneous perforators is identified. A vertical incision is made in the anterior rectus sheath lateral to the perforating vessels, creating a cuff of fascia that incorporates the perforators. The incision is then extended proximally and distally so that the entire length of the muscle to be harvested is exposed. The medial skin margin is similarly incised, and the anterior rectus sheath is exposed. The medial skin island is raised from the anterior rectus sheath for approximately 1 cm or until the medial row of perforators is encountered. To expose the superior and inferior portions of the rectus muscle, it may be necessary to elevate the abdominal skin and subcutaneous tissues from the abdominal wall above and below the skin island, depending on the vertical length of the skin island. The superior- and inferior-most portions of the rectus muscle can then be identified by splitting the anterior rectus midway between the linea semilunaris and the linea alba. The rectus is divided superiorly. The flap is carefully elevated from the posterior sheath, in a superior to inferior direction, so that the transversalis fascia is not damaged (Figure 17-6). Several intercostal nerves and vessels, which will be visible on the surface of the posterior rectus sheath, are then divided. At the level of the arcuate line, the deep inferior epigastric vessels become visible on the undersurface of the rectus abdominis muscle. To obtain adequate pedicle length, the artery and vein are traced toward their origin from the external iliac vessels. The inferior portion of the rectus muscle is transected just below the entry of the vascular pedicle.

3. Transposition and inset

Care must be taken to maintain adequate room during transposition of the flap into the pelvis so that there is no pressure over the pedicle. For positioning into the pelvis, the flap is usually rotated anywhere from 120 to 180 degrees. For vaginal reconstructions, the angle used is closer to 180 degrees, so that the flap reaches down into the vaginal region (Figure 17-7A). The flap is rotated on its DIEA pedicle and is usually tunneled in an intraperitoneal fashion into the pelvis (Figure 17-7B). There should be a smooth trajectory, with no pedicle kinking and no tension placed once the flap is down in the pelvis/vaginal region. In addition, the flap should fit without too much pressure over the muscle or the skin island. There should be a comfortable amount of room maintained in the pelvis and the vagina for the entire flap. The transversalis or peritoneal defect should have adequate dimensions to avoid flap constriction; however, it must also be adequately tight to prevent the complication of hernia.

The perineal wound can be closed in a layered fashion using interrupted 2-0 Vicryl in the Scarpa layer and 3-0 Vicryl in the dermal layer. The skin can be closed using interrupted 3-0 Vicryl sutures. Meticulous closure should be performed in the perineal incision because this is a region at increased risk for wound dehiscence.

4. Skin island design

Once the flap is mobilized and the location and orientation are conformed to the vaginal defect, the skin island can be marked out; the portion that will remain in the pelvis is de-epithelialized, and the portion that will resurface the vaginal wall is retained. The skin island that will remain is marked out, the flap is again brought back to the surface, and the abdomen and the rest of the skin are removed. This usually requires de-epithelialization of the inferior portion of the skin paddle (Figures 17-8). If the flap is used to

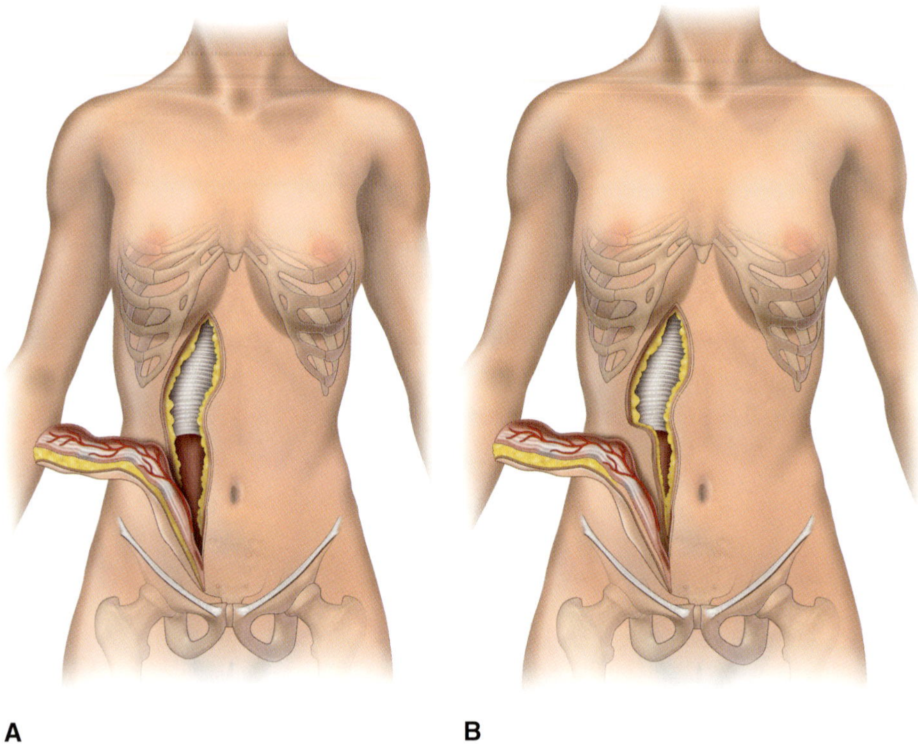

Fig. 17-6. The flap is transected at the superior muscle border and elevated from the posterior sheath, from the cranial to the caudal direction. The intercostal nerves and vessels should be ligated between the muscle and the posterior sheath. (A) Larger paddle (B) Smaller paddle

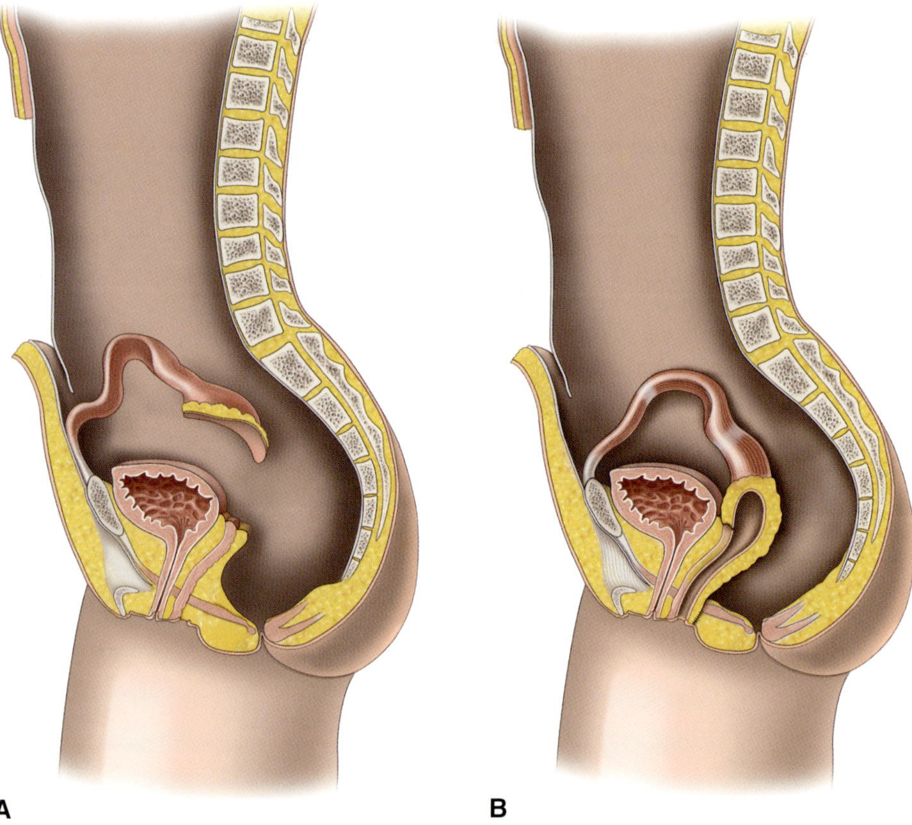

Fig. 17-7. (A) The flap is rotated 180 degrees intraperitoneally into the pelvis. (B) The flap is sutured to the residual vagina.

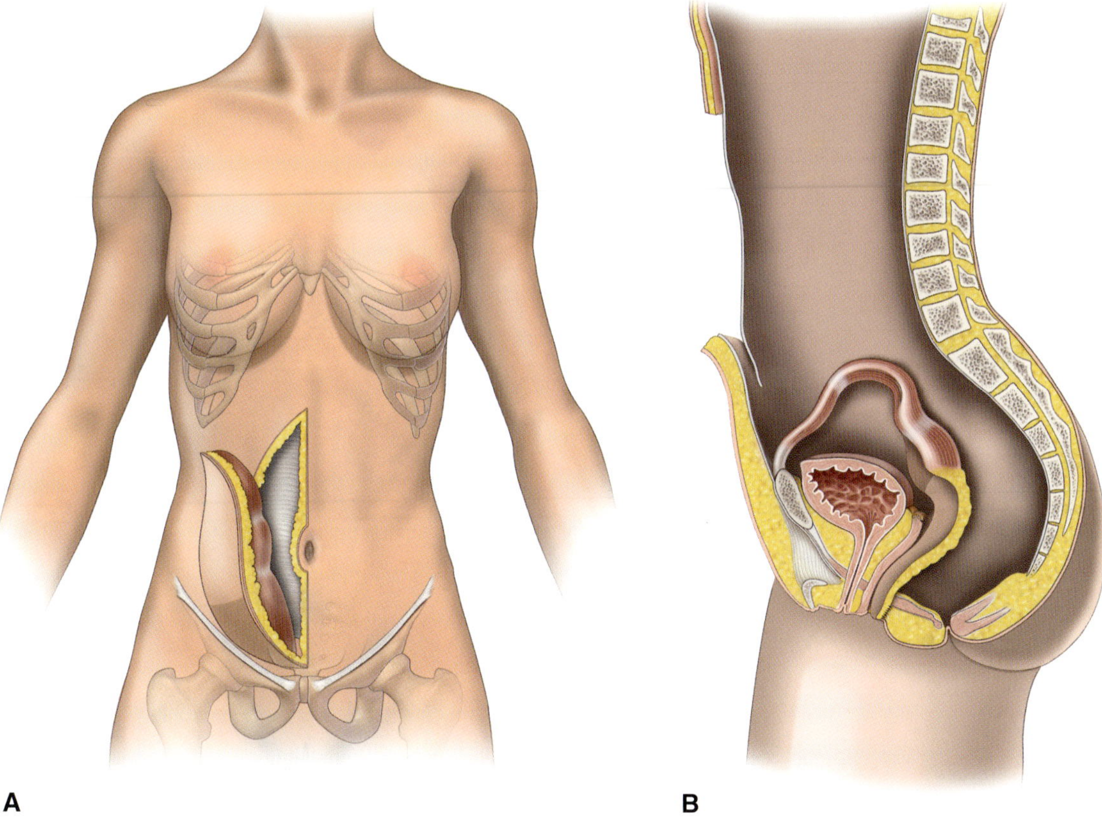

Fig. 17-8. (A) Mobilization of skin island. (B) For a posterior vaginal defect, the inferior portion of the vertical skin island is de-epithelialized. This portion will later sit in the pelvis, whereas the superior portion of the skin island will form the new posterior vaginal wall.

reconstruct a circumferential defect, it is tubed in a transverse fashion into a pouch, with no de-epithelialization, and the pouch is tunneled into the pelvis (Figures 17-9). The edge of the flap is sutured to the remaining vaginal cuff from above (Figure 17-9).

5. Donor site closure

Meticulous donor site closure is critical for avoiding future herniation and maintaining abdominal wall integrity. The anterior sheath is closed primarily with running or interrupted permanent sutures. If the fascia appears to be weak or attenuated, then mesh can be placed as reinforcement. Skin can be closed using a 2-layered closure.

SINGAPORE OR PUDENDAL THIGH FASCIOCUTANEOUS FLAP

Anatomic Considerations

The Singapore or pudendal thigh fasciocutaneous flap was originally described for vaginal reconstruction by Wee and Joseph in 1989.[13] It is well vascularized and reliable, which makes it an excellent option for type IA defects. Because of its fasciocutaneous nature, the thin flap easily conforms to the anterior/lateral wall vaginal defect.

1. Blood supply and innervation

Blood is supplied to the pudendal thigh flap by the posterior labial artery, which originates from the internal pudendal artery.[13] The pedicle is approximately 10 to 12 cm in length and 1 to 1.5 mm in diameter. The main nerve supply to the flap is the pudendal nerve (S2–S4). Only the posterior aspect of the flap is innervated by the pudendal nerve branches (the posterior labial branch and the perineal branch of the posterior cutaneous nerve of the thigh). As the posterior portion of the flap is neurovascularly intact, this flap is sensate and has the same erogenous sensation as that of the perineum and medial upper thigh.

Preoperative Preparation

The flap can be safely elevated up to 15 × 6 cm, in accordance with the original anatomic studies.[13] This also allows for primary closure of the donor site. The flap can be raised in the groin crease just lateral to the labia major and then transposed toward the midline (Figures 17-10 and 17-11). This is further modified by releasing the labia majora, which allows

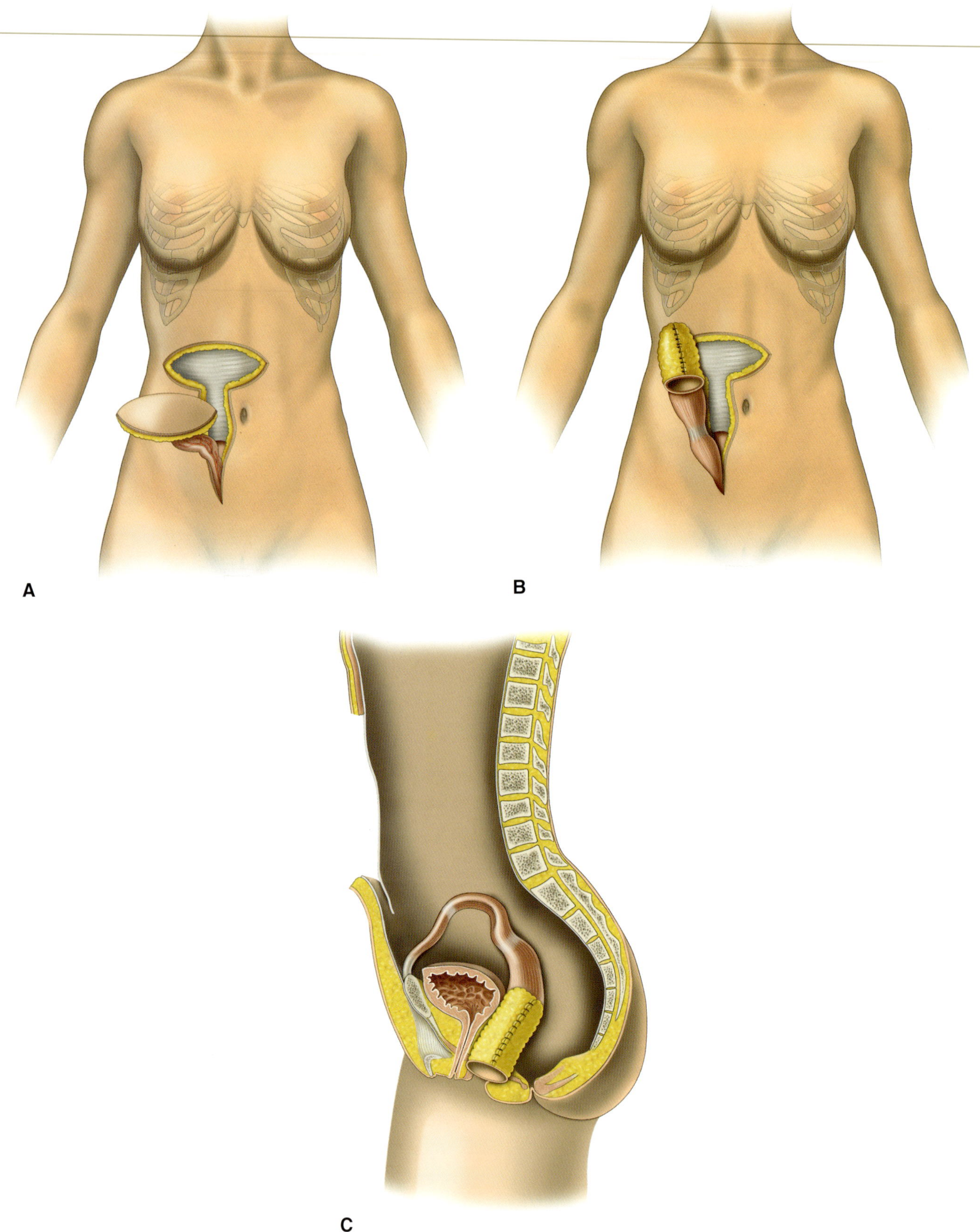

Fig. 17-9. For circumferential defects (A), a transverse skin island is designed, and (B) the flap is tubed and (C) inset into the pelvis.

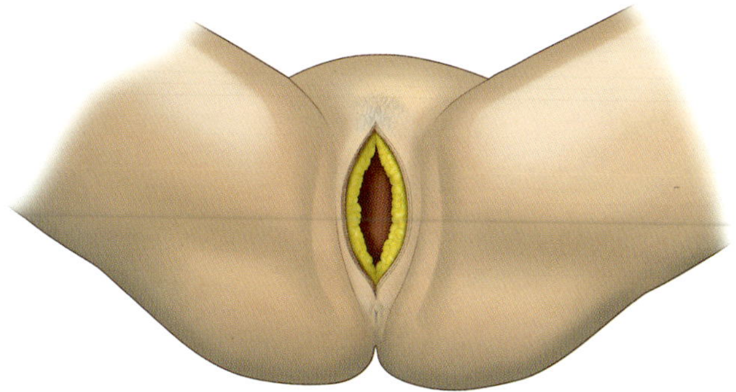

Fig. 17-10. The skin island for the pudendal thigh flap is just lateral to the groin crease. The flap is elevated in an anterior to posterior direction.

for easier rotation of the flap into position (Figure 17-12).[23] Key preoperative markings consist of the posterior border of the vagina, which marks the posterior margin and the base of the flap. The lateral border of the labia majora is the medial edge of the flap. The flap dimensions are then centered over the groin, with the distal margin of the flap in the femoral triangle region. The lateral edge of the flap is determined by the width that will allow closure of the primary donor site. Although in its native dimensions this flap is generally sufficient for reconstruction of the vagina, tissue expansion can be performed before the flap procedure if a larger skin area is needed.

This flap is a good option for patients who are obese, because the flap is thin compared with the bulkier rectus flap. It is important to note that this flap may not be feasible for patients who need vulvectomy or who have malignancy of the lower third of the vagina. In such cases, there is an increased risk of lymphatic spread to the groin and medial thigh region, making the pudendal thigh flap undesirable for transfer, as this would place potentially malignant tissue in the zone of reconstruction.

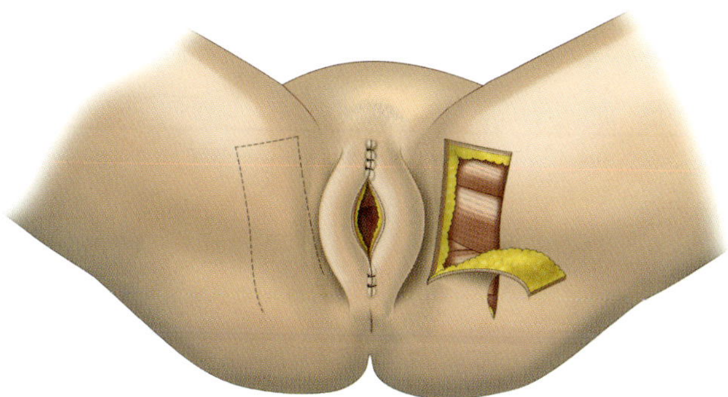

Fig. 17-11. The modified pudendal thigh flap releases the labia majora to allow better arc of rotation of the flap.

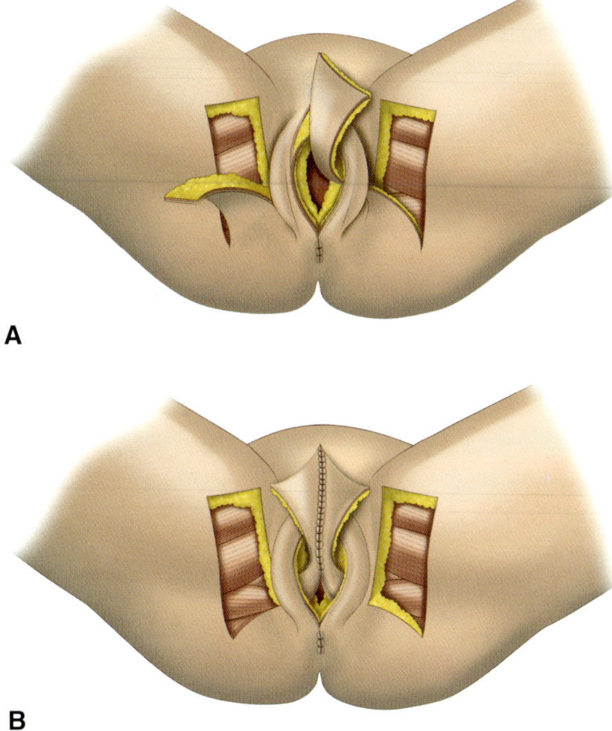

Fig. 17-12. The flaps can also be (A) tunneled under the labia majora and (B) placed into the defect.

Surgical Procedure

Box 17-3 MASTER SURGEON'S PRINCIPLES

- To prevent shearing, the deep fascia should be sutured to the skin flap.
- To facilitate flap transposition and insetting, the labia can be posteriorly divided.
- The posterior perineal wound should be closed meticulously, because this area is prone to wound breakdown.

The patient is placed in the lithotomy position. The incision is first marked along the anterior border of the flap, in the femoral triangle, and is then performed in the lateral and medial aspects. The flap is elevated starting at the distal margin, down through the subcutaneous layer, to the deep fascia. It has been postulated that inclusion of the deep fascia in the flap improves the reliability of the vascularity. The subfascial plane is developed along the flap, and the epimysia of the adductor muscles are raised, along with the flap. The posterior border of the flap is then incised, and the base of the flap is undermined at the subcutaneous layer, approximately 1 to 1.5 cm deep. This will help to make flap rotation and insetting

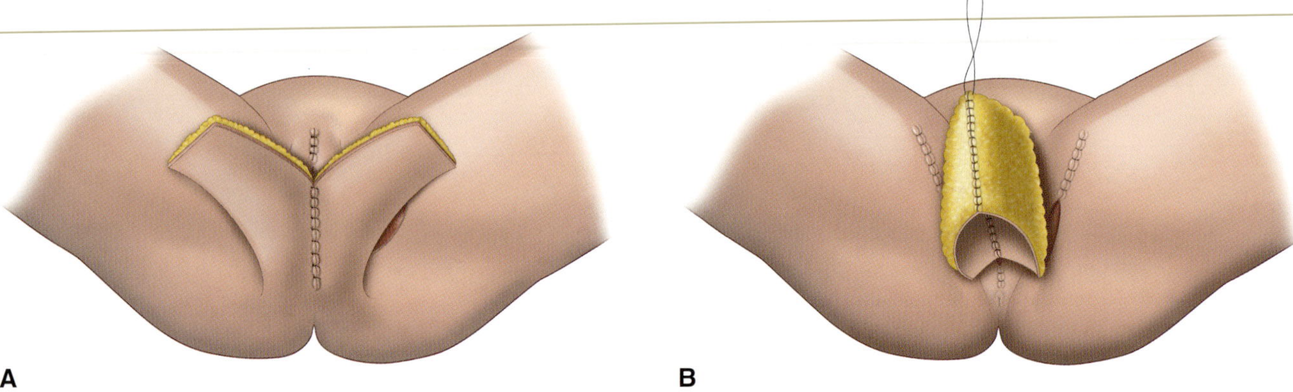

Fig. 17-13. (A) The flaps are everted, and the posterior suture line is stitched together, and (B) this is followed by suturing of the anterior aspect.

easier, as well as help to avoid the pedicle that runs deeper than this dissection.

If the size of the defect requires bilateral flaps, the other side can be raised in the same fashion.

1. Transposition and inset

The flap is next tunneled under the labia majora (Figure 17-12). The labia are elevated from the pubic rami and the perineal membrane. The labia can also be divided posteriorly to facilitate insetting, as well as to allow retraction anteriorly. If bilateral flaps are used, then they each are transposed approximately 70 to 90 degrees after tunneling to allow them to meet in the midline. They are sutured to each other to form the neovagina. The posterior suture line is performed first, from an anterior to a posterior orientation, with the flaps everted through the introitus (Figure 17-13). Once the tip of the neovagina is sutured, the anterior suture line is completed (Figure 17-13). The tip of the neovagina is then invaginated and sutured to the pelvis. This can be anchored to the sacrum or to whatever stable pelvic structures still remain from the resection. This maintains the desired vaginal depth. To complete the neovagina introitus, the posterior base of each flap is then sutured, at the skin level, to the remaining perineal skin (Figure 17-14).

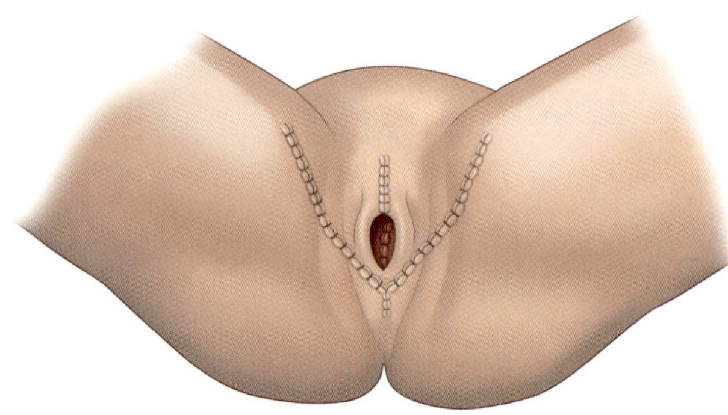

Fig. 17-14. In the completed perineal defect, the flaps are sewn circumferentially to the remaining perineal skin.

A drain is placed in the pelvis, as well as in each donor site thigh. The donor sites are primarily closed. The scars in the groin are usually well hidden.

POSTOPERATIVE CARE

Box 17-4 PERIOPERATIVE MORBIDITY

- If there is a visible skin island at the introitus, then the color, capillary refill, and turgor of the flap should be monitored to evaluate the vascularity and viability of the flap.
- Fevers, leukocytosis, and malodorous drainage from the perineal region or the pelvic drain can indicate pelvic abscess; this usually occurs 7 to 10 days following surgery. Further evaluation by computed tomography should be performed if suspicion of abscess is high.
- The risk of pelvic collection or abscess is approximately 10%.[35] This can usually be treated using drains placed by interventional radiology.
- Incisional dehiscence can occur, especially in patients with a history of radiation; its prevalence ranges from 10% to 50%.[34] This can usually be treated with local wound care, as long as there is viable muscle underneath. To avoid any pressure on the perineal wound, activity restrictions should be adhered to.
- Rectus abdominis flap loss occurs in fewer than 5% of patients.[36,37]
- Pudendal thigh flap loss occurs in fewer than 15% of patients[25]; however, these flaps are prone to tip necrosis.

Patients can be allowed to ambulate after surgery, as tolerated. However, to avoid putting pressure on the flap, they should avoid sitting for 6 weeks. For comfort, patients with a pudendal thigh flap can lie in bed with thighs adducted. To prevent pressure necrosis of the perineal incision as well as the flap, patients should have an air-fluidized therapy bed ordered before surgery. Urinary catheter drainage should be continued for approximately five to seven days, while the skin incision heals.

For patients with a rectus abdominis flap, diets can be advanced, as tolerated; this is often dictated by the intra-abdominal portion of the procedure, as bowel function returns.

Donor site drains can be removed when output is less than 30 cc during a 24-hour period. The pelvic drain can also be removed when output is less than 30 cc during a 24-hour period; however, this often occurs later than for the donor site drains. For both pelvic and donor sites, drains should be removed only once the patient is mobile, as increased mobility tends to increase the amount of output.

Early postoperative complications include wound dehiscence, hematoma, seroma, pelvic abscess, and flap loss.[34,35] Therefore, it is important to monitor the quality of drain outputs, to perform a clinical workup for any fevers, and to monitor any skin paddle changes from the flap. To protect against surgical wound infection, patients should be placed on perioperative antibiotics.

LONG-TERM OUTCOMES

Box 17-5 DELAYED COMPLICATIONS

- Hernia formation, bowel strictures, and fistulas
- Inappropriate size of neovagina—stenosis vs excessive size
- Vaginal dryness or oversecretions
- Vaginal or pelvic pain
- Flap prolapse
- Body image issues

Late complications can be both physical and psychological in nature. In the case of rectus reconstruction, there can be issues with abdominal wall weakness, resulting in visible bulges or hernia formation. The incidence of hernia is approximately 10%. Bowel strictures or fistulas can occur. Urinary or bowel complaints have also been reported.[39-41]

Although there are multiple methods and flaps available for vaginal reconstruction, a reduced number of patients return to sexual activity after reconstructive surgery. The literature shows that the percentage of survivors who return to sexual activity ranges from 30% to 70%.[36,42-45] This loss in sexual activity can be attributable to physical as well as psychological reasons. As reported by various studies, there can be vaginal dryness from inadequate secretion, and there can also be excessive vaginal secretion. Vaginal or donor site dysesthesias have also been reported. In cases with sensate pudendal thigh flaps, late complications can be associated with pelvic/neovaginal or thigh pain. The size of the neovagina can be a problem if stenosis occurs, resulting in inadequate vaginal size, which has been reported in 18% to 20% of cases. This complication has been found to have a higher incidence among patients with a pudendal thigh flap.[42] If there is difficulty in maintaining patency, requiring the use of obturators, this can be a deterrent to sexual activity. The neovagina can also have excessive size. This potential complication makes the insetting of the skin portion of the flap to the labia junction critical for maintaining an appropriate size of the new introitus, as well as the appropriate vaginal depth. Flap protrusion or prolapse can occur if the flap is not adequately fixated to stable pelvic structures. In addition, patients may complain of pelvic pain or pain with intercourse.

Overall, studies have shown that flaps decrease complications in patients who have previously undergone radiation or chemotherapy, who have other medical risk factors (eg, cancer recurrence, obesity, diabetes, smoking history), or both. When flaps are performed, there is less wound dehiscence, infection, and pelvic abscess.[48-51] Compared with fasciocutaneous flaps, myocutaneous flaps have fewer associated postoperative complications, and myocutaneous flap neovaginas have a lower rate of stenosis, compared with fasciocutaneous neovaginas.

Patients can experience body image issues and feel self-conscious of their ostomies or because of unsightly and conspicuous scarring. They may still be dealing with stressors, such as those related to their primary diagnosis and adjuvant therapies, and they may be anxious about cancer recurrence. Even with an anatomically functional vaginal reconstruction, the psychological impact of the disease and surgery is still considerable and should not be overlooked in the reconstructive process.

SUMMARY

Owing to the cancer disease process and the effect of adjuvant therapies—as well as the related psychological, sexual, physical, and emotional effects on the patient—vaginal reconstruction in the setting of oncologic resection is challenging. The goal of vaginal reconstruction is to restore not only the anatomy but also the function of the vagina. To adequately reconstruct the defect and to promote uncomplicated healing, a detailed assessment of the wound must be performed. To optimize the results of the reconstruction, an appropriate flap can be selected by use of an algorithm approach based on the type of vaginal defect.

REFERENCES

1. Crowe PJ, Temple WJ, Lopez MJ, et al. Pelvic exenteration for advanced pelvic malignancy. *Semin Surg Oncol.* 1999;17:152-160.
2. Eltabbakh GH. Recent advances in the management of women with ovarian cancer. *Minerva Ginecol.* 2004;56:81-89.
3. Bhoola SM, Alvarez RD. Novel therapies for recurrent ovarian cancer management. *Expert Rev Anticancer Ther.* 2004;4:437-448.
4. Elit L, Chambers A, Fyles A, et al. Systematic review of adjuvant care for women with stage I ovarian carcinoma. *Cancer.* 2004;101:1926-1935.

5. Frank RT. The formation of an artificial vagina without operation. *Am J Obstet Gynecol.* 1938;35:1053-1055.
6. McIndoe A. The treatment of congenital absence and obliterative conditions of the vagina. *By J Plast Surg.* 1949;2:254-267.
7. Buss JG, Lee RA. McIndoe procedure for vaginal agenesis: results and complications. *Mayo Clin Proc.* 1989;64:758-761.
8. McCraw JB, Massey FM, Shanklin KD, et al. Vaginal reconstruction with gracilis myocutaneous flaps. *Plast Recons Surg.* 1976;58:176-183.
9. Copeland LJ, Hancock KC, Gershenson DM, et al. Gracilis myocutaneous vaginal reconstruction concurrent with total pelvic exenteration. *Am J Obstet Gynecol.* 1989;160:1095.
10. Heath PM, Woods JE, Podratz KC, et al. Gracilis myocutaneous vaginal reconstruction. *Mayo Clin Proc.* 1984;59:21-24.
11. Cain JM, Diamond A, Tamimi HK, et al. The morbidity and benefits of concurrent gracilis myocutaneous graft with pelvic exenteration. *Obstet Gynecol.* 1989;74:185-189.
12. Soper JT, Larson D, Hunter VJ, et al. Short gracilis myocutaneous flaps for vulvovaginal reconstruction after radical pelvic surgery. *Obstet Gynecol.* 1989;74:823-827.
13. Wee JT, Joseph VT. A new technique of vaginal reconstruction using neurovascular pudendal-thigh flaps: a preliminary report. *Plast Recons Surg.* 1989;83:701-709.
14. Tobin GR, Day TG. Vaginal and pelvic reconstruction with distally based rectus abdominus myocutaneous flaps. *Plast Recons Surg.* 1988;81:62-73.
15. Skene AI, Gault DT, Woodhouse CR, et al. Perineal, vulval and vaginoperineal reconstruction using the rectus abdominus myocutaneous flap. *Br J Surg.* 1990;77:635-637.
16. Kroll S, Pollock R, Milburn J, et al. Transpelvic rectus abdominus flap reconstruction of defects following abdominal-perineal resection. *Am Surg.* 1989;55:632-637.
17. Wheeless CR. Neovagina constructed from an omental flap and a split-thickness skin graft. *Gynecol Oncol.* 1989;35:224-226.
18. Morton KE, Davies D, Dewhurst J. The use of the fasciocutaneous flap in vaginal reconstruction. *Br J Obstet Gynecol.* 1986;93:970-973.
19. Wang TN, Whetzel T, Mathes SJ, et al. A fasciocutaneous flap for vaginal and perineal reconstruction. *Plast Recons Surg.* 1987;80:95-103.
20. Chen ZJ, Chen MY, Chen Z, et al. Vaginal reconstruction with an axial subcutaneous pedicle flap from the interior abdominal wall: a new method. *Plast Recons Surg.* 1989;83:1005-1012.
21. Cordeiro PG, Pusic AL, Disa JJ. A classification system and reconstructive algorithm for acquired vaginal defects. *Plas Recons Surg.* 2002;110:1058-1065.
22. Pusic AL, Mehrara BJ. Vaginal reconstruction: an algorithm approach to defect classification and flap reconstruction. *J Surg Onc.* 2006;94:515-521.
23. Woods JE, Alter G, Meland B, et al. Experience with vaginal reconstruction utilizing the modified Singapore Flap. *Plas Recons Surg.* 1992;90:270-274.
24. Giraldo F, Gonzalez C. The versatility of the pudendal thigh fasciocutaneous flap used as an island flap (letter). *Plast Recons Surg.* 2001;108:2172-2174.
25. Gleeson NC, Baile W, Roberts WS, et al. Pudendal thigh fasciocutaneous flaps for vaginal reconstruction in gynecologic oncology. *Gynecol Oncol.* 1994;54:269-274.
26. Monstrey S, Blondeel P, Van Landuyt K, et al. The versatility of the pudendal thigh fasciocutaneous flap used as an island flap. *Plast Recons Surg.* 2001;107:719-725.
27. Joseph VT, Wee JTK. New technique of vaginal reconstruction using neurovascular pudendal-thigh flaps. In: Strauch B, Vasconez O, Hall-Findlay EJ, eds. *Grabb's Encyclopedia of Flaps, 2nd ed.* Philadelphia, PA: Lippincott-Raven; 1998:1466-1470.
28. Khazanchi RK, Takkar D. Vaginal depth following reconstruction with pudendal thigh flaps in congenital vagina atresia. *Plast Recons Surg.* 1997;99:592-593.
29. Bell SW, Dehni N, Chaouat M, et al. Primary rectus abdominus myocutaneous flap for repair of perineal and vaginal defects after extended abdominoperineal resection. *Br J Surg.* 2005;92:482-486.
30. D'Souza DN, Pera M, Nelson H, et al. Vaginal reconstruction following resection of primary locally advanced and recurrent colorectal malignancies. *Arch Surg.* 2003;138:1340-1343.
31. Boyd JB, Taylor GI, Corlett R. The vascular territories of the superior epigastric and the deep inferior epigastric systems. *Plast Recons Surg.* 1984;73:1-16.
32. e Costa MAC, Carriquiry C, Vasconez LO, et al. An anatomic study of the venous drainage of the transverse rectus abdominus musculocutaneous flap. *Plast Recons Surg.* 1987;79:208-217.
33. Moon HK, Taylor GI. The vascular anatomy of rectus abdominus musculocutaneous flaps based on the deep superior epigastric system. *Plast Recons Surg.* 1988;82:815-832.
34. de Haas WG, Miller MJ, Temple WJ, et al. Perineal wound closure with the rectus abdominus musculocutaneous flap after tumor ablation. *Ann Surg Oncol.* 1995;2:400-406.
35. Shibata D, Hyland W, Busse P, et al. Immediate reconstruction of the perineal wound with gracilis muscle flaps following abdominoperineal resection and intraoperative radiation therapy for recurrent carcinoma of the rectum. *Ann Surg Oncol.* 1999;6:33-37.
36. Casey WJ, Tran NV, Petty PM, et al. A comparison of 99 consecutive vaginal reconstructions an outcome study. *Ann Plast Surg.* 2004;52:27-30.
37. O'Connell C, Mirhashemi R, Kassira N, et al. Formation of functional neovagina with vertical rectus abdominus musculocutaneous (VRAM) flap after total pelvic exenteration. *Ann Plast Surg.* 2005;55:470-473.
38. Salgarello M, Farallo E, Barone-Adesi L, et al. Flap algorithm in vulvar reconstruction after radical, extensive vulvectomy. *Ann Plast Surg.* 2005;54:184-190.
39. Mirhashemi R, Averette HE, Lambrou N, et al. Vaginal reconstruction at the time of pelvic exenteration: a surgical and psychosexual analysis of techniques. *Gynecol Oncol.* 2002;87:39-45.
40. Reece GP, Kroll SS. Abdominal wall complications. Prevention and treatment. *Clin Plast Surg.* 1998;25:235-249.
41. Jakowatz JG, Porudominsky D, Riihimaki DU, et al. Complications of pelvic exenteration. *Arch Surg.* 1985;120:1261-1265.
42. Ratliff CR, Gershenson DM, Morris M, et al. Sexual adjustment of patients undergoing gracilis myocutaneous flap vaginal reconstruction in conjunction with pelvic exenteration. *Cancer.* 1996;78:2229-2235.
43. Smith H, Genesen M, Runowicz C, et al. The rectus abdominus myocutaneous flap: modifications, complications, and sexual function. *Cancer.* 1998;83:510-520.
44. Becker DJ, Massey F, McCraw J. Musculocutaneous flaps in reconstructive pelvic surgery. *Obstet Gynecol.* 1979;54:178-181.
45. Soper J, Secord A, Havrilesky L, et al. Comparison of gracilis and rectus abdominus myocutaneous flap neovaginal reconstruction performed during radical pelvic surgery: flap-specific morbidity. *Int J Gynecol Cancer.* 2007;17:298-303.
46. Scott JR, Liu D, Mathes DW. Patient-reported outcomes and sexual function in vaginal reconstruction. *Ann Plast Surg.* 2010;64:311-314.
47. Wu L, Song D. The rectus abdominus musculoperitoneal flap for the immediate reconstruction of partial vaginal defects. *Plast Recons Surg.* 2005;115:559-562.
48. Chessin DB, Hartley J, Cohen Am, et al. Rectus flap reconstruction decreases perineal wound complications after pelvic chemoradiation and surgery: a cohort study. *Ann Surg Oncol.* 2005;12:104-110.
49. Nelson RA, Butler CE. Surgical outcomes of VRAM versus thigh flaps for immediate reconstruction of pelvic and perineal cancer resection defects. *Plast Recons Surg.* 2009;123:175-183.
50. Butler CE, Gundeslioglu AO, Rodriguez-Bigas MA. Outcomes of immediate vertical rectus abdominus myocutaneous flap reconstruction for irradiated abdominoperineal resection defects. *J Am Coll Surg.* 2008;206:694-703.
51. Berger JL, Westin SN, Fellman B, et al. Modified vertical rectus abdominus myocutaneous flap vaginal reconstruction: an analysis of surgical outcomes. *Gynecol Oncol.* 2012;125:252-255.

Chapter 18. Gracilis, Tensor Fascia Lata, Vastus Lateralis, Rectus Femoris, and Gluteus Maximus Flaps

Ritu Salani, MD, MBA,
Pankaj Tiwari, MD, and
Jeffrey M. Fowler, MD

BACKGROUND

The introduction of radical vulvar surgery and pelvic exenteration in 1950s allowed for the treatment of locally advanced or recurrent cancer with improved survival outcomes.[1,2] Unfortunately, the large defects accompanying radical vulvar surgery were often complicated by significant infections and poor wound healing. In light of the significant risk of postoperative morbidity, the quality of life following radical surgery has been of great concern to both patients and surgeons. To improve these outcomes, advances in reconstructive procedures have evolved to provide coverage of defects, enhance cosmetic results, and preserve quality of life.[3]

A thorough understanding of anatomy and surgical technique is a prerequisite for reconstruction of surgical defects of the vulva and pelvic floor. When selecting the appropriate closure technique, the simplest method is usually preferred. In many cases, extensive prior treatment (eg, radiation therapy), will make primary closure impractical and require the use of myocutaneous flaps for reconstruction of the pelvic floor. The use of myocutaneous flaps has become more popular over the past several decades and may include (1) transposition flaps, which pass over a portion of normal tissue to reach the defect, (2) rotational flaps, which are turned on an arc onto the defect, and (3) advancement flaps, which are moved onto the defect along a straight axis. Myocutaneous flaps are defined by the musculature, but also include the skin, subcutaneous tissue, and fascia and receive their blood supply from a predominant subcutaneous artery. The overlying skin typically receives its blood supply from perforators coming off the axial vessels within the muscle. Appropriate flap design allows for the placement of healthy, well-vascularized tissue into a surgical defect achieving the elimination of "dead-space" and defect closure.

Although reconstruction of the pelvic floor was introduced in the nineteenth century for congenital absence of the vagina, advances in surgical understanding and techniques have led to improved outcomes. Since the 1970s, the use of myocutaneous flaps derived from the upper portion of the lower extremity have been described for reconstructive purposes. Initially, pelvic defects resulting from radical vulvovaginal surgery were repaired in a 2-step process or left to heal by secondary intention. However, over the last 2 decades, immediate reconstruction of pelvic floor defects has become the standard and resulted in favorable outcomes.[4,5] Once a decision has been made to perform reconstructive surgery, the selection of the specific procedure should be based on the principles of restoring normal anatomy, optimizing function, and minimizing the risk of postoperative morbidity. Patients and providers need to be aware of the affect of reconstructive surgery on both the transfer site and the donor site.

Vulvovaginal reconstruction following radical extirpative surgery results in superior outcomes in quality of life measures, particularly sexual function. Furthermore, when compared with patients who have not undergone reconstructive surgery, those who have undergone reconstruction have shown reduced complications such as infection and fistula formation.[6] As a result, pelvic floor reconstruction should be seriously considered as a means to reduce perioperative morbidity and enhance would healing even if the patient does not desire preservation of sexual function.[6]

Preoperative preparation for vaginal or vulvar reconstruction requires thorough surgical planning as well as extensive counseling of the patient and her caregivers. The patients should be made aware of the goals of reconstruction and understand the requirements for successful convalescence, which may include prolonged bed rest or limited mobility.

The potential effects of reconstructive surgery on sexual health and possible need for rehabilitative services should be specifically delineated. Identifying patients at high risk for vascular compromise of the flap pedicle, such as heavy smokers, diabetics and obese patients, is a priority. For example, smokers should be advised to discontinue smoking at least 3 weeks prior to operation. Similarly, diabetes control should be optimized preoperatively and maintained throughout the postoperative period.

In addition to basic preoperative considerations, such as anesthesia consultation and reservation of a critical care bed, meticulous deliberation regarding the impact of the procedure on both the transfer and the donor sites is required. The size, shape, and thickness of the defect to be covered are all important factors that must be taken into account. For example, situations where the subcutaneous component of the flap may limit or preclude creation of a neovagina, such as with morbid obesity, the muscle alone with a skin graft may be used safely. A careful review of relevant previous surgeries is critical to appropriate flap selection and may identify vascular pedicles that could be compromised. If there is a concern for the patency of the flap vasculature, then evaluation with preoperative angiography should be performed. A detailed review of prior radiation treatment records is always warranted so that flaps can be selected from outside of irradiated fields (eg, lower extremity), which may result in better neovascularization of the flap.[5] If postoperative radiation is anticipated, then the flap transfer site may also be impacted.

This chapter provides an overview of myocutaneous flaps derived from the posterior trunk and the upper portion of the lower extremity. Specific flaps along with anatomic landmarks are listed in Table 18-1, and an overview of the relevant surgical anatomy of the anterior and lateral thigh is shown in Figure 18-1.

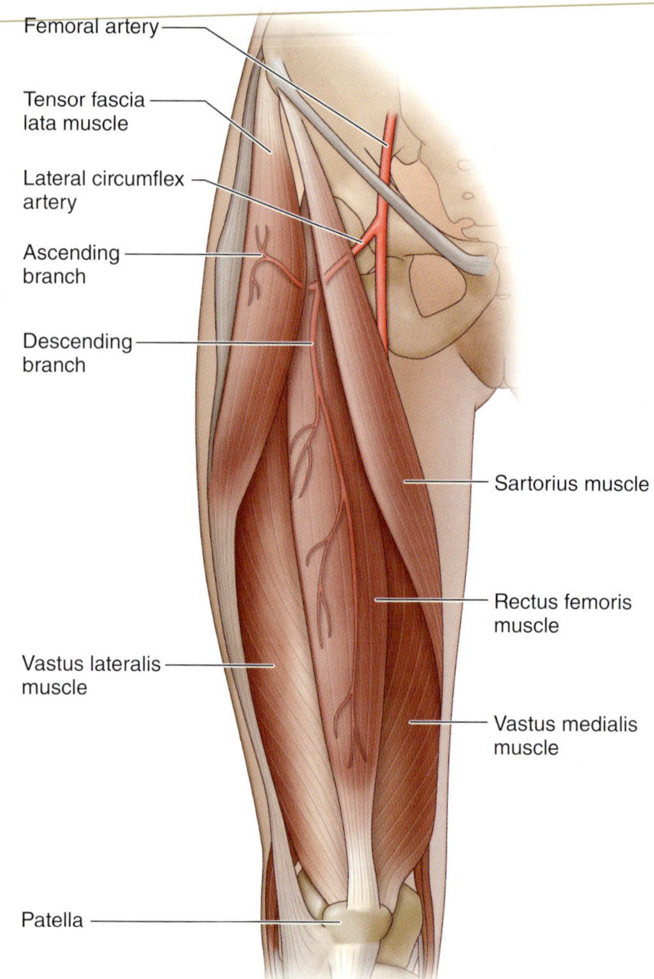

Fig. 18-1. Surgical anatomy for myocutaneous flaps from the anterior and lateral thigh.

Table 18-1. Reconstructive flaps for vulvovaginal and inguinal defects.

Flap	Blood Supply	Innervation	Origin	Insertion	Indications
Gracilis	Medial femoral circumflex	Anterior cutaneous thigh	Pubic rami	Medial condyle of tibia	Vulvar, groin defects, neovagina
Tensor Fascia	Lateral femoral circumflex	Superficial gluteal	Anterior superior iliac spine	Distal lateral fascia lata	Vulvar and groin defects
Vastus Lateralis	Lateral femoral circumflex	Femoral nerve	Greater trochanter	Patella, quadriceps tendon	Perineal defects
Rectus Femoris	Lateral femoral circumflex	Femoral nerve	Anterior inferior iliac spine	Patellar tendon	Groin and anterior perineal defects
Gluteus Maximus	Inferior gluteal	Inferior gluteal nerve	Gluteal surface of ilium, lumbar fascia	Gluteal tuberosity of the femur	Vulvar and perineal defects

GRACILIS FLAP

Indications and Clinical Applications

The gracilis muscle flap was first described in 1976 and is one of more common flaps used for reconstruction of the vagina and/or vulva.[7] The flap is quite versatile and can be used for partial or total vaginal reconstruction, suprapubic wound closure, and anal sphincter reconstruction.[6-10] The gracilis flap is a useful alternative for pelvic floor reconstruction when a rectus abdominus flap is not an option because of concurrent abdominal stoma placement accompanying exenterative surgery.

Anatomic Considerations

The gracilis muscle originates from the pubic symphysis, inserts on the medial tibial condyle, and functions as a thigh adductor. It is a thin, flat muscle that lies between the adductor longus and sartorius muscles anteriorly and the semimembranosus muscle posteriorly. Due to the presence of the abductor longus and magnus muscles, the gracilis muscle is expendable from a functional standpoint. The dominant blood supply to the gracilis flap arises from the ascending branches of the medial circumflex femoral vessels. This vascular pedicle is typically 6 cm in length and enters the gracilis muscle approximately 8 to 10 cm below the muscle origin. Additional branches of the femoral vessels also supply the muscle and enter the distal third of the muscle belly. The overlying skin is supplied by perforating vessels from the gracilis muscle.

The gracilis myocutaneous flap can be designed with either a vertically or transversely oriented skin island. The standard vertical skin island design is centered over the proximal third of the gracilis muscle with average dimensions of 8 cm in width and 15 cm in length. The transverse skin island may extend beyond the muscle edges for 4 to 5 cm and should be centered over the proximal third of the muscle. The transverse skin island can accommodate dimensions of 20 cm in width and 6 cm in length. Although the muscle has an excellent and predictable blood supply, the distal aspect of a longitudinally oriented skin paddle can be variable. In patients who are obese, the thickness of the skin paddle may limit flap mobility or result in constriction of the vascular supply. In such circumstances, a gracilis muscle-only flap combined with a skin graft may be a more prudent choice that the full-thickness myocutaneous flap.

Preoperative Preparation

Box 18-1 KEY SURGICAL INSTRUMENTATION

- Bipolar, jeweler forceps (coated): Fine-tipped forceps to allow for manipulation of the vascular adventitia without risking traumatic injury during vessel dissection
- Dissecting scissors (eg, Reynolds tenotomy): Fine-tipped dissecting scissors to allow for vascular dissection if increased pedicle length is desirable prior to flap transposition
- Microvascular clips (automatic or manual applier): Hemostatic clips during flap dissection
- Weitlaner retractors (medium, sharp): Self-retaining retractors during pedicle dissection
- Richardson retractors: Wide, right-angled retractor to facilitate flap and vascular exposure

As a thin, pliable muscle, the gracilis muscle is used for reconstruction of small-to moderate-sized defects involving the skin, soft tissue, bone and the pelvic floor. Preoperative consideration must be given to the following: need for unilateral or bilateral flaps, whether skin is to be included, and whether the skin paddle will need to be oriented transversely or longitudinally over the muscle. The operative goals with respect to elimination of "dead space," cosmesis, and amount of skin required will be the primary drivers for the type of gracilis flap designed.

The flap can be elevated as either a muscle-only or a myocutaneous flap. Preoperative markings should be made while the patient is standing and able to contract the muscle allowing for a more accurate orientation of the skin paddle (Figure 18-2). Placing the patient in the supine or lithotomy position with the hips abducted (45 degrees) allows for the muscle to easily palpated (Figure 18-3).[6] However, this position may lead to anterior displacement of the skin paddle relative to the underlying muscle. With this shift of the overlying skin inferior to the muscle, the true skin paddle lies posterior to the muscle belly. Understanding this dynamic is important to limit the potential for skin devascularization.

To mark the site, a line is drawn from the pubic tubercle, at the adductor longus tendon insertion, to the medial condyle of the femur. A second line is drawn 2 to 3 cm posterior to this original marking and represents the surface marking of the longitudinal axis of the muscle. The terminal branches of the medial circumflex femoral vessels enter the posteromedial surface of the muscle approximately 8 to 10 cm below the pubic tubercle. If a muscle-only flap is required, then an incision can be made overlying the belly of the muscle as represented by the surface skin marking. For a myocutaneous flap, the skin paddle can be oriented either transversely or longitudinally over the muscle. A 15 × 8 cm vertical skin paddle can be designed, centered over the proximal third of the inner thigh. The distance between the skin bridge from the introitus to the apex of the incision should be 6 to 8 cm.[6] The distal aspect of this skin paddle can have variable vascularity and must be designed with caution. A transverse skin paddle is generally more reliable and can be designed to measure 20 × 6 cm. Although more reliable, a transverse skin paddle limits the arc of rotation.

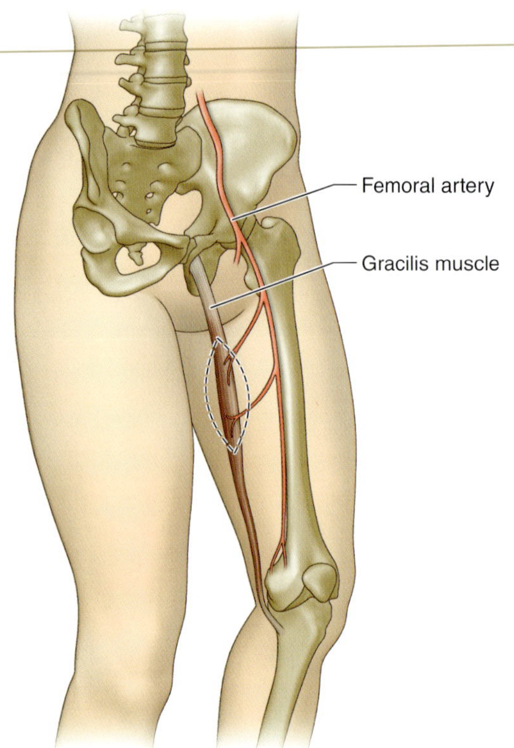

Fig. 18-2. Gracilis flap skin paddle design with the patient in the standing position.

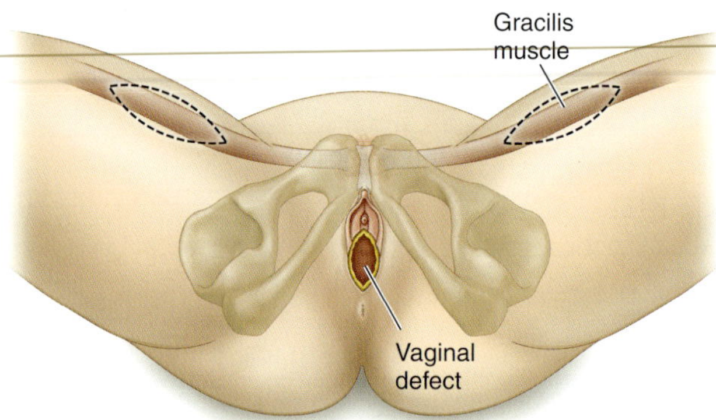

Fig. 18-3. Gracilis flap skin paddle design with the patient in dorsal lithotomy position.

Surgical Procedure

Box 18-2 MASTER SURGEON'S PRINCIPLES

- Predetermination of the size and shape of the flap to fit the defect is imperative.
- Patient positioning should be comparable to the postoperative position so that tension is not increased across the flap.
- Obese patients (body mass index [BMI] > 35 kg/m^2) may present a challenge due to a variable blood supply to the skin and decreased mobility of the flap.

The muscle-only flap can be elevated by making the skin incision along the surface marking of the longitudinal axis of the muscle. The muscle can be easily identified posterior to the adductor longus muscle. If a skin paddle is required, then it must be centered over the proximal one-third of the muscle, as this is where the cutaneous perforating vessels are primarily located. To ensure appropriate design of the skin paddle, the distal aspect of the muscle at its musculotendinous insertion is identified as the first step to muscle elevation by making a 3-to 4-cm transverse incision over the palpable gracilis tendon on the distal medial thigh. A long Kelly clamp is inserted beneath the tendinous insertion and used to place the gracilis muscle belly on traction to precisely define its location. If necessary, the skin paddle can be reoriented at this time to more closely approximate the course of the muscle belly. In developing the skin paddle, the subcutaneous tissue dissection should be beveled outward for 1 to 2 cm in order to maximize the cutaneous perforating vessels included with the flap. The incisions are then carried down through the deep muscular fascia until the anterior and posterior edges of the muscle have been identified. A layer of fascia should be left on the muscle, as this may also include vessels to the overlying skin paddle. The skin paddle should be anchored to the underlying muscle to prevent shearing forces from disrupting small perforating vessels as the flap is manipulated. The muscle is raised working in a distal to proximal direction, and the minor pedicles from the superficial femoral vessels should be ligated after the more proximal dominant primary pedicle is identified. The main vascular pedicle to the gracilis flap is identified by retracting the adductor longus muscle medially at a point approximately 10 cm below the pubic tubercle. If necessary, the muscle can be divided both proximally and distally to increase the arc of rotation. Care should be taken to avoid excessive tension on the vascular pedicle, particularly if the proximal muscle has been divided. More commonly, the proximal muscle is left intact and the distal muscle divided. The skin paddle can be designed as a "skin island" to further improve the arc of rotation into the defect. Incising the proximal fasciocutaneous portion of the flap skin paddle creates an island flap. After the extirpative operation has been completed, a subcutaneous tunnel with a skin bridge is created from the gracilis donor site to the vaginal defect. Once isolated, the flap is brought under the skin bridge with gentle traction (Figure 18-4). If further length is needed to maximize the arc of rotation, then the proximal muscle can be divided, and the flap pedicle can also be lengthened by dissection to its take-off point at the profunda femoris vessels.

A unilateral gracilis flap is usually sufficient for reconstructing a partial vaginal defect. However, reconstructing

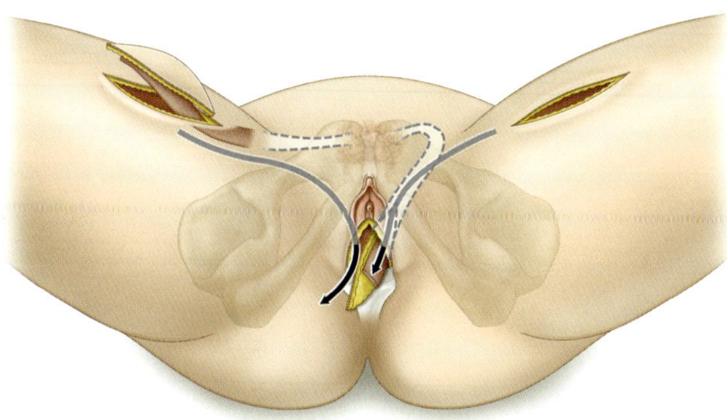

Fig. 18-4. Gracilis muscle flap elevation, rotation, and transposition into the vaginal defect.

large or complete vaginal defects or creation of a neovagina will likely require bilateral flaps. For total vaginectomy defects, the flaps are positioned so that the skin surfaces face each other and the skin edges of the flaps are sutured together using an interrupted absorbable suture, such as 3-0 delayed absorbable suture (Figure 18-5). The lateral walls of the remaining vaginal mucosa can be incised for 1 to 2 cm and are allowed to splay open to prevent vaginal stenosis near the entrance of the vagina.[11] The distal points of each flap are then inset into these incisions and the edges of the vaginal defect reapproximated using an absorbable suture. For partial vaginectomy defects, the flap is inset and the skin edges of the flap are sutured to the vaginal mucosa circumferentially, using the same suture technique. The neovaginal pouch (sutured gracilis flaps) is then sutured to the periosteum of the pubis to prevent herniation of the neovagina.

In patients who are obese, inclusion of an overlying skin paddle may make the flaps too thick to create a neovaginal vault. In this setting, skin graft placement over the muscle is preferred. The gracilis muscles are passed into the perineal aspect of the vaginal defect and sutured together along their perimeter to create a muscular pouch. Skin grafts can be harvested at 10/1000 thickness with a dermatome from the lateral aspect of the thigh. The skin grafts are then sutured (dermal side out) around a large, soft vaginal stent with absorbable chromic suture. The skin-grafted stent is placed into the muscular pouch, and the pouch and stent are placed into the vaginal defect. The labia majora are sutured together for 7 days to allow for the skin graft to take and to prevent the stent from being extruded out of the neovagina.[10]

If the gracilis muscle is utilized for "dead space" obliteration along the pelvic floor, then the skin paddle can be de-epithelialized. This technique can be used when a synthetic mesh has been placed for pelvic stability to limit the potential for a mesh-associated complication (eg, erosion).

The donor site is closed primarily. It is generally not necessary place a muscle closure layer. Placement of intermuscular sutures can lead to myonecrosis and undue tension. Dermal and skin closure is sufficient with appropriate flap design that avoids excessive tension at the closure. Drainage catheters are placed on each side of the subcutaneous perineal tunnel and alongside each gracilis muscle flap. Round, hubless closed suction drains are our preferred drain type. The skin of the gracilis donor site is closed in 2 layers using 3-0 delayed absorbable for the subcuticular layer and a running 3-0 Prolene for reapproximation of the skin. With appropriate skin paddle design that avoids excessive tension, a surface bolster overlying the incision is not necessary.

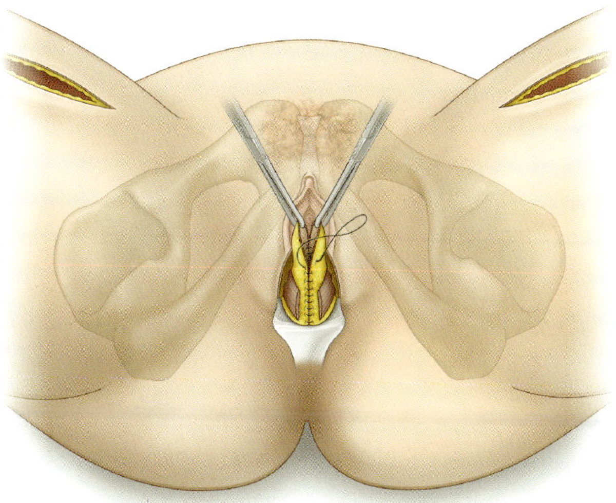

Fig. 18-5. Bilateral gracilis flap neovagina.

Postoperative Care

Box 18-3 PERIOPERATIVE MORBIDITY

- Flaps may be associated with vaginal abscess or cellulitis, which is often amenable to antibiotics and conservative measures.
- Surgical intervention/revision may be required for flap necrosis and flap prolapse.
- The flap donor site is at risk for myonecrosis or compartment syndrome and should be inspected each day.

The patient is encouraged to ambulate by the second or third postoperative day. Due to increasing edema and venous congestion of the flap, prolonged sitting should be avoided. The gracilis flap should be inspected daily for both color and capillary refill. When a gracilis flap has been used for vaginal reconstruction, the distal aspect of the flap is easily examined by retracting the labia minora. Examination of the proximal portion of the flap(s) is best performed at the time of examination under anesthesia 7 to 10 days postoperatively. Doppler signals are typically not present in a gracilis flap design and should not be used for flap monitoring. If a muscle-only flap is performed with overlying skin graft placement, then assessment of the perfusion can be difficult. The same parameters for color and capillary refill do not pertain to skin graft placement overlying muscle. Although the muscle can be evaluated for color, this can prove difficult within the reconstructed vaginal vault particularly as the muscle becomes edematous in the postsurgical period.

The most common cause of compromised flap viability is tension on the vascular pedicle. Excessive abduction of the thigh should be avoided. Persistent concern over flap viability may require a return to the operating room for exploration and takedown of the flap transfer site. The vascular pedicle may need further dissection to optimize pedicle length. Consideration should also be given to revising the subcutaneous tunnel, which should be at least 3 times as wide as the width of the muscle (3-4 fingerbreadths) to account for postoperative edema and compression of the muscle/and or vascular pedicle.

Patients and caregivers should be aware that after gracilis flap, vaginal drainage is anticipated due to sloughing of the skin and can often be treated with conservative measures. Judicious use of antibiotics and consideration of drain placement to prevent accumulation of fluid may reduce the incidence of infection or abscess formation.[4]

Although operative mortality and surgical complications have decreased markedly with improvements in technique, morbidity from gracilis muscle flaps is common.[3,7,12] Early complications requiring intervention may occur in up to 50% of patients, and flap loss rates may reach as high as 15%.[3,4,13] The most common problems include skin necrosis, which often requires debridement, and vaginal drainage and abscess, which may be a result of skin sloughing and infection.[5,6,8,13] Skin separation, dysethesias, hematoma formation, and erythema are also common, but are usually amenable to conservative measures.[4,5,13,14]

In an effort to reduce the rate of flap complications, a modification of the gracilis flap that utilizes a smaller flap size for neovagina construction has been described and is associated with improved clinical outcomes.[13,15,16] The enhanced mobility of the smaller flap design reduces the risk of wound breakdown and necrosis. Anchoring the gracilis flap to the pelvic floor can further reduce tension on the vascular pedicle as well as decrease the risk of flap prolapse.[15]

Long-Term Outcomes

Box 18-4 DELAYED COMPLICATIONS

- Enterocutaneous fistula to pelvic floor flaps can occur late, although this is less likely than if no reconstruction is performed.
- Scarring or atrophy of the neovagina or vulvar flap may affect sexual function outcomes.
- Donor site complications, such as leg weakness and scar retraction, can manifest months after flap harvesting.

Of all reconstructive flaps used in gynecologic surgery, the gracilis muscle has been in use for the longest period of time and has the most robust data on long-term outcomes.[7] Gracilis flap reconstruction of the pelvic floor or neovagina is associated with statistically and clinically significant reductions in the incidence of pelvic infection and enterocutaneous fistulae.[17,18] In addition, the use of the smaller gracilis flap design is associated with reduction in the likelihood of flap prolapse from 65% to 16%, while the proportion of patients with severe flap prolapse is decreased from 25% to just 6%.[12]

The gracilis flap neovagina generally yields satisfactory vaginal caliber and depth; nevertheless, vaginal stenosis can occur as a delayed complication in up to 20% of patients.[13,14,16] In a small study, Becker et al[19] reported that more than 80% (13/16) of patients undergoing gracilis neovagina reconstruction reported sexual satisfaction. By contrast, other investigators have found that although most patients had physically adequate vaginal length, fewer than 50% actually chose to engage in sexual activity.[6,9,14] In general, the likelihood of sexual activity after neovagina reconstruction with the gracilis muscle is comparable with that associated with a rectus abdominus flap.[5,20-22]

TENSOR FASCIA LATA FLAP

Indications and Clinical Applications

The tensor fascia lata (TFL) flap is commonly utilized for coverage of ischial and trochanteric pressure ulcers as well as coverage of locoregional defects of the groin and abdomen.[23,24] The muscle component is well suited to obliterating dead space, while the skin can be used to provide a tensionless closure over the defect. As a result, one of the chief indications for the TFL flap is reconstruction of skin defects after inguinal lymphadenectomy in an irradiated field.[25] The inclusion of fascia in the TFL flap makes it particularly well suited for closure of complex abdominal wounds where the defect includes the rectus sheath, as it can be raised as a myofascial flap or a myofasciocutaneous flap. The TFL flap has an arc of rotation that includes coverage of the lower abdomen, the groin, the anterior perineum, and the hip.

Anatomic Considerations

The TFL flap is a small, thin flat muscle, measuring approximately 5 cm in width and 15 cm in length, located laterally on the upper thigh and extending through the iliotibial tract of the fascia lata to the lateral aspect of the knee. The muscle originates at the anterior 5 to 8 cm of the outer lip of the anterior superior iliac spine (ASIS) immediately behind the origin of the sartorius muscle. The TFL inserts onto the iliotibial tract of the fascia lata and serves to flex and abduct the thigh as well as tighten the iliotibial tract of the fascia lata. Generally, the TFL is considered an expendable muscle.

The dominant vascular pedicle to the TFL is the ascending branch of the lateral circumflex femoral artery (see Figure 18-1). This vessel originates from the profunda femoris artery and has a length of approximately 7 cm. The vessel enters the muscle deep on the medial aspect at a point approximately 10 cm below the anterior superior iliac spine. The muscular and septocutaneous branches of the lateral circumflex femoral artery account for the major blood supply to the skin of the lateral thigh. The nerve supply to the TFL is from the superior gluteal nerve that enters the deep surface of the muscle. The skin territory is innervated by the lateral femoral cutaneous nerve of the thigh.

Preoperative Preparation

Supine positioning is ideal for identification of the TFL, particularly for groin reconstruction, although the flap can also be marked with the patient in the lateral position. TFL flap design can also be performed with the hip and knee in flexion with the hip internally rotated. The leg is included in the surgical prep so that position can be easily changed to maximize exposure of the surgical defect and facilitate flap insetting.

For preoperative flap design, a line between the anterior superior iliac spine and the lateral tibial condyle of the knee is drawn with a marking pen (Figure 18-6). The posterior border is approximately 5 cm cephalad to the knee and the length/width should be tailored to size and configuration of the transfer site defect. The TFL muscle lies between the biceps femoris posteriorly and rectus femoris anteriorly and the vastus lateralis muscle is attached to the deep surface. A flap that is 30 cm long can be safely raised; however, the vascular supply to the distal third of the flap can be variable. Typically, the overlying skin paddle can accommodate a width of 7 to 8 cm and still allow for primary closure without the need for skin graft placement.

Surgical Procedure

The standard TFL musculocutaneous flap includes the entire muscle and an island of overlying skin measuring 8 × 20 cm. These dimensions place the skin island just larger than the actual muscle. The incision is made along the distal border of the flap and continued downward through the fascia lata. Dissection begins distally and anteriorly, working in a caudal to cephalad direction. The dissection proceeds in a relatively bloodless plane deep to the fascia lata overlying the vastus lateralis. At a level approximately 10 cm below the anterior superior iliac spine, the terminal branches of the lateral circumflex femoral are identified. The ascending branch of the lateral circumflex femoral artery supplies the TFL, the gluteus maximus, and portions of the vastus lateralis muscles. The dissection continues above the vascular pedicles, separating the TFL from the underlying gluteal muscles. In the majority of cases, it is not essential to divide the origin of the muscle to achieve adequate flap rotation. However, to elevate a true island flap or to avoid a "dog-ear" at the point of rotation, the origin of the muscle from the iliac crest may be divided (Figure 18-7).[26]

When skin coverage is not required, the TFL musculofascial flap is useful for reconstruction of abdominal wall defects. The fascia lata is harvested with the muscle, and an incision is made along the midlateral point of the thigh extending from the ASIS to within a few centimeters of the knee. The skin is then reflected on each side and the fascia lata is identified. A very wide and long strip of fascia may be harvested that extends over the rectus femoris muscle anteriorly and the biceps femoris posteriorly.

Primary closure of the donor site is performed whenever feasible. Undermining the skin and fascia lata for additional mobility may reduce tension. The skin edges can be closed in 2 layers using 3-0 delayed absorbable suture in a subcuticular fashion followed by a running 3-0 Prolene in the skin (Figure 18-8). If the skin cannot be reapproximated, then

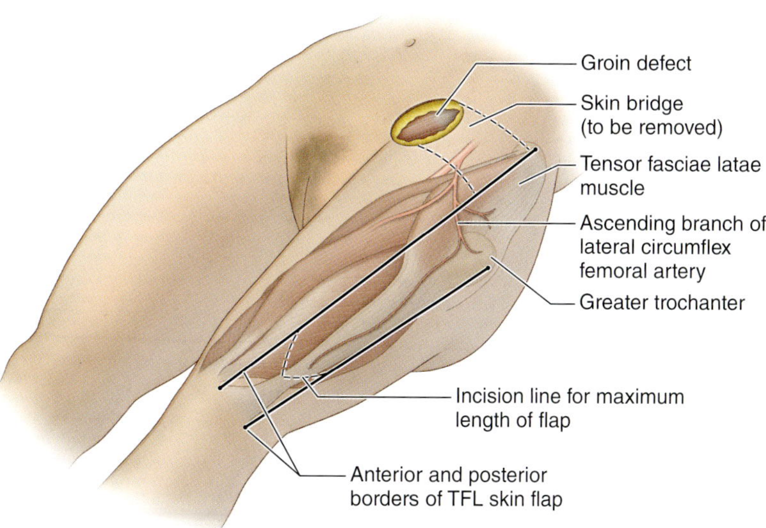

Fig. 18-6. Anatomic landmarks for designing the tensor fascia lata flap.

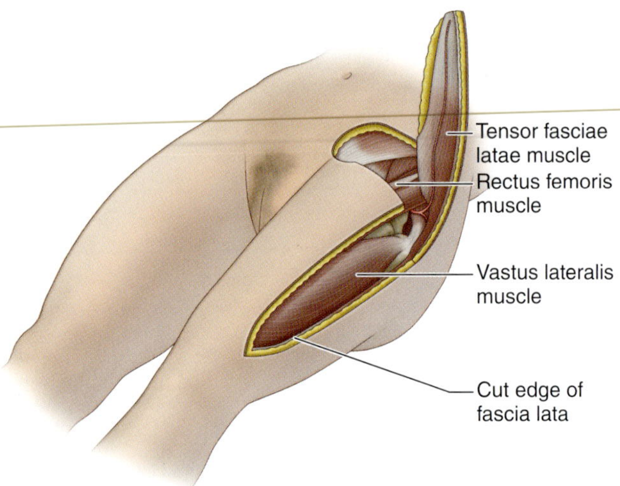

Fig. 18-7. Elevation of the tensor fascia lata flap.

the skin edges can be sutured to the underlying muscle or fascia and the remaining defect covered with a split thickness skin graft.

Postoperative Care

Following TFL flap harvesting and incision closure, the leg is placed in a dressing. Our preferred dressings are Vaseline-impregnated gauze over the incision, Kerlix (Covidien, Mansfield, Massachusetts) fluffs, and a 6-in. bandage wrap circumferentially around the thigh without excessive compression.[27] A suction drain is placed in the donor site and brought out through a separate stab incision. Drains are typically left in place until output is less than 30 mL over a 24-hour period. In contrast to other muscle flaps based in the thigh, such as the rectus femoris flap, immobilization of the knee is not a requirement with the TFL flap. If the donor site has been closed with a skin graft, then a bolster dressing should be placed to optimize skin graft "take" to the wound bed. Typically, the skin graft bolster is left in place for 7 days. A wound vacuum–assisted closure device can also be utilized in lieu of a bolster for skin graft placement.

Heat or ice packs on the incision should be avoided in the postoperative period. Due to disruption of the cutaneous sensation, such interventions can lead to a partial or full-thickness skin loss, while little is achieved in the way of symptomatic relief or edema management. When the donor site defect has been closed primarily, early ambulation is encouraged.[23]

Long-Term Outcomes

The TFL flap is associated with an excellent blood supply and heals readily, making it a safe and relatively trouble-free choice for reconstruction of groin, vulvar, or abdominal wall defects.[23] The scar at the donor site may be suboptimal, however, this is especially true if primary closure cannot be achieved and a skin graft is required. Complications related to the muscle function, such as lateral knee instability, can occur infrequently.[23]

VASTUS LATERALIS FLAP

Indications and Clinical Applications

The vastus lateralis muscle flap was original described for coverage of ischial pressure sores.[28] More recently, the vastus lateralis flap has proven useful for reconstruction of lower extremity and locoregional vulvovaginal defects following pelvic exenteration.[29-31]

Anatomic Considerations

The vastus lateralis muscle is the largest of the quadriceps muscle group, measuring 10 × 26 cm. It is located between the vastus intermedius and the biceps femoris muscles and beneath the tensor fascia lata (see Figure 18-1). It originates at the intertrochanteric line, greater trochanter of the femur, gluteal tuberosity, and lateral intermuscular septum and inserts onto the patella. Although it is a powerful leg extensor, it is a relatively expendable muscle due to the redundancy of function provided by the remaining 3 muscles of the quadriceps group.

The dominant vascular pedicle is the descending branch of the lateral circumflex femoral artery and venae comitantes, which branch from the profunda femoris vessels (see Figure 18-1). The vascular pedicle is approximately 4 cm in length and is located within the superior one-third of the muscle extending inferiorly along the medial border of the muscle belly. Perforating vessels from the lateral circumflex femoral provide a vascular supply to the skin overlying the vastus lateralis muscle. Typically, the dominant perforating vessel is located at the midpoint on a line drawn from the anterior superior

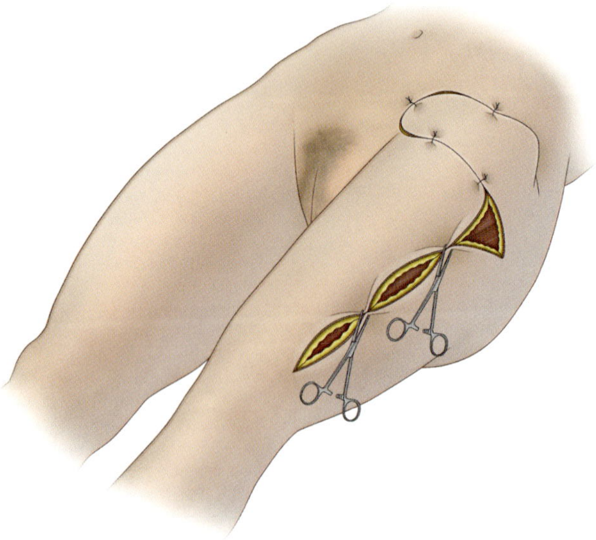

Fig. 18-8. The tensor fascia lata flap is rotated into position to cover the groin defect and the donor site is closed primarily.

iliac spine to the lateral border of the patella. The flap can be elevated as a muscle-only flap, a musculocutaneous flap, or as a "perforator flap" in which only the fasciocutaneous tissue is harvested based on perforating vessels dissected to the lateral circumflex femoral artery. The innervation to the vastus lateralis is the muscular branch of the femoral nerve. If designed with a skin paddle, the flap can be made sensate by preserving the lateral femoral cutaneous nerve.

Preoperative Preparation

To identify the vastus lateralis muscle, a line is drawn from the anterior superior iliac spine to the superior lateral border of the patella. The designated skin territory is then drawn with a marking pen and is can measure 10 cm in width × 15 cm in length (Figure 18-9). Larger skin paddles may require skin grafting for closure of the donor site. It should be noted that obese patients (BMI > 30 kg/m^2) tend to have relatively immobile anterolateral thigh skin, which may limit the width of the skin paddle design.

Surgical Procedure

The skin incision is created along the line of the vastus lateralis muscle belly for a muscle-only flap or is tailored to the skin paddle design for a musculocutaneous flap. The vastus lateralis muscle is exposed superior to the lateral condyle of the knee. Flap elevation should begin at the medial border of the flap and is carried down to the deep fascia. The dissection is carried laterally toward the intermuscular septum between the rectus femoris and the vastus lateralis muscles. Exposure of the vastus lateralis muscle is completed by deepening the lateral thigh incision from a point 10 cm below the anterior superior iliac spine at the level of the greater trochanter to the lateral condyle of the femur. The incision extends through the deep fascia at the medial edge of the tensor fascia lata muscle in the proximal one-fourth of the leg and to the iliotibial tract distally.

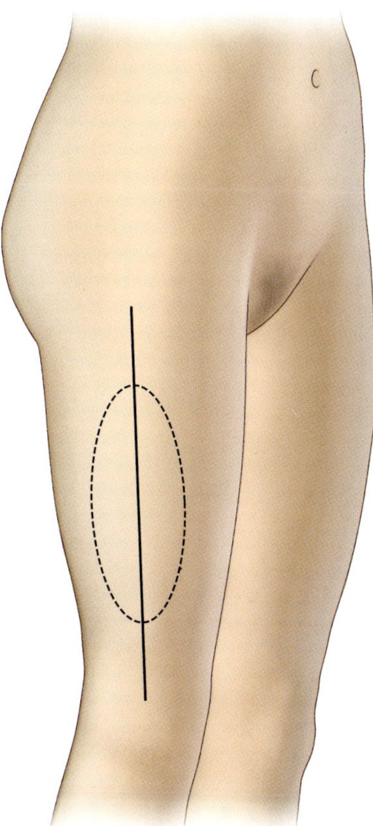

Fig. 18-9. Anatomic landmarks for the vastus lateralis flap design.

The rectus femoris is retracted medially and the descending branch of the lateral femoral circumflex artery is identified. The flap pedicle is then dissected free toward the origin of the lateral circumflex femoral artery.

Because the borders of the vastus intermedius and lateralis muscles are indistinct in the proximal three-fourths of the thigh, it is helpful to examine the distal muscle below the skin island where the 2 muscles separate before forming their respective tendons of insertion.[32] The lateral and medial extensions of the skin island are elevated with the deep fascia until the muscle borders are reached. The muscle fibers of insertion are divided and the muscle is elevated moving from distal to proximal. In the distal posterior muscle, the minor vascular pedicle from the lateral genicular artery and associated veins are also divided. The vastus lateralis muscle is then elevated from the underlying femur to the level of the greater trochanter, visualizing and carefully preserving the descending branch of the lateral circumflex femoral artery that passes beneath the rectus femoris and enters the medial aspect of the vastus lateralis muscle. At this point flap elevation is complete for a standard arc of rotation.[32] A muscle-only or musculocutaneous vastus lateralis flap can be rotated up to 90 degrees with the muscle and overlying skin then sutured to the edges of the defect (Figure 18-10). The donor site edges can usually be approximated via layered primary closure. If the donor site edges have insufficient mobility for primary closure, a split thickness skin graft is used to cover the defect and a bolster dressing or a vacuum-assisted closure device should be applied. This will optimize skin graft uptake to the wound bed and should be left in place for seven days. A suction drain is placed in the donor bed and brought out through a separate skin incision.

Postoperative Care

The flap should be inspected daily for signs of vascular compromise or flap failure. Drains are typically left in place until output is less than 30 mL over a 24-hour period. Immobilization of the knee is not a requirement with the vastus lateralis flap. It is important to note that harvesting of the vastus lateralis muscle may lead to weakness of the extensor function at the knee. Limiting disruption of the tendinous portion of the vastus lateralis will preserve the patellar tendinous insertions of the remaining quadriceps muscles and minimize leg weakness. Early postoperative ambulation of patients is advised and our recommendation is to have the patient out of bed to a chair by the first postoperative day.

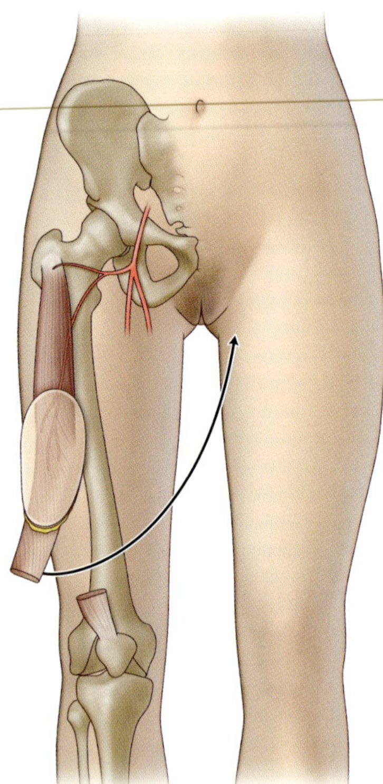

Fig. 18-10. The vastus lateralis flap is based on the descending branch of the lateral circumflex femoral artery and can be rotated as much as 90 degrees.

This is followed by increased ambulation for the remaining hospital stay, which is typically for 3 to 4 days.

Long-Term Outcomes

The vastus lateralis muscle is associated with a low rate of complications and impairment of functional morbidity. A study evaluating the anterolateral thigh fasciocutaneous flap in conjunction with vastus lateralis motor nerve division or harvest of large segments of vastus lateralis muscle demonstrated that most patients return to their preoperative level of function.[32,33] Complications include seroma (5%), hematoma (1%), infection (1%), and neuroma (1%).[33] Flap necrosis and wound dehiscence have been reported, however, total flap survival rate is excellent and exceeds 94%.[33,34] A total of 84% of patients report a sensory loss in the distribution of the lateral femoral cutaneous nerve. Weakness or instability is reported by 8% of patients at their initial postoperative visit but almost always resolves by 6 months.[33]

RECTUS FEMORIS FLAP

Indications and Applications

One of the earliest reports for use of the rectus femoris muscle flap was by Ger in 1971.[35] Though rarely used in gynecologic cancer, the rectus femoris flap can be used to reconstruct a pelvic floor defect after radical vulvar resection with or without exenterative surgery when other flaps (eg, gracilis/rectus abdominis) are not feasible due to prior surgery or anatomical limitations.[36] The rectus femoris muscle has a dense fascial layer on its deep surface that can also be used for anterior abdominal wall restoration. The chief indication for rectus femoris muscle flap in gynecologic surgery has been predominantly for the reconstruction of the lower abdomen and groin.

Anatomic Considerations

The rectus femoris is a superficial thigh muscle that is located in the middle of the anterior thigh (see Figure 18-1). The muscle extends from its origin at the ilium to the patella of the knee. It is a central muscle of the quadriceps extensor muscle group and lies between the vastus lateralis and vastus medialis muscles. The muscle takes its dominant vascular supply from the descending branch of the lateral circumflex femoral vessels, which in turn branch from the profunda femoris artery and vein. The vascular pedicle enters the proximal one-third of the muscle and has a length of approximately 5 cm. The nerve supply is from the muscular branch of the femoral nerve, which enters the muscle belly adjacent to the vascular pedicle. If overlying skin is incorporated into the flap, it can be made sensate with inclusion of the intermediate branch of the anterior femoral cutaneous nerves (L2–L3). The arc of flap rotation includes the groin, anterior perineum, and hip; the reach of the rectus femoris flap can be extended by using it as a "turn-over" flap rather than a rotational flap (Figure 18-11).

Preoperative Preparation

The rectus femoris muscle extends between the anterior inferior iliac spine and the patella. To facilitate preoperative

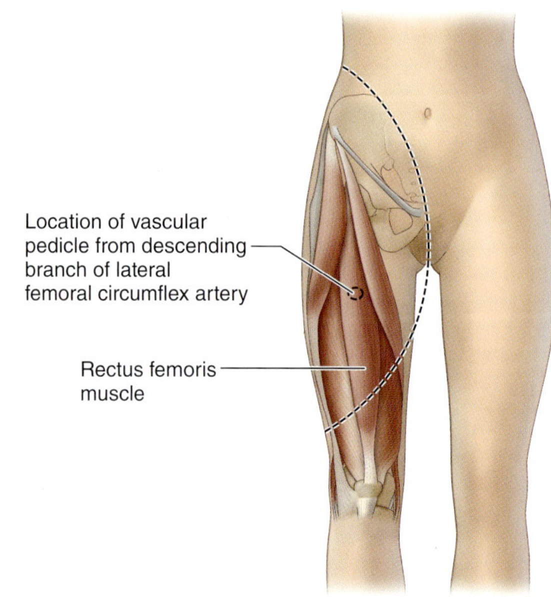

Fig. 18-11. Possible rotational arc of the rectus femoris flap.

marking, the patient can be asked to flex the quadriceps musculature, allowing the lateral border of the vastus medialis and medial border of the vastus lateralis to be visualized. The tendon of the rectus femoris muscle is located in the depression between these two muscles and is located just proximal to the patella. The axis of the rectus femoris flap can be approximated by drawing a line from the anterior superior iliac spine to the patella, as this represents the intermuscular septum between the rectus femoris and vastus lateralis muscles.

The rectus femoris flap can be designed as a muscle-only or a myocutaneous flap. When used as a myocutaneous flap, the skin paddle can measure up to 10 cm in width × 20 cm in length; even this large of a flap will usually allow for primary closure of the donor site. The majority of perforating vessels to the rectus femoris are located along the middle third of the muscle belly. The skin paddle can be extended distally over the tendinous portion of the rectus femoris muscle and proximally over the sartorius muscle.[37] The patient is positioned supine on the operating room table. The leg is prepped circumferentially and "draped free" if it is necessary to reposition the leg to facilitate exposure of the vascular pedicle.

Surgical Procedure

The skin incision is tailored to reflect either a muscle-only or a musculocutaneous rectus femoris flap. If a skin island is planned, then the muscle, tendon, or both of the rectus femoris are identified proximally and distally to the skin island. An isolated skin island that is designed over the distal muscle belly is unreliable, thus the skin paddle should be centered along the proximal one-third of the muscle belly. The medial and lateral incision margins of the skin island are extended through the skin and deep fascia and dissected to the borders of the rectus femoris muscle. The separation of the quadriceps muscles can be most easily performed by working in a distal to proximal direction, as there is a coalescence of fibers proximally that can obscure the distinct underlying inter-muscular planes.

The dissection to elevate the flap begins with the distal release of the musculotendinous insertion of the rectus femoris muscle into the patella and proceeds working from distal to proximal. The muscle should be divided at least 6 cm above the patella to preserve the integrity of the tendon and of the suprapatellar bursa, which will avoid weakening the extensor mechanism of the knee. The vastus medialis and lateralis muscles are separated from the rectus femoris muscle at this distal level. A secondary vascular pedicle from the lateral circumflex femoral artery will be encountered distally within the muscle and should be ligated in order to allow for proximal transposition of the flap. The main vascular pedicle is identified along the deep surface of the muscle and is approximately 10 cm caudal to the anterior superior iliac spine. At this level, the sartorius muscle crosses the medial border of the rectus femoris muscle. As the rectus femoris is dissected, an effort should be made to preserve the motor nerve branches from the femoral nerve to the adjacent vastus lateralis, vastus medialis, and tensor fascia lata muscles.

Primary closure of the rectus femoris donor site is usually feasible when the skin island does not exceed a width of more than 7 to 8 cm. Reapproximating the edges of the vastus lateralis and medialis muscles may help limit weakness of terminal leg extension resulting from harvesting the rectus femoris muscle. Maintaining the integrity of the quadriceps extensor mechanism is especially important for preserving functional strength. In elevating the rectus femoris flap, the distal 6 cm of tendinous insertion into the patellar tendon should be left intact (Figure 18-12). Any violation of the tendinous insertion can be repaired with simple, nonabsorbable, braided sutures reapproximating the tendinous architecture.[36] Direct closure over the distal thigh is imperative to avoid skin graft placement over the patella tendon mechanism.

Postoperative Care

Postoperatively, the donor site leg should be placed in a knee immobilizer.[36] The patient should begin ambulation with "toe-touch" weight bearing for the first week. Return to

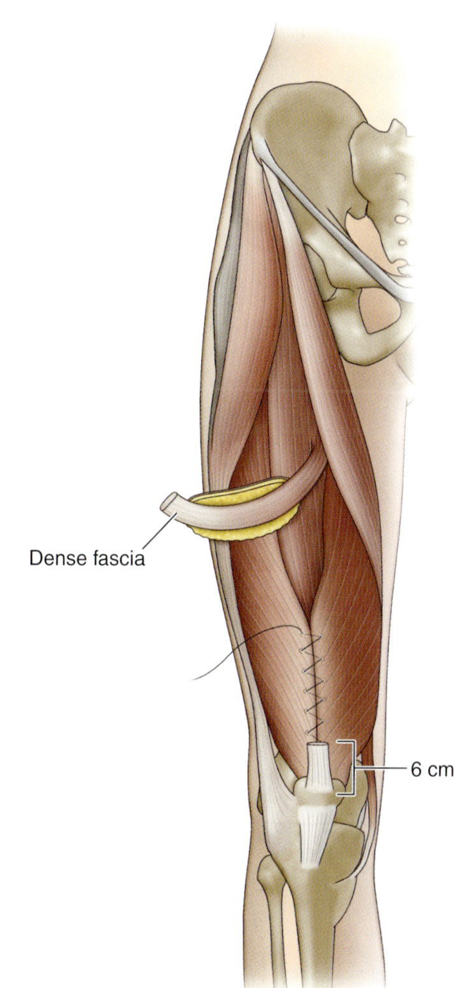

Fig. 18-12. Raising the rectus femoris flap with reconstruction of the quadriceps extensor mechanism.

regular ambulation should progress within the first 3 postoperative weeks as the patient tolerates increasing weight placement at the knee.

Long-Term Outcomes

Rectus femoris myocutaneous flaps are at higher risk for donor site-related complications than other similar flaps. A large skin defect may result in a less than favorable scar. The rectus femoris flap can result in limitation of terminal leg extension, so that this flap should not be used in patients for whom optimal knee function is critical.[36,38] As the rectus femoris is generally not considered an expendable muscle, complications, which can occur in 25% of cases, include leg weakness, loss of strength, and impaired leg extension.[38]

GLUTEUS MAXIMUS FLAP

Indications and Clinical Applications

The gluteus maximus muscle has typically been used to replace tissue defects of the posterior trunk region, including sacral and ischial pressure ulcers as well as in the closure of lumbosacral defects.[39] The muscle has a limited arc of rotation and is not appropriate for lateral and anterior defects. However, due to its proximity, the gluteus maximus flap has been successfully used for reconstruction of vulvar and perineal defects and closure of large defects in the pelvic cavity. This is accomplished by designing the flap as an extended compound myocutaneous flap based on the inferior gluteal artery with the cutaneous portion of the flap rotating at a point superior to the ischial tuberosity.[40] The flap is oriented just posterior to the defect and can provide a large amount of tissue, both muscle and adipose tissue, providing "padding" over bony promontories and obliterating dead space. Finally, the rectal sphincter has been reconstructed utilizing a gluteus maximus split muscle flap technique where the flap is based on the inferior gluteal vascular pedicle and inferior gluteal nerve.

The gluteus maximus muscle functions to extend and rotate the thigh laterally and is not an expendable muscle, as harvesting the flap may impact a patient's ability to ambulate. To reduce the risk of a negative effect when using this flap, preservation of the muscle insertion and reapproximation of the muscle origin at the posterior midline may be performed.[39] The gluteus maximus muscle can also be employed as a V-Y advancement flap. This modification releases the superior half of the muscle while the inferior half is left intact, allowing for preservation of function.

Anatomic Considerations

The gluteus maximus muscle is a large quadrilateral muscle forming the prominence of the buttocks. The muscle originates from the gluteal line of the ilium and sacrum and inserts on to the greater tuberosity of the femur and the iliotibial band of the fascia lata. The muscle has 2 dominant vascular pedicles, the superior and inferior gluteal and vessels, which originate from the internal iliac vessels. The vascular pedicles are identified relative to the piriformis muscle with the superior gluteal vessels above and the inferior gluteal vessels below (Figure 18-13). The motor nerve to the gluteus maximus muscle is the inferior gluteal nerve (L5, S1–S2), which courses through the sciatic foramen and enters the deep surface of the muscle. The skin territory receives innervation from the posterior division of S1 to S3 medially and L1 to L3 laterally. The posterior cutaneous nerve supplies the skin of the inferior buttock and posterior thigh. Therefore, the gluteus maximus flap can be elevated as a neurosensory musculocutaneous flap.

Preoperative Preparation

In designing the gluteus maximus flap, consideration must be given to the need for overlying skin as a component of the gluteus flap, as the muscle alone generally provides insufficient coverage. If a myocutaneous flap is desired, there are various skin designs that can be used. Skin flap designs include superior or inferior V-Y advancement flaps, gluteal thigh flap, and inferiorly or superiorly based rotational flaps (Figure 18-14).

Preoperative marking is most easily performed with the patient in the prone position. The muscle insertion and origin are determined by marking the lateral edge of the sacrum and greater trochanter of the femur. The posterior superior iliac spine and the ischial tuberosity are marked to determine the medial extent of the muscle. The inferior buttock fold marks the caudal extent of the muscle and the iliac crest marks the cephalad extent. The superior gluteal artery can be identified on the skin surface at a point lying 5 cm inferior to the posterior iliac spine and 5 cm lateral to the midline. The inferior gluteal artery lies approximately 3 cm inferior to the superior gluteal vessels and is marked by a point halfway along a line from the posterior superior iliac spine (PSIS) to the ischial tuberosity. The superior skin island is located inferior and lateral to the PSIS and is elevated with the superior half of the muscle based on the superior gluteal vessels.

With the patient in lithotomy position and the thighs in hyperflexion, the gluteus maximus V-Y advancement flap skin island is located on the medial half of the muscle. For reconstruction of a vulvar defect, a triangular skin island flap is outlined over the ischial prominence with the base oriented along the margin of the vulvar defect (see Figure 18-14). The flap apex should be oriented posteriorly and laterally toward the inferior border of the gluteus maximus muscle. The inferior skin island is centered above the ischial tuberosity on a line passing between the ischial and trochanteric tuberosity. The gluteal thigh flap is designed from the gluteus maximus muscle along the posterior thigh and can extend to a point 3 cm above the popliteal fossa, if necessary, and will accommodate a skin paddle measuring 7 cm in width × 35 cm in length based on the descending branch of the inferior gluteal artery (see Figure 18-14). The skin territory is innervated by the posterior cutaneous nerve of the thigh, which is centered halfway between the ischium and greater trochanter.

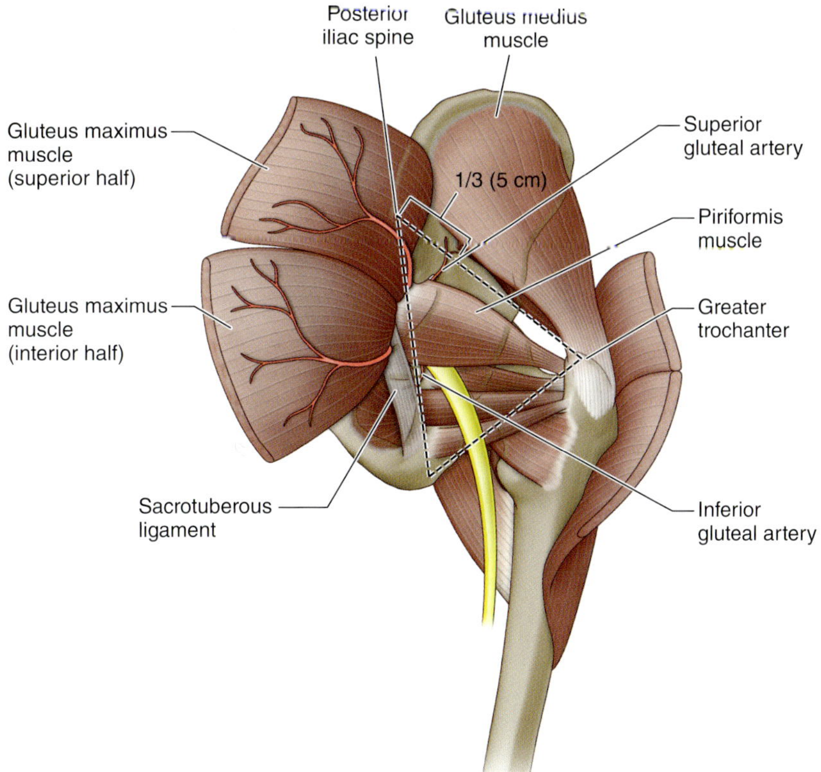

Fig. 18-13. Surgical anatomy of the gluteus maximus muscle in relation to the superior and inferior gluteal vascular pedicles.

Surgical Procedure

1. V-Y advancement flap

An incision is created delineating the skin island. The dissection is carried down to the superficial aspect of the gluteus maximus muscle and the entire muscle is exposed. The gracilis muscle can be divided, if necessary, for additional flap mobility.[41] Either the entire muscle fibers of insertion or the superior or inferior half of these fibers are divided depending on whether the flap is to be used as a segmental or complete muscle advancement flap. The fibers at the sacrum are divided, keeping the inferior and superior gluteal vessels intact, and the muscle is elevated over the sacral edge to the level of a midline defect. The skin island is advanced into the defect, and the leading edge is sutured to the margin of the vaginal introitus and perineal skin. The donor site is closed in layers, approximating the wound edges to form the stem of the Y (Figure 18-15).

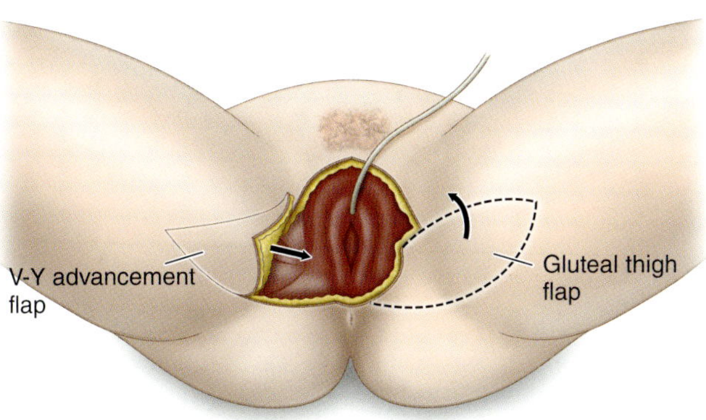

Fig. 18-14. Skin island designs for an inferior gluteal V-Y segmental advancement flap (left) and a gluteal thigh flap (right) to cover a large vulvar defect.

2. Gluteal thigh flap

An incision is made over the distal third of the gluteal thigh flap and extended through the skin overlying the gluteus maximus muscle at the level of the mid-buttock region. The superficial surface of the muscle is exposed and the inferior lateral edge of the muscle is identified and dissected toward the muscular insertion. The muscle fibers are divided, and the deep surface of the muscle is exposed and separated in a largely avascular plane from the piriformis muscle. The deep fascia is incised and the posterior femoral cutaneous nerve is kept intact. The flap is centered over the course of this nerve and the adjacent inferior gluteal vessels. The muscle can then be transposed still attached to its origin. The distal flap is elevated to the level of the gluteal crease dissecting to the

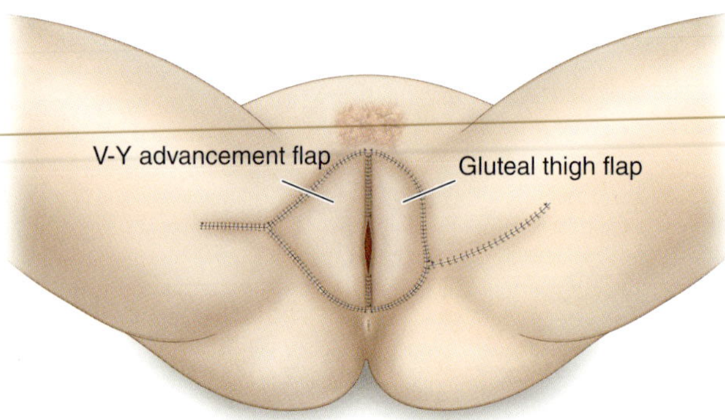

Fig. 18-15. The inferior gluteal V-Y segmental advancement flap (left) and a gluteal thigh flap (right) have been transposed into place and the donor site defects closed primarily.

deep muscular fascia. Leaving the proximal skin bridge intact, medial rotation transposes the flap into the vulvar defect and it is sutured into place (see Figure 18-15). The donor site defect is closed in layers.

Postoperative Care

Patients who are nonambulatory are generally admitted to the hospital for at least 2 weeks. Direct pressure on the flap at the site of closure must be avoided, which can be minimized with the use of an air-fluidized bed. Regardless of the postoperative bed choice, priority should be placed on minimizing postoperative compression. Patients are typically placed in a lateral decubitus position if a standard hospital bed is used. Once at home, the patient should be advised to continue to avoid compression to the flap transfer area. Avoidance of shear stress with bed-rest for a minimum of 3 days is advised.[41] To prevent moisture-related wound breakdown, the use of drains for several weeks may minimize the development of a seroma into areas of underlying dead space. Sutures are removed 3 weeks postoperatively, at which time physical therapy can be initiated.

Long-Term Outcomes

Because of the potential functional loss with the rotation of the muscle, the gluteus maximus muscle should be used with caution in ambulatory patients. Strong hip stabilization is critical for climbing stairs or walking up an incline. Furthermore, the loss of the gluteus muscle can lead to significant deformity. In a series of 20 patients, flap survival was 100% and complications, such as erythema, wound separation, or delayed healing, were conservatively managed.[41] In women undergoing this procedure for vulvar reconstruction, long-term outcomes were also favorable. Although all patients reported excellent functional activity, only 3 patients reported regular sexual activity.[41]

SUMMARY

The introduction of radical vulvar surgery and pelvic exenteration in 1950s allowed for the treatment of locally advanced or recurrent cancer with improved survival outcomes.[1,2] Unfortunately, the large defects accompanying radical vulvar surgery were often complicated by significant infections and poor wound healing. In light of the significant risk of postoperative morbidity, the quality of life following radical surgery has been of great concern to both patients and surgeons. To improve these outcomes, advances in reconstructive procedures have evolved to provide coverage of defects, enhance cosmetic results, and preserve quality of life.[3]

REFERENCES

1. Way S. The anatomy of the lymphatic drainage of the vulva and its influence on the radical operation for carcinoma. *Ann R Coll Surg Engl.* 1948;3(4):187-209.
2. Brunschwig A. Radical surgery for advanced pelvic cancer. *J Mich State Med Soc.* 1949;48(4):451.
3. Pusic AL, Mehrara BJ. Vaginal reconstruction: an algorithm approach to defect classification and flap reconstruction. *J Surg Oncol.* 2006;94(6): 515-521.
4. Epstein DM, Arger PH, LaRossa D, Mintz MC, Coleman BG. CT evaluation of gracilis myocutaneous vaginal reconstruction after pelvic extenteration. *AJR Am J Roentgenol.* 1987;148(6):1143-1146.
5. Burke TW, Morris M, Roh MS, Levenback C, Gershenson DM. Perineal reconstruction using single gracilis myocutaneous flaps. *Gynecol Oncol.* 1995;57(2):221-225.
6. Berek JS, Hacker NF, Lagasse LD. Vaginal reconstruction performed simultaneously with pelvic exenteration. *Obstet Gynecol.* 1984;63(3): 318-323.
7. McCraw JB, Massey FM, Shanklin KD, Horton CE. Vaginal reconstruction with gracilis myocutaneous flaps. *Plast Reconstr Surg.* 1976;58(2):176-183.
8. Nassar OAH. Primary repair of rectovaginal fistulas complicating pelvic surgery by gracilis myocutaneous flap. *Gynecol Oncol.* 2011;121(3): 610-614.
9. Heath PM, Woods JE, Podratz KC, Arnold PG, Irons GB. Gracilis myocutaneous vaginal reconstruction. *May Clin Proc.* 1984;59(1):21-24.
10. Evans GRD, Khoo A. Gracilis flap for perineal reconstruction and reconstruction for anal continence. In Evans GRD, ed. *Operative Plastic Surgery.* 1st ed. Norwalk: Appleton & Lange; 2000:805-813.
11. Soper JT, Berchuck A, Creasman WT, Clarke-Pearson DL. Pelvic exenteration: factors associated with major surgical morbidity. *Gynecol Oncol.* 1989;35(1):93-98.
12. Soper JT, Rodriguez G, Berchuck A, Clarke-Pearson DL. Long and short gracilis myocutaneous flaps for vulvovaginal reconstruction after radical pelvic surgery: comparison of flap-specific complications. *Gynecol Oncol.* 1995;56(2):271-275.
13. Scott JR, Liu D, Mathes DW. Patient-reported outcomes and sexual function in vaginal reconstruction. *Ann Plat Surg.* 2010;64(3):311-314.
14. Copeland LJ, Hancock KC, Gershenson DM, Stringer CA, Atkinson EN, Edwards CL. Gracilis myocutaneous vaginal reconstruction concurrent with total pelvic exenteration. *Am J Obstet Gynecol.* 1989;160(5): 1095-1101.
15. Soper JT, Larson D, Hunter VJ, Berchuck A, Clarke-Pearson DL. Short gracilis myocutaneous flaps for vulvovaginal reconstruction after radical pelvic surgery. *Obstet Gynecol.* 1989;74(5):823-827.
16. Cain JM, Diamond A, Tamimi HK, Greer BE, Figge DC. The morbidity and benefits of concurrent gracilis myocutaneous graft with pelvic exenteration. *Obstet Gynecol.* 1989;74(2):185-189.
17. Miller B, Morris M, Gershenson DM, Levenback CL, Burke TW. Intestinal fistulae formation following pelvic exenteration: a review of the University of Texas M.D. Anderson Cancer Center experience 1957-1990. *Gynecol Oncol.* 1995;56(2):207-210.
18. Becker DW Jr, Massey FM, McCraw JB. Musculocutaneous flaps in reconstructive pelvic surgery. *Obstet Gynecol.* 1979;54(2):178-183.

19. Soper JT, Secord AA, Havrilesky LJ, Berchuck A, Clarke-Pearson DL Comparison of gracilis and rectus abdominis myocutaneous flap neovaginal reconstruction performed during radical pelvic surgery: flap-specific morbidity. *Int J Gynecol Cancer*. 2007;17(1):298-303.
20. Ratliff CR, Gershenson DM, Morris M, et al. Sexual adjustments of patients undergoing gracilis myocutaneous flap vaginal reconstruction in conjunction with pelvic exenteration. *Cancer*. 1996;78(10):2229-2235.
21. Lacey CG, Stern JL, Feigenbaum S, Hill EC, Braga CA. Vaginal reconstruction after exenteration with use of gracilis myocutaneous flaps: the University of California, San Francisco experience. *Am J Obstet Gynecol*. 1988;158(6):1278-1284.
22. Reece GP, Baldwin, BB. Gracilis flap for vaginal reconstruction. In: Evans GRD, ed. *Operative Plastic Surgery*. 1st ed. Norwalk: Appleton & Lange; 2000:797-804.
23. McGregor JC, Buchan AC. Our clinical experience with the tensor fasciae latae myocutaneous flap. *Br J Plast Surg*. 1980;33(2):270-276.
24. Nahai F, Silverton JS, Hill HL, Vasconez LO. The tensor fascia lata musculocutaneous flap. *Ann Plast Surg*. 1978;1(4):372-379.
25. Gopinath KS, Chadrashekhar M, Kumar MV, Srikant KC. Tensor fasciae latae musculocutaneous flaps to reconstruct skin defects after radical inguinal lymphadenectomy. *Br J Plast Surg*. 1988;41(4):366-368.
26. Tensor fascia lata flap. In Mathes SJ, Nahai F, eds. *Reconstructive Surgery: Principles, Anatomy and Technique*. 1st ed. New York: Churchill Livingstone; 1997:1271-1292.
27. Durden F Jr, Tiwari P, Kocak E. Can the DermaClose device contribute to periwound tissue ischemia and necrosis: a case presentation and discussion? *Plast Surg Nurs*. 2012;32(3):132-133.
28. Minami RT, Hentz VR, Vistnes LM. Use of vastus lateralis muscle flap for repair of trochanteric pressures sores. *Plast Reconstr Surg*. 1977;60(3):364-368.
29. Mathes SJ, Vasconez LO, Jurkiewicz MJ. Extensions and further applications of muscle flap transposition. *Plast Reconstr Surg*. 1977;60(1):6-13.
30. Wong S, Garvey P, Skibber J, Yu P. Reconstruction of pelvic exenteration defects with anterolateral thigh-vastus lateralis muscle flaps. *Plast Reconstr Surg*. 2009;124(4):1177-1185.
31. Huang L-Y, Lin H, Liu Y-T, Chang Chien C-C, Chang S-Y. Anterolateral thigh vastus lateralis myocutaneous flap for vulvar reconstruction after radical vulvectomy: a preliminary experience. *Gynecol Oncol*. 2000;78(3 Pt 1):391-393.
32. Vastus lateralis flap. In Mathes SJ, Nahai F, eds. *Reconstructive Surgery: Principles, Anatomy and Technique*. 1st ed. New York: Churchill Livingstone; 1997:1293-1306.
33. Hanasono MM, Skoracki RJ, Yu P. A prospective study of donor-site morbidity after anterolateral thigh fasciocutaneous and myocutaneous free flap harvest in 220 patients. *Plast Reconstr Surg*. 2010;125(1):209-214.
34. Hsu H, Chien SH, Wang CH, et al. Expanding the applications of the pedicled anterolateral thigh and vastus lateralis myocutaneous flaps. *Ann Plast Surg*. 2012;69(6):643-649.
35. Ger R. The surgical management of decubitus ulcers by muscle transposition. *Surgery*. 1971;69(1):106-110.
36. Cardosi RJ, Hoffman MS, Greenwald D. Rectus femoris myocutaneous flap for vulvoperineal reconstruction. *Gynecol Oncol*. 2002;85(1):188-191.
37. Rectus femoris flap. In Mathes SJ, Nahai F, eds. *Reconstructive Surgery: Principles, Anatomy and Technique*. 1st ed. New York: Churchill Livingstone; 1997:1233-1246.
38. Caulfield WH, Curtsinger L, Powell G, Pederson WC. Donor leg morbidity after pedicled rectus femoris muscle flap transfer for abdominal wall and pelvic reconstruction. *Ann Plast Surg*. 1994;32(4):377-382.
39. Ramirez OM, Orlando JC, Hurwitz DJ. The sliding gluteus maximus myocutaneous flap: Its relevance in ambulatory patients. *Plast Reconstr Surg*. 1984;74(1):68-75.
40. Hurwitz DJ. Closure of a large defect of the pelvic cavity by an extended compound myocutaneous flap based on the inferior gluteal artery. *Br J Plast Surg*. 1980;33(2):256-261.
41. Arkoulakis NS, Angel CL, DuBeshter B, Serletti JM. Reconstruction of an extensive vulvectomy defect using the gluteus maximus fasciocutaneous V-Y advancement flap. *Ann Plast Surg*. 2002;49(1):50-54.

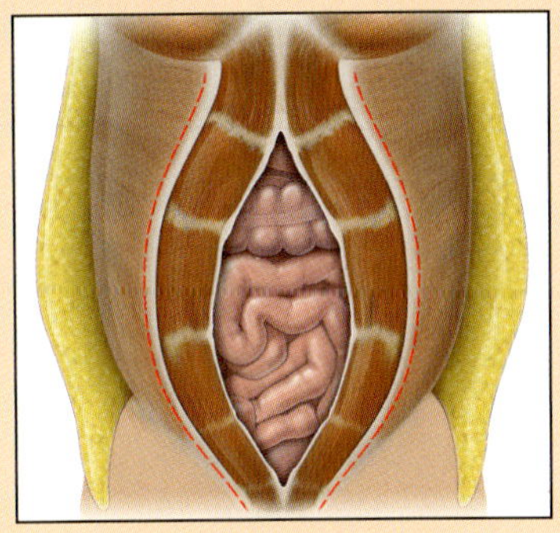

Section D Management of Complex Abdominal Wall Defects

Chapter 19. Tissue Rearrangement Techniques and Regional Flaps

Cindy Wei, MD and
Evan Matros, MD

BACKGROUND

Extirpative gynecologic cancer surgery may result in partial or full-thickness defects of the abdominal wall. Although minor defects can be repaired primarily, large or composite defects present a significant challenge requiring careful planning to obtain a successful reconstruction. A multidisciplinary team, including gynecologic oncology, urology, general, and plastic surgery, may be required for treatment of the patient with gynecologic cancer. Goals of abdominal wall reconstruction in these patients are to restore structural integrity of the abdominal wall musculofascial system and provide stable wound coverage.

Repair of complex abdominal wall defects can be divided into 2 main modalities: autologous tissue or nonautologous (prosthetics or biomaterials). Depending on the clinical situation, either or both modalities may be required. This chapter delineates preoperative and anatomic considerations that factor into reconstructive decision-making, with an emphasis on techniques of autologous tissue repair. Prosthetics and biomaterials are discussed in Chapter 20.

INDICATIONS AND CLINICAL APPLICATIONS

Functions of the abdominal wall include protection of intra-abdominal organs, provision of dynamic support for respiration and upright posture, and assistance in Valsalva for coughing, urination, and defecation. Difficulty performing these functions due to abdominal wall discontinuity will not only impact function, but health-related quality of life as well. Gross herniation of intra-abdominal contents can create obvious difficulty in social situations. By contrast, small hernias, while not as visible, are at greater risk for incarceration and strangulation. Indications for reconstruction of abdominal wall defects thus range from functional to aesthetic.

Few absolute contraindications to abdominal wall repair exist. Hemodynamically unstable patients can be temporarily closed using negative pressure wound dressings or large intravenous bag coverage with definitive closure performed at a later date. In patients desiring elective repair of chronic ventral hernias or wounds, thorough preoperative evaluation and counseling must be performed. These patients often have significant medical comorbidities; thus, the benefits of major abdominal surgery must be weighed before undertaking repair. Such procedures can cause significant cardiopulmonary embarrassment both intraoperatively and postoperatively, particularly for chronic ventral hernias with a significant loss of domain. Asymptomatic, high-risk medical patients at low risk for incarceration may be managed conservatively with observation.

Defect Etiology

Abdominal wall defects requiring reconstruction may result from tumor extirpation, incisional hernia, abdominal wound infection, or a combination thereof. Malignant pelvic tumors extending to the anterior abdominal wall may require wide resection of myofascial structures, subcutaneous tissue, and/or skin, depending on the extent of tumor invasion. Incisional hernia following prior laparotomy has a reported incidence of 2% to 11%.[1,2] Risk factors for developing this complication include elderly age, morbid obesity, malnourishment, immunosuppression, and previous abdominal surgery. Medical conditions such as connective tissue disorders and those associated with increased intra-abdominal pressure (eg, chronic cough, constipation, ascites) also predispose to incisional hernia development. Soft tissue infections of the abdominal wall may follow laparotomy or prior mesh repair. Mesh infection often necessitates removal with staged or delayed reconstruction.

ANATOMIC CONSIDERATIONS

Assessing the Wound

1. Wound bed status

The extent and timing of reconstruction depends in part on the level of bacterial contamination of the wound bed. Otherwise healthy patients with clean, stable wounds following tumor resection can have definitive reconstruction performed immediately. By contrast, if a wound is infected or heavily contaminated, or if additional abdominal surgeries are planned, then definitive reconstruction is delayed. Infected or contaminated wounds should undergo multiple irrigation and débridements until clean, at which point they can be temporarily closed. Frequently used techniques for wound temporization include applying absorbable Vicryl mesh, negative pressure wound dressings, or both followed by split-thickness skin grafting over the granulated bowel. Once the wound is epithelialized or the skin graft has matured, delayed reconstruction with hernia repair can be entertained. It is best to allow at least 6 months before reconstruction begins in order to permit resolution of local inflammation and scar maturation.

Special consideration should be given to wounds in areas with prior irradiation or extensive scar tissue following previous surgery. These wounds share in common poor vascularity with atrophic and nonpliable soft tissues. Attempts to obtain closure with local tissue advancement through undermining have a high likelihood of failure. Treatment with vascularized flaps from outside the region is required to optimize healing.

2. Characteristics of the defect

The next factor to evaluate is the extent of the skin/soft tissue deficit and the fascial defect size. Small defects of the skin and subcutaneous tissue (< 5 cm) can usually be closed primarily if undermining of the skin permits tension-free reapproximation. Larger defects require additional tissue in the form of local or regional flaps, or skin grafting. It is also important to differentiate between relative and absolute tissue deficits. Subacute or chronic wounds suffer from retraction of local tissues, whereas tumor resection results in absolute tissue loss. Knowing the etiology of the defect is helpful when planning reconstruction because a small or moderate relative tissue deficiency can often be overcome with local advancement, whereas an absolute deficiency requires additional tissue recruitment to close the defect.

Fascial and composite defects involving both skin and fascia require restoration of fascial continuity to prevent herniation of intra-abdominal contents. Small fascial defects (< 3–5 cm) can be closed primarily if the repair is tension free. Larger fascial defects require formal reconstruction using prosthetic mesh, components separation, or autologous flaps. Regardless of the reconstructive method chosen for either the skin or fascial component, the most important principle is a tension-free closure. Tension predisposes to wound dehiscence, hernia development, and abdominal compartment syndrome.

3. Position of the defect

A final aspect to consider is the location of the defect on the abdominal wall. Central defects are often amenable to closure with local skin advancement and fascial components separation from both sides. By contrast, lateral defects are more challenging to close because abdominal wall skin or fascia can only be released for advancement from one side. Defects adjacent to the costal margin or iliac crest are hindered by the rigidity of these fixed structures.

PREOPERATIVE PREPARATION

Box 19-1 KEY SURGICAL INSTRUMENTATION

- General plastic surgery trays and set-ups, including electrocautery, bipolar cautery, a variety of handheld retractors, and fine dissecting instruments such as McIndoe forceps and tenotomy scissors are sufficient for most procedures
- Dermatome if skin grafting is planned
- Doppler probe and machine if an axial pattern flap is planned

History and Physical Examination

As with all surgical candidates, preoperative assessment of the patient should begin with a thorough history and physical examination. Patients with cardiopulmonary disease or diabetes should undergo evaluation by specialists for medical optimization and clearance prior to surgery. Malnourished patients should be nutritionally optimized to promote adequate wound healing postoperatively. Smokers may be referred to smoking cessation programs and should be encouraged to quit smoking at least six weeks prior to surgery, if possible, in an effort to prevent wound healing complications.

Physical examination should take note of the patient's general condition, body habitus, and body mass index. Palpate the abdomen to identify hernias or a rectus diastasis. Knowledge of the patient's prior surgeries is helpful, as well as identifying existing scars on the trunk, abdomen, and legs. Such information is critical in determining available tissue donor sites for reconstruction. In patients with multiple prior abdominal wall scars, the vascular supply to the existing skin needs to be considered when designing additional incisions. Previous incisions can be incorporated into the design of the reconstruction to limit scar burden and minimize potential watershed areas.

Imaging Studies

For patients who have had prior abdominal procedures or chronic ventral hernias, it is helpful to obtain preoperative imaging to assist in reconstructive planning. Computed tomography (CT) scan is the preferred modality. It is helpful in evaluating the patient's intestinal anatomy, the location and size of fascial defects, and extent of prosthetic material placed during previous surgeries. CT scans obtained with intravenous contrast can clarify the presence and patency of vascular pedicles, which may be important for flap reconstruction.

Key Surgical Instrumentation

In the operative suite, general plastic surgery trays and instruments should be readily available, including standard electrocautery, bipolar cautery, a variety of handheld retractors and find dissecting instruments such as McIndoe forceps and tenotomy scissors. If a skin graft is planned as part of the procedure, then a dermatome should be made available. Similarly, if an axial pattern flap is going to be performed, then a Doppler probe and machine will help assess vascularity.

SURGICAL PROCEDURES

Box 19-2 MASTER SURGEON'S PRINCIPLES

- Thorough preoperative planning is essential
- Have a backup surgical plan available

Attempts to formulate an algorithm for abdominal wall reconstruction are difficult because of the numerous variables involved. A more useful method is to climb the reconstructive ladder starting with the simplest surgical options before proceeding to the more complex. The best reconstructive plan is one that provides a reliable, durable closure with the least potential morbidity. The surgeon should always have a secondary option planned in the event that the first option fails or is unavailable due to extended extirpation.

Reconstruction cases often benefit from coordination with other services in the event that further abdominal wall manipulation is required such as a urinary conduit or colostomy creation. The plastic surgeon may help plan skin incisions at the commencement of a major extirpative procedure to aid reconstruction and preserve flap vascular pedicles.

Repair of Fascial Defects

1. Primary closure

The simplest method of fascial repair is primary closure, which can be attempted in defects smaller than 3 to 5 cm.[3] It is recommended that the fascia is closed with nonresorbable monofilament suture in continuous fashion.[4] The benefit of continuous suture is that the tension is distributed evenly over the length of the defect, which is in contrast to interrupted or figure-of-8 sutures. The surrounding tissues should be mobilized to ensure the fascia could be reapproximated in a tension-free manner. Repairs preformed under tension result in fascial strangulation with necrosis and are more likely to fail. Large, full-thickness abdominal wall retention sutures are not a means to compensate for a tight fascial closure and contribute to both skin and fascial necrosis.

Incisional hernias repaired with hernia sac excision and primary suture closure demonstrate recurrence rates ranging from 25% to 63%, even for small defects less than 5 cm in size.[5,6] Therefore, if the fascial closure is tight, then there should be a low threshold for use of prosthetic mesh.

2. Prosthetics and bioprosthetics

Since the late 1980s, the use of prosthetic mesh for abdominal wall reconstruction has dramatically increased and has since become the standard of care for incisional hernia repair.[7] For abdominal wall defects resulting from tumor resection, the use of synthetic mesh represents a simple and readily available method of fascial replacement. Additional advantages include the absence of donor site morbidity and its ability to result in a tension-free closure. Significant disadvantages of mesh include mesh extrusion, infection, bowel adhesions, and enterocutaneous fistula formation. Its use also provides static—rather than dynamic—support for the abdominal wall, potentially leading to respiratory embarrassment. Synthetic mesh is contraindicated in infected and heavily contaminated wounds, and it should be used with caution in cases with tenuous overlying soft-tissue coverage. It is best reserved for clean wounds with fascial defects not amenable to either primary closure or component separation (discussed below).

The potential morbidity of synthetic mesh-related complications spurred the development of more biocompatible prosthetics. A variety of biologic meshes have been introduced which have gained popularity for use in many facets of reconstruction. Derived from human or animal sources, these bioprosthetic consist of a decellularized collagen-based extracellular matrix, which acts as a scaffold for host tissue ingrowth and regeneration once implanted in the body. This affords biologic mesh distinct advantages over synthetic mesh, namely the ability to resist infection and be used in contaminated fields. Disadvantages include increased expense and higher rates of hernia recurrence secondary to matrix attenuation over time.[8] High-level studies evaluating acellular dermal matrices in abdominal wall reconstruction have not yet been published, which makes their role difficult to define. At this time, the main utility of these matrices appears to be in cases where synthetic mesh is contraindicated such as in infected or heavily contaminated fields. A more detailed discussion of prosthetics and bioprosthetics is given in Chapter 20.

3. Free fascial graft

An alternative to synthetic or biologic mesh is the use of autologous fascial grafts to repair abdominal wall fascial defects. The most commonly used fascial graft is the tensor fascia lata (TFL), initially described by Kirschner in 1913.[9] The fascia lata graft is strong, versatile, and easy to harvest. Harvest is performed through a longitudinal incision along the lateral aspect of the thigh. The skin and subcutaneous tissue are elevated over the area of fascia to be harvested. Care should be taken not to injure the underlying muscle while incising and elevating the graft. The entire fascia lata can be harvested save for the posterior condensation of the iliotibial tract, which should be preserved to prevent lateral knee instability. To repair the abdominal wall, the graft is sutured in place using an inlay technique with the smooth deep surface of the fascia lata oriented toward the viscera. The graft must be covered with local or regional skin flaps for it to revascularize. Studies have demonstrated that fascial grafts retain the parallel orientation of collagen fibrils[10] and become revascularized[11] after implantation.

With the advent of synthetics and bioprosthetic meshes, use of autologous fascial grafts has fallen out of favor. The limited quantity and need for a donor site can make autologous grafts a less attractive option than readily available off-the-shelf prosthetics. Conversely, the ease of graft harvest and minimal donor site morbidity of grafts such as the fascia lata make them appealing in situations in which synthetics are contraindicated or components separation is not possible. The autologous nature of the grafts makes them a useful biocompatible tool for contaminated cases or when prior synthetic meshes have failed.

4. Components separation

A method of fascial repair that restores dynamic abdominal wall function is the components separation technique. First described by Ramirez in 1990,[12] this technique involves medial advancement of composite myofascial flaps on the abdomen, which can be performed unilaterally or bilaterally. The procedure is ideal for midline defects of the abdominal wall in which the absolute quantity of tissue loss is small, such as a chronic hernia where the abdominal musculature has retracted.

The classically described technique involves elevating the skin and subcutaneous tissue off the fascia of the anterior abdominal wall (Figure 19-1A). A vertical incision is made through the external oblique aponeurosis and muscle, 1 to 2 cm lateral to the semilunar line along the entire length of the muscle. The external oblique is dissected off the internal oblique, staying in the avascular fascial plane between the 2 muscles (Figure 19-1B). The neurovascular structures are deeper, between the internal oblique and transversus muscles. It is helpful to continue the dissection laterally to at least the level of the midaxillary line, and it can be continued to the posterior axillary line if more mobility is required. The rectus-internal oblique-transversus complex can then be advanced medially with the rectus muscles reapproximated in the midline using strong nonresorbable suture. These maneuvers permit ipsilateral advancement up to 5 cm in the epigastrium, 10 cm at the umbilicus, and 3 cm in the suprapubic region. Thus, performing bilateral components separations can provide closure of defects up to 20 cm wide in the midabdomen. If additional advancement is required, then transection of the posterior rectus sheath and dissection off the rectus muscle can provide an additional 2 to 4 cm of advancement (Figure 19-1C).

A major benefit of the components separation technique is its ability to restore dynamic abdominal wall function. By preserving lateral innervation to the abdominal wall musculature and restoring the rectus complexes to the midline, the functions of the abdominal wall in trunk flexion and extension, respiration, micturition, and defecation are restored (Figure 19-1E). Additional advantages include the avoidance of a separate donor site, the lack of a need for prosthetic materials, and low hernia recurrence rates (8%–22%) compared with primary closure.[13]

The most common complications are wound related, occurring in about 25% of cases.[13] These are related to undermining of the skin and subcutaneous tissues off the abdominal wall, which disrupts epigastric perforators supplying the overlying skin. Numerous modifications to the traditional components separation technique have been developed in an attempt to preserve the periumbilical perforators and prevent abdominal wall necrosis. Although a lack of consensus exists on the most effective variant, numerous studies have shown a decrease in wound complications using perforator-preserving approaches. In general, these approaches minimize the extent of skin and subcutaneous tissue undermining from the medial edge of the rectus to up to 4 cm.[14,15] To access the semilunar line, small lateral or subcostal incisions can be made to expose the external oblique aponeurosis. By limiting the extent of soft tissue dissection, especially around the umbilicus, these approaches preserve many of the perforators to the overlying skin. Studies have shown a decrease in wound complications from 20% with the traditional technique to 2% using modified approaches.[14] Endoscopic components separation procedures have also been developed with perforator preservation in mind; however, the need for specialized equipment and additional setup has prevented these methods from gaining widespread popularity.

Repair of Skin Defects

1. Primary closure

As mentioned previously, small skin defects (< 5 cm) may be primarily closed in many instances. This often requires undermining of the skin and subcutaneous tissues immediately above the level of the anterior abdominal wall fascia. Drawing from lessons learned from components separation, undermining should be limited to that required for a tension-free closure. Excessive undermining increases the potential for wound breakdown or seroma by disrupting blood flow to the skin and increasing raw tissue surface area.

2. Skin graft

The split-thickness skin grafting of abdominal wall defects is a temporary maneuver when delayed reconstruction is planned, particularly following a period of wound care for extensive bacterial contamination. Alternatively, if a patient is unstable or not fit for extensive reconstruction, then skin grafting can be performed as a means of definitive wound closure.

Skin grafts can be directly placed on vascularized tissue or once granulation tissue has formed. When a fascial defect is present, mesh placement to address the fascial defect is performed first using either Vicryl or a biologic mesh. Negative pressure wound dressings are applied on the mesh until a layer of granulation tissue is present followed by delayed skin grafting (Figure 19-2). If future reconstruction is desired, the skin graft can be excised once it has matured and is no longer adherent to the underlying bowel. A final alternative in the most hostile situations is to place a negative pressure wound device directly on the bowel until granulation tissue is present, followed by skin grafting. Whenever Vicryl mesh is used or a skin graft is used directly on the bowel, development of a hernia is guaranteed.

Split-thickness skin grafts can be harvested from almost any surface of the body, with the most common donor sites

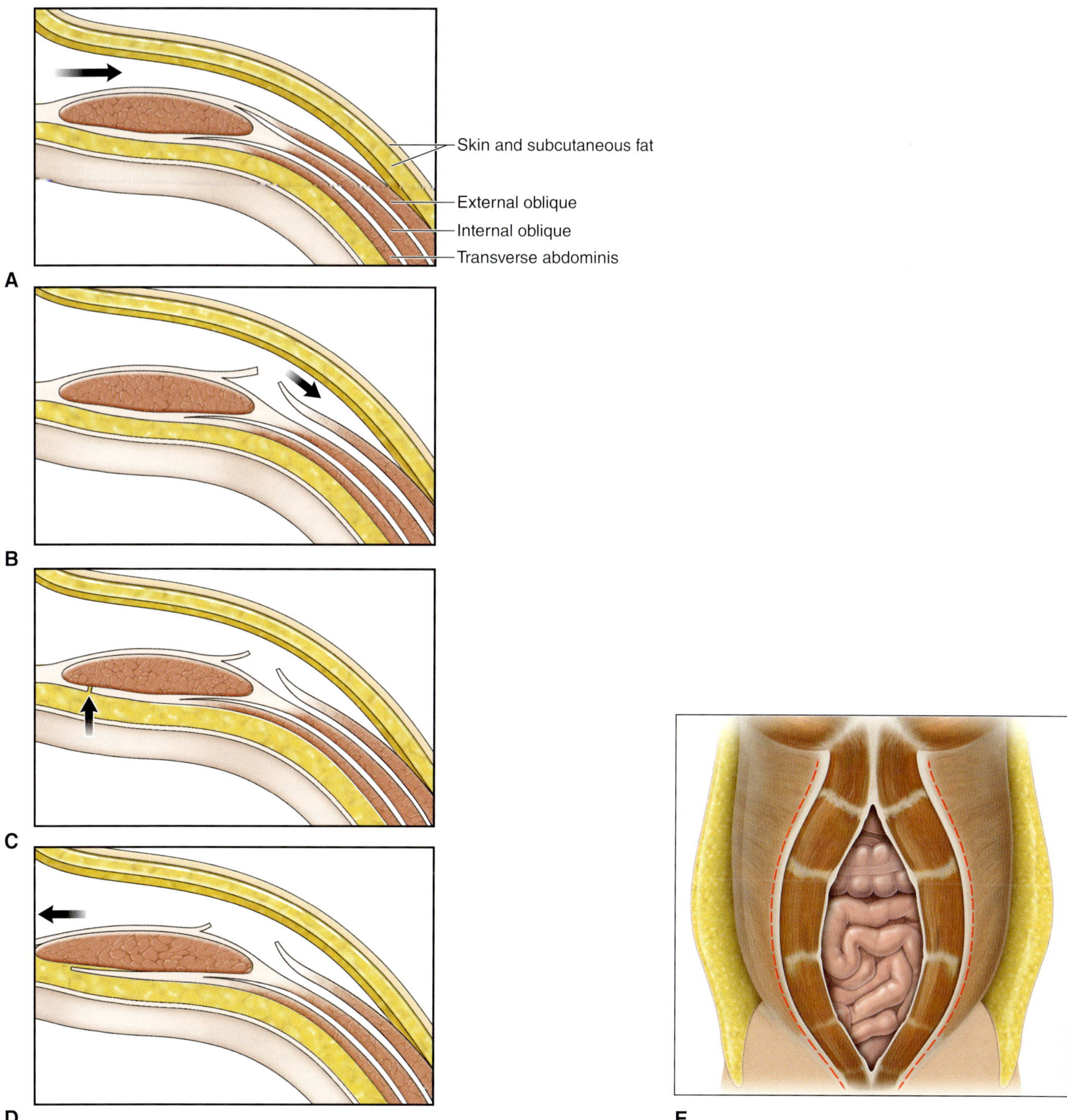

Fig. 19-1. Separation technique of the components. (**A**) Skin and subcutaneous tissue are dissected off the anterior abdominal wall. (**B**) The external oblique aponeurosis is incised 1 to 2 cm lateral to the semilunar line and dissected off the internal oblique. (**C**) The posterior rectus sheath can be divided if further advancement is needed. (**D**) The rectus complex is advanced toward the midline. (**E**) Frontal view of abdomen for components separation. Site of external oblique aponeurosis incision marked with red dashed lines. (Redrawn and modified with permission from Journal of the American College of Surgeons Vol 196(1), de Vries Reilingh TS, van Goor H, Rosman C et al. *"Components separation technique" for the repair of large abdominal wall hernias,* pages 32-7, 2003, Elsevier.)

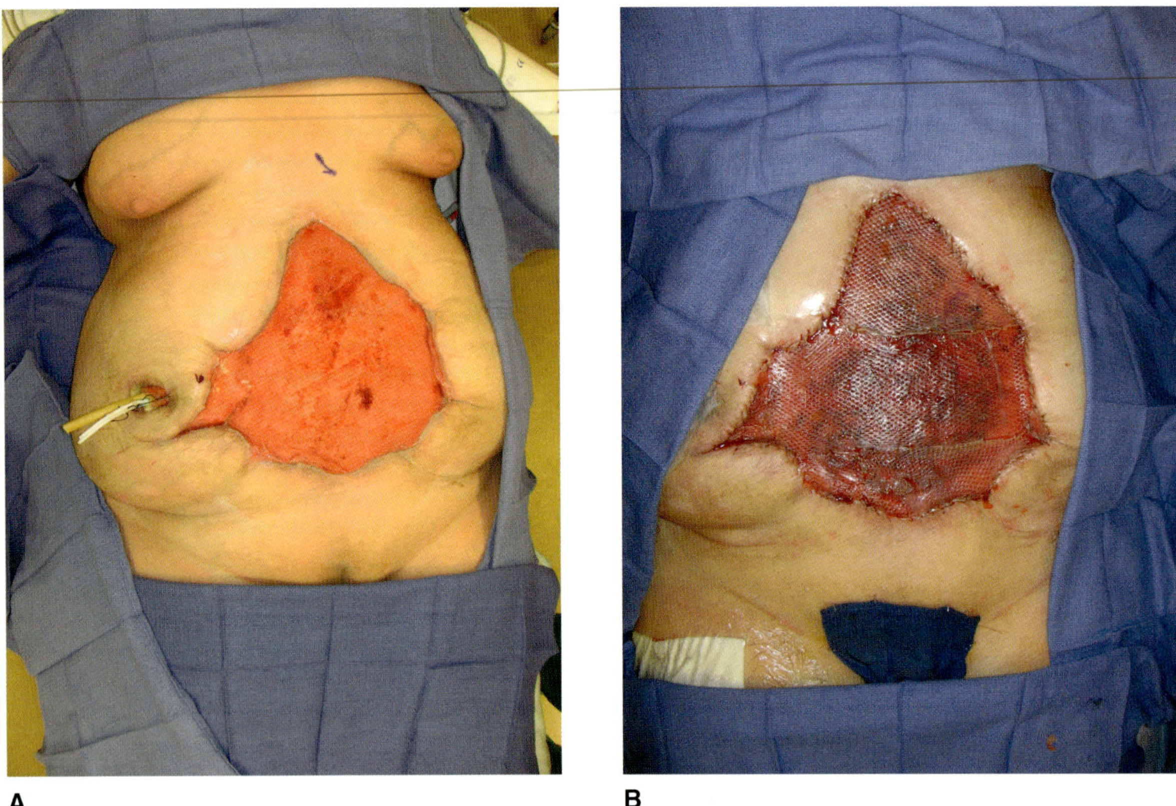

Fig. 19-2. Split-thickness skin grafting. This patient had a large chronic wound of the midabdomen with a skin and soft tissue deficit. Negative pressure wound therapy was used to encourage wound bed granulation. Once granulated (**A**), a split-thickness skin graft was applied for coverage (**B**).

being the anterior and lateral thigh, buttocks, and back. Grafts are typically harvested using an air-powered or electric dermatome at a thickness of 0.012 to 0.018 inches for a thin- or intermediate-thickness graft. If a large surface area needs to be covered, then the graft can be meshed. Typical graft meshing devices permit expansion of the graft at ratios ranging from 1:1.5 up to 1:9. Use of a meshed graft usually leads to an irregular, cobble-stoned appearance of the grafted area after healing. If meshing is not desired, then the graft can be pie-crusted using an 11-blade or fine sharp scissors to create fenestrations, which allow for egress of fluid from under the graft. The graft is then trimmed to fit the donor site and stapled or sutured in place. Placement of a bolster dressing helps appose the graft to the recipient bed, prevent shearing forces, which can disrupt graft take, and maintain a moist environment for healing. Bolsters are typically left in place for 5 to 7 days. The donor site is dressed with a semi-occlusive dressing (eg, Tegaderm, OpSite) for 7 to 21 days until re-epithelialization occurs.

3. Flap reconstruction

Regional fasciocutaneous and myocutaneous flaps can provide a large amount of skin and soft tissue for reconstruction of abdominal wall defects. In most clean cases following tumor resection, flaps are used to provide soft tissue coverage across a fascial repair performed with synthetic mesh. In select cases, the fascia harvested with the flap can be used for the fascial repair.

Rectus abdominis flap. The workhorse flap in abdominal wall reconstruction is the vertically oriented rectus abdominis myocutaneous flap. If available, it is the flap of choice due to its reliability, wide arc of rotation, and ease of harvest. The flap can be elevated with or without a skin paddle and can reach the upper and lower quadrants of the abdomen, groin, and proximal thigh. Size limitations of the cutaneous portion of the flap are dictated by the laxity of the patient's skin and the ability to close the donor site primarily. Depending on the defect location, the flap can be based either inferiorly on the deep inferior epigastric artery, or superiorly on the superior epigastric artery. The main disadvantage of the rectus flap is the sacrifice of a rectus muscle with overlying fascia, which predisposes patients to hernia development. To minimize hernia rates, the flap can be elevated on a limited number of perforating vessels thereby reducing the extent of fascial sacrifice.

Harvest of the rectus myocutaneous flap begins with designing a vertically oriented elliptical skin paddle over the rectus muscle (Figure 19-3A). The skin and subcutaneous fat

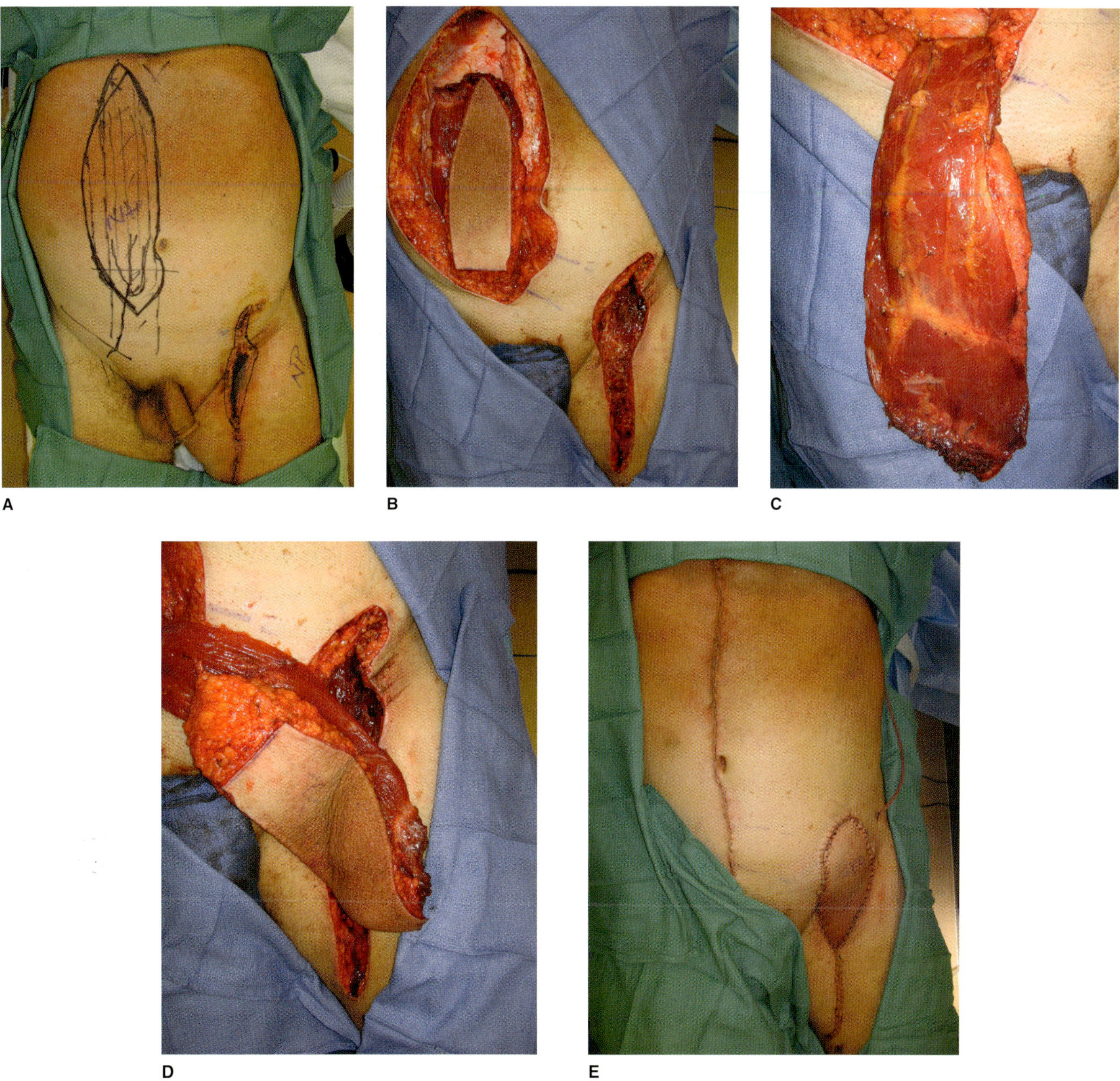

Fig. 19-3. Rectus abdominis myocutaneous flap reconstruction of groin defect. (**A**) Skin paddle designed over the right rectus muscle showing the course of the deep inferior epigastric vessels. (**B**) Inferiorly based rectus abdominis flap shown in situ. (**C**) Undersurface of flap, showing the inferior epigastric pedicle running along the posterior surface of the rectus muscle. (**D**) Flap rotated inferiorly and inset into the defect. (**E**) Flap inset and donor site closed.

are divided down to the level of the rectus sheath. To preserve as much fascia at the donor site for repair as possible, the skin paddle can be carefully dissected off the fascia until the lateral and medial rows of perforators to the skin are identified. The rectus sheath is divided around the perforators, and the fascial edges are elevated off the muscle medially and laterally. The deep inferior epigastric pedicle is identified laterally at the inferior aspect of the muscle by gently retracting the muscle. If the flap is to be based superiorly, then this pedicle can be ligated with the muscle transected near its pubic symphysis origin. The flap is then elevated off the posterior sheath from caudal to cephalad. If the flap is to be based inferiorly, then the superior end of the muscle is divided at the costal margin along with the superior epigastric vessels (Figure 19-3B). The muscle is elevated off the posterior sheath and inset into the defect (Figures 19-3C to 19-3E). The anterior rectus fascia of the donor site is closed with permanent sutures. The skin is closed in standard fashion following undermining in the subcutaneous plane to allow primary soft-tissue closure of the donor site. A drain can be placed in the subcutaneous space to minimize seroma accumulation.

Extended deep inferior epigastric artery flap. For defects exceeding the size or arc of rotation of the standard rectus abdominis flap, the extended deep inferior epigastric artery (DIEA) flap provides a reliable and versatile alternative. First described by Taylor et al in 1983,[16] the flap consists of the rectus abdominis muscle and an obliquely oriented skin paddle extending superolaterally over the chest wall toward the axilla (Figure 19-4). The length of the flap can extend from the periumbilical region to the posterior axillary line. The flap width is again determined by the laxity of the patient's tissues such that the donor site can be primarily closed. The flap has a tremendous arc of rotation, capable of covering large defects from the inferior chest down to the knee. The flap is supplied by periumbilical perforators originating from the deep inferior epigastric artery and their connections with the lateral cutaneous branches of the intercostal arteries.

The skin island of the extended DIEA flap is designed along an axis extending from the umbilicus to the angle of the scapula, roughly parallel to the ribs. Dissection begins at the superolateral tip of the flap, raising the skin flap off the chest wall and external oblique fascia until the lateral border of the rectus muscle is reached. The remainder of the flap is elevated in similar fashion as described for the standard rectus flap. To maximize flap reach, the origin of the rectus muscle can be completely divided such that the flap is entirely "islandized" on the deep inferior epigastric vessels.

Groin flap. The groin flap, also known as the superficial circumflex iliac artery (SCIA) flap, was described by McGregor in 1972.[17] Commonly used as a tubed flap for hand reconstruction, the groin flap is also widely used for reconstruction of the mid- and lower abdominal wall. The flap is centered on an axis drawn one fingerbreadth below the mid-inguinal point to one fingerbreadth below the anterior superior iliac spine (ASIS; Figure 19-5A). The width of the flap is determined by the pinch test. If the length of the flap required extends significantly beyond the ASIS, the extension is designed approximately one-third above and two-thirds below the iliac crest. This portion of the flap can be delayed 2 weeks prior to flap elevation to ensure reliable perfusion. Flap delay involves surgically interrupting a portion of the blood supply to the flap, usually by incising its borders, and

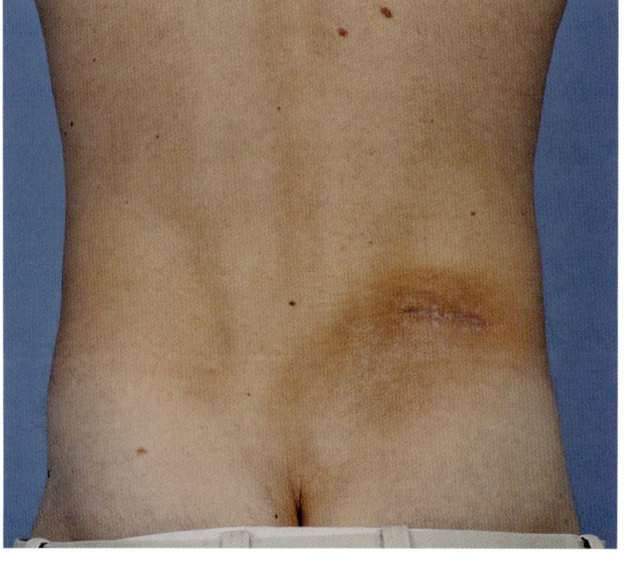
A

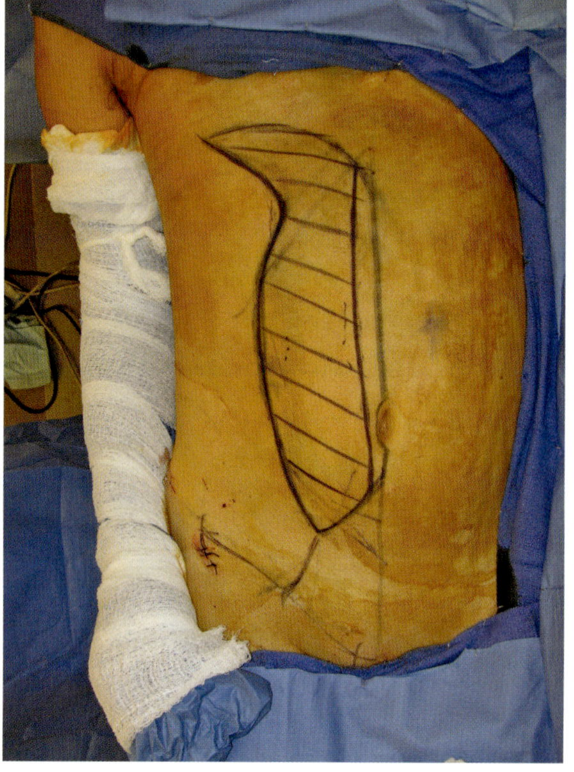
B

Fig. 19-4. Extended DIEA flap reconstruction of lumbar defect. (**A**) Patient with sarcoma involving lumbar abdominal wall. Incision marked with dashed lines. Tumor was resected with overlying skin and soft tissue and underlying bone (posterior iliac crest). (**B**) Design of extended DIEA flap with fasciocutaneous extension over inferior chest wall.

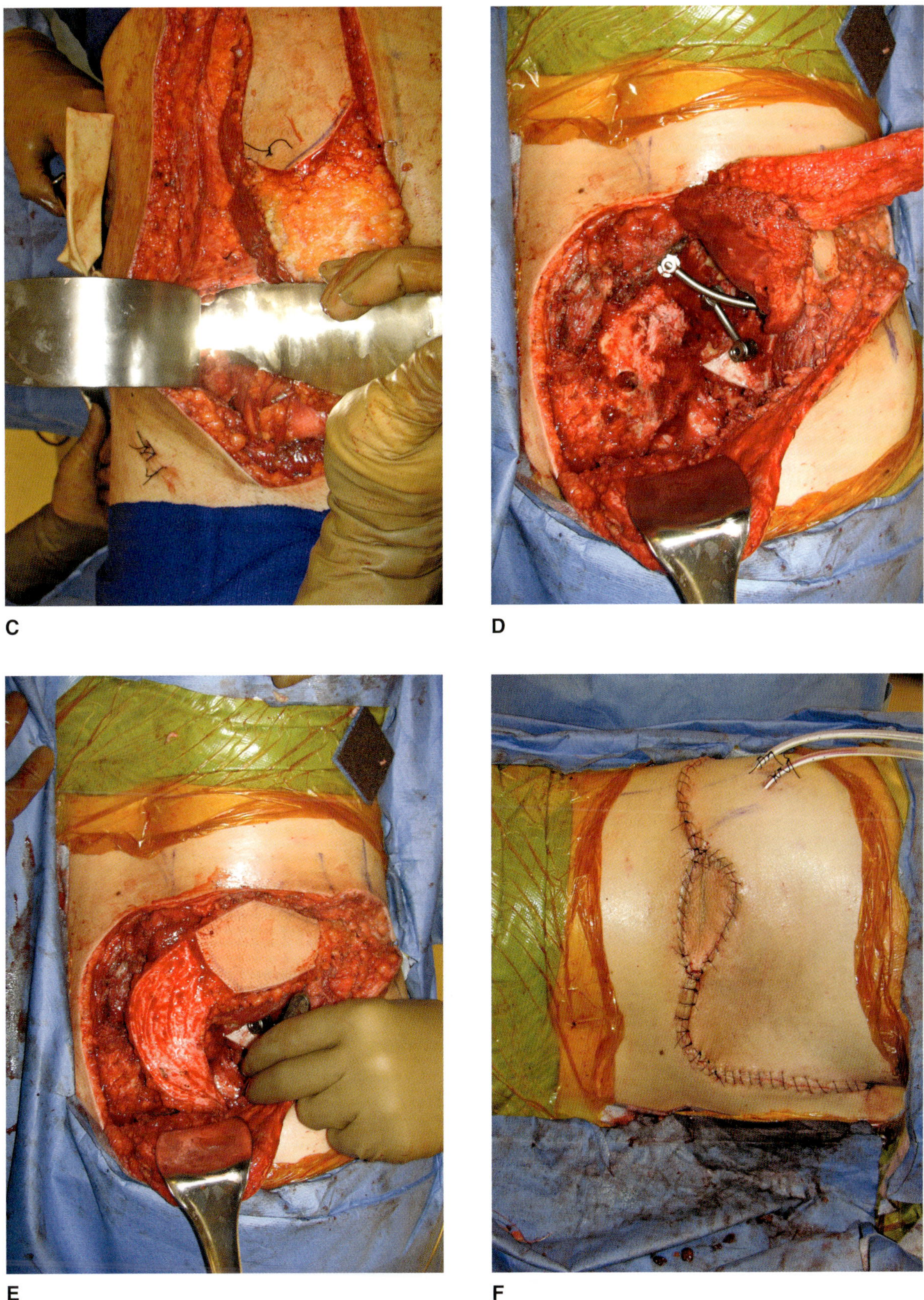

Fig. 19-4. (*Continued*) (**C**) Extended DIEA flap raised and partially de-epithelialized. Retractors show site of tunnel (black arrow) being created from anterior abdominal wall to posterior lumbar defect. (**D**) Flap tunneled through to lumbar defect. (**E**) Flap being inset to cover exposed bone and hardware. (**F**) Final flap inset and closure. DIEA = extended deep inferior epigastric artery.

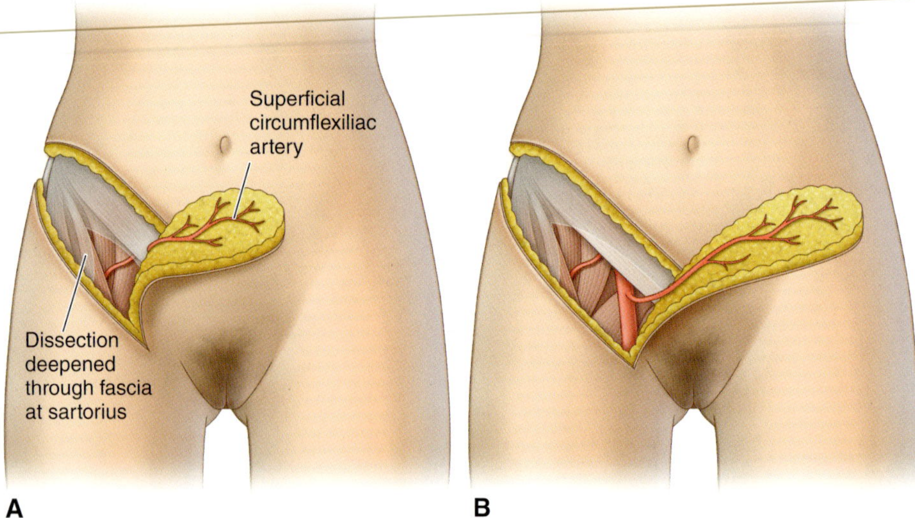

Fig. 19-5. Groin flap. (**A**) Elevation of the groin flap from lateral to medial. Flap is elevated off deep fascia until the lateral border of sartorius is encountered, when dissection is deepened to include the fascia. (**B**) Flap can be dissected back to the origin of the superficial circumflex iliac pedicle to "islandize" the flap. (Modified with permission from Zenn MR, Jones G. *Reconstructive Surgery: Anatomy, Techniques, and Clinical Applications.* St. Louis: Quality Medical Publishing, 2012.)

leaving it in situ for 10 to 14 days prior to elevation and transposition. The mechanism of flap delay is unclear, but it is thought to involve conditioning the tissue to ischemia and/or increasing tissue perfusion by dilation of choke vessels or stimulating vascular ingrowth.

Flap elevation commences laterally by elevating the skin and subcutaneous tissue off the deep fascia medially to the lateral border of the sartorius. The SCIA pierces the fascia consistently at the medial border of the sartorius; thus, the sartorius is an important landmark for identifying the pedicle during the dissection. Once the lateral border of the sartorius is encountered, the muscular fascia is incised and flap elevation continues deep to the fascia (Figure 19-5B). The superficial circumflex iliac vessels can be seen running in the fascia above the sartorius. If enough flap length and mobility have been achieved, the dissection can be stopped at the medial border of the sartorius. If additional mobility is required, the flap can be islanded on its pedicle (Figure 19-5C). The flap is then transposed into the defect and the donor site primarily closed.

Tensor fascia lata and anterolateral thigh flaps. More distant flaps that can be used for abdominal wall reconstruction include the TFL and anterolateral thigh (ALT) flaps based on the ascending and descending branches of the lateral circumflex femoral artery (LCFA), respectively. The size and reach of the TFL flap are limited compared to the ALT flap, which has led to the ALT becoming the preferred flap for abdominal wall defects in many cases.[18] Furthermore, the distal third of the TFL skin paddle has a random blood supply and is thus unreliable unless the flap is delayed. Due to the short pedicle length and the proximal bulkiness of the TFL, its arc of rotation is limited to the ipsilateral lower abdomen below the umbilicus. The reach of the flap can be increased by detaching the muscle from its origin. The main advantage of the TFL flap is the thickness of the fascia lata over the muscle, which can be used as vascularized fascia for reconstructing defects of the abdominal wall when mesh is not desired.

The ALT flap was first reported by Song et al in 1984.[19] Although often used as a free flap, a pedicled flap can easily reach defects of the lower abdomen, groin, and perineum, and reports of the flap reaching the epigastrium have been published in the literature.[18,20] The flap is extremely versatile and can be designed to include skin, fascia, and muscle, depending on the requirements of the defect. The flap is designed along the intermuscular septum running between the rectus femoris and vastus lateralis, which can be approximated by a line extending from the ASIS to the lateral border of the patella (Figure 19-6A). The middle of this line marks the area in which perforators from the descending branch of the LCFA are most likely to be found. A pencil Doppler can be used to mark the location of perforators to help design the margins of the flap. A flap measuring up to 25 × 8 cm generally allows the donor site to be primarily closed, but a much larger expanse of skin encompassing the lateral half of the thigh can be harvested if the donor site is skin grafted.

Harvest of a fasciocutaneous ALT flap begins by elevating the medial half of the flap first, deep to the investing fascia of the thigh muscles. Perforators running in the intermuscular septum are identified and preserved (Figure 19-6B). The lateral aspect of the flap is then elevated toward the septum, again noting any perforators. Once the septum has been approached from both sides, the perforators can be selected. The perforators are traced down to the descending branch of

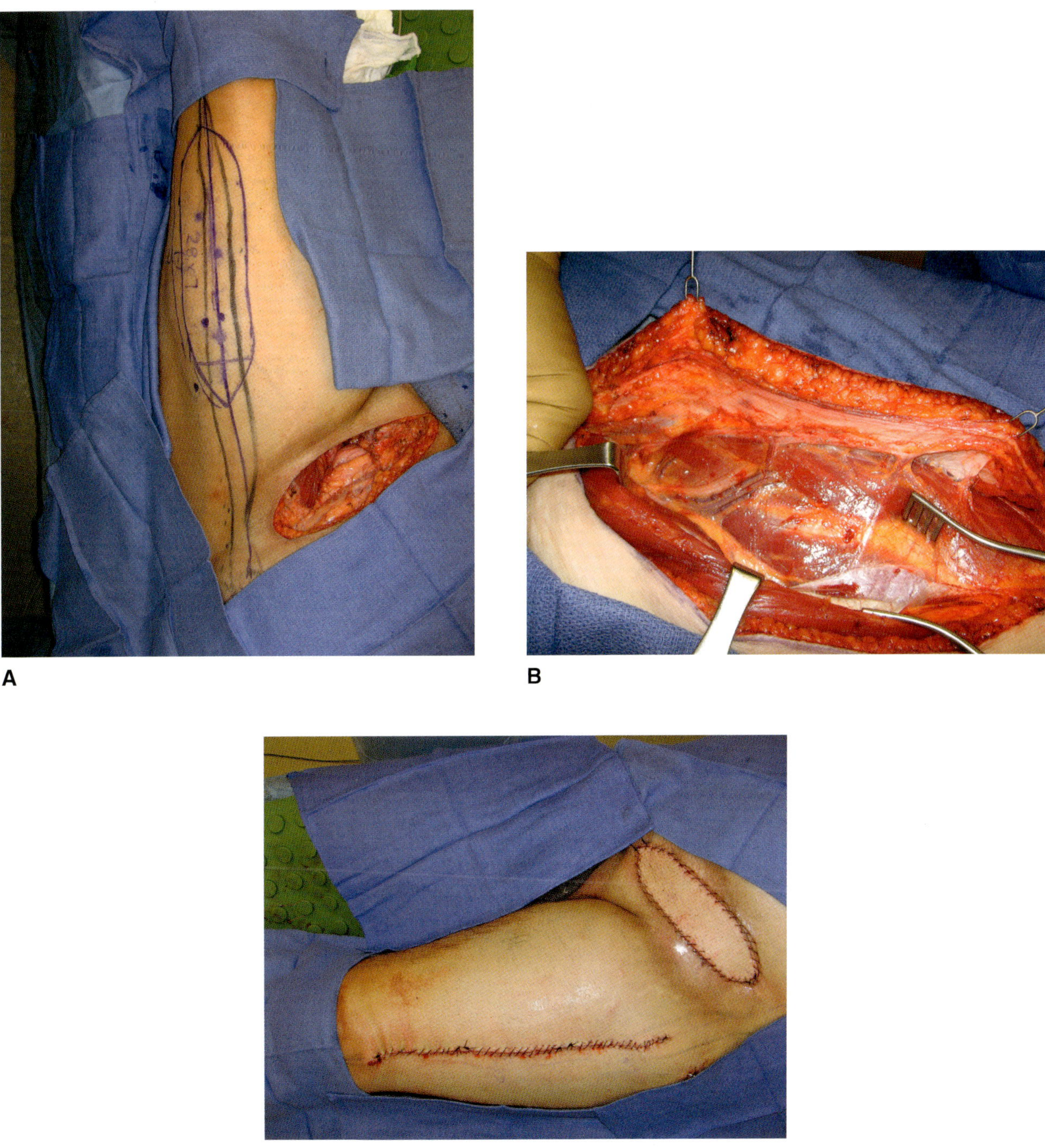

Fig. 19-6. ALT flap reconstruction of lower quadrant abdominal wall defect. (**A**) Skin paddle designed along the axis from the ASIS to the lateral patella. (**B**) Anterior border of flap is raised, showing 2 perforators supplying flap (black arrows). Retractors are placed between the rectus femoris and vastus lateralis, revealing lateral circumflex femoral vessels running between them. (**C**) Flap tunneled subcutaneously and inset into the defect. Donor site primarily closed. ALT = anterolateral thigh, ASIS = anterior superior iliac spine.

the LCFA, which is located at the base of the septum. The LCFA pedicle can be lengthened further by tracing it to its origin off the deep femoral artery. Care should be taken to preserve the nerve to the vastus lateralis, which runs in close proximity to the pedicle. If desirable, then a segment of vastus lateralis containing perforator(s) can be harvested with the flap. The flap can be tunneled subcutaneously or under the rectus femoris to reach the abdomen. The donor site is closed primarily in layers, if possible, or is covered with a split-thickness skin graft.

Overall, the versatility and advantages offered by the ALT flap make it an attractive choice for reconstruction. However, disadvantages of the flap include a more tedious dissection for those inexperienced with perforator dissection, an unsightly donor site defect if skin grafting is required, and the variability in the course of vascular perforators.

Rectus femoris flap. Like the ALT flap, the rectus femoris flap is also supplied by the descending branch of the LCFA. It is a smaller flap with a limited cutaneous component, but it has a wide arc of rotation and is useful for reconstruction of the lower abdomen. The main disadvantages of the flap are the unreliability of the distal skin paddle and donor site morbidity. Traditionally, it was thought that rectus femoris sacrifice resulted in decreased terminal knee extension and strength; however, studies have shown conflicting results.[21,22] Suture of the vastus lateralis and medialis to each other and the cut rectus femoris tendon distally may minimize problems with knee extension.

Design of the flap begins by drawing a line from the ASIS to the midpoint of the patella, which represents the longitudinal axis of the muscle (Figure 19-7A). A skin paddle can be designed centered over the long axis of the muscle. The width of the paddle is determined by the pinch test, and the length is usually limited to the middle third of the thigh to ensure adequate perfusion. The incisions are carried down through the muscular fascia to expose the rectus femoris and sartorius. The sartorius is retracted medially to expose the pedicle, which lies on the deep surface at the junction of the upper and middle thirds of the muscle. The muscle is transected distally, elevated, and transposed into the defect. If desired, the flap can be raised as an island flap by dividing it proximally. The vastus lateralis and medialis should be sutured together distally to preserve knee extension. The donor site is closed primarily in layers over a drain.

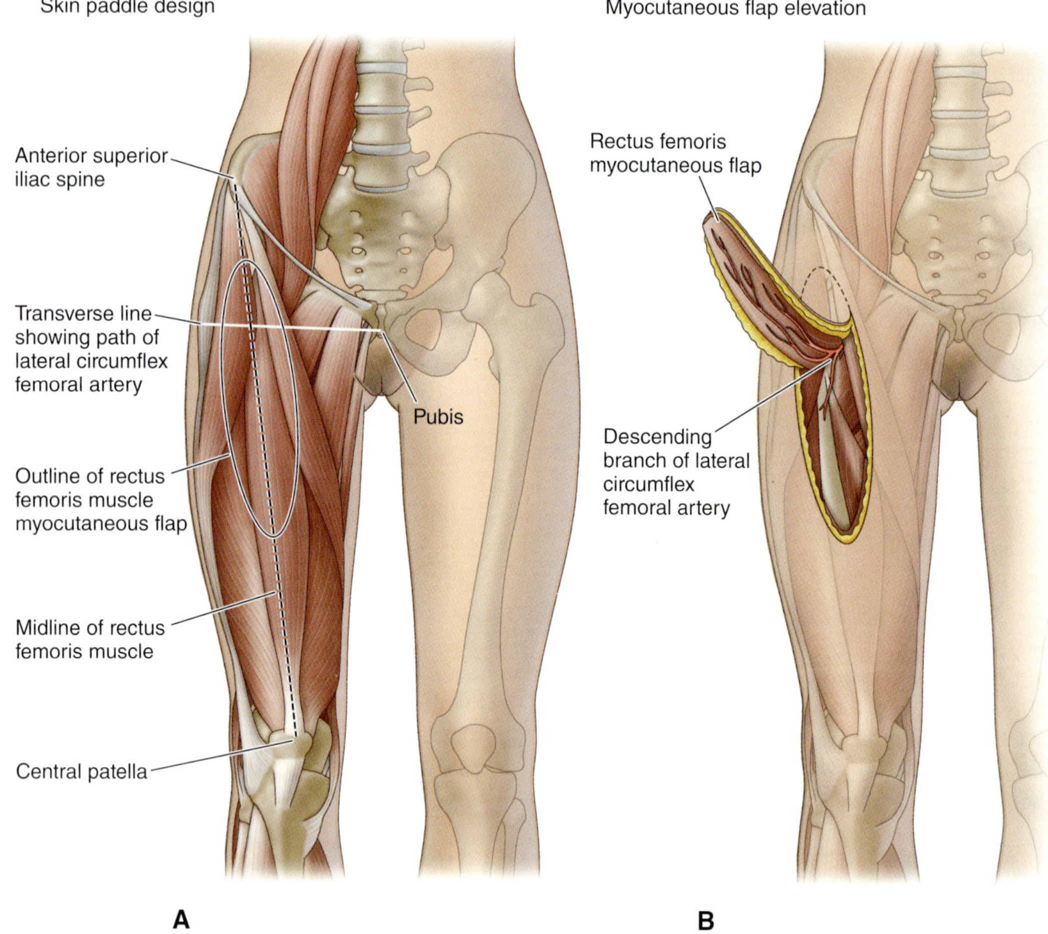

Fig. 19-7. Rectus femoris flap. (**A**) Design of skin paddle centered over muscle along the axis from the ASIS to the mid-patella. (**B**) Flap raised from inferior to superior, including the rectus femoris muscle and lateral circumflex femoral pedicle. ASIS = anterior superior iliac spine. (Modified with permission from Zenn MR, Jones G. *Reconstructive Surgery: Anatomy, Techniques, and Clinical Applications.* St. Louis: Quality Medical Publishing, 2012.)

POSTOPERATIVE CARE

Box 19-3 PERIOPERATIVE MORBIDITY

- Seroma or hematoma
- Wound infection or dehiscence
- Mesh infection or exposure
- Partial/total flap loss
- Abdominal compartment syndrome

Wound Care

Postoperative wound care following abdominal wall reconstruction varies depending on the type of reconstruction performed. In cases such as primary closure, components separation, and prosthetic fascial repair with primary skin closure, incisions should be dressed for the first 24 to 48 hours until the wound edges have epithelialized. Skin grafted wounds are immobilized with either a tie-over bolster or negative pressure wound dressing until postoperative day 5. They are kept moist with Xeroform gauze until the graft has stabilized, usually 5 to 7 days. Lower extremities with donor sites that are skin grafted should be elevated at all times with ambulation restricted until the graft has stabilized. Flap reconstructions should be monitored regularly for skin color, capillary refill, and warmth to ensure adequate perfusion. Strict instructions to avoid pressure on the flap and pedicle should be given to all staff caring for the patient. When flaps from the lower extremity have been tunneled over the groin to reach the abdomen, hip flexion should be limited to less than 60 degrees for several weeks to avoid pedicle compression.

Complications

Potential complications following abdominal wall reconstruction in the early postoperative period include seroma, hematoma, delayed wound healing, infection, ileus or bowel obstruction, abdominal compartment syndrome, and donor site complications. Mesh infection and extrusion are two of the most undesirable complications, as they often necessitate mesh removal with more complex delayed reconstruction. The rate of mesh infection is approximately 7%, with *Staphylococcus aureus* and *epidermidis* being the most common organisms isolated. Although cases of mesh salvage in the setting of infection have been reported,[23] infection is associated with significantly higher rates of hernia,[24] possibly due to weakening at the mesh-fascial interface.[25]

Abdominal compartment syndrome is another potentially devastating complication that can develop following abdominal wall reconstruction. Intra-abdominal hypertension may be more likely in patients with chronic hernias with loss of domain due to the simultaneous reduction in size of the abdominal cavity and return of the visceral contents. Intra-abdominal hypertension is defined as a pressure greater than 20 mm Hg. The increased pressure can cause respiratory difficulties, decreased cardiac output, and decreased hepatorenal perfusion with organ dysfunction. Intra-abdominal pressure greater than 25 mm Hg results in abdominal compartment syndrome, which can quickly result in multiorgan failure and death if not emergently decompressed. Abdominal pressures can be measured with a Foley catheter attached to an arterial line transducer.

LONG-TERM OUTCOMES

Box 19-4 DELAYED COMPLICATIONS

- Hernia recurrence
- Delayed wound/mesh infection

The main measure of long-term outcome following abdominal wall reconstruction is the rate of hernia recurrence. Unfortunately, hernia recurrence is difficult to quantify due to differences in reconstructive method and technique, variable follow-up, and patient-related factors. This is reflected in the disparate percentages for recurrence reported in the literature. In general, mesh repair (< 5%–32%)[5,26] and components separation (8%–22%)[13] appear to result in lower recurrence rates than primary suture repair (25%–63%)[5,6] in the long term. Recurrence following flap repair also appears to be lower, ranging from 5% to 42%.[27] The lack of controlled, high-level studies, have made attempts to develop an algorithmic approach to abdominal wall reconstruction difficult.

SUMMARY

Abdominal wall defects can result from a variety of causes and represent a reconstructive challenge. Numerous autologous, prosthetic, and combined approaches to repair have been described, but no consensus exists on the optimal method of treatment. An understanding of anatomy and dynamic function of the abdominal wall, combined with a thorough assessment of the defect and a comprehensive reconstructive plan, is essential to a successful outcome. Continued advances in the fields of gynecologic oncology, plastic surgery, and tissue engineering are necessary to improve upon the management of these defects.

REFERENCES

1. Bucknall TE, Cox PJ, Ellis H. Burst abdomen and incisional hernia: a prospective study of 1129 major laparotomies. *Br Med J (Clin Res Ed)*. 1982;284(6364):519.
2. Mudge M, Hughes LE. Incisional hernia: a ten year prospective study of incidence and attitudes. *Br J Surg*. 1985;72(1):70.
3. Korenkov M, Paul A, Sauerland S, et al. Classification and surgical treatment: results of an experts' meeting. *Langenbecks Arch Surg*. 2001;386:65.
4. Hodgson NC, Malthaner RA, Østbye T. The search for an ideal method of fascial closure: a meta-analysis. *Ann Surg*. 2000;231(3):436.
5. Luijendijk RW, Hop WC, Van den Tol MP, et al. A comparison of suture repair with mesh repair for incisional hernia. *N Engl J Med*. 2000;343(6):392.

6. Burger JW, Luijendijk RW, Hop WC, et al. Long term follow up of a randomized controlled trial of suture versus mesh repair of incisional hernia. *Ann Surg*. 2004;240(4):578.
7. Voeller GR, Ramshaw B, Park AE, et al. Incisional hernia. *J Am Coll Surg*. 1999;189(6):635.
8. Janis JE, O'Neill AC, Ahmad J, et al. Acellular dermal matrices in abdominal wall reconstruction: a systematic review of the evidence. *Plast Reconstr Surg*. 2012;130(Suppl. 2):183S.
9. Kirschner M. Uber freie Sehne- und Fascientransplantation. *Beitr klin Chir*. 1913;65:472.
10. Peacock EE Jr. Subcutaneous extraperitoneal repair of ventral hernias: a biological basis for fascial transplantation. *Ann Surg*. 1975;181(5):722.
11. Disa JJ, Goldberg NH, Carlton JM, et al. Restoring abdominal wall integrity in contaminated tissue-deficient wounds using autologous fascia grafts. *Plast Reconstr Surg*. 1998;101(4):979.
12. Ramirez OM, Ruas E, Dellon L. "Components separation" method for closure of abdominal-wall defects: an anatomic and clinical study. *Plast Reconstr Surg* 1990;86(3):521.
13. de Vries Reilingh TS, Bodegom ME, van Goor H, et al. Autologous tissue repair of large abdominal wall defects. *Br J Surg*. 2007;94(7):791.
14. Saulis AS, Dumanian GA. Periumbilical rectus abdominis perforator preservation significantly reduces superficial wound complications in "separation of parts" hernia repairs. *Plast Reconstr Surg*. 2002;109(7):2275.
15. Ko JH, Wang EC, Salvay DM. Abdominal wall reconstruction: lessons learned from 200 "components separation" procedures. *Arch Surg*. 2009;144(11):1047.
16. Taylor GI, Corlett R, Boyd JB. The extended deep inferior epigastric flap: a clinical technique. *Plast Reconstr Surg*. 1983;72(6):751.
17. McGregor IA, Jackson IT. The groin flap. *Br J Plast Surg*. 1972; 25(1):3.
18. Kimata Y, Uchiyama K, Sekido M, et al. Anterolateral thigh flap for abdominal wall reconstruction. *Plast Reconstr Surg*. 1999;103(4):1191.
19. Song YG, Chen GZ, Song YL. The free thigh flap: a new free flap concept based on the septocutaneous artery. *Br J Plast Surg*. 1984;37 (2):149.
20. Ting J, Trotter D, Grinsell D. A pedicled anterolateral thigh (ALT) flap for reconstruction of the epigastrium: case report. *J Plast Reconstr Aesthet Surg*. 2010;63(1):e65.
21. Gardetto A, Raschner C, Schoeller T. Rectus femoris muscle flap donor-site morbidity. *Br J Plast Surg*. 2005;58(2):175.
22. Caulfield WH, Curtsinger L, Powell G. Donor leg morbidity after pedicled rectus femoris muscle flap transfer for abdominal wall and pelvic reconstruction. *Ann Plast Surg*. 1994;32(4):377.
23. Kelly ME, Behrman SW. The safety and efficacy of prosthetic hernia repair in clean-contaminated and contaminated wounds. *Am Surg*. 2002;68(6):524-8.
24. Breuing K, Butler CE, Ferzoco S, et al. Incisional ventral hernias: review of the literature and recommendations regarding the grading and technique of repair. *Surgery*. 2010;148(3):544.
25. Law NW, Ellis H. A comparison of polypropylene mesh and expanded polytetrafluoroethylene patch for the repair of contaminated abdominal wall defects—an experimental study. *Surgery*. 1991;109(5):652.
26. Millikan KW. Incisional hernia repair. *Surg Clin North Am*. 2003;83(5):1223.
27. Shell DH, de la Torre J, Andrades P, et al. Open repair of ventral incisional hernias. *Surg Clin North Am*. 2008;88(1)61.

Chapter 20. Bioprosthetic and Prosthetic Materials in Abdominal Wall Reconstruction and Hernia Repair

Mary S. Brady, MD, FACS

BACKGROUND

Prosthetic materials for abdominal wall reconstruction and hernia repair have been available to surgeons for repair of the groin and abdominal wall since the mid-twentieth century. Indeed, use of these materials by either an open or laparoscopic technique is the standard method of repairing incisional or groin hernia in most centers in North America and Europe. The first prosthetic materials used for hernia repair were synthetic meshes made of polypropylene or polyester.[1,2] They were introduced in an attempt to decrease the high risk of recurrent hernia observed in patients undergoing direct suture repair. Eventually, prospective randomized trials were conducted that demonstrated repair of even small incisional hernias without the use of mesh (primary closure repair) was associated with a significantly higher risk of recurrence (Figure 20-1), and nonmesh repair of all but the smallest abdominal wall defects was abandoned.[3-5]

Initially, mesh repair of abdominal wall defects was accomplished by sewing the edges of the defect to the prosthetic material, which served to "bridge" the defect, much as a cloth patch repairs a defect in a garment (Figure 20-2). Although this was an improvement compared with primary closure, recurrence rates remained high. In the 1980s, surgeons in Europe and then in the United States began to place the mesh in a "sublay" position, allowing a generous underlay of mesh beyond the fascial defect, usually posterior to the rectus abdominus muscle of the abdominal wall (Figure 20-3). This placement utilized the physical forces of the abdominal wall and peritoneal cavity to hold the prosthetic in place, resulting in an effective repair, and dramatically lower rates of recurrence. An additional advantage of this technique, the "Stoppa" repair (named for Rene Stoppa, a French surgeon), was that the mesh was placed in an extraperitoneal position, essentially replacing the transversalis fascia in the pelvis or abdomen.[6] In this setting bowel loops were not in contact with the mesh, and the risk of fistula and/or bowel adhesion and subsequent obstruction was minimized. In addition, the "Stoppa" or "Stoppa repair," or giant prosthetic repair of visceral sac (GPRVS), was popularized in the United States by Wantz[7] and could be applied to reconstruction of large groin hernias, particularly when bilateral or recurrent. This was accomplished by placing mesh in the extraperitoneal pelvis posterior to the pubis, anterior to the bladder, and extending into the iliac fossa bilaterally. Again, the extraperitoneal location of the mesh allowed a large sheet to be placed and minimized the potential for complications related to bowel adhesion to the mesh.[8]

The problem of bowel adhesion to synthetic mesh was further addressed with the development of "composite" synthetic meshes. These meshes were designed for placement within the peritoneal cavity with the parietal surface designed to minimize bowel adhesion. This development expanded the complexity of hernias that could be successfully repaired and facilitated hernia repair using minimal access techniques, which are almost exclusively intraperitoneal.

More recently, bioprosthetic implants have been created that are even less likely to cause adhesions or fistulas when placed in the peritoneal cavity. In addition, these materials can often be used to repair hernias or reconstruct the abdominal wall when bowel resections or contaminated procedures preclude the use of a synthetic mesh because the risk of infection is too high. They are expensive and associated with a higher risk of recurrent hernia, but if their use spares the patient a subsequent reconstructive operation, they are worth consideration at the time of oncologic resection.

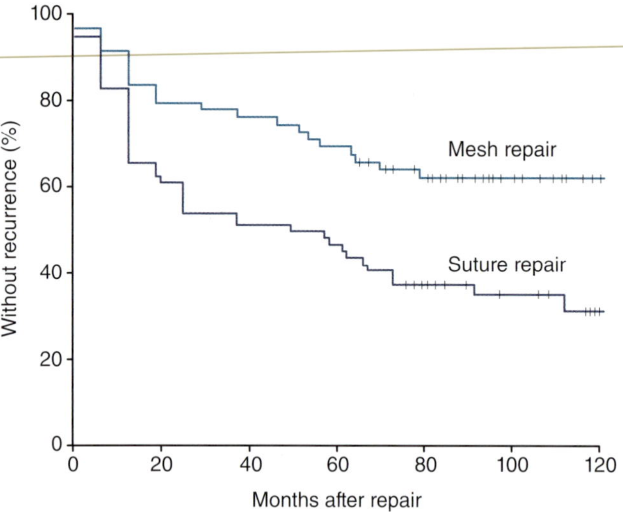

Fig. 20-1. Prospective randomized trial of 181 patients with primary or initial recurrent midline incisional hernia were randomized to undergo repair with mesh or by primary suture without mesh. The 10-year cumulative rate of recurrence was 63% for suture repair and 32% for mesh repair ($P < .001$). (Reprinted with permission from: Burger JW, Luijendijk RW, Hop WC, Halm JA, Verdaasdonk EG, Jeekel J. Long-term follow-up of a randomized controlled trial of suture versus mesh repair of incisional hernia. *Ann Surg.* 2004;240:578-83.)

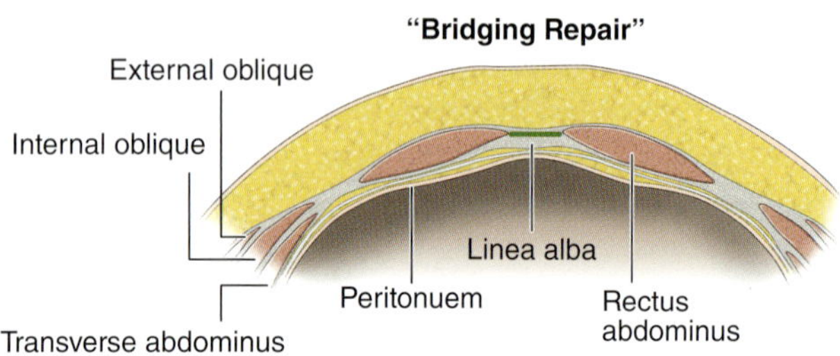

Fig. 20-2. Cross-section of the abdominal wall demonstrating a "bridging repair" with mesh (green) reapproximating the edges of the external oblique aponeurosis. The mesh is sewn to the edges of the hernia defect. This was a standard approach used in the mid-twentieth century but was associated with an unacceptably high rate of eventual failure.

The oncologic surgeon must have a fundamental understanding of reconstructive materials available for patients with abdominal wall defects. The decision to proceed with repair of these defects or to hold off has important implications for quality of life and cancer treatment, and these competing concerns require a knowledgeable and experienced surgeon or surgical team. Selection of the appropriate mesh or biologic implant for use is important to facilitate post-treatment recovery. A reasonable understanding of the advantages, disadvantages, and appropriate use of synthetic mesh and biologic implants will facilitate optimal care of these often complex surgical patients.

INDICATIONS AND CLINICAL APPLICATIONS

Abdominal wall reconstruction should be undertaken in most patients with structural defects undergoing radical cancer surgery. Clearly, if a patient is at high risk for infection secondary to gross contamination, excessive blood loss, morbid obesity, or some combination of high-risk clinical features, then delaying reconstruction may be more prudent. In most patients undergoing elective surgery; however, reconstruction of the abdominal wall or inguinal defect at the time of resection is preferable. Definitive repair of an incisional or groin hernia will add 1 to 3 hours to the operative procedure, depending on patient factors and prior surgical history. Done well, it can provide the patient with a significantly improved postoperative recovery and quality of life and avoid future operative procedures.

Preoperative Incisional Hernia

The most common clinical scenario faced by the gynecologic cancer surgeon is the patient who requires operation and has a preexisting incisional hernia. Consideration of repair after cancer resection should be made as part of preoperative planning. In most settings, repair can be safely undertaken, although the technique used and the type of prosthetic material placed requires considerable judgment. Although it is tempting to close a midline incision if it is feasible without the use of mesh, in a patient with an incisional hernia, recurrent hernia will almost always ensue.[3,4]

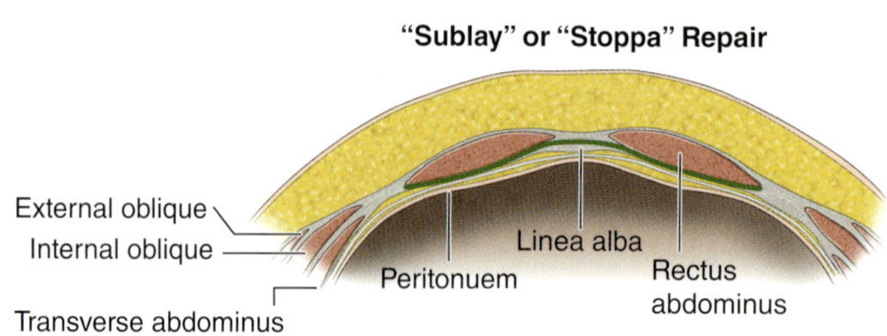

Fig. 20-3. Cross-section of the abdominal wall demonstrating a "sublay " or "Stoppa" incisional hernia repair with mesh (green) placed in the retrorectus position within the anterior abdominal wall. The mesh lies posterior to the rectus muscle and anterior to the posterior sheath and/or transversalis fascia, and is, thus, extraperitoneal.

Table 20-1. Examples of synthetic mesh available for hernia repair and abdominal wall reconstruction.

Material	Trade Name	Shrinkage	Strength	Features
Standard polypropylene	Marlex C.R. (Bard, Inc, Murray Hill, New Jersey)	Marked	Strong	Marked abdominal wall "stiffness" with healing
Intermediate weight Polypropylene	Prolite (Atrium Medical Corporation, Hudson, New Hampshire)	Mild	Strong	Less shrinkage Less "stiffness"
Lightweight polypropylene	Prolene Soft Mesh (Ethicon, Johnson & Johnson, New Brunswick, New Jersey)	Minimal	Less strength	Minimal shrinkage Minimal "stiffness"
Polyester fiber	Mersilene (Ethicon, Johnson & Johnson, New Brunswick, New Jersey)	Moderate	Strong	Conforms well Abdominal wall "stiffness"
Polyglactin	Vicryl (Ethicon, Johnson & Johnson, New Brunswick, New Jersey)	Temporary	Temporary	Useful as temporizing buttress/support

All of these, except for Vicryl mesh, are used as permanent synthetic extraperitoneal repair implants.

1. Choice of prosthetic and surgical placement

Synthetic Prosthesis. Patients undergoing incisional hernia repair without large bowel resection, or with a limited small bowel resection, urinary tract procedure, or both can often be repaired with a synthetic prosthesis. Several examples of synthetic meshes for use in an extraperitoneal location are listed in Table 20-1. In addition, Vicryl (Ethicon, Johnson & Johnson, New Brunswick, New Jersey) mesh is listed, a slowly absorbable mesh composed of a polymer of glycolic and lactic acids, which can be used intraperitoneally as a temporary mesh to reconstruct the peritoneal sac or serve as a temporary repair when the use of a permanent mesh is too hazardous. Permanent synthetic meshes are used when the risk of mesh infection is low. The advantage of synthetic mesh is that it is associated with a significantly lower risk of hernia recurrence than a biologic implant. In addition, the cost of synthetic mesh is very low compared to a biologic implant. Synthetic extraperitoneal mesh is easy to work with and requires relatively few sutures to be placed in order to hold it in place. This is particularly true in pelvic reconstruction, where placement of a large sheet of synthetic mesh in the retropubic, extraperitoneal position with extension into the iliac fossa bilaterally (the Stoppa repair[9]) requires little fixation because the peritoneal sac holds the mesh in place with the patient in the upright position (Figure 20-4).

If used in the extraperitoneal position (ie, within the abdominal wall), then a lightweight polypropylene single layer mesh is ideal. These wide-weave meshes are less prone to shrinkage and may cause less sensation of abdominal wall stiffness compared to the traditional heavyweight standard weave polypropylene mesh. In patients with recurrent hernia, obesity, or other risk factors for recurrence, an intermediate weight polypropylene mesh is a reasonable choice and may provide more strength. Polypropylene or polyester mesh is always placed in an extraperitoneal location, so that the peritoneal sac must be closed in order to exclude bowel loops from the mesh and prevent bowel obstruction or fistula. Vicryl mesh (see Table 20-1) is a temporizing, absorbable mesh that can be used to reapproximate the peritoneum to exclude it from a permanent synthetic mesh. This is particularly true when the risk of adhesions is low, namely when the omentum is preserved, and when there has been no extensive adhesiolysis and the bowel has not been previously radiated.

Composite Mesh. When the repair is undertaken with a mesh within the peritoneal cavity, a composite mesh may be used (Table 20-2). The composite mesh is used in an intraperitoneal "underlay" position (Figure 20-5). Any intraperitoneal mesh must be secured to the undersurface of the abdominal wall with sutures placed circumferentially every 1.5 to 2 cm, to prevent interposition of bowel loops between the mesh or implant and the abdominal wall. If a composite synthetic mesh is used, then the parietal surface is composed of material designed to minimize bowel adhesion, while the side facing the abdominal wall promotes adhesion and adherence to secure the mesh and discourage mechanical displacement. There are many composite meshes available for use in hernia repair. Because they are more expensive than noncomposite synthetic mesh and must be secured with more suture fixation, they are almost always restricted to use in an intraperitoneal underlay repair. A few examples among many available products are listed in Table 20-2.

Biologic Implant. The third category of prosthetic that may be used for hernia repair and abdominal wall

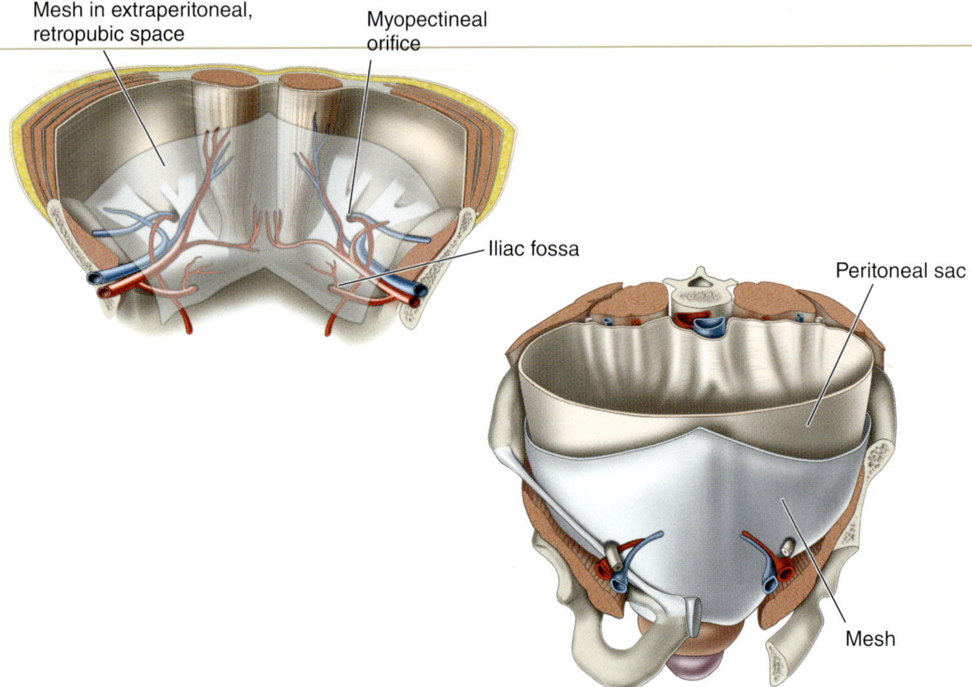

Fig. 20-4. Preperitoneal repair of bilateral inguinal hernia using Stoppa technique (giant prosthetic repair of visceral sac). The synthetic mesh is placed between the myopectineal orifice and the peritoneal sac, and envelops the sac, which holds it in place with the patient in the upright position. Extension of the mesh into the retropubic space and into the iliac fossa bilaterally is also a crucial component of repair of a lower abdominal incisional hernia. (Adapted and reproduced with permission from Wantz GE. *Atlas of Hernia Surgery*. New York, NY: Raven Press, 1991.)

reconstruction is a biologic implant. These can also be used when patients are at very high risk for bowel adhesion to intraperitoneal composite mesh because of extensive adhesiolysis, prior radiation therapy, fistula, or omentectomy. Similar to composite mesh, biologic implants are designed for use within the peritoneal cavity. Biologic implants are composed of xenografts or allografts of acellular collagen and elastin that serve as a scaffold and allow for tissue ingrowth. Biologic implants come in different sizes, thicknesses, and have very different handling characteristics, and several examples are

Table 20-2. Selected examples of composite mesh commercially available for hernia repair and abdominal wall reconstruction.

Mesh	Adhesive Surface	Parietal Surface	Features
C-Qur (Atrium Medical Corporation, Hudson, New Hampshire)	Polypropylene impregnated with omega-3 fatty acids	Omega-3 fatty acid cross-linked absorbable gel	May be cut, easy to use Fatty acids decrease inflammatory response
Parietex (Covidien Corporation, Mansfield, Massachusetts)	Polyester	Hydrophilic film	Cannot be cut Film comes off with handling
Proceed (Ethicon, Johnson & Johnson, New Brunswick, New Jersey)	Lightweight polypropylene	Oxidized regenerated cellulose	Cannot be cut Cellulose comes off with handling
Ultrapro (Ethicon, Johnson & Johnson, New Brunswick, New Jersey)	Lightweight polypropylene	Poliglicaprone-25 (Monocryl™)	Partially absorbable lightweight mesh Useful for parastomal reinforcement

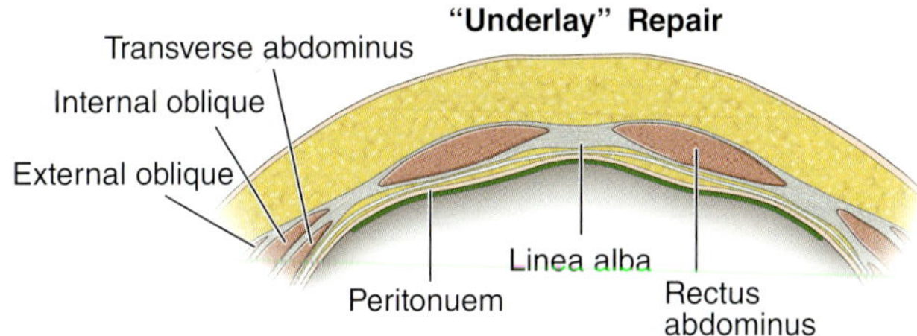

Fig. 20-5. Cross section of the abdominal wall demonstrating an "underlay" incisional hernia repair with intraperitoneal composite mesh or biologic implant (green) placed within the peritoneal cavity.

listed in Table 20-3. Because they promote capillary ingrowth and appear to be more resistant to infection, xenografts and allografts can be used in cases where a synthetic mesh may be considered too risky because of the potential for infection. Perhaps the greatest advantage of the prosthetics is that, if they do become infected, they often break down and are less likely to require explant, at least theoretically. Biologic implants take much longer to adhere to the patient's abdominal wall, so that they rely on the mechanical strength of the suture and the positioning of the mesh to hold the implant in place. In addition, they must be used with great caution in patients who will require postoperative radiation therapy, as their safety in this setting is unknown.

Another use for biologic implants is to reconstruct the peritoneal sac so that the bowel loops can be excluded from a synthetic mesh repair. A thin piece of allograft or xenograft can be very useful in this setting.

Biologic implants may be used in many similar circumstances as composite synthetic meshes. Although recurrence rates may be higher, risks of infection and adhesion are lower; therefore, careful patient selection is critical to optimal outcomes.

Patients With Groin Hernia Undergoing Cancer Resection

Many patients with primary or recurrent groin hernia should undergo repair at the time of pelvic surgery, although these defects can be more commonly ignored when appropriate and usually do not interfere with closure of the abdominal wall. In a patient at relatively low risk for infection, placement of a large sheet of synthetic single layer mesh in the extraperitoneal retropubic space after reduction of a groin hernia is a safe and effective method of inguinal hernia repair using the preperitoneal approach (see Figure 20-4). Patients who should be strongly considered for repair at the time of cancer surgery include those who are symptomatic preoperatively, and those with femoral hernias, which are associated with a higher risk of incarceration than direct or indirect inguinal hernias. In addition, patients with recurrent groin hernia, or bilateral groin hernia, are ideal candidates for a pelvic preperitoneal repair at the time of cancer resection. This will decrease the potential risk of incarceration postoperatively and preclude the necessity of a subsequent operation.

After radical gynecologic cancer resection, a preperitoneal mesh repair may no longer be technically feasible. The peritoneal sac may not be able to be closed, and thus the bowel loops will lie against the mesh. In this setting, a composite mesh may be placed over the myopectineal orifice with the parietal side facing the peritoneal cavity and the abdominal wall side opposed to the anterior abdominal wall/retropubic space/myopectineal orifice. The mesh is secured to the fascia behind the pubic bone and extends across the defect laterally (see Figure 20-4).

Patients With Extensive Adhesions and Prior Pelvic Radiation or Bowel Resection

Many patients undergoing pelvic cancer surgery will have large bowel resection, or undergo extensive adhesiolysis, and many may have had prior pelvic radiation. In this setting, an

Table 20-3. Biologic implants available for hernia repair and abdominal wall reconstruction.

Implant	Source	Process	Thickness	Cost	Features
AlloDerm (Lifecell Corporation, Bridgewater, New Jersey)	Cadaveric dermis	Proprietary	0.23–3.3 mm	High	Easy to use, supple
Surgimend (TEI Biosciences, Boston, Massachusetts)	Acellular porcine dermal collagen	Non x-linked	1–4 mm	Moderate	Easy to stitch, soft and pliable
Permacol (Covidien Corporation, Mansfield, Massachusetts)	Acellular porcine dermal collagen	Chemical x-linked	0.5–1.5 mm	Moderate	Stiffer, more difficult to suture, strong

intraperitoneal pelvic mesh should be avoided, and a simultaneous anterior repair or subsequent anterior repair of an inguinal hernia(s) may be a safer approach.

Patients Undergoing Permanent Stoma Placement

Strong consideration should be given to mesh placement as a prophylactic measure in patients undergoing creation of a permanent abdominal wall stoma. Parastomal hernia is a debilitating and common complication of stoma creation. Prospective randomized trials have demonstrated that preemptive mesh placement can prevent parastomal hernia and is associated with no higher risk of infection in patients undergoing elective surgery.[10,11] Synthetic mesh is used and is placed in the extraperitoneal retrorectus position following stoma creation. Partially absorbable synthetic mesh, such as composite Vicryl/polypropylene (Ultrapro [Ethicon, Johnson & Johnson, New Brunswick, New Jersey]) in the retrorectus sublay, can be used for this purpose (see Table 20-2).

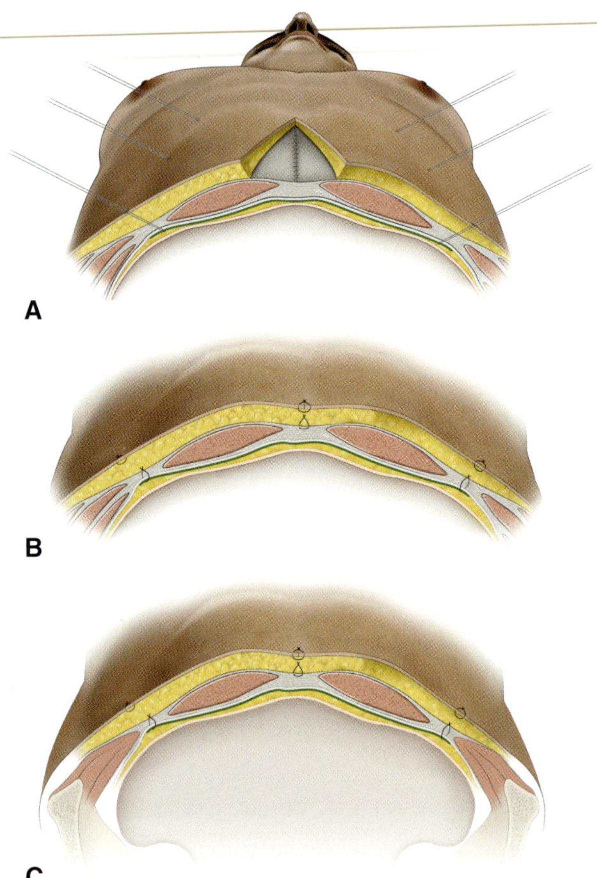

Fig. 20-6. Incisional hernia repair using Stoppa technique. Upper abdominal incisional hernias can be repaired with mesh extending above the coastal margins. Transfascial sutures secure the mesh circumferentially (**A, B**). Lower incisional hernias extend into the pelvis and the visceral sac holds the lower aspect of the mesh in place with the patient in the upright position; only a retropubic suture secures the lower aspect of the mesh (**C**). (Adapted with permission from: Wantz GE. *Atlas of Hernia Surgery.* New York, NY: Raven Press; 1991.)

ANATOMIC CONSIDERATIONS

Synthetic Mesh Repair of Abdominal Wall Hernia

Patients are suitable candidates for repair of incisional or groin hernia if they are undergoing elective surgery and there is no gross contamination, and if the procedure has gone well (ie, without excessive blood loss or hemodynamic instability). Essential components of repair include (1) a suitable sublay mesh to accomplish the repair, (2) closure of the peritoneal sac to exclude the bowel from the mesh, and (3) reconstruction of the external oblique with a bridging mesh or primary fascial closure over the sublay repair.

1. Synthetic repair of the mid/upper abdominal incisional hernia (Figure 20-6A and B)

Stoppa Repair. The ideal location for mesh placement to repair a primary or recurrent incisional hernia is the retrorectus position. This requires dissection of the retromuscular plane bilaterally followed by placement of a sublay prosthetic mesh fixed with transfascial sutures to the abdominal wall (Figure 20-7). The epigastric artery and vein traverse this space and care must be undertaken to ligate branches of the vessels when necessary throughout the dissection. Sometimes dissection of this plane results in bleeding from the main trunk of the vascular pedicle, and ligation can be accomplished without sequelae. This plane is identified by entering the rectus sheath at the midline, then retracting the rectus muscle anteriorly. The posterior rectus sheath above the arcuate line and the transverses abdominus fascia below the arcuate line provide a layer on which the mesh rests excluding the mesh from the peritoneal cavity. A synthetic intermediate weight mesh is placed and secured with transfascial sutures. The mesh should extend to the lateral border of the rectus sheath bilaterally, and at least 6 to 8 cm beyond the hernia defect superiorly and inferiorly. A defect can be cut in the midline at the cephalad and caudad ends of the mesh to allow it to extend above and below the hernia in the midline.

2. Synthetic repair of lower midline incisional hernia

Most incisional hernias occur in the periumbilical area, and for patients with prior gynecologic procedures these often extend into the lower abdominal midline. Repair of incisional hernias that occur in the lower abdomen and involve the area just above the pubis can be particularly problematic in the reoperative setting. Adhesions from prior surgery make retropubic dissection treacherous and a sufficient underlay of mesh behind the pubis extending into the iliac fossa bilaterally—the ideal approach to these defects—are

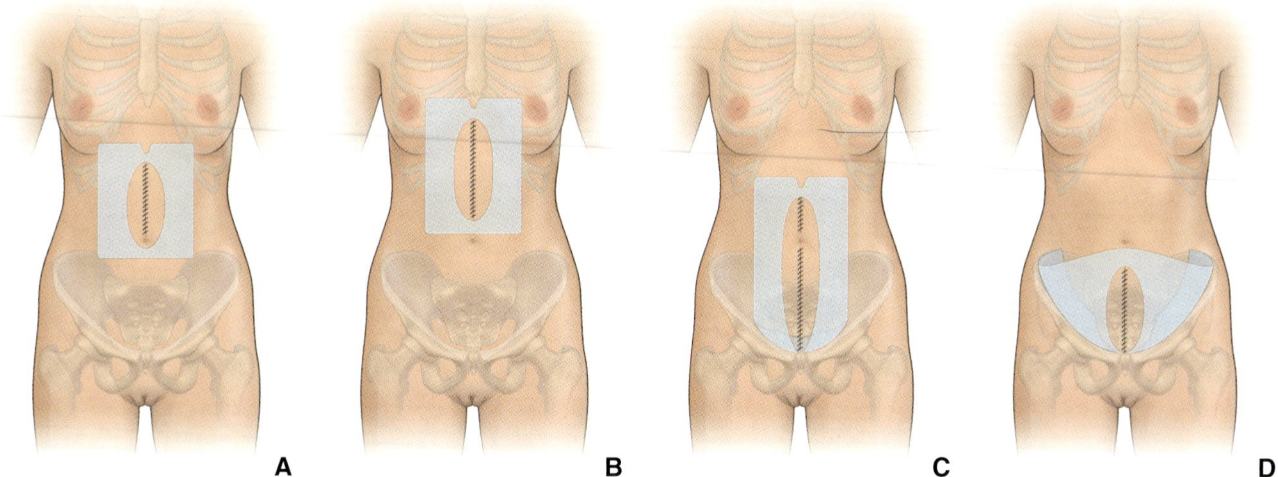

Fig. 20-7. Schematic demonstrating placement of transfascial sutures lateral to the rectus muscle securing the mesh in place (Stoppa repair). (**A**) Upper abdominal hernia repair: slit in mesh on either side of linea alba. (**B**) High upper abdominal hernia repair: mesh extends over lower rib cage. (**C**) Lower abdominal hernia repair: inferior mesh deep into retropubic space. (**D**) Infraumbilical incisional hernia repair: similar to Stoppa repair (GPRVS). (Adapted with permission from: Wantz GE. *Atlas of Hernia Surgery.* New York, NY: Raven Press; 1991.)

required so that recurrence at the lower aspect of the repair does not occur (Figures 20-6C and D). These defects can be challenging in patients who have extensive pelvic adhesions or prior pelvic radiation, and use of a preformed "ventral patch" (C-Qur [Atrium Medical Corporation, Hudson, New Hampshire] or Proceed [Ethicon, Johnson & Johnson, New Brunswick, New Jersey] are 2 examples) at the retropubic portion of the incision after optimal dissection and mesh placement can be very helpful.

Bioprosthetic Repair of Incisional Hernia

In select patients, use of a bioprosthetic implant may be preferable to a synthetic mesh. The advantages are that it can be used in less than optimal operative conditions with less risk of infection, and it can be placed in the peritoneal cavity with less concern about adhesion to bowel or other viscera. The disadvantages are that because it integrates slowly, sutures are more important to fix the mesh and prevent bowel loop interposition; therefore, more sutures need be placed. In addition, recurrence rates are higher. Another disadvantage of a bioimplant is that seroma formation around the mesh is very common and can be quite dramatic, necessitating prolonged postoperative surgical drainage. Nonetheless, for the patient in whom a retrorectus dissection is not feasible or a synthetic mesh is not safe, use of a biologic implant for incisional hernia repair can prevent the patient from having to undergo a subsequent hernia repair at another time.

Careful consideration should be given to patients who require postoperative radiation therapy. There are no data regarding the safety of an intraperitoneal bioprosthesis in this setting, and it may be more prudent to defer hernia repair, abdominal wall reconstruction, or both in patients who will require pelvic irradiation. Whether radiation therapy diminishes capillary ingrowth or changes the characteristics of the implant and therefore promotes adhesion of bowel to the graft is unknown.

Synthetic Repair of Groin Hernia, Unilateral or Bilateral

1. Stoppa repair (GPRVS)

Pelvic cancer surgery often involves exposure of the myopectineal orifice as the peritoneal sac is dissected away from the pelvic organs. This exposure provides an ideal opportunity to undertake a groin hernia repair with mesh in the appropriate setting. The repair requires reduction of the hernia sac from the inguinal canal, a step that must be completed for successful mesh placement between the myopectineal orifice and peritoneal sac. This will prevent migration of the sac back into the inguinal defect. The round ligament is usually divided and the hernia sac is dissected free from the myopectineal orifice. The mesh is then interposed between the peritoneal (visceral) sac and the myopectineal orifice/pubis. The mesh essentially envelops the peritoneal sac, and extends with it into the iliac fossa (see Figure 20-4).

A bilateral hernia is repaired by reducing both sides and then fashioning a mesh to extend across the retropubic space/myopectineal orifice and into the iliac fossa bilaterally. As described by Wantz,[14] it measures almost as wide as the iliac crests and envelops the sac, extending anteriorly along the lower midline. Because the peritoneal sac essentially holds the mesh in place, only 1 retropubic suture is generally used for fixation. The mesh envelops the sac along the colic gutters as well (see Figure 20-4). Because the peritoneal sac is closed, excluding the bowel loops from the mesh, a synthetic mesh such as polypropylene or polyester can be used for the repair (see Table 20-1).

Parastomal Hernia

Most patients with a parastomal should undergo repair, as these defects enlarge with time and can cause dysfunction of the fecal or urinary conduit. Prior to repair, the hernia contents are reduced from the soft tissue of the abdominal wall, taking care not to devascularize the stoma by disrupting the mesentery supplying the conduit. Once the hernia is reduced, the fascial edges are defined. The defect is then reapproximated with interrupted, 0-Polydiaxanone (PDS) suture. There are several techniques described for repair of parastomal hernia, but these are best undertaken by surgeons with experience and special expertise because recurrence rates are high. Prevention is essential, and patients undergoing permanent stoma creation should be considered for stoma reinforcement with partially absorbable synthetic sublay mesh at the time of stoma creation. Prospective randomized trials have demonstrated that it is a safe and effective method to reduce parastomal hernia occurrence.[10,11] Alternatively, intraperitoneal placement of a mesh around the stoma loop can be accomplished, with careful fixation of the mesh to the undersurface of the abdominal wall. A composite mesh or biologic implant may be chosen and used as an underlay in this setting (see Tables 20-2 and 20-3).

PREOPERATIVE PREPARATION

Box 20-1 KEY SURGICAL INSTRUMENTATION FOR EXTRAPERITONEAL REPAIR

- Synthetic, noncomposite mesh, both intermediate (for underlay) and lightweight (bridging) for external oblique closure
- Endo Close device for transfascial suture placement
- 0-Vicryl sutures for transfascial suture and retropubic fixation
- Headlights
- Wide and narrow Deaver retractors
- Wide and narrow malleable retractors

Most of the preoperative planning in patients undergoing cancer surgery involves planning the primary procedure. The surgeon planning abdominal wall reconstruction, hernia repair, or both will need to wait until the cancer operation has been completed prior to determining precisely how to reconstruct or repair the abdominal wall. Preoperative discussions with the patient and family should involve these uncertainties, and specific approaches or specific discussion about the prosthetic material to be used should be limited as these decisions can only be made once the cancer operation has been accomplished. In addition, if the cancer surgery has been particularly difficult or associated with significant blood loss or bowel contamination, then proceeding with hernia repair or reconstruction with a prosthetic may best be deferred.

Patients who smoke present an extraordinary risk for complications following incisional hernia repair with mesh. They have a very high risk of recurrence following repair,[12] and a high risk of wound complications, including infection, dehiscence, necrosis, and chronic mesh infection requiring explant. In patients who will require postoperative adjuvant chemotherapy, it may be more appropriate to forgo repair of an incisional hernia with a prosthetic mesh in a person who smokes, because of the risk that wound complications would prevent the patient from timely treatment with chemotherapy.

The surgeon should ensure that a reasonable variety of mesh is available to accomplish repair. There should be access to synthetic mesh, both polypropylene alone (intermediate and lightweight) and composite mesh suitable for intraperitoneal use. Intermediate and lightweight synthetic mesh shrink less than standard heavyweight polypropylene, and both are suitable for the extraperitoneal underlay repair and/or the bridging mesh sometimes required to reapproximate external oblique over an underlay or sublay repair. In addition, the surgeon should have access to allograft or xenograft for use in case intraoperative events necessitate use of these materials. Hernia repair and abdominal wall reconstruction represent an unpredictable science, and while much preoperative planning can facilitate repair, unexpected circumstances require the availability of a variety of synthetic meshes, composite meshes, and biologic implants in order to perform efficient, safe, and successful abdominal wall reconstruction. Mechanical bowel prep is important prior to hernia repair. This will avoid unnecessary strain on the abdominal wall postoperatively.

SURGICAL PROCEDURES

Box 20-2 MASTER SURGEON'S PRINCIPLES

- Repair incisional hernias using a sublay, ideally a synthetic, extraperitoneal mesh
- If a biologic implant is used, then more suture fixation is required and an intraperitoneal underlay is performed
- Reconstruct the peritoneal cavity, when possible, with an absorbable mesh (Vicryl) in low-risk patients with omentum, or a bioprosthesis in patients at higher risk for adhesions/fistula
- Always reconstruct the external oblique over the sublay or underlay incisional hernia repair, either with primary closure (sometimes facilitated by component separation) or an additional bridging mesh

Stoppa Repair of Midline Hernia

At completion of the cancer resection, the hernia surgeon assesses the abdominal wall. In patients with an intact rectus muscle and posterior rectus sheath/transversalis fascia, the

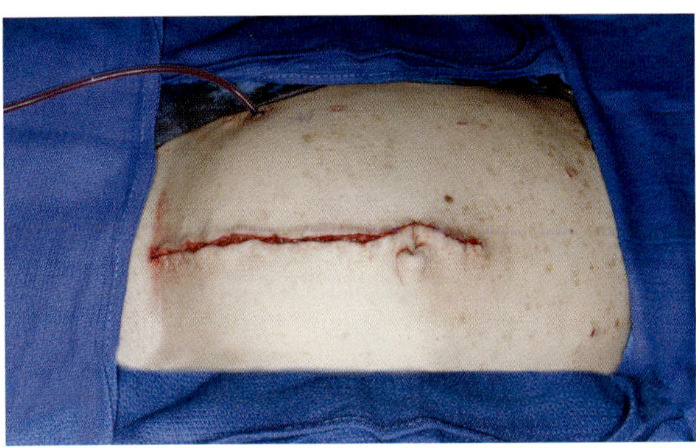

Fig. 20-8. The completed Stoppa repair of a midline hernia.

Stoppa repair should be considered the "gold standard" open repair (Figure 20-8). The hernia sac itself can be dissected from the soft tissue of the abdominal wall and used to facilitate closure of the peritoneal sac. If the sac cannot be closed, a small piece of Vicryl mesh may be used to reapproximate the peritoneum. In patients at high risk for adhesions (ie, those with prior enteric fistula, radiated bowel, or multiple adhesions without omentum), a thin piece of allograft may be used instead.

The surgeon enters the rectus sheath at the midline, identifies the rectus muscle, and dissects the plane posterior to the muscle and anterior to the posterior rectus sheath/transversalis fascia. This plane extends from the midline to the lateral border of the sheath, and for a sufficient distance cephalad and caudad from the fascial defect to allow the mesh to extend well above and below the edges of the hernia. Branches of the epigastric vessels must be clipped or ligated as encountered during this dissection, and the LigaSure device can be very useful, as is a headlight. For a large defect, the rectus sheath can be dissected from the costal margin to the iliac crest and down into the pelvis. Each side of the abdominal wall is dissected, and then a decision is made whether to perform a "component release" to medialize the rectus muscles and external oblique aponeurosis.[13] A synthetic mesh is shaped, and circumferential, interrupted 0-Vicryl sutures are placed (see Figure 20-6) to correspond with small circumferential incisions made in the abdominal wall, which approximate the edges of the mesh in situ.

When the defect is very large and the rectus muscle is so displaced that there is little lateral space present for the mesh, a "component release" procedure can be performed to extend the space available for the mesh and "medialize the rectus muscles." I prefers a "posterior" component release because it does not violate the anterior sheath and create a defect in the anterior fascia (ie, another hernia). This is performed by (1) dissecting all the way to the lateral border of the rectus sheath, (2) retracting the muscle cephalad, (3) entering the space between the internal and external oblique muscles with cautery or by sharp dissection, and (4) opening the length of the lateral border or the rectus sheath from the costal margin to the pelvic brim. This can be performed on one side or on both sides of the abdominal wall, as required.

Once the space for the mesh has been created, then the peritoneal sac is closed with a running suture. If it cannot be closed primarily, a bioprosthesis such as AlloDerm (Lifecell Corporation, Bridgewater, New Jersey; in patients at high risk for adhesion) or Vicryl (when there is omentum over the bowel loops) is used. The surgeon then determines where the transfascial sutures will be placed to secure the mesh. Because the mesh is synthetic, and extraperitoneal, only about 6 transfascial sutures are needed on each side to secure the mesh. The mesh is fashioned, remembering that the retro-rectus space is smaller than the same space as visualized on the anterior abdominal wall, and that the anterior fascia and rectus muscle will be pulled medially prior to completion of the repair. Once the mesh has been cut, the surgeon determines the optimal sites for placement of the transfascial fixation sutures and marks these on the abdominal wall. An eleven blade is used to incise the skin at these sites, creating small stab wounds for passage of the Endo Close device (Figure 20-9). 0-Vicryl sutures are then placed in the mesh at the points for fixation, and the needles removed. The rectus muscle is then retracted anteriorly, and the Endo Close is passed through the anterior stab wounds and used to grab and pull the suture up through the abdominal wall (Figure 20-10). It is passed a second time to grasp the other end of the suture so that separate transfascial passes are performed. These sutures are circumferentially secured, and in this way the mesh is fixed in place. For patients with defects involving the lower abdominal wall in the midline, the mesh is placed down into the retropubic space and extends into the iliac fossa bilaterally. A Vicryl suture in the retropubic fascia to secure the mesh at this point is generally all that is required inferiorly.

Drains are placed bilaterally, and maintained for at least 5 days. They are removed once the volume is 40 cc or less for 24 hours. Seroma accumulation around the mesh can disrupt the repair by displacing the mesh and must be avoided.

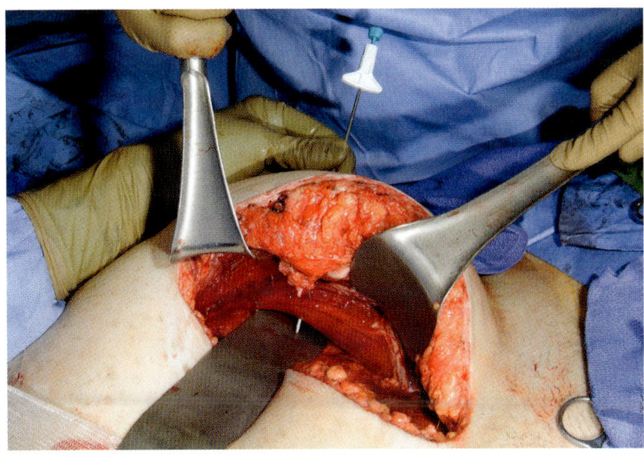

Fig. 20-9. Use of an 11-blade to incise the skin, creating small stab wounds for passage of the Endo Close device.

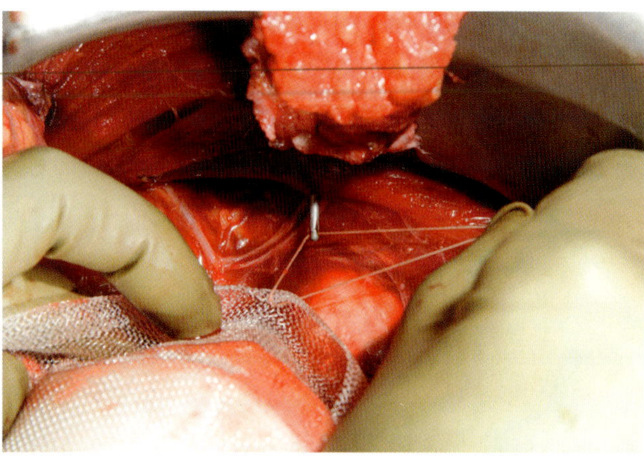

Fig. 20-10. The Endo Close device is passed through the anterior abdominal wall to grab the suture.

Groin Hernia Repair

When the cancer procedure is complete, the surgeon can proceed with groin hernia repair. Once the peritoneal sac is reduced from the myopectineal orifice and retracted cephalad, a large piece of polypropylene mesh is fashioned into the shape of a chevron, with the two extensions of the V placed into the iliac fossa bilaterally. The apex of the V should be secured with an absorbable stitch to the retropubic fascia, and the mesh should extend above the sac for 10 to 18 cm and extend around the sac bilaterally, essentially enveloping it (see Figure 20-4).

Either intermediate or lightweight polypropylene mesh can be used for repair of groin hernia using this approach. If bowel loops cannot be excluded from the mesh, then composite mesh (in patients at low risk for adhesions/infection) or a biologic implant (in patients at higher risk for adhesions or infection) can be used. Use of a biologic intraperitoneal prosthesis requires more fixation because the sutures hold the mesh in place until the mesh integrates into the surrounding tissue.

POSTOPERATIVE CARE

Box 20-3 PERIOPERATIVE MORBIDITY

- Bleeding
- Wound infection
- Mesh infection

A surgical binder can be useful postoperatively by providing the patient with some degree of abdominal wall support. Excessive pulmonary toilet should be avoided (ie, excessive coughing), and ambulation encouraged. Drains should be monitored carefully, and not discontinued until significant drainage ceases.

Surgical drains are essential in patients undergoing placement of synthetic mesh or a biologic implant. Drains should be left in place until the volume diminishes to less than 40 cc for 24 hours, and should be maintained for the first 3 days postoperatively even if the volume is low. Drainage will increase as the patient becomes more active. Postoperative seromas complicate mesh or bioprosthesis integration, and when unattended, they can disrupt the repair and increase the risk of a mesh infection.

Ambulation is essential for recovery, and patients who undergo incisional hernia repair should be encouraged to increase their distance daily, especially after hospital discharge. This will facilitate return of normal bowel function, aid in pain control, and promote optimal wound healing.

Most of the perioperative morbidity experienced by patients undergoing hernia repair or abdominal wall reconstruction can be attributed to the cancer operation. Abdominal wall bleeding following retrorectus mesh placement can occur, and this is manifested by fullness and bruising of the soft tissues of the abdominal wall. It is uncommon to return to the operating room for control. The epigastric vessels course along the posterior/lateral border of the rectus muscle, particularly in the lower abdominal wall. Care must be taken to avoid or ligate these as encountered, especially during drain placement and mesh fixation.

Many patients with abdominal wall hernias are obese, and wound infection can be both a cause and a result of incisional hernia. The triad of obesity/infection/hernia is well known to experienced surgeons. We have found that a negative pressure dressing on a closed wound (Prevena, KCI, San Antonio, Texas) may decrease the risk of wound infection in these high-risk patients. Our initial experience has been promising. This wound covering is left on for 5 to 6 days and can be used on a wound closed with staples or suture. Surgical glue is not applied to the wound if use of this wound covering is planned.

There is considerable confusion in the literature regarding the issue of mesh infection. Polypropylene mesh is a useful synthetic, and can usually be salvaged in the setting of a deep wound infection, with careful attention to drainage of all collections and timely and appropriate use of antibiotics. It is distinctly unusual, in my experience, to have to remove a polypropylene mesh in a patient with a deep wound infection. In patients with exposed bridging mesh (external oblique reconstruction), debridement of the superficial mesh may be required, but the underlay or sublay mesh is usually salvageable. In a patient who continues to have a nonhealing wound, fever, or wound drainage, complete or subtotal mesh removal may be required. Prolonged courses of antibiotic therapy should be avoided, as these inevitably lead to the development of resistant organisms and delay the eventual therapy required, which is foreign body (ie, mesh) removal.

One of the most important advantages to a biologic implant is that it is less susceptible to infection. In addition, if infection occurs, the biologic implant will often disintegrate without having to be surgically removed. If removal is necessary, the nonadherent parts of the biologic implant can be removed, and if the other portions are integrated and vascularized, these can be left in place. However, infection may occur with any mesh or implant, and considerable judgment is required to recognize an underlying mesh infection that will require explant from one that can be addressed with antibiotic therapy and drainage of associated collections.

LONG-TERM OUTCOMES

Box 20-4 DELAYED COMPLICATIONS

- Recurrence
- Delayed mesh infection
- Bowel obstruction or fistula

The retrorectus synthetic mesh repair of incisional hernia is the "gold standard" repair of incisional hernia. Traditionally, a standard polypropylene mesh was used. Over time, it became clear that this mesh would shrink and stiffen, leading to abdominal wall discomfort in some patients. The use of this standard polypropylene mesh has largely been replaced by more "lightweight" meshes. These include the wider weave intermediate weight mesh and even wider weave "lightweight" mesh. Both options are suitable for repair of incisional or groin hernia; though in patients at very high risk for recurrence, this author prefers the intermediate weight mesh. However, it is important to remember that surgical technique is probably more important than tensile mesh strength. When placed carefully and secured without tension, a lightweight mesh with a wide weave is an excellent choice.

Recurrence following initial repair of an incisional hernia in a reasonable risk patient using the Stoppa technique is about 10% to 15%. Most recurrences will become apparent in the first 2 years, but some occur 5 or more years after repair. Often the area of recurrence is small, and the patient may elect not to undertake repair. If the recurrence is symptomatic and the patient requests repair, a smaller procedure with an intraperitoneal, preformed "patch" is often sufficient. It is not necessary or advisable to remove the previously placed retrorectus mesh. Preformed meshes that are useful for small defects include the C-Qur V-Patch or Proceed Ventral Patch. These come in several sizes depending on the size of the defect to be repaired.

Delayed mesh infection is becoming more common, for reasons that are somewhat unclear. When it occurs, it is highly likely that removal of the mesh will be required because it represents an infection of the mesh itself and not contamination of a portion of the mesh from a deep wound injection. Drainage of all localized collections and a trial of antibiotic therapy are the mainstays of initial care, but if this strategy fails, the mesh should be surgically removed. If the patient has had a prior polytetrafluoroethylene mesh placed and this has become infected, there is no need for antibiotics. The mesh must be removed, and the infection will never be eradicated without complete removal of the implant. I do not use mesh composed of polytetrafluoroethylene because of the risk of infection requiring explant.

As discussed, extraperitoneal placement of the repair mesh is ideal. This will make a bowel fistula related to the mesh nearly impossible. When extraperitoneal placement is not feasible, an intraperitoneal composite mesh is used. Despite the best efforts of surgeons and bioprosthetic engineers, a foreign body within the peritoneal cavity provides an opportunity for bowel adhesion. This is particularly true of patients without to act as a layer between the bowel and the mesh or implant, as well as patients at risk for bowel adhesion because of extensive lysis of adhesions, prior radiation, and/or bowel resection. In a patient at high risk for adhesions to an intraperitoneal mesh, a biologic implant should be used either as the repair mesh or to reconstruct the peritoneal cavity prior to synthetic sublay repair. This will minimize, but not eliminate, the risk of this difficult complication. If obstruction occurs, then fistula risk increases, as dilated loops of bowel press up against the intraperitoneal foreign body. A fistula may ensue and manifest as enteric drainage into the wound. Management with bowel rest and parental nutrition will usually result in resolution, and removal of the mesh may subsequently eventually be required.

MINIMALLY INVASIVE SURGICAL APPLICATIONS

Minimally invasive techniques can be employed for the repair of incisional hernia. The disadvantage of these techniques is that the mesh is always intraperitoneal, an issue whose implications we have discussed. However, careful selection of patients will identify those in whom this approach is appropriate.

SUMMARY

Reconstruction of the groin, abdominal wall, or both following cancer surgery is an essential component of the care of the patient with a gynecologic malignancy. Abdominal wall defects create significant problems for patients recovering from surgery and negatively impact on their quality of life. Cancer surgeons should understand how to repair these defects and be familiar with the array of synthetic and biologic prosthetics available to accomplish repair or reconstruction of the abdominal wall. This will ensure that their patients will enjoy optimal oncologic and functional outcomes.

REFERENCES

1. Usher FC, Fries JG, Ochsner JL, Tuttle LL, Jr. Marlex mesh, a new plastic mesh for replacing tissue defects. II. Clinical studies. *AMA Arch Surg*. 1959;78:138-145.
2. Usher FC, Gannon JP. Marlex mesh, a new plastic mesh for replacing tissue defects. I. Experimental studies. *AMA Arch Surg*. 1959;78:131-137.

3. Burger JW, Luijendijk RW, Hop WC, Halm JA, Verdaasdonk EG, Jeekel J. Long-term follow-up of a randomized controlled trial of suture versus mesh repair of incisional hernia. *Ann Surg*. 2004;240:578-585.
4. Arroyo A, Garcia P, Perez F, Andreu J, Candela F, Calpena R. Randomized clinical trial comparing suture and mesh repair of umbilical hernia in adults. *Br J Surg*. 2001;88:1321-1323.
5. Luijendijk RW, Hop WC, van den Tol MP, et al. A comparison of suture repair with mesh repair for incisional hernia. *N Engl J Med*. 2000;343:392-398.
6. Stoppa RE, Rives JL, Warlaumont CR, Palot JP, Verhaeghe PJ, Delattre JF. The use of Dacron in the repair of hernias of the groin. *Surg Clin North Am*. 1984;64:269-285.
7. Wantz GE. Giant prosthetic reinforcement of the visceral sac. The Stoppa groin hernia repair. *Surg Clin North Am*. 1998;78:1075-1087.
8. Stoppa RE. The treatment of complicated groin and incisional hernias. *World J Surg*. 1989;13:545-554.
9. Yaghoobi Notash A, Yaghoobi Notash A, Jr., Seied Farshi J, Ahmadi Amoli H, Salimi J, Mamarabadi M. Outcomes of the Rives-Stoppa technique in incisional hernia repair: ten years of experience. *Hernia*. 2007;11:25-29.
10. Janes A, Cengiz Y, Israelsson LA. Randomized clinical trial of the use of a prosthetic mesh to prevent parastomal hernia. *Br J Surg*. 2004;91:280-282.
11. Serra-Aracil X, Bombardo-Junca J, Moreno-Matias J, et al. Randomized, controlled, prospective trial of the use of a mesh to prevent parastomal hernia. *Ann Surg*. 2009;249:583-587.
12. Sorensen LT, Hemmingsen UB, Kirkeby LT, Kallehave F, Jorgensen LN. Smoking is a risk factor for incisional hernia. *Arch Surg*. 2005;140:119-123.
13. Ramirez OM, Ruas E, Dellon AL. "Components separation" method for closure of abdominal-wall defects: an anatomic and clinical study. *Plast Reconstr Surg*. 1990;86:519-526.
14. Wantz GE. *Atlas of Hernia Surgery*. New York, NY: Raven Press; 1991.

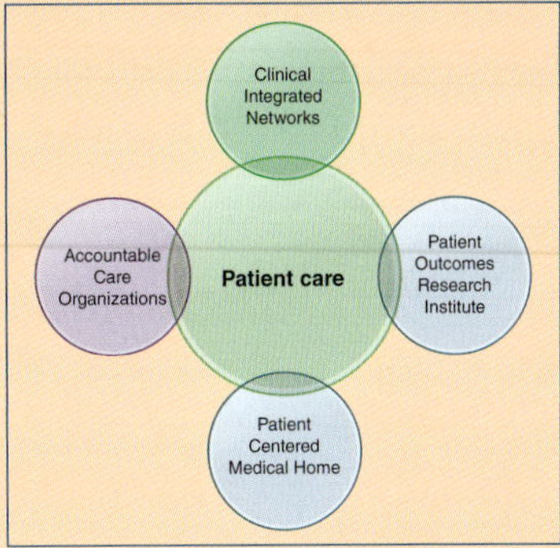

Section E Supportive Care

Chapter 21. Rehabilitation, Quality of Life, and Symptom Management

Michele L. McCarroll, PhD,
G. Dante Roulette, MD, and
Vivian E. von Gruenigen, MD

INTRODUCTION

According to the American Cancer Society (ACS), almost one-third of women in the United States will develop cancer. Most of these women will survive their cancer diagnosis yet face an uphill battle of maintaining their health as well as to reduce the risk of cancer recurrence. To help women in coordinate, there is a shift toward patient-centered approaches to survivorship with Clinical Integrated Networks (CIMs), Patient-Centered Medical Homes (PCMHs), Accountable Care Organizations (ACOs), and the Patient-Centered Outcomes Research Institute (PCORI; Figure 21-1). The focus of these emerging concepts is to help women make informed health care decisions, improve health care delivery, and implement plans of care using evidence-based information. Ultimately, survivorship is guided by patients, caregivers, and the broader health care community.[1] Ideally, patients as well as members of the public have the information they need to make decisions with their health care professional that reflect desired health outcomes. As health care professionals, we must hear the call of our patients' desires to improve survivorship through rehabilitation, quality of life (QOL), and symptom management. As the nation moves from physician-centric care to a patient-centered team approach, our patients deserve more active roles in their survivorship.

Cancer survivorship can be improved by participating in rehabilitation, improving QOL, and managing symptoms. With new national guidelines putting the patient at the center of communication between oncologists and primary care providers, we need to ensure all survivorship options are available to them.

REHABILITATION

Definitions

Gynecologic cancer diagnosis can play havoc on a woman's body. Oncologists typically use various conventional therapies for treating gynecologic cancers to facilitate a positive prognosis. Unfortunately, these therapies along with a list of comorbidities can reduce the functional ability and QOL of women in survivorship. Rehabilitation is defined as restoring the body for use in life. Oncology rehabilitation specifically addresses a patient's debilitating adverse events as a result of the therapeutic interventions.[2] Evidenced-based oncology rehabilitation includes physical strengthening, flexibility, functional assessments, QOL improvement strategies, stress management, lifestyle changes, and nutrition/dietary interventions. While still fairly new, oncology rehabilitation is still underutilized as a tool in survivorship, even as we face a future of patient-centered health care.

Although the potential benefits of oncology rehabilitation are obvious, the optimal frequency, intensity, type, and timing of rehabilitation for patients undergoing treatment or in survivorship still remain unclear.[3,4,5,6] Clinicians struggle to find the balance of challenging gynecologic cancer survivorship and encouraging one to make lifestyle changes all at once. However, can patients really afford to be inactive? Encouraging patients to be physically active can improve glucose metabolism, digestive function, immune function, and cardiovascular risk factors.[7,8] The balancing act between cancer recovery and thriving in survivorship can be tricky. Nevertheless, the literature remains clear that physical activity/rehabilitation is necessary to reduce the decline of a patient's health status and support a full recovery. In fact, several health care practitioner groups have developed oncology survivorship-specific toolkits to help serve as guidance documents to ensure the well being of patients with cancer. These toolkits highlight the conventional approaches to rehabilitation for improving physical capacity as well as encouraging healthy lifestyles. Regardless of the cancer diagnosis, exercise/physical activity is the most important thing that a survivor can do in reducing cancer-related fatigue, cancer-related stress, and reoccurrence.[9]

The American Physical Therapy Association (APTA) provides basic guidelines for treating the adult cancer survivor (Table 21-1). Mainly, the plan of care includes improving physical function (metabolic equivalents of tasks [METs]) during or after various treatments of cancer. Typically, a

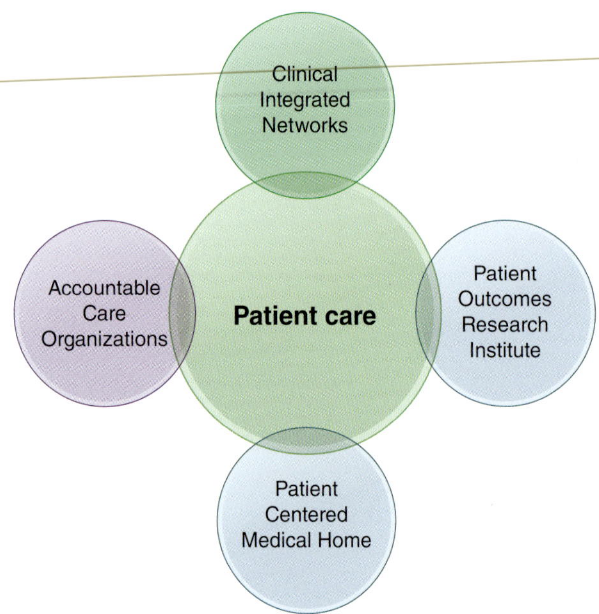

Fig. 21-1. Approach to patient care with the dawn of health care reform.

multisystem approach of improving cognitive, physical, and psychosocial arenas of a patient's life is also included in the standard plan of care. Specifically, oncology rehabilitation can be beneficial to gynecologic oncology patient at any place on the spectrum of survivorship in various settings of outpatient or inpatient venues.[10] These highly specialized rehabilitation programs have produced promising outcomes in reducing symptoms and in improving physical and psychosocial functioning.[11,12] For example, in a recent Cochrane review on the effects of rehabilitation and cancer-related fatigue,[13] 56 studies demonstrated a significant impact on the aerobic system and reducing fatigue for patients undergoing oncology rehabilitation compared to controls. However, evidence for increased muscle strength was not significant in regards to overall resistance training and other alternative exercises. Alternatively, targeted resistance training such as strengthening the pelvic floor muscles after pelvic surgery due to gynecologic cancer has been shown to improve muscle strength, QOL, and urethral function. In a prospective, randomized, controlled trial of pelvic-floor exercises (PFRPs) in gynecologic cancer survivors, the intervention group significantly improved pelvic-floor function and QOL domains.[14] The PFRP program consisted of one 45-minute exercise session and a 30-minute counseling session per week for 4 weeks. Overall, the stance of the APTA is to optimize activity by improving functional METs with reduced perception of fatigue allowing for improved activities of daily living (ADLs), knowledge through education, range of motion, and general strength training for ADLs.

The Society of The Society of Gynecologic Oncology (SGO) recently developed recommendations for rehabilitation for cancer survivors to help guide survivorship treatment.[15] With similar goals to the APTA, the SGO recommends evidence-based cancer rehabilitation to be a standard of care for survivors. Unfortunately, this is not always the case even though it is widely accepted that exercise and lifestyle changes achieved in rehabilitation will improve survivorship. Specifically, the SGO encourages a healthy lifestyle that engages a healthy diet, stress management, tobacco cessation, and whole system approaches to wellness (see Table 21-1).

The American College of Sports Medicine (ACSM) and the ACS have joint guidelines, which establish detailed exercise prescriptions for cancer survivorship during and after treatment.[16] This is the first time where guidelines have been implemented for survivorship just as emphatic as cancer prevention. Our patients need to have a priority of being physically active and eating a healthy diet in survivorship. The ACSM follows 2008 federal *Physical Activity Guidelines for Americans*, which states at least 150 minutes per week of moderate-intensity aerobic activity.[17] Generally, moderate-intensity aerobic exercise, resistance exercise, neurocognitive training, and/or combined programs are the most successful.[18] The art and science of exercise prescription in this population should be tailored to each individual's needs and provide progression using the frequency, intensity, time, and type (FITT) principles of fitness (see Table 21-1).

Overall, the general recommendations of the APTA, ACSM, ACS, and SGO demonstrate that a comprehensive oncology rehabilitation program is a crucial part of recovery for cancer survivors. The balancing act between thriving and surviving should be approached with precaution and a good understanding of contraindications to rehabilitation (Table 21-2). Data from randomized clinical trials indicate that unpleasant symptoms such as fatigue are the largest barrier to exercise and can affect exercise adherence.[19] As a result, the APTA, ACSM, ACS, SGO, and National Comprehensive Cancer Network (NCCN) emphasize the importance of oncology rehabilitation on the management of cancer-related fatigue to assist patients in overcoming this barrier.[20,21] To that end, the benefits of performing rehabilitation should be considered when contraindications do not exist (Table 21-3). With the mulitdisplnary approach, medically supervised oncology rehabilitation can provide a safe atmosphere for a patient and ensure adherence to lifestyle changes in survivorship.

Lifestyle Approaches to Survivorship Rehabilitation

Today, the majority of research done on rehabilitation programs for oncology patients supports mixed-interventions using strategies to improve body image, aerobic fitness, strength, dietary compliance, weight-loss, stress management, cognitive function, and QOL in concert with reduced fatigue.[14-21] However, in gynecologic cancer survivorship, weight-loss and weight management are at the forefront of a successful prognosis, yet endometrial cancer survivors are not likely to modify nutritional intake and exercise without supervision or direct intervention.[22] Studies conducted in gynecologic cancer survivors using a broad

Table 21-1. Summary of oncology rehabiltation guidelines.

	Aerobic	Muscle Strength	Flexibility	Cognitive	Education
ACSM and ACS	Overall volume of weekly activity of 150 minutes of moderate-intensity exercise or 75 minutes of vigorous-intensity exercise or an equivalent combination	Perform 2–3 weekly sessions that include exercises for major muscle groups	Flexibility guidelines are to stretch major muscle groups and tendons on days that other exercises are performed		Maintain a healthy weight Healthy diet Exercise Tobacco use Healthy bones Regular physician check-ups Survivor support Cancer surveillance
APTA	Optimize general physical activity for activities of daily living	Light resis-tance training	Range of motion	Incoporate coordination activities inline with occupational duties and activities of daily living	Energy conservation Nutrition Weight control Compensatory techniques Lymphadema managenemt Sensory re-education
SGO	A relaxed pace for 10–15 minutes, and then gradually buidling up more minutes. Ideally, be physically active for at least 30 minutes of moderate activity every day. Maximum health benefits, aim for 60 minutes or more of moderate activity every day, or 30 minutes or more of vigorous activity	None mentioned	None mentioned	None mentioned	Maintain a healthy weight Healthy diet Exercise Tobacco use Healthy bones Regular physician Check-ups Survivor support Cancer surveillance

ACS = American Cancer Society, ACSM = American College of Sports Medicine, AICR = American Instittue for Cancer Research, APTA = American Physical Therapy Association, SGO = Society of Gynecologic Oncology.

Table 21-2. Precautions and contraindications to rehabilitation.

Anemia	Exercise may need to be scaled back and possibly avoided
Neutropenia	Exercise should be avoided if there is a fever above 100.4°F (> 38°C)
Thrombocytopenia	Avoid contact sports or activities with high risk of injury or falling
Side effects	Vomiting, diarrhea, swollen ankles, unexplained weight loss/gain, or shortness of breath with low levels of exertion may make exercise unsafe

Reproduced with permission from American College of Sports Medicine. *ACSM's guidelines for exercise testing and prescription*. 8th ed. Philadelphia: Lippincott Williams and Wilkins, 2009.

lifestyle management rehabilitation approach demonstrate reduced stress, which, in turn, decreases stress hormone release and improved weight loss. Studies using the cognitive-behavioral intervention (CBI; eg, relaxation exercises, guided imagery, nature sound recordings) in cancer patients (colorectal, lung, prostate, and gynecologic cancers) had immediate symptom improvements from the beginning of the session to the end of the session.[23] Research indicates that elevated levels of stress hormones, such as cortisol and norepinephrine, sustained overtime affect the rate of abdominal fat deposition and the adiponectin-leptin ratio.[24] Specifically, Diaz et al[24] found that the adiponectin-leptin ratio is significantly linked to disease-specific survival in ovarian cancer patients. Furthermore, in endometrial cancer studies, most women with a larger waist and hip circumferences suffer more than those of normal proportioned survivors.[25] When stress hormones are present, weight control appears to be an uphill battle when trying to make lifestyle changes, especially in survivorship. Thus, tackling issues of stress, physical activity, and weight management demonstrates the need for a multidisciplinary approach in oncology rehabilitation.

The National Cancer Institute (NCI) recognizes the need to define patterns of weight, physical activity, and nutrition that contribute to survivorship. From current data, we know the majority of obese cancer survivors are not meeting public health exercise and/or nutrition recommendations. Furthermore, overweight and obese cancer survivors are susceptible to diabetes, coronary heart disease, and premature death.[26] Cardiovascular (CVD) comorbidities are the leading cause of death among endometrial cancer survivors. The risk of death from CVD-related causes begins to exceed the risk from cancer-related causes 3.5 years after diagnosis (Figure 21-2).[27] Specifically, obesity is the greatest CVD-related risk factor for endometrial cancer. In the prospective study by Ward et al,[20] the researchers examined the relationship between cancer, body mass index (BMI), and risk of

Table 21-3. Benefits to rehabilitation.

Weight	Helps maintain body weight for not only overweight survivors but even those of normal weight
Physical functioning	Maintaining or improving metabolic equivalents can improve morbidity and mortality
Cancer recurrence	Improves overall mortality among multiple cancer-survivor groups, including breast, colorectal, prostate, and ovarian cancers
Dietary compliance	Patients obtain support in dietary interventions to improve compliance to a diet high in fruits, vegetables, whole grains, poultry, and fish

Reproduced with permission from American College of Sports Medicine. *ACSM's guidelines for exercise testing and prescription*. 8th ed. Philadelphia: Lippincott Williams and Wilkins, 2009.

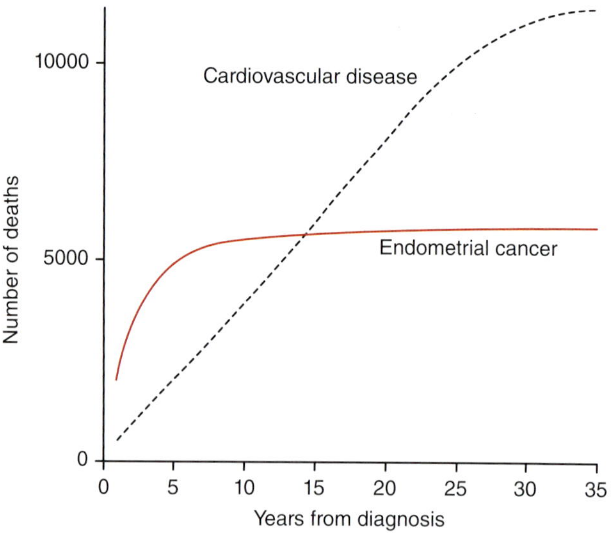

Fig. 21-2. Endometrial cancer cardiovascular death rates following diagnosis. (Reproduced with permission from Ward KK, Shah NR, Saenz CC, McHale MT, Alvarez EA, Plaxe SC.. Cardiovascular disease is the leading cause of death among endometrial cancer patients. *Gynecol Oncol.* 2012 Aug;126(2):176-9. doi: 10.1016/j.ygyno.2012.04.013. Epub 2012 Apr 13. PMID:22507532.)

death, demonstrating a significantly increased risk of death in obese women with endometrial cancer. The relative risk of death for obese endometrial cancer women with a BMI between 30 and 34 kg/m^2 was 2.53, and BMI above 40 kg/m^2 was 6.25; the highest of all cancers. It is well established that prevalence of obesity is higher in endometrial cancer survivors than of all the US cancers caused by excess body fat. More than 85% of endometrial cancer patients are overweight and approximately 70% are obese—this number is double the percentage of women with breast cancer.[28] Conversely, in a large population-based study of 1423 invasive epithelial ovarian cancer survivors, there were no significant associations between height, weight, or BMI and ovarian cancer-specific mortality.[29] However, in a cohort study of 1400 women diagnosed with invasive epithelial endometrial cancer prediagnosis, BMI was associated with a higher risk of all-cause 5-year mortality and an increased risk for 10-year CVD mortality.[30] Thus, there are mixed data on the relationships of BMI and gynecologic cancer survivorship. Then again, what we do know from a variety of studies is that obesity is related to an overall decline in survival and increases the risk of CVD-death. These authors conclude that obesity is linked to prognosis and overall survival in gynecologic cancer survivors and medically supervised programs to encourage weight loss is essential.

Several studies have explored the relationship between BMI and gynecologic malignancies, yet evidence surrounding nutrition and diet still remain inconclusive. Using the Health Eating Index, ovarian cancer patients scored very similar to controls identifying no differences in consumption of whole fruit, dark green and orange vegetables, and whole grains.[24] The only significant difference between groups was related to meat and beans, which were slightly higher in controls.[31] Thus, a multidisciplinary approach using nutrition and physical activity seems to be the combination for successful survivorship. von Gruenigen et al[32] used a whole systems approach in a randomized clinical trial where early stage overweight and obese (BMI ≥ 25 kg/m^2) endometrial cancer survivors followed a 6-month lifestyle intervention program supporting physical activity, dietary compliance of fruits/vegetables, and counseling to improve self-efficacy and QOL. The lifestyle program demonstrated significant increases in physical activity, daily intake of fruits/vegetables, and significant weight loss compared with controls in several cohort studies.[33,34] Maintaining a healthy lifestyle and routine examinations are also key components to fighting recurrence and improving one's prognosis. Dietary change and increased exercise together are effective for weight loss and improving CVD risk factors. Several concerns have been raised regarding the safety and efficacy of oncology rehabilitation due to increased oxidative stress generation and free radicals from exercise impairing cellular functions (Figure 21-3).[35] However, in a systematic review by Ballard-Barbash et al,[36] they identified cancer survivors with higher levels of activity were more likely to reduce risk of death from any cause and there may even be a dose-related response to physical activity.

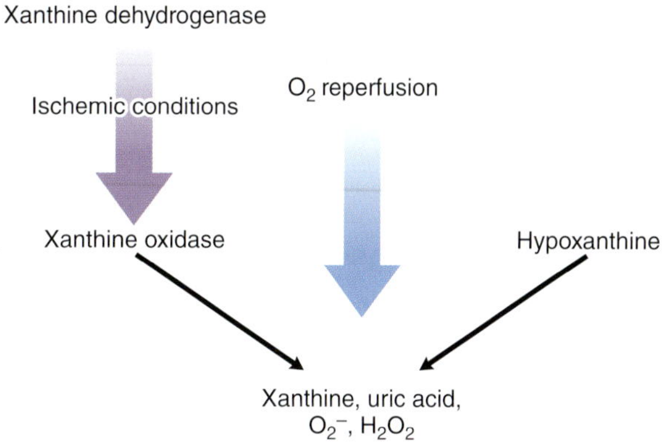

Fig. 21-3. Suggested mechanism for the production of free radicals upon reoxygenation of ischemic or hypoxic tissues (Reproduced with permission from Gomes EC, Silva AN, Oliveira MR. Oxidants, Antioxidants, and the Beneficial Roles of Exercise-Induced Production of Reactive Species. *Oxid Med Cell Longev*. 2012; 2012: 756132. Published online 2012 June 3. doi: 10.1155/2012/756132.)

Studies encompassing survivors of breast, colon, prostate, gastric, ovarian, endometrial, and brain cancer report that physical activity is associated with a reduction of all-cause mortality.

Exercise is medicine and can provide a protective shield for gynecologic cancer survivors. From a landmark study conducted by Blair and Cooper in 1998,[30] morbidity and mortality rates were directly related to physical functioning or metabolic capacity. Most notably, they demonstrated a linear reduction of risk with increasing levels of maximal METs achieved on functional capacity evaluations. Based on these data, the goals of oncology rehabilitation should be to improve patient functional capacity to be between 5 and 8 METs. These moderate-to-high activity levels will double the odds of survival compared with those individuals who have lower maximal MET levels.[37] Gynecologic cancer survivors are no exception. In a small study of obese endometrial cancer patients, functional capacity was significantly worse compared with normal obese controls.[38] In this instance, regardless of the cancer status, self-reported exercise for both groups was associated with improving health status. This emphasizes the point that peak exercise capacity is a stronger predictor of death than any other risk factors, such as hypertension, diabetes, obesity, heart arrhythmia, high cholesterol, and even smoking.

Oncology rehabilitation does not only provide benefits to maximal oxygen consumption, it also reduces the risk of frailty, especially after cancer treatments. In a study of frail elderly women recovering from gynecologic cancers, BMI was significantly different (P = .02) between groups women who were categorized as not frail (26.1 kg/m^2), intermediately frail (31.5 kg/m^2), and frail (36.0 kg/m^2).[39] The risk of frailty is directly related to the excess weight of most gynecologic cancer patients as a result of not meeting public health guidelines for physical activity. The importance for survivors to engage in regular physical activity is plentiful even in various forms of rehabilitation. For example, in a randomized control study of 110 patients, the intervention group performed supervised, home-based training program shortly after chemotherapy. The program included flexibility training, both low- and moderate-intensity exercises over several months after treatment. As a result, the intervention group significantly improved cancer-related fatigue and increased maximal functional capacity compared with the control group.[40] Therefore, it is feasible and beneficial for cancer survivors to engage in supervised home-training programs or medically based supervised rehabilitation programs.

Research evidence suggests that individuals with cancer who follow recommended guidelines and observe specific precautions can safely exercise during cancer treatment and in survivorship. However, is there an optimal dose of physical activity to improve survivorship prognosis? Studies show that physical activity and obesity may predict cancer survivorship. There is some evidence suggesting a dose–response effect of increasing risk reduction with increasing physical activity levels.[41] In a review by Litterini et al,[42] patients are likely to benefit from an oncology rehabilitation exercise program approximately 12 weeks long; however, studies revealed a wide variety of frequency, duration, and intensity of exercise. In these studies, most oncology rehabilitation programs took a multiple mode approach along with a healthy lifestyle education curriculum. Further research is needed to determine the best type, timing, and intensity of exercise for the different types and stages of cancer. Despite these limitations, for the most part, exercise prescriptions have closely followed the published guidelines of the ACSM and ACS joint recommendations. Without reservation, gynecologic cancer survivors should be referred to oncology rehabilitation programs to assist women in making lifestyle changes. It is important to get survivors into supervised exercise and lifestyle programs because most gynecologic cancer survivors do not make spontaneous lifestyle changes. The effectiveness of interventions such as oncology rehabilitation among cancer survivors has demonstrated long-term health benefits and survival.[43] In addition, research studies testing the effectiveness of various types of rehabilitation and training regimens for cancer survivors found that exercise was effective in preventing or reducing cancer-related fatigue.[44] Thus, physicians have a responsibility to ensure patients get referred to rehabilitation programs to assist a patient's well being and provide support on the journey of survivorship.

PSYCHOSOCIAL FACTORS

Quality of Life

The NCI recognizes that there are few national measures available to accurately measure health-related QOL for cancer survivors.[45] The American Association for Cancer Research (AACR) states that obesity can interfere with a survivor's recovery and subsequent QOL. QOL measures, an example of patient-reported outcomes (PROs), are becoming a common component in patient-centered approaches to survivorship with CIMs, PCMHs, ACOs, and the PCORI. QOL encompasses subjective and objective life conditions as well as personal aspirations and values.[46,47] The multiple dimensions of QOL include physical, mental, social, emotional well-being, and development/activity. Within the last 4 decades, QOL has become an important end point relating to the treatment of cancer. Specifically, QOL in endometrial cancer patients are at the forefront of cancer-related QOL due to the early age of diagnosis and number of survivors. Obesity is not only the most significant risk factor for the development of endometrial cancer; obesity also reduces the QOL of endometrial cancer survivors. In a prospective ancillary analysis of women with endometrial cancer, results revealed that increasing BMI correlated with decreasing health-related QOL scores, specifically physical and functional well being.[48] Previous work in a meta-analysis from 30 randomized controlled trials in the European Organization for Research and Treatment of Cancer (EORTC) confirmed that QOL could predict survival.[49] Thus, QOL measures can provide significant prognostic value of cancer survivors and interventions such as oncology rehabilitation can influence QOL in survivorship.

Recently, a review of the most commonly applied QOL tools for women with ovarian, cervical, endometrial, and vulvar cancers revealed that disease-specific questionnaires are available, but there is little evidence to support the superior sensitivity and responsiveness of cancer-specific versus generic QOL questionnaires.[50] Several studies explored this point of QOL symptom-specific and cancer-specific questionnaire to more accurately reflect the QOL domains directly related to survival.[49] One study attempted to advance the understanding of QOL in ovarian cancer patients by assessing the top 10 symptoms important to women and their related QOL scores.[51] Symptom management, the preservation of functionality, a sense of hope, sleep quality, and the maintenance/improvement of QOL all emerged as important components; however, choosing the right QOL tool is essential to capture the multidimensional experience of ovarian cancer patients stages of their survival. Thus, the specificity of symptoms for each patient should be carefully correlated with an appropriate QOL tool (eg, FACT-O, FACT-G, EORTC QLQ-C30). The psychometric properties of these tools can be beneficial when assessing a woman for QOL concerns, especially after pelvic surgery—meaning that not all QOL tools are created equal. Most notably, a small study of women (n = 50) who underwent pelvic surgery for vulvar, cervical, or endometrial cancer reported significant reduction in sexual frequency, vaginal lubrication, and ability to achieve orgasm; in spite of these results, no differences were noted in QOL/depression between sexual dysfunction groups.[52] The results of these studies indicate the importance of engaging women in oncology rehabilitation programs that focus on QOL improvement initiatives specific to each woman guided by a multidisciplinary team of health care professionals. A Cochrane review of 40 trials with 3694 cancer patients revealed positive effects on QOL, specifically body image/self-esteem, emotional well-being, sexuality, sleep disturbance, social functioning, anxiety, fatigue, and pain for those patients participating in a formal intervention program.[53] Consequently, interventions facilitating women to improve QOL can greatly benefit women in any stage of treatment for gynecologic cancers.

Self-Efficacy

Often, QOL and self-efficacy are mentioned hand in hand; conversely, they represent 2 separate entities of patient approach to survivorship. Self-efficacy may actually influence the QOL of cancer survivors. Particularly, if a woman feels a sense of confidence toward her survivorship whether it be exercise self-efficacy, weight loss self-efficacy, or self-efficacy toward stressful situations, the more likely she is to have a better prognosis. Limited studies are available to assess the level and type of self-efficacy in women with endometrial, cervical, and ovarian cancers. Principally, because most endometrial and ovarian cancer patients struggle with obesity comorbidities, self-efficacy toward weight loss should be at the forefront of intervention programs. Interventions designed to enhance a woman's self-efficacy will have a larger impact on her cancer journey. In a randomized intervention study of endometrial cancer survivors by von Gruenigen et al,[54] the study demonstrated weight loss and increased exercise correlating to a positive effect on QOL and self-efficacy. The key ingredient in the intervention focused on improving the survivors Weight Efficacy Life-Style (WEL) self-efficacy. An earlier pilot study (n = 45) examining the effects of 6-months of lifestyle interventions on QOL, depression, self-efficacy, and eating behavior change revealed improved self-efficacy and changes in eating behaviors.[55] In a randomized control study by Rejeski,[56] a positive correlation between weight loss and WEL scores was observed. Patients (n = 288) were randomized to a physical activity only group, a weight loss plus physical activity group, or a successful aging health education program. Those individuals in the combination group of weight loss and physical activity lost 8.6% of their body weight and had significant higher scores for all domains on the WEL questionnaire when compared with the other groups. Mainly, the positive impact of supervised interventions led to increased self-efficacy in the health domains of weight loss, exercise, and nutrition. Ultimately, there is a balancing act that must occur between self-efficacy and QOL (Figure 21-4). The role of the physician after surgical intervention may be foggy to some patients and the even the physician themselves. The follow-up care after reconstruction or treatment typically involves an overview of symptom management postsurgery. Unfortunately, in a review by Lajer et al[57], studies showed no evidence of a positive effect on survival in women followed up after primary treatment of endometrial or ovarian cancer. Follow-up after treatment should have a clearly defined and evidence-based purpose. The physician should now take the opportunity to include self-efficacy support and QOL interventions recognizing the important of the psychometric roles of cancer survival.

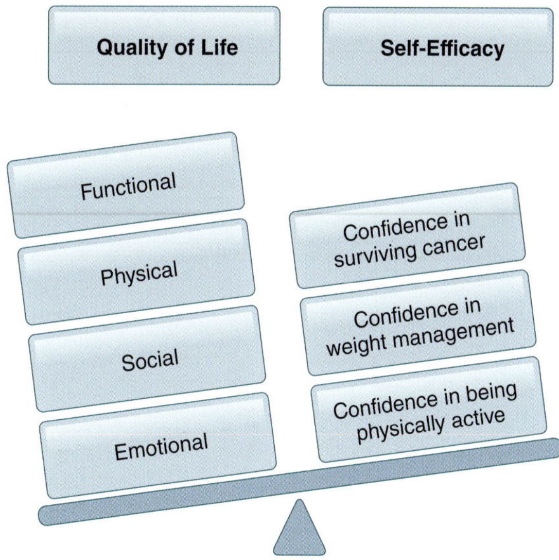

Fig. 21-4. There must be a balance of quality of life and self-efficacy for treatment to be successful.

SEXUAL FUNCTION

Sexuality can include sexual response, sexual roles, and relationships. The World Health Organization defines sexuality as a central aspect of being human throughout life that encompasses sex, gender identities and roles, sexual orientation, eroticism, pleasure, intimacy, and reproduction. It is experienced and expressed in thoughts, fantasies, desires, beliefs, attitudes, values, behavior, practices, roles, and relationships. Not all these dimensions are experienced or expressed at the same time. Each is influenced by the interaction of biologic, psychological, social, economic, political, cultural, ethical, legal, historical, religious, and spiritual factors.[58]

Historically, sexual health in women has been little researched and poorly understood. A general increase in interest in sex-specific outcomes has led to increased interest in sexual functioning after surgical procedures. To date, our understanding of the impact has been limited by lack of validated tools and retrospective studies. The original, 4-stage description of the human sexual response cycle by Masters and Johnson has since been modified, and represents a linear continuum from desire, through arousal, orgasm, ending with resolution.[59] Although this model accurately represents the objective physical changes in sexual function, the full spectrum of psychological components is discounted. Unlike male sexuality, which can in part be objectively measured, in the setting of a mature relationship, female sexuality relies on both physical and psychosocial factors.[60] Body image is a component of women's sexual self-concept related to feeling feminine and attractive, and a high number of sexual problems are associated with impaired body image.

Radical extirpative surgery as a procedure is discussed in its various forms elsewhere in detail. Since initial descriptions of these procedures in the first half of the twentieth century, there have been advances in understanding and technique. When coupled with advances in nonsurgical treatment, as well as perioperative care, morbidity and mortality rates have markedly improved. Indeed, the postoperative mortality rates have been approximately halved over the last 60 years.[61] This growing cohort of women postextirpative therapy has led directly to a need for discussion and research in QOL domains, specifically sexual function.

In 1997, Hawighorst-Knapstein et al began reporting on the impact of extirpative therapy on QOL outcomes.[62] A prospective cohort of 28 women undergoing pelvic exenteration were interviewed extensively preoperatively (T1), and at 4 (T2) and 12 (T3) months postoperatively using the Cancer Rehabilitation Evaluation System (CARES). In addition, a validated questionnaire developed by Strauss and Appelt[60] was used for subject assessment of body image. Significantly, analysis of results was performed based on no ostomy (n = 10), one ostomy (n = 10), or 2 ostomies (n = 8). A separate analysis of women with vaginal reconstruction (n = 11) and without vaginal reconstruction (n = 17) was performed. For patients with 2 ostomies, sexual (P = .039) and marital (P = .027) problems increased significantly from T1 to T2. This group had significantly more problems than patients with 1 ostomy 12 months postoperatively. Compared with the group with no ostomy, the group with 2 diversions had significantly more problems in the sexual (P = .008), and marital (P = .046) domain at T3. When looking at body image, the group with 2 ostomies reported significantly less attractiveness/self-confidence (P = .011) at 12 months than before surgery. In addition, the group with 2 ostomies had significantly higher uncertainty/discomfort compared with patients with no (P = .002) or 1 (P = .028) ostomy at 12 months. Women with colpectomy reported significantly more problems than women with vaginal capacity related to the physical (P = .023) and sexual (P = .010) QOL at T2. These groups also differed significantly in terms of sexual function (P = .015) and marital interaction (P = .017) at 12 months. Women without vaginal reconstruction felt less attractive and self-confident at 4 (P = .046) and 12 months (P = .017) when compared with preoperative states. In a follow-up after 10 years of experience, the same authors presented data on 129 patients and reported similar results.[63] In addition, a subset of women who underwent the somewhat less radical Wertheim's procedure was included in the analysis. Sexual problems were significantly lower for women with a Wertheim's procedure (T2, P = .010 and T3, P = .032). All patients reported significantly less attractiveness or self-confidence (P = .000) and more sexual uncertainty (P = .001). This effect was exacerbated by adjuvant therapy.

In 2008, da Silva et al[56] published prospective data on female sexual function, body image, and self-esteem after colorectal surgery for 93 patients. Significantly, many of these patients underwent surgery for a malignant process, with two-thirds receiving a stoma at the time of the procedure. Using the Female Sexual Function Index (FSFI), EORTC, and sexual function (SF) -36 tools, prospective information was collected preoperatively, and at 6 and 12 months. Sexual function declined significantly at 6 months, with partial recovery at 12 months (P = .02). There was an 8% increase in dyspareunia, with declines in lubrication (9.8%), arousal (8.1%), orgasm (7.9%), libido (4.9%), and sexual satisfaction (4.8%).[64] While sexual desire, satisfaction, and dyspareunia improved at 12 months, arousal, lubrication, and orgasm did not. Better sexual function was associated with good body image and self-esteem prior to surgery.

Rezk et al[57] confirmed these results among patients undergoing radical procedures for gynecologic malignancy in 2013. In this article, prospective information on the QOL of 16 women was collected preoperatively and at 3, 6, and 12 months after pelvic exenteration. Their results did show a decrease in QOL measures at 3 months, with rebound to near baseline at 12 months (P = .02).[65] A similar trend was noted in the sexual function among these patients with a rebound toward baseline seen 12 months postoperatively.

In general, the available prospective data seem to suggest that short-term declines in sexual function are to be expected after extirpative therapy. Fortunately, these declines are reversed to varying degree approximately 12 months after surgery, though it should be noted there is not a full return to baseline. Many patients undergoing extirpative therapy do not have alternative, less invasive options, if cure is the intent. Currently available data suggest part of the counseling process for these procedures should include discussion of the impact on sexual function, with positive emphasis on improvements to near baseline 1 year after treatment.

SYMPTOM MANAGEMENT

Pain Management

Pain is frequently inadequately addressed and is a common symptom in cancer patients that can affect both QOL and other systems. In the setting of inadequately controlled pain, analgesics should be given on a schedule rather than when requested or on demand, eg, every 2 to 6 hours. The WHO advocates following a "3-step management ladder." When possible, there should be prompt oral administration of drugs in the following order: (1) nonopioids (NSAIDs and acetaminophen), then (2), mild opioids as necessary, and then (3), strong opioids until the patient is free from pain. Adjuvant analgesics may also be used, which include those medications with a primary indication other than pain that have analgesics properties. Some adjuvant analgesics are useful in several painful conditions and are described as multipurpose adjuvant analgesics (eg, antidepressants, corticosteroids, alpha-2-adrenergic agonists, neuroleptics), whereas others are specific for neuropathic pain (eg, anticonvulsants, local anesthetics, N-methyl-D-aspartate antagonists), bone pain (eg, bisphosphonates, calcitonin, radiopharmceuticals), musculoskeletal pain (eg, muscle relaxants), or pain from bowel obstruction (eg, octreotide, anticholinergics). Nonpharmaceutical adjuvant therapy can be considered for oncology patients. In a multisite, randomized clinical trial of 400 patients with advanced cancer, both massage and simple touch were shown to improve pain and mood, with massage found to be superior.[66]

Nausea and Vomiting

Nausea and vomiting in the gynecologic oncology patient may be disease or treatment related. Nausea associated with slowing of the gut should respond to gastrokinetic antiemetics, such as metoclopramide, that promote gastric emptying and increase gut motility. However, bowel obstruction must be considered in patients with intra-abdominal disease; in these patients, stimulating agents may worsen symptoms. Chemotherapy-induced nausea and vomiting (CINV) is influenced by a number of factors, with the intrinsic emetogenicity being dominant and the factor that most influences antiemetic treatment regimen. Other important factors include sex and age, with female patients and younger patients more affected, as well as dosage. A number of chemotherapy regimens for gynecologic oncology patients include medications of high and moderate risk of emesis, as defined by expert consensus (Table 21-4).[67] CINV is classified into 4 subcategories: acute, delayed, breakthrough, and anticipatory. Acute nausea occurs 1 to 2 hours after administration, resolving after 24 hours. Delayed nausea occurs after 24 hours, peaking 48 to 72 after chemotherapy administration, with resolution by day 6 or 7. Anticipatory nausea and vomiting is a conditioned response based on prior experience with chemotherapy. Finally, breakthrough CINV can occur when a patient experiences symptoms despite appropriate treatment. The physiologic pathways that lead to CINV have been elucidated over time, and the central nervous system appears to be the primary site in these afferent and efferent pathways.

Table 21-4. Emetogic potential of common chemotherapeutic agents by (incidence).

High (> 90%)	Cisplatin Cyclophosphamide ≥ 1500 mg/m^2
Moderate (30%–90%)	Oxaliplatin Carboplatin Cyclophosphamide < 1500 mg/m^2 Doxorubicin Ifosfamide
Low (10%–30%)	Paclitaxel Docetaxel Liposomal doxorubicin Topotecan Etoposide Methotrexate Mitomycin Gemcitabine
Minimal (< 10%)	Bevacizumab

Treatment of CINV is based on the chemotherapeutic agent with the most emetogenic potential, and the incidence of delayed emesis. First-line agents, classified as having a high therapeutic index, include 3 main classes of drugs: 5-hydroxytrptophan (5-HT_3) receptor antagonists, corticosteroids, and neurokinin-1 receptor antagonists (Aprepitant, Fosaprepitant, Merck and Company, Whitehouse Station, New Jersey). Agents of low therapeutic index include metoclopramide, phenothiazines, butyrophenones, and cannabinoids. These can be used for chemotherapeutic agents with low emetogenic potential, or for control of breakthrough nausea and vomiting.[68] The incidence of anticipatory emesis is decreasing as adequate treatment of CINV is increasing. When anticipatory CINV does occur, benzodiazepines and behavioral therapy are suggested. A Cochrane review of the literature supports the efficacy of acupuncture point stimulator for acute CINV as well as for postoperative nausea.[69] In a randomized study of ovarian cancer patients, all of whom were receiving a standard antiemetic regimen, the combination of vitamin B6 and acupuncture led to significantly fewer emesis episodes and a greater proportion of emesis-free days when compared with acupuncture or vitamin B6 alone. In a randomized, double-blind crossover study in nearly 50 gynecologic cancer patients receiving cisplatin-based chemotherapy, ginger in capsule form was found to be equivalent to metoclopramide for delayed nausea.[70]

Bowel Obstruction

Bowel obstruction in gynecologic oncology patients is a complicated and heterogeneous clinical entity. According to a 2010 Cochrane review, 25% to 50% of ovarian cancer patients will experience a bowel obstruction.[71] The causes can be related to benign conditions (eg, surgical adhesions, hernia, or fibrosis after radiation or intra-abdominal chemotherapy), or directly related to the underlying malignancy. Median survival at time of presentation is 4 months.[72] Management of bowel obstruction can be medical or surgical and decisions related to bowel obstruction should be based on the prognosis, performance status, and goals of care.

Physiologically, bowel obstruction is the pathologic cycle of distention from gas and nonabsorbed secretions. The resulting damage leads to an inflammatory response and release of vasoactive intestinal peptides, resulting in increase secretions. The patient may present symptomatically with any combination of bloating, pain, cramping, nausea, and vomiting, with severity based on location and degree of obstruction.[73] Surgical management may involve bypassing, or resecting, the affected bowel or stenting the stricture. For patients focusing on managing discomfort, a combination of methods can be used, including pain management, antiemetics, corticosteroids, percutaneous gastrostomy placed endoscopically or by interventional radiology, and medications for decreasing intestinal secretions. Octreotide for this purpose has been shown to control emesis and to improve QOL and decrease hospitalization. Care should be taken to evaluate the patient with respect to symptom control, fluid status, and correction of any underlying electrolyte abnormality related to the obstruction. A review of the literature by the Cochrane Collaboration in 2010 found only low-quality evidence comparing medical and surgical treatment of bowel obstruction in ovarian cancer patients. Only one article, Mangili et al,[74] was of sufficient quality for inclusion, and was limited by a lack of randomization and QOL measurements. In the article 47 women received either palliative surgery or medical management with octreotide, and overall survival and perioperative morbidity and mortality were reported. Multivariate analysis found that women receiving surgery had significantly better survival when compared with medical management, although 6 (22%) surgical patients had serious complication from the operation, and 3 (11%) died of complications. Women with low performance status were excluded in this group, potentially biasing the result. A recent, prospective report on symptomatology in a small highly selected group of patients with ovarian cancer undergoing palliative endoscopic of operative procedures is available. The researchers noted symptomatic improvement or resolution within 30 days in 23 (88%) or 26 patients, with 1 (4%) post-procedure mortality. At 60 days, 10 (71%) of 14 patients who underwent operative procedures and 6 (50%) of 12 patients who had endoscopic procedures had symptom control. Median survival from the time of the palliative procedure was 191 days for those undergoing an operative procedure and 78 days for those undergoing an endoscopic procedure. For large bowel obstruction, less invasive strategies like colorectal stenting can help patients with recurrent disease. Caceres et al[75] have demonstrated the feasibility of this strategy in acutely ill gynecologic cancer patients who had successful stent placement. Like bowel obstruction, constipation is a frequent complaint, and may be related to the disease process, or an adverse effect of pharmacotherapy (ie, 5-HT_3 antagonists, narcotics). Constipation that is pharmacologic in nature is best controlled through anticipation, and hydration. Consideration should be given to use of stool softeners, peristaltic agents, and osmotic laxatives. Bulking agents may not be appropriate in patients who are not able to hydrate, have radiation-related dysfunction, or extensive intra-abdominal disease. A presenting complaint may be constipation when the mesenteric plexus is involved with extensive intra-abdominal disease. Treatment is aimed at increasing bowel peristalsis with prokinetic agents (eg, metoclopramide), and avoidance of constipation and impaction with hydration and appropriate laxatives.

Oral and Intestinal Mucositis

Oral and intestinal adverse events can be related to chemotherapy, radiation, or disease progression, presenting as oral and esophageal ulceration, diarrhea, and tenesmus. These morbid side effects are collectively termed alimentary mucositis. The underlying physiologic causes of alimentary mucositis are incompletely understood. However, advances in the understanding of the pathophysiologic basis of mucositis have led to the characterization of oral and gastrointestinal mucositis as a continuum of injury rather than distinct clinical entities.[76] Frequently, patients present with mouth and oropharyngeal pain, and impaired swallowing. These complaints can be significant and may require intravenous opioid administration for palliation. When accompanied with mucositis of the gastrointestinal tract, nausea, vomiting, abdominal pain, tenesmus and bleeding may be present. Gynecologic cancer patients with diarrhea and tenesmus need to be evaluated for disease progression. Infection as a causative etiology should be investigated. When infection and disease progression are excluded, pharmacologic intervention (eg, loperamide, octreotide) may improve symptoms of radiation or chemotherapy-induced diarrhea. Tenesmus usually responds to anticholinergic agents, corticosteroids, and opioids, often used in combination. In severe cases of radiation enteritis and proctitis, surgical intervention may be required. This clinical entity is important, and advances in understanding and clinical application ongoing at a rapid pace. Historically, the treatment and interventions aimed at prevention have been variable and largely dependent on local practice. The evidence for these interventions has been varied and often conflicting. In 2011, Cochrane reviewers update their publication on the range of preventative interventions for mucositis, now including 131 studies in their meta-analysis.[77] There is evidence of benefit for ice chips (cryotherapy) and keratinocyte growth factor (Palifermin, Amgen, Thousand Oaks, California) for all categories of mucositis, including moderate and severe. It should be noted that Palifermin is approved for hematologic malignancies and patients undergoing stem cell transplantation.[78] In the previous recommendations, there was limited and weak evidence for granulocyte-colony stimulating factor, honey, amifostine, intravenous glutamine, and PTA (polymyxin B, tobramycin, amphotericin B) lozenges; this is unchanged. Evidence for low-level laser remains weak; however, benefit was seen in the prevention of severe mucositis.[79] Based on expert opinion, a multidisciplinary approach to the care of patients at risk for mucositis may be beneficial. Ongoing preventive and therapeutic oral care should be standardized into the plan of care.

Ascites

Ascites is a frequent complaint in ovarian cancer patients and can have a significant negative impact on QOL, especially in cases of treatment refractory ascites. Current research points to high concentrations of vascular endothelial growth factor as a cause of ascites due to increased peritoneal permeability.[80] Treatment is largely practitioner dependent, though many favor repeated large volume peritoneal paracentesis, which can result in infection. Patient's QOL is impacted by abdominal distention, anorexia, and pain associated with accumulation of the ascites as well as fatigue, dizziness, and nausea associated with large volume paracentesis, in addition to the physical and emotional morbidity associated with the practice. Diuretics and diet restriction may have a role in treatment of ascites related to portal hypertension, as well as placement of a permanent indwelling catheter. Placement of indwelling intraperitoneal catheters has been studied retrospectively and found to be an effective strategy for palliation of symptoms related to refractory ascites. In 2012, Tapping et al[68] reported on retrospective evaluation of 28 patients who had tunneled peritoneal drains placed for the treatment of refractory ascites. Over a 4-year period, 28 patients had tunneled catheters placed, with 5 cases of nonsystemic infection successfully treated with oral antibiotics. Patency was maintained for a mean of 113 days, and the authors report increased patient satisfaction though validated objective measurements were not taken.[81] Successful management of refractory ascites using indwelling IP (intraperitoneal) catheters without overwhelming infection has been reported by other researchers, and appears to be an effective and safe means of palliation.[82] Case reports have studies showing the successful use of bevacizumab in palliative treatment of ascites in ovarian cancer patients with manageable toxicity profiles.[83] New biologic therapeutics may be an option in future treatment of refractory ascites. Further prospective trials should consider evaluation of these agents as a tool for palliation treatment of ascites during the EOL.

Hypercalcemia

Hypercalcemia of malignancy occurs in 10% to 30% of patients with cancer, and etiologies include humoral hypercalcemia of malignancy, which may or may not be mediated by the paraneoplastic secretion of parathyroid hormone-related peptide, and local osteolytic hypercalcemia in the setting of bone metastasis. In gynecologic cancer, hypercalcemia has been reported with ovarian small-cell carcinoma, papillary serous carcinoma, clear cell carcinoma, and dysgerminoma, as well as with uterine leiomyosarcoma and endometrial, cervical, and vulvar carcinomas. A review of more than 5000 gynecologic cancer patients identified 25 patients with hypercalcemia (5%).[84] Most patients (82%) had mild hypercalcemia. Severity of hypercalcemia was associated with disease stage, use of hypercalcemia treatment, and survival duration. A review of the published cases in the literature identified 34 patients with humoral hypercalcemia of malignancy that was parathyroid hormone-related peptide mediated, of whom 22 had ovarian cancer, 6 had uterine cancer, 3 had vulvar cancer, and 3 had cervical cancer. Clear cell carcinoma was the predominant histology. Mild hypercalcemia may be asymptomatic, while moderate-to-severe hypercalcemia can be associated with life-threatening neurologic, cardiac, gastrointestinal, and renal events. The treatment of hypercalcemia depends on the level, chronicity, and origin of the condition. General measures to treat hypercalcemia include combining aggressive saline volume replacement and forced dieresis (with loop diuretics), and inhibitors of bone resorption such as bisphosphonates and calcitonin. Glucocorticoids and oral phosphates may also be given, while renal replacement therapy is reserved for severe hypercalcemia with concomitant renal failure. Response is monitored clinically and with serum calcium levels.

Respiratory Symptoms

Dyspnea is the "subjective experience of breathing discomfort that consists of qualitatively distinct sensations that vary in intensity," not necessarily related to hypercapnia or hypoxia.[85] Respiratory symptoms, when present, may be related to metastatic disease or from pleural effusion. In addition to baseline comorbidities cancer-related cachexia, malnutrition, fatigue, anemia, and metabolic acidosis may also contribute to dyspnea. When contributing medical morbidities have been optimally treated, interventions should be made based on performance status, prognosis, and goals of care for the patient. In broad categories, interventions may be pharmacologic (eg, opioids, benzodiazepines), physical (eg, thoracentesis, chemical pleurodesis, or placement of indwelling catheter), and emotional (eg, cognitive behavior therapy, breathing training, relaxation exercises). The use of supplemental oxygen was evaluated for relief of dyspnea as indicated in Currow et al,[86] where no significant qualitative difference in dyspnea was found with the use of supplemental oxygen. It is important to note, there may be significant safety and cost issues that accompany the presence of oxygen in the home. Absent true hypoxia, the use of supplemental oxygen should be reserved. Nonpharmacologic interventions such as counseling, relaxation, and teaching coping strategies may provide benefit to oncology patients.

Urinary Tract Infection

Urinary tract symptoms in the gynecologic oncology patient may be disease or treatment related. Women with both early and late stage ovarian cancer may present with urinary urgency and frequency. Cervical cancer patients may have symptoms related to obstruction or extension of tumor into the bladder. Ureteral obstruction may justify mechanical measures including ureteric stent insertion or nephrostomy based on clinical presentation, and consideration of prognosis and goals of care. Treatment-related symptoms include bladder dysfunction after radical hysterectomy, radiation cystitis, or fistula between pelvic structures. Radiation for cervical and endometrial cancer can cause urinary tract symptoms, including immediate effects (bladder irritation or cystitis) and late effects (hematuria, fibrosis, contraction, or fistulas). The increased risk is attributed to disruptions in the uroepithelial barrier secondary to radiation therapy. In cervical cancer, the 10-year bladder complication rate in a series from the MD Anderson Cancer Center was 3%.[87] On multivariate analysis, a central pelvic dose of external beam radion higher than 50 Gy, black race, smoking, and obesity were significantly associated with increased bladder complications. In a 2012 Cornell study, among 581 patients with endometrial cancer, treatment with vaginal brachytherapy plus 3-dimensional conformal radiation therapy was associated with higher rates of UTI when compared with vaginal brachytherapy plus intensity modulated radiation therapy, 37.3% versus 9.3%, although both were higher than vaginal brachytherapy alone (2.8%).[88] Bladder symptoms may be treated with nonsteroidal anti-inflammatory medications for detrusor irritability or drugs with anticholinergic action to reduce bladder contractility. Infection, and the need for treatment, should also be assessed. Fistulas are ideally treated surgically; however, in the setting of limited prognosis, less invasive options, such as urinary catheterization, may ameliorate symptoms.

Venous Thromboembolism

Thromboembolic disease, lymphedema, and severe nutritional deficiency can contribute to acute and chronic edema in the gynecologic oncology patient. In addition, recurrent or progressive tumor may contribute to edema. A diagnosis of cancer confers a 4- to 6-fold increase in risk of venous thromboembolism (VTE).[89] Age, abdominopelvic surgery, obstructing lesions, and treatment with thrombogenic chemotherapy regimens are additional risk factors for VTE. The risk of VTE remains elevated in the postoperative period, as high as 10 to 50 times higher in the 7 to 12 weeks following surgery, with rates for PE (pulmonary embolism) in ovarian cancer patients as high as 7%. Cancer patients being treated for VTE have a higher risk of recurrence when treated with oral vitamin K antagonists (VKAs). Perioperative prevention of VTE is essential. We support the 2012 recommendations of the American College of Chest Physicians of dual prophylaxis with mechanical and pharmacologic measures, and extended duration pharmacologic prophylaxis (4 weeks) for cancer patients.[90] Treatment with a low-molecular-weight heparin is preferred over oral VKAs for patients with VTE.

Lymphedema

According to the National Lymphedema Network and the International Consensus Best Practice for the Management of Lymphoedema, lymphedema is an accumulation of lymphatic fluid in the interstitial tissue that causes swelling, most often in one or more limbs, but can occasionally occur in the trunk, breast, genitalia, head, or neck.[91] Lymphedema can develop (Table 21-5) when lymphatic vessels are missing or impaired (primary), or when lymph vessels are damaged or lymph nodes removed (secondary).[92,93] If lymphatic fluid exceeds the lymphatic transport capacity, then an abnormal amount of protein-rich fluid collects in the tissues of the affected area. Left untreated, this stagnant, protein-rich fluid not only causes tissue channels to increase in size and number, but it also reduces oxygen availability in the transport system, interferes with wound healing, and provides an environment for bacteria that can result in infection. People who develop infections may require numerous hospitalizations and a dependence on antibiotics. Lymphedema can produce physical and psychological issues that may affect mobility and body image. Lymphedema is a chronic condition that is not curable at present, but may be alleviated by appropriate management; if ignored, it can progress and become difficult to manage. It has been reported that 28% to 47% of patients treated for gynecologic cancer develop lymphedema. According to findings from Beesley et al,[94] gynecologic lymphedema was more prevalent among vulvar cancer survivors. Cervical cancer survivors who had radiotherapy or who had lymph nodes removed also had higher odds of developing swelling. Uterine and ovarian cancer survivors who had lymph nodes removed or who were overweight or obese had higher odds of developing swelling as well.[95] There may be many factors that predispose an individual to developing lymphedema or that predict the progression, severity, and outcome of the condition (Table 21-6). Lymphedema treatment should include components based on the complex decongestive therapy method, which consists of:

(a) Manual lymphatic drainage,
(b) Bandaging,
(c) Proper skin care and diet,
(d) Compression garments (sleeves, stockings, devices such as ReidSleeve® Peninsula Medical, Inc. Scotts Valley, CA, CircAid® Medical Products, Inc. San Diego, CA, Tribute Solaris, Freedom to Live, West Allis, WI, as well as other alternative approaches),
(e) Remedial exercises,
(f) Self-manual lymphatic drainage and bandaging, if instruction is available, and
(g) Continue to follow prophylactic methods at all times.

Table 21-5. Possible causes of lymphedema.

Unilateral Limb Swelling	Symmetric Swelling
Acute deep venous thrombosis	Congestive heart failure
Post-thrombotic syndrome	Chronic venous insufficiency
Arthritis	Dependency or stasis edema
Baker cyst	Renal dysfunction
Presence or recurrence of carcinoma	Hepatic dysfunction Hypoproteinemia Hypothyroidism/myxedema Drug-induced (eg, calcium channel blockers, steroids, nonsteroidal anti-inflammatory drugs) Lipedema

Data from Lymphoedema Framework. *Best Practice for the Management of Lymphoedema*. International consensus. London: MEP Ltd, 2006.

SUMMARY

As the nation moves from physician-centric care to a patient-centered team approach, our patients deserve more active roles in their survivorship. As health care professionals, we must hear the call of our patients desires to improve survivorship through rehabilitation, QOL, and symptom management. Research evidence suggests that individuals with cancer who follow recommended guidelines during and after treatment may be able to attain the highest quality of survivorship. With new national guidelines putting the patient at the center of communication between oncologists and primary

Table 21-6. Factors that predispose an individual to developing lymphedema.

Surgery with inguinal lymph node dissection
Recurrent infection in the same site
Varicose vein stripping and vein harvesting
Intrapelvic or intra-abdominal tumors that involve or compress lymphatic structures
Orthopedic surgery
Thrombophlebitis and chronic venous insufficiency, particularly post-thrombolytic syndrome
Chronic skin disorders and inflammation
Unresolved edema
Poor nutritional status
Concurrent phlebitis, hyperthyroidism, kidney or cardiac disease
Advanced cancer
Genetic predisposition/family history of chronic edema
Obesity
Postoperative pelvic radiotherapy
Prolonged limb dependency
Air travel

Data from Lymphoedema Framework. *Best Practice for the Management of Lymphoedema.* International consensus. London: MEP Ltd, 2006.

care providers, we need to ensure all survivorship options are available to them.

REFERENCES

1. Patient Centered Outcomes Research Institute. Http://Www.Pcori.Org/About/Mission-And-Vision/. Accessed February 9, 2013.
2. Oncology Rehab Partners. Http://Www.Oncologyrehabpartners.Com/. Accessed February 9, 2013.
3. Luoma ML, Hakamies-Blomqvist L, Blomqvist C, Nikander R, Gustavsson-Lilius M, Saarto T. Experiences of breast cancer survivors participating in a tailored exercise intervention—a qualitative study. *Anticancer Res*. 2014;34(3):1193-1199.
4. Bourke L, Homer KE, Thaha MA, Steed L, Rosario DJ, Robb KA, Saxton JM, and Taylor SJ. Interventions to improve exercise behaviour in sedentary people living with and beyond cancer: a systematic review. *Br J Cancer*. 2014;18:110(4):831-841. doi: 10.1038/bjc.2013.750. Epub 2013 Dec 12.
5. Seo Y, Oh H, Seo W. Causal relationships among factors associated with cancer-related fatigue. *Eur J Oncol Nurs*. 2010;14(5):380-386. doi: 10.1016/j.ejon.2009.09.008. Epub 2009 Nov 27.
6. Gilchrist LS, Galantino ML, Wampler M, Marchese VG, Morris GS, Ness KK. A framework for assessment in oncology rehabilitation. *Phys Ther*. 2009;89(3):286-306. doi: 10.2522/ptj.20070309. Epub 2009 Jan 15.
7. US Department Of Health And Human Services Office of the Assistant Secretary for Planning And Evaluation. *Physical Activity Fundamental to Preventing Disease*. 2002.
8. US Department of Health and Human Services. *2008 Physical Activity Guidelines For Americans Be Active, Healthy, And Happy! Fact Sheet*. http://www.health.gov/paguidelines/factsheetprof.aspx. Accessed February 9, 2013.
9. Schwartz AL. Exercise in cancer survivorship: building your base. *Oncology (Williston Park)*. 2012;26(10):994.
10. Shin KY, Guo Y, Konzen B, Fu J, Yadav R, Bruera E. Inpatient cancer rehabilitation: the experience of a National Comprehensive Cancer Center. *Am J Phys Med Rehabil*. 2011;90(suppl):S63YS68.
11. Courneya KS, Segal RJ, Mackey JR, et al. Effects of aerobic and resistance exercise in breast cancer patients receiving adjuvant chemotherapy: a multicenter randomized controlled Trial. *J Clin Oncol*. 2007;25: 4396-4404.
12. Courneya KS, Mackey JR, Bell GJ, et al. Randomized controlled trial of exercise training in postmenopausal breast cancer survivors: cardiopulmonary and quality of life outcomes. *J Clin Oncol*. 2003;21:1660Y8.
13. Cramp F, Byron-Daniel J. Exercise for the management of cancer-related fatigue in adults. *Cochrane Database Syst Rev*. 2012;11:CD006145.
14. Yang EJ, Lim JY, Rah UW, Kim YB. Effect of a pelvic floor muscle training program on gynecologic cancer survivors with pelvic floor dysfunction: a randomized controlled trial. *Gynecol Oncol*. 2012;125:705-711.
15. Society of Gynecological Oncology. Survivorship toolkit. Https://Www.Sgo.Org/Clinical-Practice/Management/Survivorship-Toolkit/. Accessed February 19, 2013.
16. American Cancer Society. Http://Www.Cancer.Org/Cancer/News/News/Guidelinesaddress-Diet-Exercise-And-Weight-Control-For-Cancer-Survivors. Accessed February 19, 2013.
17. 2008 physical activity guidelines for Americans. Accessed February 19, 2013. Http://Health.Gov/Paguidelines/Pdf/Paguide.Pdf.
18. American College of Sports Medicine. Roundtable statement for exercise and cancer patients. 57th Annual Meeting in Baltimore. Available at: http://www.acsm.org/about-acsm/media-room/acsm-in-the-news/2011/08/01/new-guidelines-strongly-recommend-exercise-for-cancer-patients-survivors. Accessed May 19, 2014.
19. Shang J, Wenzel J, Krumm S, Griffith K, Stewart K. Who will drop out and who will drop in: exercise adherence in a randomized clinical trial among patients receiving active cancer treatment. *Cancer Nurs*. 2012;35(4):312-322.
20. Barsevick AM, Newhall T, Brown S. Management of cancer-related fatigue. *Clin J Oncol Nurs*. 2008;12(5 Suppl):21-25. doi:10.1188/08.CJON.S2.21-25.
21. Tomlinson D, Diorio C, Beyene J, Sung L. Effect of exercise on cancer-related fatigue: a meta-analysis. *Am J Phys Med Rehabil*. 2014;16. [Epub ahead of print]
22. von Gruenigen VE, Gil KM, Frasure HE, et al. Complementary medicine use, diet and exercise in endometrial cancer survivors. *J Cancer Integrative Medicine*. 2005;3:3-18.
23. Kwekkeboom KL, Abbott-Anderson K, Wanta B. Feasibility of a patient-controlled cognitive-behavioral intervention for pain, fatigue, and sleep disturbance in cancer. *Oncol Nurs Forum*. 2010;37(3):E151-E159.
24. Diaz ES, Karlan BY, Li AJ. Obesity-associated adipokines correlate with survival in epithelial ovarian cancer. *Gynecol Oncol*. 2013;Pii:S0090-8258(13)00077-2.
25. Friedenreich CM, Langley AR, Speide TP, et al. Case–control study of markers of insulin rResistance and endometrial cancer risk. *Endocr Relat Cancer*. 2012;19(6):785-792.
26. National Cancer Institute. Research-Tested Intervention Program (RTIPs). Moving science into programs for people. Http://Rtips.Cancer.Gov/Rtips/. Accessed February 19, 2013.
27. Ward KK, Shah NR, Saenz CC, Mchale MT, Alvarez EA, Plaxe SC. Cardiovascular disease is the leading cause of death among endometrial cancer patients. *Gynecol Oncol*. 2012;126(2):176-179.
28. National Institutes Of Health (NIH). Obesity Research. Last updated March 30, 2011. Http://Www.Obesityresearch.Nih.Gov/About/Strategic-Plan.Aspx.
29. Kotsopoulos J, Moody JR, Fan I, et al. Height, weight, BMI and ovarian cancer survival. *Gynecol Oncol*. 2012;127(1):83-87.
30. Arem H, Park Y, Pelser C, et al. Prediagnosis body index, physical activity, and mortality in endometrial cancer patients. *J Natl Cancer Inst*. 2013 Jan 7. [Epub ahead of print]

31. Chandran U, Bandera EV, Williams-King MG, Paddock LE, Rodriguez-Rodriguez L, Lu SE, Faulkner S, Pulick K, Olson SH. Healthy eating index and ovarian cancer risk. *Cancer Causes Control.* 2011;22(4):563-571.
32. von Gruenigen V, Frasure H, Kavanagh MB, et al. Survivors of Uterine Cancer Empowered By Exercise And Healthy Diet (SUCCEED): a randomized controlled trial. *Gynecol Oncol.* 2012;125(3):699-704.
33. von Gruenigen VE, Waggoner SE, Frasure HE, et al. Lifestyle challenges in endometrial cancer survivorship. *Obstet Gynecol.* 2011;117:93-100.
34. von Gruenigen VE, Courneya KS, Gibbons HE, Kavanagh MB, Waggoner SE, Lerner E. feasibility and effectiveness of a lifestyle intervention program in obese endometrial cancer patients: a randomized trial. *Gynecol Oncol.* 2008;109:19-26.
35. Gomes EC, Silva AN, de Oliveira MR. Oxidants, antioxidants, and the beneficial roles of exercise-induced production of reactive species. *Oxid Med Cell Longev.* 2012;2012:756132.
36. Ballard-Barbash R, Friedenreich CM, Courneya KS, Siddiqi SM, McTiernan A, Alfano CM. Physical activity, biomarkers, and disease outcomes in cancer survivors: a systematic review. *J Natl Cancer Inst.* 2012;104(11):815-840.
37. Blair SN, Cooper KH. Dose of exercise and health benefits. *Arch Intern Med.* 1997;157(2):153-154.
38. Modesitt SC, Geffel DL, Via J, L Weltman A. Morbidly obese women with and without endometrial cancer: are there differences in measured physical fitness, body composition, or hormones? *Gynecol Oncol.* 2012;124(3):431-436.
39. Courtney-Brooks M, Tellawi AR, Scalici J, et al. Frailty: an outcome predictor for elderly gynecologic oncology patients. *Gynecol Oncol.* 2012;126(1):20-24.
40. Thorsen L, Skovlund E, Strømme SB, Hornslien K, Dahl AA, Fosså SD. Effectiveness of physical activity on cardiorespiratory fitness and health-related quality of life in young and middle-aged cancer patients shortly after chemotherapy. *J Clin Oncol.* 2005;23(10):2378-2388.
41. Schmitz KH, Courneya KS, Matthews C, et al. American College of Sports Medicine Roundtable on Exercise Guidelines for Cancer Survivors. *Med Sci Sports Exercise.* 2010;42(7):1409-1426.
42. Litterini AJ, Jette DU. Exercise for managing cancer-related fatigue. *Phys Ther.* 2011;91:301-304.
43. Schmitz KH, Holtzman J, Courneya KS, Mâsse LC, Duval S, Kane R. Controlled physical activity trials in cancer survivors: a systematic review and meta-analysis. *Cancer Epidemiol Biomarkers Prev.* 2005;14(7):1588-1595.
44. Watson T, Mock V. Exercise as an intervention for cancer-related fatigue. *Phys. Ther.* 2004;84:736-743.
45. National Cancer Institute. *Cancer Trends Progress Report 2011/2012 Update.* Http://Progressreport.Cancer.Gov/Doc.Asp?Pid=1&Did=2011&Mid=Vcol&Chid=105. Accessed February 19, 2013.
46. Felce D. Defining and applying the concept of quality of life. *J Intellect Disabil Res* 1997;41:126-135.
47. Felce D, Perry J. Quality of life: its definition and measurement. *Res Dev Disabil* 1995;16:51-74.
48. Fader AN, Frasure HE, Gil KM, Berger NA, von Gruenigen VE. Quality of life in endometrial cancer survivors: what does obesity have to do with it? *Obstet Gynecol Int.* 2011;2011:308609.
49. Quinten C, Coens C, Mauer M, et al. EORTC Clinical Groups. Baseline quality of life as a prognostic indicator of survival: a meta-analysis of individual patient data from EORTC clinical trials. *Lancet Oncol.* 2009;10(9):865-871.
50. Luckett T, King M, Butow P, Friedlander M, Paris T. Assessing health-related quality of life in gynecologic oncology: a systematic review of questionnaires and their ability to detect clinically important differences and change. *Int J Gynecol Cancer.* 2010;20(4):664-684.
51. Jensen SE, Rosenbloom SK, Beaumont JL, et al. A new index of priority symptoms in advanced ovarian cancer. *Gynecol Oncol.* 2011;120(2):214-219.
52. Aerts L, Enzlin P, Verhaeghe J, Vergote I, Amant F. Sexual and psychological functioning in women after pelvic surgery for gynaecological cancer. *Eur J Gynaecol Oncol.* 2009;30(6):652-656.
53. Mishra SI, Scherer RW, Geigle PM, et al. Exercise interventions on health-related quality of life for cancer survivors. *Cochrane Database Syst Rev.* 2012;15;8:CD007566.
54. von Gruenigen V, Frasure H, Kavanagh MB, et al. Survivors of uterine cancer empowered by exercise and healthy diet (SUCCEED): a randomized controlled trial. *Gynecol Oncol.* 2012;125(3):699-704.
55. von Gruenigen VE, Gibbons HE, Kavanagh MB, Janata JW, Lerner E, Courneya KS. A randomized trial of lifestyle intervention in obese endometrial cancer survivors: quality of life outcomes and mediators of behavior change. *Health Qual Life Outcome.* 2009;7:17.
56. Rejeski WJ, Mihalko SL, Ambrosius WT, et al. Weight loss and self-regulatory eating efficacy in older adults: the cooperative lifestyle intervention program. *J Gerontol B Psychol Sci Soc Sci.* 2011;66(3):279-286.
57. Lajer H, Jensen MB, Kilsmark J, et al. The value of gynecologic cancer follow-up evidence-based ignorance? *Int J Gynecol Cancer.* 2010;20:1307Y1320.
58. World Health Organization. Sexual and reproductive health. http:/S/www.who.int/reproductivehealth/topics/sexual_health/sh_definitions/en/index.html. Accessed August 7, 2013.
59. Li C-C, Rew L. A feminist perspective on sexuality and body image in females with colorectal cancer: an integrative review. *WOCN.* 2010;37(5):519-525.
60. Basson R. The female sexual response: a different model. *J Sex Marital Ther.* 2000;26(1):51-65.
61. Carter J, Chi DS, Abu-Rustum N, Brown CL, McCreath W, Barakat RR. Brief report: total pelvic exenteration—a retrospective clinical needs assessment. *Psycho-oncology.* 2004;13(2):125-131.
62. Hawighorst-Knapstein S, Schönefussrs G, Hoffmann SO, Knapstein PG. Pelvic exenteration: effects of surgery on quality of life and body image—a prospective longitudinal study. *Gynecol Oncol.* 1997;66(3):495-500.
63. Hawighorst-Knapstein S, Fusshoeller C, Franz C, et al. The impact of treatment for genital cancer on quality of life and body image—results of a prospective longitudinal 10-year study. *Gynecol Oncol.* 2004;94(2):398-403.
64. da Silva GM, Hull T, Roberts PL, et al. The effect of colorectal surgery in female sexual function, body image, self-esteem and general health: a prospective study. *Ann Surg.* 2008;248(2):266-272.
65. Rezk YA, Hurley KE, Carter J, et al. A prospective study of quality of life in patients undergoing pelvic exenteration: interim results. *Gynecol Oncol.* 2013;128(2):191-197.
66. Kutner JS, Smith MC, Corbin L, et al. Massage therapy versus simple touch to improve pain and mood in patients with advanced cancer: a randomized trial. *Ann Intern Med.* 2008;149(6):369-379.
67. Roila F, Herrstedt J, Aapro M, et al. Guideline update for MASCC and ESMO in the prevention of chemotherapy- and radiotherapy-induced nausea and vomiting: results of the Perugia consensus conference. *Ann Oncol.* 2010;21:232-243).
68. Hesketh PJ. Chemotherapy-induced nausea and vomiting. *N Engl J Med.* 2008;358(23):2482-2494.
69. Lee A, Fan LT. Stimulation of the wrist acupuncture point P6 for preventing postoperative nausea and vomiting. *Cochrane Database Syst Rev.* 2009;2:CD003281.
70. Basch E, Prestrud AA, Hesketh PJ, et al. Antiemetics: American Society of Clinical Oncology clinical practice guideline update. *J Clin Oncol.* 2011.
71. Kucukmetin A, Naik R, Galaal K, Bryant A, Dickinson HO. Palliative surgery versus medical management for bowel obstruction in ovarian cancer. *Cochrane Database Syst Rev.* 2010;(7):CD007792.
72. Pothuri B, Montemarano M, Gerardi M, et al. Percutaneous endoscopic gastrostomy tube placement in patients with malignant bowel obstruction due to ovarian carcinoma. *Gynecol Oncol.* 2005;96(2):330-334.
73. Tradounsky G. Palliation of gastrointestinal obstruction. *Can Fam Physician.* 2012;58(6):648-652-e317-21.
74. Mangili G, Franchi M, Mariani A, Zanaboni F, Rabaiotti E, Frigerio L, Bolis PF, Ferrari A. Octreotide in the management of bowel obstruction in terminal ovarian cancer. *Gynecol Oncol.* 1996;61(3):345-348.

75. Cáceres A, Zhou Q, Iasonos A, Gerdes H, Chi DS, Barakat RR. Colorectal stents for palliation of large-bowel obstructions in recurrent gynecologic cancer: an updated series. *Gynecol Oncol.* 2008;108(3):482-485. [Epub 2008 Jan 10]
76. Keefe DM, Schubert MM, Elting LS, et al. Updated clinical practice guidelines for the prevention and treatment of mucositis. 2007;109:820-831.
77. Worthington HV, Clarkson JE, Bryan G, et al. Interventions for preventing oral mucositis for patients with cancer receiving treatment. *Cochrane Database Syst Rev.* 2011;(4):CD000978.
78. Radtke ML, Kolesar JM. Palifermin (Kepivance) for the treatment of oral mucositis in patients with hematologic malignancies requiring hematopoietic stem cell support. *J Oncol Pharm Pract.* 2005;11(3):121-125.
79. Worthington HV, Clarkson JE, Bryan G, et al. Interventions for preventing oral mucositis for patients with cancer receiving treatment. *Cochrane Database Syst Rev.* 2011;(4):CD000978.
80. Sugiyama M, Kakeji Y, Tsujitani S, Harada Y, Onimaru M, Yoshida K, Tanaka S, Emi Y, Morita M, Morodomi Y, Hasegawa M, Maehara Y, Yonemitsu Y. Antagonism of VEGF by genetically engineered dendritic cells is essential to induce antitumor immunity against malignant ascites. *Mol Cancer Ther.* 2011;10(3):540-549. [Epub 2011 Jan 5]
81. Tapping CR, Ling L, Razack A. PleurX drain use in the management of malignant ascites: safety, complications, long-term patency and factors predictive of success. *Br J Radio.* 2012;85(1013):623-628.
82. Fleming ND, Alvarez-Secord A, Gruenigen Von V, Miller MJ, Abernethy AP. Indwelling catheters for the management of refractory malignant ascites: a systematic literature overview and retrospective chart review. *J Pain Symp Manage.* 2009;38(3):341-349.
83. Eskander RN & Tewari KS. Emerging treatment options for management of malignant ascites in patients with ovarian cancer. *Int J Womens Health.* 2012;4:395-404. Published online Aug 3, 2012.
84. Jaishuen A, Jimenez C, Sirisabya N, et al. Poor survival outcome with moderate and severe hypercalcemia in gynecologic malignancy patients. *Int J Gynecol Cancer.* 2009;19(2):178-185.
85. American Thoracic Society Dyspnea. Mechanisms, assessment, and management: a consensus statement. *Am Thor Soc.* 1999;159:321-340.
86. Currow DC, Agar M, Smith J, and Abernethy AP. Does palliative home oxygen improve dyspnoea? A consecutive cohort study. *Palliat Med.* 2009;23(4):309-316.
87. Eifel PJ, Jhingran A, Bodurka DC, Levenback C, and Thames H. Correlation of smoking history and other patient characteristics with major complications of pelvic radiation therapy for cervical cancer. *J Clin Oncol.* 2002;20(17):3651-3657.
88. Boothe D, Patel SH, Stessin A, Parashar B. Comparing the rates of urinary tract infections among patients receiving adjuvant pelvic intensity modulated radiation therapy, 3-dimensional conformal radiation therapy, and brachytherapy for newly diagnosed endometrial cancer. *Pract Radiat Oncol.* 2013;3(4):269-274.
89. Akl EA, Labedi N, Barba M, et al. Anticoagulation for the long-term treatment of venous thromboembolism in patients with cancer. *Cochrane Database Syst Rev.* 2011:(6):CD006650.
90. Antithrombotic Therapy and Prevention of Thrombosis, 9th Ed. American College of Chest Physicians Evidence-Based Clinical Practice Guidelines. Methodology for the development of antithrombotic therapy and prevention of thrombosis guidelines: antithrombotic therapy and prevention of thrombosis, 9th ed: American College of Chest Physicians Evidence-Based Clinical Practice Guidelines. *Chest.* 2012;141(2 suppl):53S-70S.
91. Lymphoedema Framework. *International Consensus: Best Practice for the Management of Lymphoedema.* London: MEP Ltd; 2006. http://ewma.org/fileadmin/user_upload/EWMA/Wound_Guidelines/Lymphoedema_Framework_Best_Practice_for_the_Management_of_Lymphoedema.pdf.
92. Gordon K. A guide to lymphedema. *Exp Rev Dermatol.* 2007;2(6): 741-752.
93. Lymphoedema Framework. *International Consensus: Best Practice for the Management of Lymphoedema.* London: MEP Ltd; 2006. http://ewma.org/fileadmin/user_upload/EWMA/Wound_Guidelines/Lymphoedema_Framework_Best_Practice_for_the_Management_of_Lymphoedema.pdf.
94. Beesley V, Janda M, Eakin E, Obermair A, Battistutta D. Lymphedema after gynecological cancer treatment: prevalence, correlates, and supportive care need. *Cancer.* 2007;109(12):2607-2614.
95. Beesley V, Janda M, Eakin E, Obermair A, Battistutta D. Lymphedema after gynecological cancer treatment: prevalence, correlates, and supportive care need. *Cancer.* 2007;109(12):2607-2614.

Index

Note: Page numbers followed by f, t, and b indicate figures, tables, and boxes, respectively.